Review of
General
Psychiatry

a LANGE medical book

Review of
General
Psychiatry

THIRD EDITION

Edited by

Howard H. Goldman, MD, MPH, PhD

Professor of Psychiatry
Institute of Psychiatry and Human Behavior
University of Maryland, Baltimore

Research Associate
Center for Health Services Research and Development
School of Hygiene and Public Health
Johns Hopkins University, Baltimore

APPLETON & LANGE
Norwalk, Connecticut/San Mateo, California

0-8385-8428-4

Notice: The authors and the publisher of this volume have taken care to make certain that the doses of drugs and schedules of treatment are correct and compatible with the standards generally accepted at the time of publication. Nevertheless, as new information becomes available, changes in treatment and in the use of drugs become necessary. The reader is advised to carefully consult the instruction and information material included in the package insert of each drug or therapeutic agent before administration. This advice is especially important when using new or infrequently used drugs. The publisher disclaims any liability, loss, injury, or damage incurred as a consequence, directly or indirectly, of the use and application of any of the contents of this volume.

92 93 94 95 96 / 10 9 8 7 6 5 4 3 2 1

Prentice-Hall International (UK) Limited, *London*
Prentice-Hall of Australia, Pty. Limited, *Sydney*
Prentice-Hall Canada, Inc., *Toronto*
Prentice-Hall Hispanoamericana, S. A., *Mexico*
Prentice-Hall of India Private Limited, *New Delhi*
Prentice-Hall of Japan, Inc., *Tokyo*
Simon & Schuster Asia Pte. Ltd., *Singapore*
Editora Prentice-Hall do Brasil Ltda., *Rio de Janeiro*
Prentice Hall, *Englewood Cliffs, New Jersey*

ISBN: 0-8385-8428-4
ISSN: 0894-2404

PRINTED IN THE UNITED STATES OF AMERICA

*To my family
four generations
but especially my wife Debra
and our children Ilana and Ari*

Table of Contents

Authors

Bruce Africa, MD, PhD
Associate Clinical Professor of Psychiatry, Langley Porter Institute, University of California, San Francisco.

Renee L. Binder, MD
Professor of Psychiatry, Department of Psychiatry, University of California, San Francisco.

Emmett J. Bonner, PhD
Assistant Clinical Professor of Psychiatry, Department of Psychiatry-Medical Sociology, University of California, San Francisco.

Edward L. Burke, PhD
Clinical Professor of Psychiatry, Department of Psychiatry, University of California, San Francisco.

James David, MD
Assistant Director of Education, Albert Einstein College of Medicine/Montefiore Medical Center, The Bronx, New York.

Glenn C. Davis, MD
Chairman, Department of Psychiatry, Henry Ford Hospital, and Clinical Professor of Psychiatry, University of Michigan School of Medicine, Detroit.

Kathryn N. DeWitt, PhD
Assistant Research Psychologist, Department of Psychiatry, University of California, San Francisco; Lecturer in Psychiatry, Stanford University Medical School, Stanford, California.

Bernard L. Diamond, MD
Clinical Professor of Clinical Psychiatry, Department of Psychiatry, University of California, San Francisco; Professor of Law Emeritus, University of California, Berkeley, California.

Stuart J. Eisendrath, MD
Associate Professor of Clinical Psychiatry, Department of Psychiatry, University of California, San Francisco; Director, Psychiatric Consultation /Liaison Programs, Joseph M. Long Hospital and Herbert C. Moffitt Hospital, San Francisco.

Howard L. Fields, MD, PhD
Professor of Neurology and Physiology, Departments of Neurology and Physiology, University of California, San Francisco.

Louis M. Flohr, MD
Assistant Clinical Professor of Psychiatry, University of California, San Francisco.

Steven A. Foreman, MD
Assistant Clinical Professor, Department of Psychiatry, University of California, San Francisco.

Nelson B. Freimer, MD
Research Fellow, Department of Psychiatry, Columbia University College of Physicians and Surgeons, New York City.

Evalyn S. Gendel, MD
Clinical Professor of Psychiatry, Department of Psychiatry, and Director of Sex Counseling Clinic and Education Program, University of California, San Francisco.

Richard J. Goldberg, MD
Professor, Department of Psychiatry and Human Behavior, and Professor, Department of Medicine, Brown University, Providence, Rhode Island; Psychiatrist-in-Chief, Rhode Island Hospital and Women and Infants Hospital, Providence, Rhode Island.

Beth Goldman, MPH, MD
Medical Director, Preferred Health Care, Ltd., Southfield, Michigan.

Howard H. Goldman, MD, MPH, PhD
Professor of Psychiatry, Institute of Psychiatry and Human Behavior, University of Maryland, Baltimore; Research Associate, Center for Health Services Research and Development, School of Hygiene and Public Health, Johns Hopkins University, Baltimore.

Gary L. Gottlieb, MD. MBA
Associate Professor of Psychiatry, University of Pennsylvania School of Medicine, Philadelphia; Director, Section of Geriatric Psychiatry, Hospital of the University of Pennsylvania, Philadelphia.

Jack A. Grebb, MD
Research Scientist, Nathan S. Kline Institute for Psychiatric Research, Orangeburg, New York; Assistant Professor, Department of Psychiatry, New York University Medical Center, New York City; Guest Investigator, Laboratory of Molecular and Cellular Neuroscience, The Rockefeller University, New York City.

John H. Greist, MD
Professor of Psychiatry, Department of Psychiatry, University of Wisconsin Medical School, Madison, Wisconsin.

Gerard J. Hunt, PhD
Associate Professor, Department of Psychiatry, University of Maryland School of Medicine.

James W. Jefferson, PhD
Professor of Psychiatry, Department of Psychiatry, University of Wisconsin Medical School, Madison, Wisconsin.

Nancy B. Kaltreider, MD
Director, Medical Student Education in Psychiatry, and Clinical Professor of Psychiatry, Department of Psychiatry, University of California, San Francisco.

Nick Kanas, MD
Professor and Director, Group Therapy Training Program, Department of Psychiatry, University of California, San Francisco; Assistant Chief, Psychiatry Service, Veterans Administration Medical Center, San Francisco.

Ralph J. Kiernan, PhD
Assistant Clinical Professor of Medical Psychology, Department of Psychiatry, University of California, San Francisco.

Mim J. Landry
Medical Writing Consultant, Training and Education Project, Haight Ashbury Free Clinics, San Francisco.

J.W. Langston, MD
Senior Scientist, Institute for Medical Research, and Director, Parkinson's Research & Clinical Programs, Institute for Medical Research, Santa Clara Valley Medical Center, San Jose, California.

Hanna Levenson, PhD
Clinical Associate Professor of Psychiatry, Department of Psychiatry, University of California, San Francisco; Director of the Brief Psychotherapy Program, Veterans Administration Medical Center, Palo Alto, California. Director of the Brief Psychotherapy Program, California Pacific Medical Center, San Francisco.

Roland Levy, MD
Associate Clinical Professor of Psychiatry, Department of Psychiatry, University of California, San Francisco.

Charles R. Marmar, MD
Associate Professor of Clinical Psychiatry, Department of Psychiatry, and Director, Post-Traumatic Stress Disorder Program, Veterans Administration Medical Center, San Francisco.

Edward L. Merrin, MD
Associate Clinical Professor of Psychiatry, Department of Psychiatry, University of California, San Francisco; Chief, Psychiatric Inpatient Unit, Veterans Administration Medical Center, San Francisco.

Aubrey W. Metcalf, MD
Clinical Professor of Psychiatry and Senior Supervising Child and Adolescent Psychiatrist, Department of Psychiatry, University of California, San Francisco.

Jonathan Mueller, MD
Assistant Professor of Psychiatry, Department of Psychiatry, University of California, San Francisco.

Kim Norman, MD
Assistant Clinical Professor of Psychiatry, Department of Psychiatry, University of California, San Francisco.

Irving Philips, MD
Professor of Psychiatry, Department of Psychiatry, and Director of Child and Adolescent Psychiatry, University of California, San Francisco.

Kenneth S. Pope, PhD
Diplomate in Clinical Psychology, Los Angeles.

David Preven, MD
Director of Education, Department of Psychiatry, Albert Einstein College of Medicine /Montefiore Medical Center, The Bronx, New York.

Stephen D. Purcell, MD
Assistant Clinical Professor of Psychiatry, Department of Psychiatry, University of California, San Francisco.

David E. Reiser, MD
Associate Clinical Professor of Psychiatry and Family Medicine, Department of Psychiatry, University of Colorado Health Sciences Center, Denver.

Victor I. Reus, MD
Professor of Psychiatry, Department of Psychiatry, and Medical Director, Langley Porter Hospital, University of California, San Francisco.

Gary M. Rodin, MD
Associate Professor of Psychiatry, Department of Psychiatry, University of Toronto; Physician in Chief, The Toronto Hospital.

Stuart R. Schwartz, MD
Professor of Clinical Psychiatry, Department of Psychiatry, and Director of Postgraduate Education, University of Medicine and Dentistry of New Jersey, Piscataway, New Jersey.

Rodney J. Shapiro, PhD
Clinical Professor of Psychiatry, Department of Psychiatry, University of California, San Francisco; Director, Family Therapy Clinic, California Pacific Medical Center, San Francisco.

David E. Smith, MD
Founder and Medical Director, Haight Ashbury Free Medical Clinics, San Francisco; Research Director, Merritt Peralta Institute, San Francisco; Associate Clinical Professor of Occupational Medicine and Clinical Toxicology, University of California, San Francisco; Visiting Associate Professor of Behavioral Pharmacology, Department of Pharmacology, University of Nevada Medical School, Reno, Nevada.

Craig Van Dyke, MD
Professor of Psychiatry, Department of Psychiatry, University of California, San Francisco; Chief, Psychiatry Service, Veterans Administration Medical Center, San Francisco.

Robert S. Wallerstein, MD
Emeritus Professor of Psychiatry, Department of Psychiatry, University of California, San Francisco; Supervising and Training Analyst, San Francisco Psychoanalytic Institute, San Francisco; Immediate Past President, International Psychoanalytical Association.

Daniel S. Weiss, PhD
Associate Professor of Medical Psychology, Department of Psychiatry, and Director of Research, Posttraumatic Stress Disorders Program, Veterans Administration Medical Center, San Francisco.

Preface

Review of General Psychiatry, 3rd edition, is designed for medical students—for course adoption, to supplement course syllabus materials, to complement readings in the literature, and to use as a companion text with more comprehensive works. The book originated in the extensive program of psychiatric education offered by the University of California, San Francisco. Written by psychiatric educators, this text serves the needs of medical students in most settings. In addition, it can serve as a review text for psychiatric residents and other trainees, and as a reference for physicians and other health professionals.

Psychiatry is a discipline of observation and probing inquiry, a basic science of behavior, and a clinical science of mental disorder and emotional responses to physiologic change, somatic illness, and life events. Critics in neuroscience characterize psychiatry as brainless; critics within psychologic medicine fear that psychiatry will become mindless. Students everywhere are concerned that the medical curriculum not be witless. Our aim is to present psychiatry with the proper mix of brain, mind, and wit.

NEW TO THIS EDITION

In response to students' need for brevity and conciseness, the text has been rigorously revised and reorganized with that goal in mind. Wherever possible, chapters have been combined to eliminate overlap; all chapters have been pared to essential content and updated throughout.

New to this edition are the following chapters:

Theoretical Foundations of Psychiatry
Social & Cultural Aspects of Health, Illness, & Treatment
Introduction to Psychiatric Treatment
Somatic Therapies
Geriatric Psychiatry

CONTINUING FEATURES

- Material on basic biologic and psychosocial science as well as clinical material on diagnosis and treatment.
- Full range of disorders with complete diagnostic criteria as described in the *Diagnostic & Statistical Manual of Mental Disorders,* 3rd edition, as revised in 1987 (DSM-III-R).
- Updated neuroscience and psychopharmacology.
- Clinical vignettes illustrating the features of most mental disorders and comprehensive clinical assessment.
- Glossary of psychiatric signs and symptoms.
- Seven chapters on psychiatric assessment.
- Consistent, readable format, permitting efficient use in multiple clinical settings.
- Selected references for further investigation.
- Information useful to the nonpsychiatrist physician and the medical student and resident in psychiatry.

ACKNOWLEDGMENTS

Review of General Psychiatry represents more than the work of its title page editor and its named contributors. I would like to acknowledge the assistance of other contributors to our text.

Although the third edition bears little resemblance to the original course materials prepared at UCSF prior to the first edition, I wish to thank my predecessors and colleagues in San Francisco for setting the initial direction for this text. I would also like to thank the publisher and the editorial staff at Appleton & Lange, in particular, Nancy Evans and Jim Ransom. Special acknowledgment is offered to David Preven, MD, for his very careful critique of the second edition and to my sister, Beth Goldman, MD, for her assistance with the reorganization of this edition.

We continue to solicit comments and recommendations for future editions of this textbook. Correspondence should be addressed to us at Appleton & Lange, 2755 Campus Drive, Suite 205, San Mateo, CA 94403.

Howard H. Goldman, MD
Baltimore, Maryland
October, 1991

NOTICE

Section I. Theory & Concepts

Review of General Psychiatry: Introduction

1

Howard H. Goldman, MD, PhD

Review of General Psychiatry undertakes to examine and discuss the two major domains of the medical specialty field of psychiatry: mental disorder and individual behavior in health and sickness. Both areas are characterized by a degree of scientific uncertainty that may be puzzling to students drawn to medicine by the prospect of effecting cures by extirpating tumors or disrupting bacterial cell membrane formation. The patients being treated by psychiatrists are apt to have "idiopathic" disorders, "functional" disorders, whose causes are unknown and often cannot be corrected with instruments and drugs. The patients have behavior problems, aberrations; they are "deviant." Their disorders are "real," however, and will be described in the clinical chapters of this book. When, as occasionally happens, the etiological roots of these "idiopathic" diseases are found, psychiatry loses most or at least some of its professional dominion over them, as happened when general paresis of the insane was identified as a neurological disorder of infectious (syphilitic) origin and pellagra as a metabolic disorder attributable to niacin deficiency. Complaints with no discoverable organic cause thus always arouse a suspicion of "mental disease" and consideration of psychiatric referral. Pain or weakness with no clear pathophysiological basis is psychogenic, hysterical, a "conversion" phenomenon. The term "residual deviance" has been applied to problems left over when "real" diseases have been ruled out.

This is not to suggest that all mental diseases are "orphans" for whom parental etiologies may yet be found, though of course that can happen in many cases and surely will in some. The mood disorders (depression, mania) are obvious examples of severe incapacitating mental diseases that are beginning to give way to conventional diagnostic and therapeutic medical management. The mental disorders are not simply "residual"; they have specific diagnostic criteria and often have biological markers.

Just as the subject matter of psychiatry is different in kind from the subject matter of ophthalmology, rheumatology, and other medical and surgical specialties, the literature in which its concepts and theories are conveyed from teacher to student and to successive generations of readers is different in kind from the literature of medicine generally. In order to say different kinds of things, we need different kinds of communication. The writer's first task here will be to decide how best to convey the grays and off-whites of the subject matter in the plain black medium of print. Especially when writing for medical students, who are taught to anticipate documentation and distrust speculation and "anecdotalism," one is forever aware that some of the ground being covered is sandy soil. The psychiatrist with some years in practice occupies these areas comfortably enough—there is no choice, since that is where the patient is—but many times in the following pages the reader will be called on for that "willing suspension of disbelief . . . that constitutes poetic faith." A willful unbeliever will not be persuaded that a 5-year-old boy would really want to slay his father so he might lie with his mother. But the good-faith unbeliever will acknowledge the pragmatic utility of that concept when it is used successfully to help a young man tormented by career misfortunes brought on by arguments with his boss, a gray-haired man the age of his father, and by a marriage in trouble because of an affair with the boss's secretary. An unbeliever might reject the notion that medication could relieve the terrible agony of depression—after all a "natural" element of the human condition—or that a placebo could really relieve the pain of cancer, much less accomplish physiological anesthesia by suggestion. Yet the unbeliever might be convinced by the dramatic results of clinical trials of antidepressant drugs and by the demonstration that a narcotic antagonist can block placebo-induced analgesia. These comments do not exempt the claims of psychiatry from close scrutiny or its theorists from the rigors of systematic criticism. Their purpose is rather to encourage the reader on the way with appropriate notice about what *not* to expect in the pages that follow. Much of clinical psychiatry, like much of medicine, is not a "hard science," and *it does not need to be in order to be clinically effective*.

Uncertainty may make psychiatry difficult to "understand" in the straightforward sense of that word and certainly makes it impossible to reduce psychiatry to a catechism of verified truths. But it is still possible to think clearly in psychiatry, and one may tease out the known from the unknown and certainty from conjecture. And psychiatry is undeniably a clinically effective discipline, a healing profession, a growing body of useful knowledge based on careful observation and practical research, and a capacious receptacle of *theories!* It is the *theories* that are the special language of psychiatry and the source of its growth. Fundamentally a science of individual behavior, thought, and emotion, psychiatry is often scornfully contrasted with the sciences of basic laws, empirical truths, and reductionistic categories and typologies. In psychiatry, the domain of the mental disorders *does* share a common heritage with the reductionistic "hard sciences" of fundamental laws and empirical data; but the domain of individual behavior has been a "soft science" of human motivation, personal meaning, and individual difference. Ultimately, psychiatry is a *human* science, a clinical science—seen at its best in the personal interaction between doctor and patient. Simply stated, one need not know the "truth‘—the reducible facts—to be helpful, but one does need to have at hand a rich resource of theories and hypotheses and must be prepared to test them on every patient—to use them when they work and move along when they do not. Most importantly, the psychiatrist must be a good listener, waiting for the patient to suggest—in speech, affect, and behavior—what hypotheses may be tested with brighter hope of success. *The psychiatrist must know how to lead where the patient goes.*

THE BIOPSYCHOSOCIAL MODEL

The biopsychosocial model is a defense against uncertainty, an approach to thinking about mental disorder and individual behavior. The psychiatrist may view both domains from biomedical and psychosocial perspectives and consider specific problems and potential solutions from each viewpoint. The biopsychosocial model is a perspective, not a theory— a way of organizing disparate data that permits clinicians and scientists to consider various points of view and integrate them into a coherent approach to the patient. For example, the busy medical student with peptic ulcer is not viewed as the passive victim of familial defects in gastrointestinal function *or* the angry combatant in a competitive profession, living a stressful life-style. *Both* views are correct, potentially helpful, and not mutually exclusive. The model, championed by George Engel (1977) and discussed again in other chapters, is introduced below in a clinical case and in a summary of some current neuroscience research to demonstrate its breadth and utility.

What do the old couple in the illustrative case (below) and the animal model of anxiety in the snail *Aplysia* have in common? How does the biopsychoso-

cial model help us to appreciate these shared features? There is substantial agreement that clinical biomedical problems (eg, heart attacks) are in part influenced by psychosocial factors (eg, the sudden death of a loved one) and that biomedical problems (eg, a stroke) may cause secondary behavioral and psychosocial problems (eg, loss of a job or dissolution of a marriage). It is more difficult to appreciate the specific effect of social and psychological factors on anatomic structures and physiological functions. The clinical case of the old couple will show how the biopsychosocial model facilitates understanding of the interactions of biomedical and psychosocial factors. The animal model of anxiety in *Aplysia* illustrates the use of the biopsychosocial model in basic research. In particular, it examines the mechanism by which *learned* responses (eg, anxiety) may cause specific neurochemical and neuroanatomic changes.

Illustrative Case

A couple in their mid 80s had been married for 65 years and continued to live together in an apartment in spite of their increasing infirmities. The husband had severe emphysema and cardiac arrhythmia and was becoming forgetful; his wife had mild hypertension and was becoming impaired by senile dementia. On the eve of his 85th birthday, the old man became acutely short of breath and anxious. Fearful that he was going to die, he called his married daughter and was taken to the hospital in acute respiratory distress. He was later found to have inoperable lung cancer for which only palliative treatment could be offered.

While the patient was hospitalized, his wife went to live with their daughter and son-in-law. At night she wandered the rooms of the house, looking for her husband. She was argumentative and confused, not seeming to know where she was or what she should do. Her children and grandchildren had been aware of her increasing mental problems, but she was much more disturbed than they had realized or perhaps had wanted to realize. Her apparently dramatic change could be explained in two ways. She was undergoing a period of acute situational stress, and her deteriorated functioning had not been obvious as long as she was part of a functioning couple. Her husband had been helping her at home, nursing her, and covering up her deficits so that the family would not see. He was no longer available to do these things and never would be again. Plans were made to discharge him to a nursing home where he could continue to live with his wife in a double room. Although he was depressed, he adjusted to the nursing home, accepting the fact that this was where he would live out his days. He lived to see his granddaughter married, and then he died. The wife never adjusted, and her mental condition continued to deteriorate. She still expected her husband to come home each evening from the hospital, having concluded that she never saw him because he left early each day before she awakened and returned while she was asleep.

The interaction of biomedical and psychosocial factors in disease and illness is illustrated by this case. The husband's illness had precipitated a change in the delicate balance of the couple's independence. The wife needed nursing care, and his illness kept him from providing it. Many people die or become ill upon achieving certain milestones—an anniversary, a holiday, or, as in this case, a birthday. This man's 85th birthday had special significance. His driver's license, the key to his independence and his ability to care for his wife at home, expired on his birthday. He had been preparing for the test with great difficulty and was afraid he would not pass. Going to a nursing home gave him the comfort of knowing that when he died, his wife would be taken care of without being a burden to the family. His cancer had been growing for a long time, but clinically obvious illness began on his birthday.

A keen awareness of the interplay between biomedical and psychosocial factors is the essence of clinical medicine. Knowledge of the nuances of this interaction can help to answer two of the most important questions in medicine: Why did the patient become ill *now* (and not yesterday or a week or month ago)? And how can we treat this *individual* with an established diagnosis (that may be incurable)?

The mechanisms by which stress precipitates and exacerbates illness, lowers host resistance, and perhaps causes some diseases are currently being investigated. It would be useful also to learn how coping and adaptation work to prevent illness or reduce its severity. Learning how symbolic events, thoughts, and feelings influence behavior and initiate pathological processes in humans is a challenge for future research. Some early work in this area has been reported by Eric Kandel (1983) and his associates studying an animal model of anxiety in the marine snail *Aplysia*, whose nervous system is simple, well understood, and accessible to investigation.

Research Example: Animal Model of Anxiety

Using the sea snail *Aplysia* as a research subject, Kandel (1983) describes an animal model of anticipatory anxiety and chronic anxiety reflected in two forms of learned fear produced by classic conditioning and sensitization. Each form of fear is associated with distinguishable cellular and molecular changes.

Aplysia demonstrates a defensive "fear response" when presented with a noxious stimulus, such as an electric shock to its head. The response includes an increase in movement away from the stimulus ('escape locomotion'), an increase in other defensive behaviors (eg, withdrawal of the head and siphon into the shell, releasing ink), and a decrease in feeding behavior. This fearful response may be learned by the snail in

two ways: *Aplysia* may be conditioned, like Pavlov's dog (see Chapter 2), to respond fearfully to a neutral stimulus, such as shrimp extract, without the electric shock. If the snail is repeatedly given an electric shock each time shrimp extract is presented to it, the snail eventually responds with fear to the shrimp extract alone. This classic conditioning is similar to human anticipatory anxiety (and phobic anxiety). *Aplysia* can also be sensitized by random, unpredictable electric shocks, resulting in generally heightened responsiveness, so that almost any stimulus produces fearful behavior, as seen in chronic anxiety in humans.

In a series of elegant experiments, Kandel and his colleagues explored the cellular and molecular mechanisms associated with these two forms of learned fear. The sensitization model of chronic anxiety has been studied more extensively and appears to be due to presynaptic facilitation. The repeated head shocks lead to an "enhancement of the connections made by the sensory neurons on their target cells: the interneurons and the motor neurons . . ." (Kandel, 1983:1285), resulting in increased escape behavior. This enhancement is due to increases in a serotonin-like neurotransmitter in the presynaptic sensory neurons that produce an increase in cAMP. In turn, cAMP leads to an increase in neurotransmitter release from terminals in the synapse connecting the sensory neurons and motor neurons. The resulting neurotransmission activates "escape locomotion" and other defensive behaviors in response to a wide array of stimuli. The investigators found that the molecular mechanism involved enhanced protein phosphorylation and increased influx of calcium and resulted in morphological changes in the presynaptic neurons, detectable by electron microscopy. They speculate that the functional and structural changes associated with sensitization may be caused by alterations in gene expression: ". . . the possibility of gene regulation by experience suggests a class of molecular regulatory defects that might be caused by learning" (Kandel, 1983:1287).

The conditioning model for anticipatory anxiety is not as well described but seems to be similar in many ways to sensitization. Also producing presynaptic facilitation, conditioned fear appears to "augment" the process by "activity-dependent enhancement." This means that the learned association between the conditioned stimulus (the shrimp extract) and the fear response is produced by the increased release of neurotransmitter when the snail senses the presence of shrimp extract. The increased neurotransmission in response to the conditioned stimulus then sets in motion the same enhanced fear response mechanism seen in the sensitization model of chronic anxiety.

This research suggests that "normal learning, the learning of anxiety and unlearning it through psychotherapeutic intervention, might involve long-term

functional and structural changes in the brain . . .''
(Kandel, 1983:1291). Investigations such as these
demonstrate the interaction of biomedical and psychosocial phenomena, brain and behavior, in everyday
life and clinical medicine.

THE PLAN OF THE TEXTBOOK

Review of General Psychiatry is divided into four
sections: theories and concepts, psychiatric assessment, the mental disorders, and treatments and special
interventions.

The first section presents the basic science of psychiatry, material usually included in first-year psychiatry courses. This section introduces the biopsychosocial model and explores its various aspects, including
psychoanalytic and behavioral concepts (Chapter 2),
psychosomatics (Chapter 3), human development
(Chapter 4), neuroscience (Chapters 5 and 6), and
social science in medicine (Chapter 7). The section
concludes with an introduction to psychopathology,
the clinical science of psychiatry, and the study of
mental disorder (Chapter 8).

The second section concerns clinical assessment.
It can serve as a basic text for introductory courses
in interviewing and clinical psychiatry, including a
clerkship in psychiatry. Chapter 9 is a character sketch
of a patient admitted to a hospital for psychiatric
evaluation and treatment. His ''case'' is presented
formally in Chapter 15 after the intervening chapters
describe the components of a complete psychiatric
evaluation: psychiatric interviews (Chapter 10), mental status examination (Chapter 11), physical and laboratory examination (Chapter 12), intelligence and neuropsychological tests (Chapter 13), and personality
assessment (Chapter 14).

The third and fourth sections may be used as a
text for introductory courses in clinical psychiatry

and for the core clerkship in psychiatry. Some of
the chapters are also designed for use in a consultation-
liaison psychiatry course and for courses in the psychiatric aspects of medical practice.

The third section presents the mental disorders,
for the most part as they are classified in the third
edition of *Diagnostic and Statistical Manual of Mental
Disorders Revised (DSM-III-R)*. Chapter 16 introduces psychiatric classification and *DSM-III-R*. Chapters 17–29 discuss the clinical manifestations, diagnostic criteria, differential diagnosis, epidemiology,
etiology and pathogenesis, and treatment of each of
the mental disorders. An illustrative case is provided
for many of the disorders presented in each chapter.
Chapter 26 discusses the personality disorders from
the dual perspectives of psychiatry and general medicine. For the disorders of childhood and adolescence
(Chapter 30), clinical vignettes are presented to familiarize the reader with the wide range of childhood
psychopathology.

The fourth section discusses psychiatric treatment
methods and presents some material on special topics
in psychiatry. Following an introduction to psychiatric
treatment (Chapter 31), somatic treatments are presented in Chapter 32. The psychotherapies are discussed (Chapters 33–37), including psychoanalysis
and its derivative techniques, behavior and cognitive
therapy, group therapy, and family and marital therapy. Techniques in behavioral medicine are presented
in Chapter 38 and therapy with chronically ill and
dying medical patients in Chapter 39. Geriatric psychiatry is the subject of Chapter 40, and consultation-
liaison psychiatry is the subject of Chapter 41. Chapter
42 deals with forensic psychiatry. Psychiatric emergencies are discussed in Chapter 43.

Although the text was designed for use in general
medical and psychiatric education, we hope that trainees and practitioners in other health, mental health,
and social welfare disciplines will find *Review of
General Psychiatry* helpful and stimulating.

REFERENCES

Dubos R: *Man Adapting.* Yale Univ Press, 1980.
Eisenberg L: Interfaces between medicine and society.
Compr Psychiatry 1979;20:1.
Eisenberg L: Psychiatry and society. N Engl J Med
1977;296:903.
Engel G: The need for a new medical model: A challenge
for biomedicine. Science 1977;196:129.

Foucault M: *The Birth of the Clinic.* Random House, 1974.
Goldman H: Integrating health and mental health services.
Am J Psychiatry 1982,139:616.
Kandel E: From metapsychology to molecular biology: Ex-
plorations into the nature of anxiety. Am J Psychiatry
1983;140:1277.

Theoretical Foundations of Psychiatry

2

David Preven, MD, & James David, MD

This chapter will touch upon the history of psychiatry and move quickly through the major theories and treatment methods that comprise modern practice. These subjects are discussed in greater detail in later chapters. The purpose here is to provide a skeletal framework of the field to be fleshed out by further readings and clinical experiences.

The field of psychiatry, in concert with the allied mental health professions, has come to encompass virtually the entire spectrum of human mental, instinctual, and behavioral experience—mood disorders, eating disorders, sexual disorders, phobias, etc. It is no wonder, considering the sheer size of the territory, that a great many theories have evolved, with at times conflicting views about the causes, mechanisms, and proper treatment of mental disorders. The student in search of a unifying conceptual framework—a unified field theory of psychiatry—will be disappointed. *The student is urged to take it on trust that the various theories that comprise modern psychiatry each has its own place in the unfinished mosaic of knowledge in this field.*

HISTORY OF PSYCHIATRY BEFORE FREUD

The earliest civilizations frequently attributed the cause of madness to magical or divine forces. Early attempts at treatment were administered mostly by priests and were grounded in religious beliefs and ritual.

Greek and Roman societies then began to apply the medical knowledge of their day to psychiatric symptoms, with hypotheses stemming from the effects of imbalances of the essential humors (blood, phlegm, yellow bile, and black bile) and other derangements of vital processes. Hippocratic doctrine considered hysteria a consequence of a physically wandering uterus. (The word "hysteria" is derived from the Greek word for womb.) Galen (c130–c201) attributed melancholia to an excess of black bile.

Asylums for the mentally ill were first established in medieval times. The Renaissance ushered in a notably barbaric time for the insane. Many of these unfortunates, believed to be possessed by the devil, were condemned by the ecclesiastical authorities and tortured as witches. Even the greatest physicians of the day advocated that they be burned. It is worth noting that this age-old stigmatization of the mentally ill, with its attendant fear and discrimination, is still very much with us in spite of the scientific progress that has been made since that time.

Seventeenth and eighteenth century asylums, with some exceptions, were dreadful places where patients were kept in chains and whipped as a form of treatment. Toward the latter part of this period—and notably around the time of the French Revolution—reforms in treatment of the insane began in earnest. Phillipe Pinel (1745–1826) in France and William Tuke (1732–1822) in England were influential advocates for humane treatment of the mentally ill. The chains and cruelty began to give way to decent living conditions and to early attempts at rehabilitation.

In the late 1700s, Franz Mesmer (1734–1815), an Austrian physician, pioneered work now considered by some to be the earliest example of psychotherapy. He would establish rapport and work with an individual patient, practicing what was at the time called Mesmerism—later modified and renamed hypnosis.

The 19th century heralded the beginning of the age of a more scientific approach to psychiatry. Many detailed descriptions of psychiatric syndromes were recorded, and the basis of the modern classification of different types of mental disorders was established. Emil Kraepelin (1856–1926) is best known for his contribution to differential diagnosis in psychiatry. He suggested two major categories of severe mental disorders: **manic-depressive illness** and **dementia praecox.** Kraepelin's manic-depressive category generally corresponds to the modern mood disorders (bipolar disorder, recurrent major depression, and others discussed in Chapter 22), and he further noted the cyclical course of this type of illness, with recovery following symptomatic episodes. Dementia praecox is the forerunner to the current classification of schizophrenia and related syndromes (Chapters 20 and 21)—and Kraepelin noted the long-term deteriorating course of this type of illness, in contrast to the fluctuating course of manic-depressive illnesses. Eugen Bleuler (1857–1939), a Swiss psychiatrist, further studied and described dementia praecox and renamed the syndrome schizophrenia to distinguish it from true dementia.

In the latter part of the 19th century, Jean Charcot (1825–1893), a French neurologist, was treating hysteria with hypnosis. This treatment technique was, for a time, adopted by an obscure Austrian physician who had been impressed with Charcot's work. The emergence (under hypnosis) of psychic material not readily ascertained in the normal waking state contributed to this practitioner's later revelations regarding mental functioning. His name was Sigmund Freud.

FREUD'S CONTRIBUTION

Few men in the 20th century loom as large as Sigmund Freud (1856–1939), both as a founder of modern psychiatry and as a cultural force. His impact on the arts, literature, and education was profound and far-reaching. Much of his wide appeal can be attributed to the masterful way he described his theories and case histories, often linking them to references in the Bible, classical literature, and Renaissance culture. His role in the development of American psychiatry and culture in the mid 20th century was such that every student of medicine should know something about Sigmund Freud and his theories—regardless of recent controversies about their place in contemporary psychiatric treatment.

Although Freud trained and worked as a neurologist, he was barred from professional advancement in that discipline in part because of Viennese anti-Semitism. That professional crisis provided Freud with an unexpected opportunity. Prevented from practicing traditional neurology, he began to consult with patients whose symptoms were not explained by the traditional approaches of the discipline. Freud's work with these patients inspired him to formulate the theories and practice of psychoanalysis. The word psychoanalysis, then and now, refers both to the theory which Freud developed and the treatment itself (see Chapter 33).

Psychoanalysis as Theory

Psychoanalysis as a theory provides a comprehensive approach to understanding psychic development, emotion, and behavior as well as psychiatric illness. As Freud developed his ideas, he posited a **psychic apparatus** with three parts: **id, ego,** and **superego**. This **structural theory,** as it was called, defined the superego as the conscience, the id as the repository of raw impulses and drives such as sex and aggression, and the ego as the rational mediator between the expectations of the superego and the pressures for gratification of the id. Freud believed that the three structures related to each other in a dynamic equilib-

rium. If the ego failed to keep the demands of the id and superego in balance, the individual experienced psychological distress and symptoms.

Another fundamental concept of psychoanalysis—the **psychosexual stages of development**—postulated that a person must accomplish a series of tasks from infancy to adulthood in order to achieve psychological health (see Chapter 4). Freud associated each of these psychosexual stages with a part of the anatomy as well as with physiological and psychological functions. For example, the **oral stage,** up to the first 18 months of life, was anatomically represented by the mouth, physiologically by eating (symbolically sucking at the breast), and psychologically by being loved and nurtured. The **anal phase,** at around 2 years, focused on the anus anatomically with bowel control as the physiological function and autonomy and self control as the psychological task. Finally, the **genital phase,** at ages 3–5, defined the genitals as pleasure-providing organs psychologically linked to the then-prevalent notion that males were active (phallic) and females passive (receptive). As Freud listened to his patients' childhood histories, he hypothesized that failure to complete the task of a certain psychosexual phase would impair adult psychological health in the associated area of psychological functioning. For example, problems of inadequate nurturing during the oral stage could produce an adult who feels unloved and suffers dependency problems in relationships.

It is implicit in the concept of psychosexual stages that early experience shapes the adult's self-image and potential for success in work and relationships. *It is one of Freud's pivotal contributions to modern understanding of mental diseasse that trauma during development causes psychopathology in adult life.* Therefore, a successful psychoanalysis must include a detailed history of the patient's early life as well as current difficulties.

Psychoanalysis as a Form of Treatment

Psychoanalysis is not synonymous with psychotherapy but is a type of psychotherapy. It is practiced by a minority of practicing therapists who must receive specialized analytic training in addition to their more generalized therapeutic training. Psychoanalysis as a specific treatment method requires some explanation because its techniques are unusual and often misunderstood. The patient lies on a couch while the analyst sits out of the patient's line of sight. The analyst attempts to present himself as a neutral figure to the extent possible. In order to proceed with the major task of analysis—an examination of the patient's inner life—the analyst responds to many of the patient's comments with silence or with an explanation (**interpretation**) aimed at uncovering their deeper, latent meaning. Called the **rule of abstinence,** this seemingly asocial means of communication is designed to help the patient overcome the natural reluctance of exposing intimate details.

As unnatural in normal communication as this technique appears, Freud felt that it was essential in order to achieve the major objective of a psychoanalysis: the uncovering of the patient's hidden psychic life, the **unconscious**. He defined the unconscious as a layer of mental life that existed out of awareness but which nevertheless influenced emotions and behavior. Freud emphasized that the analyst's central task was to help the patient discover the secrets of his or her unconscious. Once aware of these hidden feelings and thoughts, the patient would be able to examine the role they played in the development of symptoms.

Symptom Formation

Freud hypothesized that mental symptoms arose when conflicting emotions such as hate or love, assertiveness or passivity produced unmanageable distress. Borrowing from popular scientific notions about conservation of energy, he posited that psychic conflict created an energy imbalance in the psychiatric apparatus. The patient was warned of this imbalance of psychic energy by experiencing anxiety. This psychological alert, called **signal anxiety,** induced the psychic apparatus to relieve distress by transferring awareness of the conflict into the unconscious. The

mechanism by which such information is assigned to the unconscious is called **repression.** However, repression often fails to bury the conflict totally. Elements of awareness leak into consciousness, again causing anxiety. Then, in another attempt to diminish distress, the psychic apparatus further disposes of the anxiety by transforming it into a neurotic symptom **(symptom formation).** Freud posited **psychic defenses** against intrapsychic conflict and anxiety—and, simply put, considered symptom formation largely a consequence of the failure of the **mechanisms of defense** (see Table 2-1).

Working With Unconscious Material

In his intensive work with patients, Freud discovered phenomena and developed techniques that allowed the analyst to observe the unconscious. These include slips of the tongue, the dream analysis, free association, transference, and resistance. These subject will be described and illustrated by means of clinical material.

Slips of the Tongue

Slips of the tongue, commonly called **Freudian slips,** were one of Freud's earliest discoveries. Clues to unconscious material were evident when a person misused a word that might seem a trivial error but

Table 2–1. Mechanisms of defense.

Denial	The unconscious literally deletes from awareness an unpleasant or anxiety-provoking reality. *A patient told of a terminal diagnosis has "forgotten" being so informed.*
Sublimation	The redirection of an unacceptable impulse into an acceptable form of behavior. *An individual with intense unconscious voyeuristic impulses becomes a sex therapist.*
Reaction formation	The redirection of an unacceptable impulse into its opposite. *A former smoker zealously enforces the new "no smoking" law.*
Displacement	An impulse toward a given person or situation is redirected toward a "safer," less distressing object. *A resident is humiliated by an attending physician and becomes enraged at his subordinate interns and medical students.*
Projection	An acceptable or anxiety-provoking impulse or affect is transplanted to another individual or situation. It is then "out there" rather than in oneself. *A parent becomes preoccupied with his adolescent daughter's alleged promiscuity, thereby projecting his own impulses onto the teenager.*
Rationalization	An unacceptable explanation for a feeling or behavior is used to camouflage the unacceptable underlying motive or impulse. *An obese man thinks he overate at the party so as not to offend his hostess.*
Intellectualization	The avoidance of "feeling" by taking refuge in "thinking." *A defeated quarterback avoids feelings of self-reproach and inadequacy by meticulously and logically explaining the details of his strategic errors.*
Repression	Disturbing psychological material is secondarily removed from consciousness or primarily prevented from becoming conscious. *Repressed memories and feelings associated with childhood sexual abuse are unleashed into consciousness when, as an adult, the patient is taken to a movie about a woman who had been raped.*
Isolation of affect	The removal of disturbing affect from an idea or event, with the dispassionate details or description remaining. *A combat veteran recounts seeing a friend killed but speaks in a cold and distant tone. He has "isolated" and "repressed" the intense fear and horror (affect) that might accompany the memory.*
Suppression	Intentional repression of unpleasant conscious material. *A medical student exits the Part I examination with a sense that he has failed. He decides not to worry about it until the scores arrive in the mail because it will accomplish nothing to do so.*
Humor	A conscious and unconscious defense which allows material that stirs unpleasant affects to be better tolerated in consciousness. *A screaming patient is the subject of laughter and mimicry in the privacy of the doctor's lounge.*

in fact revealed the patient's inner feelings. A typical Freudian slip is demonstrated by the following:

> An unattached young man, envious of a couple who are in love, remarks as they go off to the beach, "Have a nice lay" (instead of "nice day"). Before this slip, if asked directly, the young man would have been unaware that he had a fantasy about the couple's love life. But the slip suggests otherwise.

Dreams

Dreams have been described as the royal road to the unconscious. Freud believed they had a **manifest** or apparent content which disguised the **latent** or **unconscious** content. According to analytic theory, dream work allows sleep to be uninterrupted by transforming the distressing latent content of the dream into the merely perplexing manifest content.

For example, an adolescent describes a dream in which an angel appears and holds his arm. In discussing the dream, the teenager reveals he is troubled by the angel's presence. An exploration of the dream through **free association**—the process of allowing random thoughts to come to mind and be expressed verbally—reveals that the young man associates the dream image with hands, sheets, and ultimately masturbation. When fully analyzed, the angel holding his arm, preventing masturbation, symbolically represents religious values that conflict with his sex impulses. Thus, the analysis of the dream brings to his awareness conflicts about masturbation which then can be explored therapeutically. With this insight, he can then decide how to manage the conflict between sexual impulses and religious rules.

Vignette of an Analysis

The following vignette of an analysis illustrates **free association, transference, resistance,** and **symptom formation.**

> A 33-year-old single woman consults an analyst because her right arm is paralyzed and anesthetic. Previous neurological examinations have failed to explain her disability. Although the patient's family expresses concern about the symptoms, the patient herself appears remarkably calm about it (*la belle indifférence*). In the course of treatment, the analyst discovers that the patient's elderly father, a widower, has suffered a paralytic stroke, leaving him unable to feed himself. The patient's two older sisters decide that all three should take turns feeding their father. Hours before the patient was to take her first turn, the paralysis occurred. Given that the patient's impairment is not explained physically, the analyst attempts to uncover its psychological origins. He instructs the patient to verbalize whatever comes to mind (**free association**) and to report any dreams. These techniques of free association and **dream interpretation** enable the analyst to see glimpses of the patient's unconscious. The data from free association and dreams will be pieced together like the parts of a puzzle to construct a picture of the relevant unconscious material.

Over several sessions, the analyst learns that the patient has conflicting emotions about her father. For example, while free associating, the patient reports the suspicion that the analyst is staring at her breasts and wishing to touch them. Exploration of this fantasy leads to her long-term feelings of sexual vulnerability in the presence of an older man. The analyst now—and her father in her past—are thus linked (**transference**). With considerable distress, the patient then recalls episodes as a teenager when her father teased her about and playfully touched her developing breasts. This painful memory was only recovered after much reluctance by the patient, even to the point that she considered discontinuing treatment. This phenomenon, called **resistance,** occurs when a patient attempts to avoid a topic that may lead to awareness of unconscious material. Such material is shunned because of the emotional pain caused by its discovery.

As the treatment progresses using dreams, free association, transference, and resistance, the analyst discovers that the patient is unconsciously in conflict about caring for her dying father. She speaks about him with hostility as she recalls his teasing behavior but remembers him warmly for his support in later life. Now aware that she harbors the heretofore unconscious impulse to vengefully torment her now defenseless father, she understands how her **conflict** over nurturing and aggression has produced a paralysis which allowed reprieve from a difficult situation. The nature of this conflict was unconscious and, therefore, unknown to the patient before the analysis.

Once the patient has been able to recall her adolescent trauma in the safe environment of the analysis, she resolves to **work through** her conflicting hostile and loving feelings. In other words, her incompletely repressed feelings over caring for her father were converted to a paralysis. Now, with insight into these conflicts, she can work through or accept the fact that ambivalent feelings are a nonthreatening part of human experience. Once unburdened by the conflict, the anxiety disappears, the conversion symptom resolves, and the arm functions again.

> In summary, the paralysis provides an escape from an unresolved dilemma. The symptom eliminated her anxiety (now **converted** to a paralysis) because it precluded either striking or feeding her father (**primary gain**). The **conversion disorder** also elicits support and sympathy from the family (**secondary gain**) (see Chapter 24).

Hysterical paralysis is an especially dramatic symptom, but one might consider that an intrapsychic paralysis (eg, in the areas of intimacy or sexual functioning) will be less conspicuous—but perhaps no less distressing to the afflicted patient. *Unresolved unconscious conflicts may lead to a multitude of varied symptoms.*

Mind & Body

Students in the preclinical phase of medical school often find it difficult to accept the concept that mental states have influence on bodily functions. The intriguing phenomenon of hypnosis provides a familiar example of the mind's power over the body. During a state of hypnotic suggestion, if a subject is asked to make his arm "as stiff as a board," it cannot be passively flexed by another person with any amount of effort. If the subject were not in a hypnotized state, he would not be able to resist forceful flexion even if strongly motivated. Moreover, hypnotized persons can experience standardized painful stimuli without apparent distress.

SCHOOLS OF PSYCHOANALYSIS & LATER PSYCHOTHERAPIES

Psychoanalytic theory was for a time virtually synonymous with the writings and teachings of Sigmund Freud. However, over the years, divergent schools of psychoanalytic theory and psychotherapy evolved. An inner circle of practitioners had gathered around Freud, and, ironically, it was these very disciples who broke with strict freudian principles to found the major nonfreudian schools of psychoanalytic psychology.

Carl Jung and Alfred Adler are perhaps the best known of this group and are briefly discussed below. Other early psychoanalysts who became influential in the history of psychiatry and psychology include Wilhelm Reich, Otto Rank, Erik Erikson, Anna Freud, and Karen Horney.

Carl Jung (1875–1961) differed with and ultimately left Freud to found a separate school of psychology and psychotherapy. He is well known for numerous concepts, one of which was his conception of the unconscious as composed of both the personal unconscious and the collective unconscious. The **collective unconscious** was posited as an inherited commonality of all mankind, the repository of **archetypes**—universal images and concepts found repeatedly in the mythologies of diverse cultures. It is contrasted with the **personal unconscious,** which is based in one's own early experience and individual memories. Jung postulated that all humans face life with a common heritage of images and preprogrammed patterns, ie, the collective history of the human race.

Jung is also known for his schema for describing personality types according to three axes; extroversion-introversion, sensation-intuition, and thinking-feeling. He believed that individual personality styles tend toward one of the two polarities in each of these three axes and that there is benefit in reclaiming one's capacity for wholeness, ie, to actualize personality characteristics that are less developed. He asserted the importance of integrating the opposing aspects found within one's self.

Alfred Adler (1870–1937) also split with Freud after years of collaboration to found his own school of psychology. He was the first of the inner circle to do so. Adler gave less weight to unconscious psychosexual material and focused rather on socially me-diated phenomena. He discussed **feelings of inferiority,** grounded in the infant's experience of helplessness; and of a **will to power** (as a compensatory drive) influencing one's social interactions. Adler is also known for his observations regarding the role of **birth order** in personality development, and he described personality styles typical of first-borns, youngest sibs, etc.

Karen Horney (1885–1952) was an influential analyst who also founded her own school. Her views took more account of the cultural context in which we develop, in particular with regard to sex roles. She felt that character traits commonly considered feminine (dependency, submissiveness, etc) were derived from cultural influences rather than biologic ones. Horney, in general, reflected a move away from the more individualized, psychosexual origins of mental illness toward an emphasis on social and interpersonal forces in development.

Harry Stack Sullivan (1892–1949), an American who did not train with Freud, founded a school of psychoanalytic psychology with its focus turned to **interpersonal relations** as the central theme—with less emphasis on Freud's psychosexual stages. He introduced theories of later stages than Freud's, placing importance on **preadolescence** and the **juvenile** stages, viewing **peer relations** as critical to one's development. Sullivan considered close friendships ('chumships') during preadolescence and early adolescence as laying essential groundwork for the later development of love relationships with the opposite sex.

The **humanistic/existential** schools of psychology emerged later in this century and represented the field's increasing eclecticism and gradual broadening of theories away from the original freudian principles. Axiomatic to these schools are a more philosophical bent, with attention to concepts such as authenticity, taking responsibility for one's life, successful individuation, and the attainment of self-actualization. These schools tended toward the view that all persons have the full potential for mental health and the capacity to live vigorously and with meaning.

•   •   •

The progression has been from Freud to the schools of his followers and colleagues and to a widening array of psychological theories until most practicing psychotherapists consider themselves somewhat eclectic with regard to the nonsomatic treatments—and apply an amalgam of psychological constructs in their work with patients. Many psychotherapists continue to identify themselves with a specific technique or school of thought—but this is becoming the exception rather than the rule.

SOCIAL LEARNING THEORY

The development of the theories underlying modern behavioral treatments took place concurrently with the historical development of the psychoanalytic treatments. The two schools of thought evolved independently, with seemingly little common ground. The pivotal distinction arises from the early behaviorist's primary focus on **observable events,** with little, if any attention paid to the subjective reporting of such nonobservables as feelings or thoughts. In time, behavioral theories and treatments have expanded to encompass less easily quantified phenomena such as cognition and anxiety—yet *the central dogma of the behaviorists remains focused on behavioral change and not on insight, self-reflection, or unconscious mental activity.*

The principles related to the behavioral model—called **social learning theory**—assert that behaviors are **externally determined** and that even complex behaviors are learned and maintained by environmental consequences such as reward and punishment—and are not so much the result of internal psychological processes.

The history of behavioral theory begins with the experiments of Ivan Pavlov (1849–1936), best known for his paradigm of **classical conditioning,** wherein a dog that naturally salivates at the sight of meat is then conditioned to salivate at the sound of a bell when no food is present. This example illustrates several key terms in social learning theory. The **unconditioned stimulus** is the food, the original **stimulus** that led to the **response** of salivation. This unconditioned stimulus is then paired with a **conditioned stimulus,** the sound of a bell. In time the salivation response is elicited by the conditioned stimulus (the bell) even in the absence of the unconditioned stimulus (the food). This simple classical conditioning process has its role in more complex human behaviors.

Modern addictionologists know that their patients are at special risk for relapse when exposed to stimuli that were at one time closely paired with the substance of abuse. The sight of a familiar liquor store or a dealer-haunted street corner can elicit powerful craving for the abused substance in individuals whose ''high'' was closely associated with these stimuli. The abused substance in this example is the unconditioned stimulus, which elicits craving in a drug-dependent person—craving being the homologue of Pavlov's dog's salivating.

J.B. Watson (1878–1958), an American psychologist influenced by Pavlov, conducted a famous experiment in which an 11-month-old boy, Albert B., was the subject. Albert would cry and become frightened in response to loud noises, an **unconditioned stimulus.** Watson paired the loud noise with the sight of a white rat, the **conditioned stimulus.** Albert quickly learned to avoid the rat, which he had not previously feared. Furthermore, Albert also avoided other objects with appearances similar to the white rat—this being an example of **stimulus generalization**.

Edward Thorndike (1874–1949) and B.F. Skinner (1904–1990) were prominent pioneers in the field of behaviorism. Thorndike postulated the law of effect—ie, that the consequences of a behavior determine the frequency of that behavior. Skinner, a truly central figure in the development and exposition of behavioral theory, is known particularly for his work in operant conditioning.

Operant conditioning is the manipulation of behaviors through consequences structured to follow the targeted behaviors. **Positive reinforcers** increase the frequency of a behavior, and, conversely, **punishment** decreases the frequency of a behavior. This behavioral definition of punishment requires an accompanying decrease in target behavior frequency. Scolding a child, if it does not lead to a decrease in the targeted behavior—is *not* technically defined as punishment. **Negative reinforcement** is reward by the removal or avoidance of an undesirable consequence and serves, as does positive reinforcement, to increase the frequency of a targeted behavior. These terms are illustrated in the following example:

A pigeon may peck at a bar in its cage every now and then. If pecking on the bar is now **positively reinforced** by immediately rewarding the behavior with food, the frequency of bar-pecking will increase. This is **operant conditioning.** If, subsequently, bar-pecking no longer leads to a food reward, the conditioned increase in the frequency of bar-pecking will gradually be **extinguished.** The time course of this **extinction** of a conditioned response varies considerably depending on the nature of the conditioning that initiated the behavior.

In the case of pigeon, if food was forthcoming *every time* the bar was pecked **(continuous reinforcement),** the behavior would be extinguished rather quickly after the food reinforcement is discontinued. If food was given only *some of the times* the bar was pecked **(intermittent reinforcement)**, extinction of the pecking behavior would occur much more slowly. The power of **intermittent positive reinforcement** is graphically demonstrated at casinos and race tracks, where the relatively rare jackpot drives a high frequency of unrewarded plays despite the cost of each play. This is an example of the importance of the **schedule of reinforcement** on the persistence of behaviors. Behaviors conditioned by strong positive reinforcers on an intermittent reinforcement schedule are slow to extinguish.

Complex behaviors can be conditioned through shaping, wherein successive approximations of the desired behavior are reinforced in turn. Encouraging a withdrawn, hospitalized patient to interact with peers might involve initially rewarding simply sitting near peers, then rewarding an occasional ''thank you'' or ''excuse me,'' the intervention moving in stepwise fashion toward the desired complex behavior of interacting fully with peers.

Behavioral principles are often used in the treatment of phobias, including agoraphobia, and frequently employ a combination of **relaxation training** and **systematic desensitization,** a combination of techniques pioneered by Joseph Wolpe (1915–). The patient is trained to self-induce a relaxed state by serially tensing and then relaxing the muscles, working through the major muscle groups, usually from head to toe or vice versa. The patient is then instructed to imagine the phobic situation, beginning with only a mild stimulus, and to simultaneously remain in the relaxed state.

For example, a man with a fear of flying would first learn the relaxation exercise and then be directed to imagine purchasing a plane ticket while maintaining the relaxed state. The next step might be remaining relaxed while imagining arriving at the airport with his luggage, and so on, until the relaxed state can persist even while vividly imagining a turbulent flight in a crowded aircraft. The patient is thus **systematically desensitized** to a stimulus that once elicited a phobic response. A more comprehensive discussion of behavioral treatments is found in Chapters 35 and 38.

NEUROBIOLOGY & SOMATIC TREATMENTS

The somatic treatments (Chapter 32) are considered nonpsychological in nature and consist essentially of psychotropic medications and electroconvulsive therapy (ECT). The history of the somatic treatments is one of empirical and at times fortuitous advances. Preexisting nonpsychiatric medications, were in several instances discovered to have efficacy in the treatment of a mental disorder. This clinically observed effect of a new medication on a psychiatric syndrome would inevitably lead to hypotheses regarding the neurobiological basis of the drug effect.

If, for example, a medication efficacious in the treatment of delusional thinking is known to decrease central nervous system dopamine neurotransmission—a hypothesis implicating excessive dopamine neurotransmission as the cause of delusional thoughts is generated. This example is somewhat oversimplified but illustrates the concurrent evolution of somatic treatments and the science of neurobiology. The medications have helped elucidate biological mechanisms of mental illness, as has research with chemical probes structurally similar to the medications. *Modern psychopharmacology is the science of influencing central nervous system neurotransmission.*

As yet, the detailed mechanisms mediating most psychiatric illnesses are not fully understood, but modern theories are centered primarily around dysfunctional neurotransmission. For example, the medications used to treat the symptoms of schizophrenia are thought to do so via their effect on dopaminergic neurotransmission. The antidepressant medications (and ECT) affect neurotransmission mediated by norepinephrine or serotonin. Obsessive-compulsive disorder is treated with medications that affect serotonergic neurotransmission, and so on. These treatments and their hypothesized mechanisms of action are discussed in greater detail in Chapters 6 and 32 and in the chapters devoted to specific types of mental disorder.

Further light is shed on the neurobiology of mental illness by research in the fields of genetics and molecular biology. As illustrated in the following discussion and examples, *it is generally accepted that with regard to mental illness, the answer to questions about the relative influence of nature versus nurture is that both contribute to the development of psychiatric disorders*. It is often stated, in discussions of the causes of the major psychiatric disorders, that they result from the confluence of an inherited genetic vulnerability to the disorder *plus* environmental factors, ie, developmental experiences (the so-called stress-diathesis model).

A powerful tool in evaluating genetic versus environmental factors in mental illness is the study of family pedigrees and especially the study of twins. Monozygotic (identical) twins have virtually identical genomes, whereas dizygotic (fraternal) twins, on average, share only half their genes. *One can therefore predict that genetically based illnesses will show a higher concordance rate in monozygotic twins than in dizygotic twins.*

For example, in schizophrenia, the concordance rate in monozygotic twins is approximately 50%. This indicates that if one member of a pair of monozygotic twins has schizophrenia, there is a 50% likelihood that the other twin will also have the illness. In dizygotic twins the concordance rate is approximately one-fourth that found in monozygotic twins, thus supporting the role of heredity in this illness. This 50% concordance rate in genetically identical individuals argues eloquently for both the genetic contribution to the illness and for the nongenetic, environmental contribution—as the **discordance** rate is also 50%. Recent studies suggest that schizophrenic patients with the worst long-term outcome may have greater genetic loading for schizophrenia (ie, genetic relatives also have the disorder) than do schizophrenics with more favorable outcomes (Keefe et al, 1987).

Recent advances in the field of molecular genetics have also contributed to our understanding of the neurobiology of psychiatric illness, as in the following example:

A recent study probed a specific gene fragment on chromosome 11 in alcoholic versus nonalcoholic subjects, using postmortem tissue samples. This particular gene is known to code for one subtype of dopamine receptor, and two different alleles were identified as possible occupants of this particular gene locus: the A1 and A2 alleles. It was found that 69% of the alcoholic subjects possessed the A1 allele, whereas only 20% of the nonalcoholic subjects possessed the A1 allele. This research supports family pedigree studies that have suggested a hereditary component in alcoholism and further suggests that dopaminergic neurotransmission has a role in this disorder. One must note, however, that 31% of the alcoholic subjects did not possess the A1 allele (yet still developed alcoholism) and that 20% of the nonalcoholic subjects did not become alcoholics despite having the A1 allele. Again, both nature and nurture are etiologic with respect to the development of mental illnesses. The above study is not referenced as a definitive genetic model of alcoholism but to illustrate the role and techniques of molecular genetics in psychiatry.

THE CHALLENGE OF INTEGRATION

By any measure, the preceding sections have covered considerable ground—from primitive religion to molecular genetics, from Freud to Skinner, from the collective unconscious to electroconvulsive therapy. At some point, one must acknowledge and grapple with the difficulty of integrating this body of information; across disciplines and across theoretical frameworks within the field of psychiatry.

Quality patient care is ultimately an interdisciplinary and integrative endeavor. Throughout this text, several case studies will be presented to illustrate the principle that all problems involving the complexity of human beings require a broadly based integrative approach. What is called for is the simultaneous application of medical science and psychology and an appreciation of the sociological context of a patient's illness.

Specialization is the reality of modern medicine and indeed of contemporary society in general. Even within the traditional medical and surgical specialties there are subspecialists. In the face of a burgeoning biomedical database, this trend is both rational and inevitable with one proviso: *All specialists and subspecialists must avoid thinking that an effective doctor-patient relationship falls into the realm of "someone else's specialty."* And it must be emphasized also that any effective clinical relationship involves more than treating a disease or symptom. Treating a complex person requires attention to the psychological aspects of the predicament and to the social context of the patient's life (family, work, etc). The following case is reported as a narrative delivered by the patient, a 41-year-old construction foreman.

"I had to go for an insurance physical because I got a new job. This young doc noticed something suspicious on one of my testicles, and he said it was probably nothing but that I should go see a urologist to get it checked out. He says this to me and is out the door ten seconds later. Busy guy.

"So I get home, and I start to worry—but I couldn't feel anything wrong down there. So I wonder if whatever it was might be serious, like cancer, and it crosses my mind that, God forbid, I might need surgery and that I'd lose my testicles or never get hard-ons, or something. Now that really scared me—so I didn't tell my wife and just tried to forget the whole thing. She was trying to get pregnant and I figured I'd wait until after that.

"Nearly two years go by, and she's not pregnant. My wife's gynecologist sends home a plastic container for me to give a sperm sample, and then drop it off at a lab. Okay. I've been checking myself, and my testicles feel just like always, so I tell myself not to worry. But I am anyway.

"To make a long story short, it turns out that she's not getting pregnant because my sperm count is too low. I go to a urologist and he says I have an extra vein that's causing the problem, that he can fix it, and maybe my sperm count will get higher.

"He tells me that it's not cancer even though I didn't even ask him that. He says there's basically no chance I'd lose anything, and he drew some pictures on a piece of paper. He was great and I said okay to the operation. He said the insurance doctor made a good pick-up and that a lot of doctors would've missed it. My wife was pregnant about four months after the operation. I just wish sometimes that I would've gotten it checked out sooner."

Comment: As noted by the urologist, the original discovery of the varicocele was a "good pick-up" from a biomedical viewpoint—but the doctor-patient contact was nonetheless inadequate and allowed for significant distress in the psychological and social spheres of the patient's illness.

In a landmark article in 1977, George Engel elucidated the **biopsychosocial model,** a framework based in the integrative, whole person approach to patient care. Engel coined this term with the intent of distinguishing this more holistic approach from the prevalent **biomedical model.** As the field of medicine evolves, so must our awareness of the body-mind interface become more sophisticated. Terms such as "neuroendocrine," "psychoneuroimmunology," and "neuropsychiatric" have entered the lexicon of medicine as we further elucidate the actual integrative biology in the human body and brain. This is discussed further in Chapter 3.

REFERENCES

Alexander F, Selesnick S: *The History of Psychiatry.* New American Library, 1966.

Bandura A: *Social Learning Theory.* General Learning Press, 1971.

Benson H: *The Relaxation Response.* Morrow, 1975.

Blum K et al: Allelic association of human dopamine D^2 receptor gene in alcoholism. JAMA 1990;263:15. *Diagnostic and Statistical Manual of Mental Disorders (DSM-III-R),* 3rd ed, rev. American Psychiatric Association, 1987.

Engel G: The need for a new medical model: A challenge for biomedicine. Science 1977;196:129.

Engel GE: *Psychological Development in Health and Disease.* Saunders, 1962.

Engel GE: The clinical application of the biopsychosocial model. Am J Psychiatry 1978;137:535.

Farber SL: *Identical Twins Reared Apart: A Reanalysis.* Basic Books, 1981.

Fine R: *A History of Psychoanalysis.* Columbia Univ Press, 1979.

Freud A: *The Ego and the Mechanisms of Defense.* International Univ Press, 1946.

Freud S: *Standard Edition of the Complete Psychological Works of Sigmund Freud.* Hogarth Press, 1959.

Gilman AG et al (editors): *Goodman and Gilman's The Pharmacological Basis of Therapeutics,* 8th ed. Pergamon, 1990.

Hall C, Lindzey G: *Theories of Personality.* Wiley, 1957.

Horney K: *The Neurotic Personality of Our Time.* Norton, 1937.

Jung CG: *Memories, Dreams and Reflections.* Random House, 1961.

Kaplan HI, Sadock BJ (editors): *Comprehensive Textbook of Psychiatry/V,* 5th ed. Williams & Wilkins, 1989.

Keefe RSE et al: Characteristics of very poor outcome schizophrenia. Am J Psychiatry 1987;144:889.

Kubler-Ross E: *On Death and Dying.* Macmillan, 1969.

Leigh H, Reiser MF: *The Patient: Biological, Psychological, and Social Dimensions of Medical Practice.* Plenum Press, 1980.

Meltzer HY et al (editors): *Psychopharmacology: The Third Generation of Progress.* Raven Press, 1987.

Michels R et al (editors): *Psychiatry.* Lippincott/Basic Books, 1986.

Piel G et al (editors): *The Brain: A Scientific American Book.* Freeman, 1979.

Reich W: *Character Analysis.* Farrar, Straus & Young, 1949.

Skinner BF: *Science and Human Behavior.* Macmillan, 1953.

Thorndike EL: *The Psychology of Learning.* Teachers College, 1913.

Strayhorn JM: *Foundations of Clinical Psychiatry.* Year Book, 1982.

Vaillant G: *Adaptation to Life.* Little, Brown, 1977.

Weiner H: *Psychobiology and Human Disease.* Elsevier-North Holland, 1977.

Wolpe J: *The Practice of Behavior Therapy.* Pergamon, 1973.

Yalom I: *Existential Psychotherapy.* Basic Books, 1980.

3

The Mind & Somatic Illness: Psychological Factors Affecting Physical Illness

Stuart J. Eisendrath, MD

Example: A 60-year-old woman entered a hospital emergency room complaining of light-headedness and chest palpitations. Shortly thereafter, she suffered a cardiac arrest that was successfully treated, and she was transferred to the coronary care unit. When she was examined, she was not only anxious but also depressed. On questioning, she revealed that the date of her cardiac arrest was the 1-year anniversary of her husband's death from cardiac arrest.

Example: A 40-year-old businessman underwent a traumatic divorce and became seriously depressed. The wife to whom he had been devoted had left him for a 25-year-old tennis instructor. Two months later, the businessman was found to have an aggressive lymphoma, and he died 3 months later after several unsuccessful trials of chemotherapy.

Example: A 4-year-old boy had always had excellent health. Two weeks after his only sibling was born, however, he developed persistent cough and fever. He eventually required hospitalization for treatment of pneumonia.

The above are examples of typical clinical situations in which attentive and alert clinicians may see the influence of psychosocial factors on physical health. Physicians have been aware of this relationship since ancient times. The study of this relationship, usually termed **psychosomatic medicine,** has undergone marked conceptual shifts in the past decade. Today, theorists believe that there are no "psychosomatic" diseases per se and that all physical diseases have psychosocial components. These components may predispose to illness, initiate it, or maintain it. This chapter focuses on the development of theories of psychosomatic medicine in the 20th century.

Mind/Body & Stress

Before the 1900s, the philosophy of Cartesian dualism viewed the mind and the body as separate entities. Organized religions claimed the mind and spirit as their domain, while physicians were ceded the body. This dichotomy was heightened by scientific progress in the late 1800s. The discovery that bacteria were causative agents of disease emphasized the physical aspects of medicine and also led to the concept of linear causality: one type of bacterium directly causes one disease. This oversimplified concept of a unitary cause of disease—one factor directly causes one specific disease—influenced the development of psychosomatic theory for several decades.

Cannon was one of the pioneers working in psychosomatic medicine. He performed intricate laboratory experiments that studied the effects of fear and rage on animals. Cannon saw that animals responded to emergencies with adaptive changes in physiology that prepared them for "fight or flight." Cannon theorized that the mechanism involved an inhibition of anabolic (parasympathetic; cholinergic) functions and an activation of catabolic (sympathetic; adrenergic) functions. This combination of processes supplied the animals with energy needed to meet the emergency.

Selye (1974) extended the work of Cannon. He postulated that the entire organism responded to stress; eg, blood flow might be shunted from the gastrointestinal tract to the heart, brain, and musculature during stress. Such an adaptation would help the organism deal with stress over the short term, but if the stress was prolonged, the adaptation might result in increased friability of the gastrointestinal mucosa and eventual ulceration. Selye proposed that responses to stress could be triggered in inappropriate situations if the organism had been accustomed to react in that way. Later research in autonomic conditioning suggests that such inappropriate reactions may be difficult to extinguish.

Personality & Medical Illness

In the 1940s, Dunbar (1942, 1946) began developing her "personality profiles" of specific diseases. She felt that each disease was associated with a specific cluster of symptoms, and she therefore reviewed psychological data about patients with diseases such as hypertension, diabetes, rheumatoid arthritis, and myocardial infarction and from these formulated typical behavior patterns, family histories, and patterns of onset of illness that seemed to be associated. She suggested, for example, that people with myocardial infarction tend to be compulsive and to overwork and that the infarction tends to follow exposure to shock, particularly at work.

The idea that a specific personality may be associated with a certain disease is most evident in current research into the behavior of people with coronary disease. Friedman and Rosenman (1974) labeled the behavior of these patients type A. Their work suggested that these patients chronically feel the pressure of time and a sense of hostile competitiveness.

A major deficit in the "specific personality" approach to understanding the relationship between psychological makeup and disease is that almost all of the data rely on retrospective analysis. People who already have a certain disease are studied psychologically in an attempt to discern whether certain personality traits caused the disease. But specific psychological profiles are of limited value. Researchers following the model of direct linear causation derived from Koch's postulates tended to adopt the approach in the 1930s and 1940s that personality might "cause" disease. Treatment techniques (chiefly psychoanalysis) that tried to eradicate the precipitating psychological factor were notably unsuccessful, however.

It therefore became clear that direct, unitary causation did not operate in the development of diseases. Dunbar herself was careful to avoid implications of cause and effect in her work. Alternative explanations of the behavior associated with certain diseases were formulated. Perhaps the behavior resulted from the disease, or perhaps the behavior and the physical illness were both phenotypic expressions of some common gene. These theories suggested that psychological treatments that attempted to change behavior might not "cure" disease. Current research is evaluating how changes in type A behavior traits affect a person's chances of incurring myocardial infarction. Prospective studies in progress avoid the deficits of earlier work. Current studies of the effects of behavioral intervention on myocardial infarction are showing positive results. Data on recurrence are inconclusive. The hypothesis that psychological factors cause disease will still not be proved, however, even with behavioral treatments demonstrating effectiveness in preventing recurrences.

In contrast to Dunbar's personality-specific research, Alexander (1950) explored the relationship between specific psychological conflicts and disease states. He investigated seven diseases regarded as classic psychosomatic disorders: peptic ulcers, bronchial asthma, rheumatoid arthritis, ulcerative colitis, essential hypertension, thyrotoxicosis, and neurodermatitis. His work attempted to answer the main question in psychosomatic medicine in the 1930s and 1940s—why does the individual have these specific symptoms?

Alexander believed that psychosomatic diseases developed out of "visceral neurosis." Physiological changes accompanied unresolved emotional conflicts and eventually resulted in pathological derangements in the organ system. For example, Alexander hypothesized that individuals with peptic ulcer disease suffered from infantile desires for others to supply love, support, advice, and money. When frustrated, these desires intensified but then produced guilt and shame in these patients, who wanted to appear as capable, independent adults. The desire to be cared for was equivalent to the infantile wish to be fed, and the conflicting drives for independence and dependence were expressed as increased gastric secretions. The secretions in turn led to formation of ulcers.

Alexander advanced the theory of psychosomatic medicine significantly by abandoning a model of disease based on unitary, direct causation. He postulated a three-part constellation of factors necessary to produce disease: (1) The individual must have a specific set of psychological conflicts; (2) a specific situation that triggers the onset of disease must occur; in ulcer disease, this might be the loss of a person on whom the patient depended; and (3) the individual must have a constitutional vulnerability, an "X factor," that biologically predisposes the patient to that specific illness.

Alexander's work suffered because it was based on retrospective analysis. Mirsky (1958) investigated Alexander's ideas in an ingenious prospective study that used army recruits who were entering basic training. The recruits were divided into two groups on the basis of high or low levels of serum pepsinogen, a genetically determined trait that correlates with some types of ulcer formation. Those recruits with high levels of serum pepsinogen were found to have the infantile features suggested by Alexander; moreover, they could be identified from their responses to psychological testing by independent raters who did not know their serum pepsinogen levels. The recruits who subsequently developed ulcers associated with the stress of basic training proved to be from the group who had high levels of serum pepsinogen.

Further Development of Theories of Psychosomatic Medicine

The Mirsky study tended to confirm many of Alexander's ideas but left many questions unanswered. How did stress lead to formation of ulcers? Why did the psychotherapeutic approaches have such variable success in treatment of psychosomatic disorders such as ulcers?

Mirsky's study opened a new area of inquiry in psychosomatic medicine. Could an inherited biological tendency toward gastric hypersecretion lead to psychological sequelae? For example, a newborn with high rates of gastric secretion might biologically require hourly feedings to diminish gastric acidity. If the mother fed the newborn at "average" intervals of once every 3 hours, conflict concerning dependence on others for attention and nurturance might be created in the newborn's personality. The genetic predisposition to gastric hypersecretion could lead to somatopsychic effects. Personality development could therefore be a result of physiological events, rather than the reverse.

Grinker et al (1973) began integrating such possibilities into a unified field theory of psychosomatic medicine. This approach was basically a general systems model of illness. This theory emphasized that each element of the human "system" (eg, personality or genetic constitution) had multiple reverberating connections throughout the system. Biological and psychosocial forces could interact with each other to produce disease. The effect of this theory was to clearly point out the inadequacy of the unitary, direct causation model of disease.

At the same time, the work of Engel directed psychosomatic theory toward less specific but broader concepts of the production of illness. Engel (1975) noted that loss of an important person in the patient's life frequently preceded the onset or exacerbation of illness. Engel himself described how he suffered a myocardial infarction on the last day of a mourning period for his twin brother.

Engel (1967) believed that loss led to several phases of response. At first, the individual was aroused to search for the lost object. If the search failed, the person entered a state of "conservation withdrawal" and ceased to search; physiological processes (eg, gastric secretion) became hypoactive. Engel believed that such a sequence could lead to a giving up-given up state, in which the individual felt helpless to change his or her situation and hopeless about receiving aid from others. Such a condition predisposed a person to development of illness. Engel did not believe that this condition was in itself sufficient to cause illness, nor did he feel that this condition had to exist before illness occurred. Such a condition could make the person vulnerable to illness, however.

Animal experiments lent support to Engel's position. Kaufman and Rosenblum (1969) used different species of monkeys to study the physiological response of an infant who was separated from its mother. The infant's patterns of behavior tended to follow the series of responses outlined by Engel, and the incidence of illness increased. Among certain species, however, the pattern was moderated if the deprived young monkey was provided with social support.

Epidemiological studies have also supported Engel's work. Holmes and Rahe (1967) evaluated the effects of stressful events on the occurrence of physical illness. In both retrospective and prospective studies, they found that the number and magnitude of life changes (eg, bereavements, new jobs, moving to another place) correlated with the onset and severity of disease. Their work suggests that changes in life may encourage the development of disease, but in a nonspecific way.

Other researchers have evaluated bereavement as one specific and powerful type of life change. Rees and Lutkins (1967) noted that the number of deaths among relatives of patients who had died was seven times higher than in the general population. Parkes and Brown (1972) found similarly elevated mortality rates in another population of bereaved individuals. These findings have been reproduced in many countries. It is clear that loss of an emotionally important person is associated with increased incidence of both illness and death, particularly in young widowers.

Reiser (1975) believed that there are three phases related to illness. During the period before illness develops, the patient is shaped by genetic constitution and early psychosocial experiences. When the illness appears, the prior "programming" is activated by nonspecific psychosocial stresses, such as bereavement. Other factors, such as environmental exposure to viruses or malignant transformation in cells, may then challenge the stressed individual and produce disease. In the third phase, after the onset of disease, psychosocial forces operate to modulate the course of the disease.

Biopsychosocial Model of Disease

Engel (1977) synthesized the advances in psychosomatic medicine by developing the biopsychosocial model of disease, which recognizes that *all* diseases have biological, psychological, and social components. Engel's model emphasizes the view that each individual is composed of systems and is in turn part of larger outside systems. Each person is composed of molecules, cells, and organs; each person is also a member of a family, community, culture, nation, and world. Every individual has a biological, psychological, and social structure that may affect other levels of the system and vice versa. As an example, Engel (1980) described a patient undergoing cardiac arrest, an account paraphrased here and used to illustrate how Engel's theory may be applied:

A patient suffers chest pain and goes to a hospital emergency room. Because he has had one previous myocardial infarction, he suspects that he is having another. He is examined by a new intern, who also suspects an infarction and who attempts to insert an intravenous line. After several unsuccessful attempts, the intern leaves the patient alone in his cubicle and goes to get assistance. While unattended, the patient continues to feel pain and also feels alone and worried about the competence of his caretakers. He suffers a cardiac arrest and is immediately resuscitated successfully by the emergency team.

If the viewpoint adopted by the clinician is a biomedical model based on linear causality, the successful resuscitation of the patient is a laudable event. If psychosocial factors are taken into account, however, important information is revealed about the patient and the incident; namely, that the patient's pain, fear, and doubts most likely affected the physical disease process, possibly through direct vagal effects, increased levels of circulating catecholamines, or other physiological responses. If medical personnel had considered psychosocial factors and started appropriate treatment—eg, ensuring constant attention by the nursing staff or using anxiolytic medications–the cardiac arrest might not have occurred at all. The biopsychosocial model does not simplistically assert that the myocardial infarction was a direct result of the patient's psychology. It does provide a broader understanding of disease processes, and it encourages physicians to think about truly comprehensive treatment that considers both the physical and the psychosocial elements of disease.

The model also includes sociocultural factors in its conception of disease. It has been widely demonstrated, for example, that pain as a presenting symptom is affected by sex, race, and ethnic origin. The biopsychosocial model holds that a stoic New England Yankee may be experiencing as much pain as an expressive Italian patient with the same disease.

CURRENT CONCEPTS
IN PSYCHOSOMATIC MEDICINE

The biopsychosocial model provides one approach to study of the relationship between disease and psychosocial factors. Current research in psychosomatic medicine has shifted from the "why" questions so common in earlier decades to the "how" questions— eg, how does the bereavement experience become translated into physical illness? In other words, how are psychological experiences transduced into bodily changes?

Work in the field of type A behavior and psychoimmunology highlights current approaches aimed at understanding the transduction process. In extension of Friedman and Rosenman's work, a number of prospective studies have demonstrated that type A behavior is indeed a risk factor for the development of coronary heart disease. These prospective studies corrected a major weakness of the earlier retrospective research. In the more recent studies, one of the key toxic elements in type A behavior appears to be hostility, particularly when associated with conscious suppression of anger (Barefoot, 1983). In attempting to understand how type A behavior might produce coronary heart disease, several studies investigating physiological changes in type A individuals found they had higher plasma norepinephrine, epinephrine, and cortisol levels than type B individuals when challenged with a stressful task (Williams, 1982). Such changes might be expected to be important in terms of promoting atherogenesis through a variety of mechanisms, including lipid mobilization and blood pressure changes.

Psychoimmunology is another area of research that is trying to elucidate the relationship between psychological processes and physiological events. Some research has already demonstrated profound effects of

psychological events on an individual. Bartrop et al (1977) studied the spouses of survivors of an Australian train wreck and found that 5 weeks postbereavement, these individuals had lymphocyte T cell responses to mitogens that were tenfold less than in a control group. Similarly, Schliefer et al (1983) studied the spouses of women dying of breast cancer. They discovered depressed lymphocyte response to mitogens peaking at 2 months postbereavement and gradually returning to normal over the remainder of the postbereavement year for most subjects. This carefully designed study demonstrated that the immune abnormalities were a direct result of the bereavement process and not due to factors such as nutrition, activity, or sleep.

Animal experimentation has demonstrated marked effects of stress on illness. Riley (1975) exposed two groups of mice to the Bittner virus, which usually causes mammary tumors. One experimental group was kept in a stress-free setting. The other group was placed in a high-stress, crowded environment. At the end of the experiment, the incidence of tumor was 7% in the first group and 92% in the second group. In an innovative study, Ader and Cohen (1975) induced immunosuppression in rats as a conditioned response. They exposed rats to saccharin along with the immunosuppressant drug cyclophosphamide. Subsequent reexposure of the rats to saccharin alone produced immunosuppression at significant levels and demonstrated that immunosuppression may be a learned behavior.

In an extension of this approach to humans, Smith and McDaniel (1983) raised the possibility of a similar conditioned response in humans. They tuberculin skin-tested subjects on a monthly basis five times, utilizing a saline injection on the opposite arm. On the sixth trial, unbeknownst to the subject or the nurse administering the test, the injections were reversed. A markedly decreased cutaneous reaction was found in the arm where tuberculin skin test antigen was injected but saline was expected. Such experimentation demonstrates that psychological states, including expectations, can affect the immune response.

Various authors have suggested possible mechanisms of action for psychological effects on the immune system. Rogers et al (1979) suggested three possibilities. One mechanism may involve the hypothalamic-pituitary-adrenal axis. It has been known for years that stress can cause an acute increase in cortisol production. This increase, in turn, may lead to impaired cell-mediated immunity. The issue is complicated, however, because prolonged stress may not have the same effects as short-term stress and may actually be associated with enhanced cell-mediated immunity.

A second possible mediator of stress is the autonomic nervous system. For example, single lymphocytes are known to have β-adrenergic receptors, so release of catecholamines by the sympathetic nervous system would be expected to affect lymphocyte function.

A third possible mechanism is that the nervous system may be directly linked to the immune system. The conditioned response in Ader and Cohen's work might be explained by such a mechanism, since the increased amounts of cortisol alone cannot fully explain their findings of immunosuppression. In addition, Besedovsky (1977) has immunized rats and found increased electrical activity immediately afterward in the ventromedial hypothalamic nuclei. Researchers therefore speculate that there must be some afferent link between antigen stimulation and hypothalamic function. The idea is supported by experimental studies showing that anaphylactic reactions may be prevented by experimentally inducing hypothalamic lesions. In addition, antigen-stimulated lymphocytes secrete substances that may directly affect the hypothalamus (Smith, 1982). An efferent link has been suggested by the demonstration of nerve endings in the thymus and spleen as well as lymph nodes (Williams, 1980).

SUMMARY

The field of psychosomatic medicine has shifted from theories of unitary psychogenic causes of disease to an approach that integrates psychosocial and biological factors. Current research is examining how psychological factors are transduced into physiological changes.

The biopsychosocial model may be applied to all diseases and is especially useful in helping to decide which treatments to use; eg, the clinician who realizes that peptic ulcer disease has psychological and social components as well as physical elements will consider not only cimetidine but also psychotherapy as possible treatments. Treatment based only on biological considerations may be useless in coronary artery disease unless the patient's psychosocial characteristics are taken into account. Even if type A behavior is discounted as an influence on disease, the patient's compliance with medication requirements and changes in exercise, smoking habits, and diet may all affect progression and disease.

As Lipowski (1977) noted, the cause of disease remains a focus of interest in psychosomatic medicine. Another major interest is the investigation of how psychological processes are mediated in the production of disease. As this relationship is elucidated, new types of treatment are sure to follow.

REFERENCES

Ader R, Cohen N: Behaviorally conditioned immunosuppression. Psychosom Med 1975;37:333.

Alexander F: *Psychosomatic Medicine. Its Principles and Applications.* Norton, 1950.

Barefoot JC, Dahlstrom G, Williams RB: Hostility, CHD incidence, and total mortality: A 25 year follow-up study of 255 physicians. Psychosom Medic 1983;45:59.

Bartrop RW et al: Depressed lymphocyte function after bereavement. Lancet 1977;1:834.

Besedovsky H et al: Hypothalamic changes during the immune response. Eur J Immunol 1977;7:323.

Dembroski TM et al: Stress, emotions, behavior, and cardiovascular disease. In: *Emotions in Health and Illness: Theoretical and Research Foundations.* Temoshok L, Van Dyke C, Zegans L (editors). Grune & Stratton, 1983.

Dunbar HF: *Emotions and Bodily Change,* 3rd ed. Columbia Univ Press, 1946.

Dunbar HF: The relationship between anxiety states and organic disease. Clinics 1942;1:879.

Engel GL: The clinical application of the biopsychosocial model. Am J Psychiatry 1980;137:535.

Engel GL: The death of a twin: Mourning and anniversary reactions. Fragments of 10 years of self-analysis. Int J Psychoanal 1975;56:23.

Engel GL: The need for a new medical model: A challenge for biomedicine. Science 1977;196: 129.

Engel GL: A psychological setting of somatic disease: The giving up-given up complex. Proc Roy Soc Med 1967;60:553.

Friedman M, Rosenman RH: Type A Behavior and Your Heart. Knopf, 1974.

Greene WA et al: Psychosocial factors and immunity: Preliminary report of the annual meeting. American Psychosomatic Society, March 31, 1978.

Grinker RR: *Psychosomatic Concepts,* 3rd ed. Jason Aronson, 1973.

Holmes TH, Rahe RH: The social readjustment rating scale. J Psychosom Res 1967;11:213.

Kaufman IC, Rosenblum L: Effects of separation from mother on the emotional behavior of infant monkeys. Ann NY Acad Sci 1969;159:60 1.

Lipowski, ZJ: Psychosomatic medicine in the seventies: An overview. Am J Psychiatry 1977;134:233.

Locke SE: Stress adaptation and immunity. Gen Hosp Psychiatry 1982;4:49.

Locke SE et al: The influence of stress on the immune response: Preliminary report of the annual meeting. American Psychosomatic Society, March 31, 1978.

Mirsky IA: Physiologic, psychologic, and social determinants in the etiology of duodenal ulcer. Am J Dig Dis 1958;3:285.

Parkes CM, Brown RJ: Health after bereavement: A controlled study of young Boston widows and widowers. Psychosom Med 1972;34:449.

Rees WD, Lutkins SG: Mortality or bereavement. Br Med J 1967;4:13.

Reiser MF: Changing theoretical concepts in psychosomatic medicine. Pages 477–500 in: *American Handbook of Psychiatry,* 2nd ed. Vol 4. Basic Books, 1975.

Riley V: Mouse mammary tumors: Alteration of incidence as apparent function of stress. Science 1975;189:465.

Rogers MP, Dubey D, Reich P: The influence of the psyche and the brain on immunity and disease susceptibility: A critical review. Psychosom Med 1979;41: 147.

Rose RM: Endocrine responses to stressful psychological events: Advances in psychoneuroendocrinology. Psychiatr Clin North Am 1980;3:251.

Schliefer SJ et al: Suppression of lymphocyte stimulation following bereavement. JAMA 1983;250:374.

Selye H: *Stress Without Distress*. Lippincott, 1974.

Smith EM, Meyer WJ, Blalock JE: Virus-induced cortico-sterone in hypophysectomized mice: A possible lymphoid adrenal axis. Science 1982;218:1311.

Smith RG, McDaniel SM: Psychologically mediated effect on the delayed hypersensitivity reaction to tuberculin in humans. Psychosom Med 1983;45:65.

Weiner H et al: Etiology of duodenal ulcer. Psychosom Med 1957;19:1.

Williams RB et al: Type A behavior and elevated physiological and neuroendocrine responses to cognitive tasks. Science 1982;218:483.

Williams JW et al: Sympathetic innervation of murine thymus and spleen: Evidence for a functional link between the nervous and immune system. Brain Res Bull 1980;6:83.

Wolff HG, Wolf S, Hare CE (editors): *Life Stress and Bodily Disease*. Williams & Wilkins, 1950.

4

Child, Adolescent, & Adult Development

Aubrey W. Metcalf, MD*

CONCEPTS OF CHILD DEVELOPMENT

An understanding of the processes of growth and development has become indispensable for the study of human biology and behavior; the field is now a basic science in all clinical curricula. Recent advances in knowledge have revealed a striking orderliness and continuity in the immensely complicated, mysterious, and beautiful transformations that occur from conception to old age. These advances provide clues to how we come to be the way we are. Much detailed study has yet to be done, but the main mechanisms of biological development are well understood in animals and young humans, and their links to behavioral development are rapidly being clarified. As research on personality in later life accumulates, it becomes apparent that changing phases and developmental tasks may be characteristic not only of the early years but of the entire life cycle. For the clinician, an understanding of the orderliness of development serves as a framework within which each individual patient can be assessed and understood.

THE HISTORY OF INQUIRY INTO GROWTH & DEVELOPMENT

Phylogeny & Ontogeny

Phylogeny is the study of the successive forms of life that have evolved on the earth. We assume that many of the behaviors that evolved to ensure the survival of young mammals for 60 million years are directly carried over into human life—especially the first few months and years of it. This mammalian heritage appears to affect development, with decreasing influence, throughout the life cycle.

Ontogeny is the study of the succession of forms each individual passes through in a lifetime. The ancients were aware of the continuous and progressive changes in the organism from earliest life through maturity, but their concept was not "developmental" as the word is used today. Their idea of embryology

---

* The author is indebted to Nancy B. Kaltreider, MD, for the material on Erikson's adult stages.

was founded on the homunculus theory of "preformationism," first proposed by a Greek philosopher in the fifth century BC. This was a linear model of development—what we now call growth, ie, increase in the number and size of cells (technically, hyperplasia and hypertrophy). This notion was unchallenged for more than 2000 years until microscopic study revealed that older embryos had organs and tissues not present in younger ones of the same species. This showed that development was not simple linear enlargement but a progression through successive stages.

In the development of behavior, the genes are responsible for certain primitive reflex patterns that in turn act as organizers of further responses. These combinations (stimulus plus response) alter the organism in specific ways in accordance with natural laws. As a result, the organism learns and develops different behaviors.

For some functions, there are **critical periods** in time after which behavioral differentiation is incomplete or impossible. For example, cats blindfolded from birth lose the ability to see properly if their eyes are not uncovered before the end of the critical period. These timetables are more or less fixed genomically, depending on the species and the age of the organism.

THE CAUSES OF DEVELOPMENT: "INSTINCTS" & "LEARNING"

The Development of Individuals: Ontogeny

When we consider the forces that drive individual development, it is obvious that ontogeny does not rely entirely on chance conditioning by environmental stimuli. Examples are numerous of animals acting in ways they have had no opportunity to learn. We ordinarily call such behavior instinctive (unlearned) and conclude that it represents some internal system fixed by inheritance.

For both the one-celled animal and the infant human, the *causes* of individual development are those stimuli to which the young organism is sensitive at each level of its developmental cycle.* The natural element of infant humans is the **caregiving situation** within which development and learning occur, so long as the experiences are not too discrepant from the environment of evolutionary adaptedness. The infant's delight at seeing the mother is not at first connected to the conscious experience of needing her physical or nutritional support but a response to specific stimuli for which the infant is primed. This appears to be an instinctive mechanism for achieving attachment in infants and caregivers.

Human Behavior: Instinctual & Noninstinctual

"Behavior" in the human fetus begins with characteristic simple reflex responses to sensory input. After birth, and within the environment of evolutionary adaptedness, these constitutional tendencies extend to form the first-step behaviors of normal development-in newborns, eye and head orientation, rooting, sucking, grasping, and swallowing. The new behaviors become the substrates for the next step in development. The infant's actions may themselves evoke the environmental response necessary for a succeeding developmental step. The baby's smile, for example, provokes and sustains the positive social responses the infant needs to develop normally.

Behavioral maldevelopment may of course result from heritable defects, noxious intrauterine influences, maternal illnesses, or birth trauma; but the chief cause of behavior disorders with onset in early infancy is interference with the interpersonal processes necessary for normal behavior. Social interaction is as essential as physical development in the making of an intact human individual (Rutter, 1986).

In higher animals of the class Mammalia, instinctive behavior is not ready at birth as it is in insects. What is inherited is the *potential* for developing certain sorts of behavior systems, given the experiences that the young of that species can expect. This capacity permits greater individual adaptability than other animals possess, but it also imposes a risk of distorted or destructive behavior if the environment during development differs significantly from the environment to which the species is adapted. The current concern with the importance to bonding of interaction between mother and infant immediately after birth reflects awareness that there may be limits to the capacity of human infants to adapt to variations in the caregiving environment.

Social experiences of humans in their natural environment are linked in infancy with nurturing by the caregivers. Indeed, for humans, the social behaviors

are now held to be more important than the more "primary" motivators of behavior such as pain, hunger, or response to physical danger. From the first bond with the caregiver, interpersonal relationships are major factors in the growth of personality, and disturbed or inadequate relationships underlie much unhappiness and mental illness in humans.

THE DEVELOPMENTAL PERSPECTIVE

Almost all modern theories of personality and psychopathology thus have what is called a developmental perspective, whose main characteristics have been well described by Breger (1974): (1) The progression of behavioral maturation is from the less complex to the more complex; (2) what emerges in the immediate (and even the distant) future is relatively dependent upon what has already arisen; and (3) above all, the effect of any experience will often depend upon the stage at which it occurs in the development of the individual.

The third characteristic is of the greatest importance in our understanding of the ontogeny of personality and mental function. Environmental stresses may lead to very different results in a growing child depending upon the child's stage of development. Imagine the consequences for a daughter of her mother's death if the daughter is a 4-month-old baby, a 4-year-old child, or a 40-year-old adult. The birth of a sibling has different consequences for a 1-year-old or 6-year-old than for a 2-year-old. Understanding the normal progression of the individual s ability to cope with and understand the environment helps the clinician differentiate pathological social maturation from normal variations and will help the therapist decide what treatment is likely to be beneficial.

The most important aspect for medical practice of any theory of psychology or psychopathology is its usefulness in the prediction of future development and in suggesting means of altering the course of existing maldevelopment in the direction of health. Unfortunately, no single theory is adequate to explain the diversity of human individuals and cultures, although neurophysiological, behavioral, and ethnological research is beginning to merge with more sophisticated observations of human feelings and behavior.

THEORIES OF DEVELOPMENT

A number of theories of human development are derived from clinical experience and experiments with animals and humans. Many of them contribute useful

---

* For every organism, there is an environment within which its physiological and behavioral systems operate best at any one point in its ontogeny. This has been given the somewhat cumbersome name "environment of evolutionary adaptedness" by John Bowlby (1983).

perspectives, and several aspire to the status of general theories of behavior. The two best-known systems used by clinicians today are those derived from classic psychoanalysis and piagetian developmental psychology (Piaget and Inhelder, 1969). The former has been criticized as being excessively intrapsychic and unyielding to systematic validation; the latter because it takes no account of emotions or the biological mechanisms of development. Both are closed systems and products of Western culture, but they have long histories of clinical usefulness and serve as appropriate instruments for further research and validation. Recently, general systems theory and research in animal ethology have provided tools that are improving and expanding the study of infancy and early childhood.

Piaget's and two other influential theories are discussed here because of their special relevance to child development. These are Erickson's psychoanalytic view and Bowlby's attachment theory.

JEAN PIAGET
(1896–1980)

Piaget is the best-known child psychologist in the world, and his theory of cognitive development has been the most influential. His hypotheses have formed the basis of an entire discipline (he called it *épistemologie génétique*, ''the nature of development') and have provided a formal philosophic stimulus for clinical research in a number of other fields in psychology. For Piaget, the *intellectual* functions are the core of personality formation and serve to coordinate development in all spheres. He did not offer a theory of development of emotional life in childhood, though he acknowledged its importance

Piaget was the first modern theorist to emphasize that the infant is active from the beginning in exploring the world and striving for a more gratifying mastery of it. The process is genomically inherited and proceeds in all children through a series of fixed developmental phases and subphases. It is epigenetic in that mastery of each phase is dependent on success in mastering the elements of the preceding one and forms the basis for future refinement.

Piaget holds that there are two fundamental processes by which the organism adapts: assimilation and accommodation. **Assimilation** is the absorption ('taking in') of an experience as a whole, insofar as the individual understands it. It consists of fitting an experience into an existing cognitive structure. An analogy is assimilation of food by the gut, which is limited by the extent to which the organism is able to digest it. **Accommodation** is the process of changing the existing cognitive structure in order to adjust to new experiences. The digestive tract of a species may evolve so that individuals of the species can digest new foods, or a theory may be modified to explain contradictory data. Learning proceeds by assimilating new perceptions in terms of the existing cognitive capacity and refinement of the cognitive structure to accommodate new perceptions.

Piaget describes four stages of development of cognition (Table 4–1): the **sensorimotor stage** and **stage of preoperational thought,** in early childhood; the **stage of concrete operations,** roughly the grammar school years; and the **stage of formal operations,** the teenage years. Some children reach and master the oncoming stage a bit sooner than others, but this is not a function of intelligence. Very intelligent children in the preoperational stage are unable to perform ordinary tasks of the concrete stage even though they may be able to read, write, and speak far in advance of their peers. Each stage reinterprets previous understanding and experience according to new ways of thinking and organizing information.

Sensorimotor Stage
(Age 0–16/24 Months)

During the sensorimotor stage, the biological apparatus determines the experience of the child. The senses receive stimuli, and the motor apparatus responds in a stereotyped or reflex way: stimulus in, response out. A feedback loop is formed, and the result is the first cognitive structure beyond the reflexes. Piaget calls this structure (stimulus-response-awareness) a **schema.** The schema is a cognitive behavioral unit that can be used, together with other schemas, as a building block to construct more complex structures that he called **schemata**—through circular reactions, first accidental and then purposeful. For example, as the reflex grasp becomes purposeful, what is grasped finds new uses beyond simply being mouthed. As development proceeds in this manner, children become aware that they can influence the environment.

At the end of the sensorimotor stage (during the second year), children begin to become aware that material objects have an existence apart from the uses to which they are put. They can, for a time, maintain a mental image of the object. Piaget calls this **object permanency.** This ability will lead children to look for a lost toy in the place where they saw it disappear. In the latter part of this stage, which corresponds to the beginning of language use (symbolization), children are able to imagine a familiar object in a context of new action or a familiar action involving a new object—without having to discover everything by trial and error. Piaget holds that when symbolization starts to occur with some frequency, the child leaves the sensorimotor stage and begins to function intelligently.

Stage of Preoperational
Thought (Age 2–6)

The child begins to use symbols and language during the preoperational stage. This is the time of greatest active exploration of the surrounding world. Increasingly, language and thought processes replace solely physical sensations and activities. Children in this stage are egocentric and perceive themselves as the center of the universe. There is little objectivity or awareness of the self as a separate entity. Events are judged by their superficial impact without regard for logic or hidden possibilities. Early in this period, children may believe that everything that moves is alive and may impute magical powers to parents and other adults. They are unable to reverse a thought process. Shown a picture of a result, they cannot reconstruct the starting point. They do not rank things relatively except in terms of opposites, eg, "bad" or "good." Moral laws exist as indivisible parts of certain types of behavior. To obey adults is to be "good"; to disobey is to be "bad," even if doing so is accidental or unavoidable.

Stage of Concrete Operations (Age 6–12)

The name Piaget gave to this stage (concrete operations) exemplifies the manner of functioning now possible; the child employs **operational thinking.** Impressionistic intuition is replaced by small, logical steps in reasoning, and the data used are **concrete;** that is, they are constant, reproducible, and communicable. Concrete operations still depend on perception, but the perceptions are no longer egocentric. Rather, they are external and susceptible to validation by thinking through or acting through. Children of this age are able to organize data as parts of a whole and to keep the whole and the parts in mind at the same time. Even the brightest preoperational 5-year-old is unable to say whether there are more crows in the world or more birds, whereas the 8-year-old has no difficulty with the question. Still, both children will be unable to distinguish moral judgments from physical processes. The concept of infection can be understood but will also be connected with morality. Thus, being "bad" may be seen to be the cause of illness.

Although children in this stage of development are limited in what they can achieve intellectually by the literal quality of their understanding, they are able to order their lives according to rules and do so with enthusiasm. There is a general decrease in egocentrism, and the moral authority of the parents begins to be less magical and absolute. The child occasionally can see things from someone else's point of view.

Stage of Formal Operations (From Age 12 Onward)

At some time between age 12 and 15, some (not all) children acquire a capacity for abstract reasoning. When in the concrete stage, children live in the present, doing what they know best and reacting to the world in an immediate, superficial way without much thought about the past or future. During adolescence,

children become able to think ahead and hypothesize from here and now to a number of different outcomes elsewhere and in the future. They also learn to think backward to analyze why a present situation exists, and they develop the capacity to "think about thinking." Fantasy, which in earlier developmental periods focused on wish fulfillment, now becomes a powerful instrument for experimental manipulation of ideas and essences.

Regression During Stress & Illness

Physicians and others caring for sick or injured people have noted that stress is often accompanied by regression of cognitive functioning. An adult is apt to become as "concrete" and egocentric as a child of 8 when health is threatened. Even well adolescents and adults may have ideas about illness that fall short of their cognitive mastery of other nonstressful subject matter. Piaget's special importance has been that he emphasized clinical *developmental* psychology. For decades before it became popular to do so, he was insisting that the child understands the world differently from adults and learns in a different way. Everyone who works with children (and with adults under stress) is in Piaget's debt for these insights. Comments on how children's cognitive powers affect their responses to illness are included in the descriptions of the developmental phases in the next section of this chapter.

ERIK ERIKSON (1902–)

Erik Erikson was born in Germany and trained in Vienna as the first male Montessori teacher. He then became a psychoanalyst with a special interest in the problems of children. He relocated in the USA in 1933 and has had a distinguished career as a writer on anthropology, personality development, and psychohistory. His first book, *Childhood and Society* (1950; second edition 1963) provided a synthesis of human development from his unique point of view.

Erikson expands basic psychoanalytic theory to include social and cultural dimensions. In his theory, there are two basic drives working in opposite directions—one, an outgoing vector, tending toward expansion and life; and the other, a backward-turning vector, tending toward retreat from life. The tension between these drives gives rise to the several normal crises of the life cycle. Erikson gives prominence to the ego and to interpersonal relationships as the foundation of emotional life and the principal forces in shaping of development. The child affects the parents and through them the society. Thus, development is psycho*social* as well as psycho*sexual*.

Erikson has distilled **modes of operation** from the psychosexual **zones** and **phases** of classical psychoan-

Table 4–1 Summary of human development from multiple perspectives.

	DEVELOPMENTAL LANDMARKS Performance Levels (A. Gesell, etc)	PSYCHODYNAMIC DEVELOPMENT			INTELLECTUAL DEVELOPMENT Cognitive Stages (J. Piaget)
		PSYCHOSEXUAL STAGES (S. FREUD) Ego Defense Mechanisms (G. Vaillant)	PSYCHOSEXUAL STAGES Psychosocial Modes Tasks and VALUES (E. Erikson)	ATTACHMENT THEORY (J. BOWLBY) Psychologic Characteristics (A. Freud)	
INFANCY					
Birth	Reflex smile/grimace. Develops eye/head control.	ORAL "Narcissistic" defenses Projection (delusional in older persons) Denial (psychotic in older persons) Distortion	ORAL-RESPIRATORY-SENSORY-KINESTHETIC Incorporative mode Trust versus mistrust HOPE	1. PREATTACHMENT: (0 TO 8–10 WEEKS) Orientation to signals without discrimination of a figure	SENSORIMOTOR STAGE I. Reflex (0–2 months) II. Primary circular reaction (2–6 months) III. Secondary circular reaction (2–8 months) IV. Secondary schemes (8–12 months) V. Tertiary circular reaction (12–16 months) VI. Invention of new means through mental combinations (16 months on)
2 mo	Social smile. 180-degree visual pursuit.			II. ATTACHMENT-IN-THE-MAKING: (8–10 WEEKS TO 6 MONTHS) Orientation and signals directed toward one (or more) discriminated figures	
3 mo	Reaches for objects; rolls over.				
6 mo	Transfers objects; raking grasp.			III. CLEAR-CUT ATTACHMENT: (6 MONTHS TO END OF LIFE) Maintenance of proximity to a discriminated figure by means of local motion as signals	
9 mo	Sits up well; purposeful release; prehension deft; cruises at rail.				
1 yr	Walks unassisted; uses 3–4 words; builds towers of 2 cubes.	ANAL "Immature" defenses Projection Schizoid fantasy Hypochondriasis Passive-aggressive behavior Acting out	ANAL-URETHRAL-MUSCULAR Retentive-eliminative mode Autonomy versus shame and doubt WILL	Exuberant exploration Realizes omnipotence is limited, becomes conservative Oppositional behavior Messiness Parallel play Pleasure in looking and being looked at	
18 mo	Scribbles with crayon; uses 10–20 words; builds towers of 5–6 cubes; names a few pictures.				
2 yr	Runs and falls; uses 3-word sentences; names several body parts; uses appropriate personal pronouns.				
PRESCHOOL					
3 yr	Rides tricycle; copies a circle; can stand on one foot; talks of self and others.	PHALLIC/INFANTILE GENITAL "Neurotic" defenses Intellectualization Repression Displacement Reaction formation Dissociation	GENITAL/OEDIPAL Intrusive-inclusive mode Initiative versus guilt PURPOSE	IV. GOAL-CORRECTED PARTNERSHIP: Disgust Orderliness possible Fantasy play Masturbation begins Curiosity heightened Cooperative play Imaginary companion Task perseverance Rivalry with parent of same sex Problem solving Games with rules begin	STAGE OF PREOPERATIONAL THOUGHT (PRELOGICAL) (1) Development of symbolic Functions (2) Differentiation between signs and symbols (3) Use of language (4) Observational learning, representation versus direct action (5) Egocentrism (6) Thinking by intuition
4 yr	Buttons clothes; throws ball overhand; copies square; draws a person; says ABCs.				

Developmental chart (rotated). Reading with ages in the left column and the center "psychodynamic" columns matched to theorists' systems.

Age	Milestones	Defenses (Freud)	Psychosexual / Psychosocial (Erikson)	Social/Behavioral	Cognitive (Piaget)
SCHOOL AGE					
5 yr	Copies triangle and diamond; ties knots in string; complete toilet self-help.	**LATENCY** — Continues "neurotic" defenses (see Preschool) and begins "mature" defenses (see Adolescence)	**PSYCHOSEXUAL MORATORIUM** — Industry versus inferiority — *SKILL*	**LATENCY** — *Hobbies, Ritualistic play, Rational attitudes about foods, Enjoys friends and "best friends", Invests self in teachers and older leaders*	**STAGE OF CONCRETE OPERATIONS** — Child begins to be rational and more stable in thought. An orderly conceptual framework is applied in understanding the world. Physical quantities such as weight and volume are now viewed as constants despite changes in shape and size.
6 yr	Can roller-skate; prints name; ties shoelaces.				
7 yr	Knows seasons of year; rides 2-wheeled bike.				
8 yr	Shares ideas; names days of week; repeats 5 digits forward.				
9 yr	Can define such words as sympathy and foolish.				
10 yr	Able to rhyme; repeats 4 digits in reverse.				
11 yr	Understands pity, grief, surprise; knows where sun sets.	PREADOLESCENCE			
ADOLESCENCE					
12 yr	Can comprehend definitions of scientific words of great complexity such as entropy.	EARLY ADOLESCENCE — "Mature" defenses: Altruism, Humor, Suppression, Anticipation, Sublimation	**PSYCHOSOCIAL MORATORIUM** — Identity vs role confusion — *FIDELITY*	**ADOLESCENCE** — *Rebelliousness, Loosens family ties, Runs in cliques, Responsible independence emerges in fragments, Work habits solidify, Obvious heterosexual interests (girls usually before boys)*	**STAGE OF FORMAL OPERATIONS** — Child can now deal deductively not only with the reality the child sees but also with abstractions and propositional statements. The adolescent uses deductive reasoning and can evaluate the logic and quality of his or her own thinking. Increased powers of abstraction enable him or her to deal with laws and principles. Although egocentrism is still evident, balanced idealistic attitudes emerge in late adolescence. Some "normal" people do not advance this far in intellectual development; many do not lose their essential egocentrism at all. Egocentrism returns at senescence.
13 yr					
14 yr	Can divide small number in head.		**YOUNG ADULTHOOD** (age 20–30) — Intimacy vs isolation — *LOVE*		
15 yr	Can repeat 6 digits forward and 5 digits backward.	MIDDLE ADOLESCENCE			
16 yr			**ADULTHOOD** (age 30–65) — Generativity vs self-absorption or stagnation — *CARE*		
17 yr		LATE ADOLESCENCE			
18 yr			**LATE MATURITY** (65 and older) — Integrity vs despair — *WISDOM*		

*In each of the 3 center columns on psychodynamic development, the different styles of printing are vertically matched to the names and systems of the theorists in the heading box.

alysis and shows how these modes are reflected in typical behaviors throughout life (Table 4–1). Although we quickly outlive the "oral" phase of psychosexual development, for example, we never outlive the need for food or the tasks mastered during this phase of development. Our style of "getting" or "taking in" will reflect the adequacy of our resolution of that phase, and it provides a pattern of behavior that may include regression to infantile behaviors.

Erikson conceives of normal development as a succession of eight stages from birth to old age. These stages are **epigenetic** in that the success of each subsequent stage is partially dependent on how well the previous one has been mastered. Each stage is represented by a personal, intrapsychic balance (the psychosexual) and an outer, interpersonal balance (the psychosocial). The balance is dynamic and much affected by personal relationships and by the culture in which the child is reared. Each successive stage presents a new challenge to be met if normal development is to continue, but each stage also presents opportunities for new and more adaptive solutions to inadequately mastered previous stages. This is true because all modes of operation are still present in each stage.

Erikson uses somewhat different terms to characterize Freud's psychosexual stages. These appear in capitals at the top of each stage in Table 4–1. Underneath, in regular type, is what Erikson considers the **mode** of that stage (incorporative mode for the oral stage, retentive-eliminative mode for the anal stage, etc). The next characterization is the polarity implicit in that stage, printed in italic type (eg, trust versus mistrust for the oral stage). These are the **psychosocial tasks** of the stage. Finally, Erikson characterizes his view of development as a crucible for fundamental human values. In each stage, one of the eight human values is established or lost (HOPE in the oral stage, WISDOM in late adult life). These are in italic capitals in Table 4–1.

More will be said of Erikson's life cycle description when adult development is taken up later in this chapter (Erikson, 1959).

JOHN BOWLBY (1907–1990)

The body of thought that has come to be called **'attachment theory'** begins with the 1958 publication of "The Nature of a Child's Tie to His Mother," by British psychoanalyst John Bowlby. In this and in subsequent major works, Bowlby reinterprets psychoanalytic understanding of early development in terms of animal ethology and modern evolutionary theory. In addition, he takes into account the newer ideas of control systems and the model of information processing.

Bowlby emphasizes Darwin's explicit view that every feature of anatomy, physiology, and behavior

in an animal species contributes—or once contributed to the survival of that species in its natural environment. The behaviors underlying mating, the care of infants, and the attachment of young to their caregivers are obviously of the greatest importance to survival and are so stable across human cultures that they have come to be numbered among the few instinctual systems of the species. Survival through years of helpless dependency is not left to chance or to the dedication of caregivers alone. A behavioral system evolved to make certain that the infant itself would be motivated to remain with its caregivers. Protection from predators, Bowlby maintains, is the evolutionary purpose of attachment behaviors. In general, attachment behaviors are those observable actions of a child that promote an appropriate nearness to the attachment figure so that dangers may be avoided. From the first, strong stimuli are frightening. Shortly after birth, looming figures or a sensation of dropping from a safe (held) position causes distress. By age 2 or 3 months, being alone or in strange surroundings elicits obvious fear. By the time attachment to caregivers begins (between 3 and 6 months), fearful behavior and attachment behavior are aroused by the same stimuli; the child is alarmed by the danger, and this alarm precipitates action to increase proximity to the caregiver. If adequate proximity cannot be achieved quickly, the child will then feel distress that is both more severe and qualitatively different from the original sense of alarm. Bowlby called this different kind of distress anxiety.

The infant experiences minor degrees of anxiety (awareness of not being close enough to the attachment figure) repeatedly and learns to master anxiety if ready access to the attachment figure is maintained. After about 6 months, the infant will anticipate the discomfort of anxiety on seeing its caregiver preparing to leave and will activate its attachment behaviors and protests in an attempt to prevent departure. The more consistent the caregiver's behavior is in the mind of the child, the more separation the child is likely to tolerate. In the presence of the attachment figure, the child is likely to feel the opposite of anxiety—security—unless fearful that the attachment figure will unexpectedly leave or become unresponsive. The very young baby explores the body of the attachment figure, so that the attachment and exploration systems coincide; this favors the development of a strong bond. Later, the caregiver serves as a secure base from which to explore at some distance, so that exploration behavior is balanced by attachment behavior. A child who feels secure is able to explore; when security is threatened by alarm or separation, attachment behavior predominates. If security is threatened much of the time, the child's capacity for learning and for developing social relationships is impaired.

The stages of attachment are described in detail in the next section. Attachment behavior must be distinguished from the **attachment bond** implied by the behavior. Once formed, the attachment bond persists and is manifested by the emotional consequences of long separations. Anger, apparent indifference, or cold behavior in a child separated from its attachment figure by death or desertion is the child's emotional and cognitive reaction to the trauma of separation and not a sign of absence of attachment.

Bowlby's approach to the dawn of social relations has clarified the essentially social origins of the child's tie to its caregiver. Earlier theories from psychology and psychoanalysis held that infants become attached to their caregivers only secondarily, out of a primary need for nourishment. Attachment, as it seems to Bowlby, although overlapping the nutritional behavioral system, is itself a separate and essential social behavioral system.

SUMMARY OF THEORIES OF CHILD DEVELOPMENT

Table 4–1 summarizes five perspectives on human development. They are, of course, not the only views on the subject. The psychodynamic approaches of the psychoanalytic schools are heavily represented in this table because they are most used in clinical psychiatric practice. For a modern psychoanalytic view of child and adolescent development, informed in other disciplines, see Lewis and Volkman (1990), Theories of personality and psychopathology derived from nonanalytic psychology and philosophy, especially the modern humanistic theories, are mentioned in other chapters in this text.

CHILD DEVELOPMENT FROM BEFORE BIRTH TO ADOLESCENCE

THE PREPSYCHOLOGICAL PERIOD: CONCEPTION THROUGH AGE 2 MONTHS

Prenatal Life

Cerebral processes and responses can be demonstrated in utero (such as conditioning of the fetal electroencephalogram to a sound), but it is not known whether the gestating infant must have any specific sensory experiences in order to develop properly, nor do we know what (if any) noxious sensory input distorts or impedes that development. Excess or deficiency of maternal circulating hormones (eg, thyroid, pituitary, adrenocortical, and sex hormones) are known to adversely affect physical development, especially of the central nervous system; but damage to the fetus occurs only as a result of physical and

chemical agents—directly through trauma and disease, and indirectly through ill health of the mother. There is no evidence that the mother's emotional state, attitudes, thoughts, or conflicts have any direct effect on the fetus. Aside from obstetric complications, the chief dangers to the fetal nervous system are maternal viral infections and severe protein malnutrition. Chronic alcoholism in the mother during pregnancy results in several types of abnormality. Central nervous system metaplasia (increases in number and complexity of cells) is maximal during the first 3 months of pregnancy, and protein starvation during this period is devastating for future intellectual development. Unlike most of the rest of the body, if brain tissue fails to receive adequate nourishment in this period, repair cannot be achieved by proper feeding later. This vulnerability continues, but to a lesser extent, throughout gestation and the first few years of life.

Birth & the Neonatal Period

Much creative energy has been expended in contemplating the physical act of obstetric delivery as a possible factor in emotional development. Despite eloquent conjectures, current evidence indicates that birth is an experience of negligible psychological importance to the infant. However, it is of major psychological importance to the mother and her supporters, which means that even if it is never shown that favorable conditions at delivery are directly crucial to the *child's* psychological future, they certainly may be to the mother and others and thus indirectly to the child. A satisfied mother and father and a smiling baby are more likely to form early and strong bonds with each other. This common sense assumption has led some progressive obstetric units to provide a more homelike atmosphere in labor and delivery rooms and to allot a more active role to the parents, including the presence of the father (or other supporting adult) during the birth process and afterward.

One thing that is certain is that the infant even at the moment of delivery is not a "tabula rasa" on which experience writes all. In the delivery room, some infants are observed tracking with their eyes certain colors and shapes of light while ignoring others. Within a few days, and without much experience, this skill improves markedly. What appears to be happening is that the infant is already seeking a pattern. At this point, it is a relatively nonspecific pattern, but it is definitely not indiscriminate. With time, what infants seek becomes shaped by what they actually get and how satisfying it is; but from the first there are inclinations to react in predictable ways to certain patterns of sight, sound, and touch.

Mutually satisfying caregiver-child interactions, the result of the caregiver's speedy and contingent responses to the infant's signals, consolidate the rhythms of the baby's life and lead to more awake-alert times within which learning takes place before physical tensions such as hunger or other discomforts stimulate the child to cry. The act of being satisfied serves as an early prototype of a future feeling of trust or security. If needs are satisfied efficiently and empathetically, a sense of trust and security begins to take form; if not, the result is mistrust and distress, the forerunners of insecurity, anxiety, and psychic conflict in later life.

The Dawn of Psychological Awareness

The prenatal and early neonatal period appears to be dominated by biological needs and responses. The mother or other caregiver is the "auxiliary ego" who makes life not only bearable but possible, and it is mostly through her—the rhythms of her body during gestation and her physical interventions and social stimulations after birth—that the child experiences the world. The caregiver's physical ministrations bridge the physiological gaps that delivery creates in the systems of breathing, feeding, elimination, regulation of body temperature, etc. Up to this point, it is doubtful if any experience is appreciated in a psychological way by the child. For an event to have psychological meaning for an infant, one must assume the existence of rather sophisticated mental processes and the ability to discriminate between external and internal stimuli. These hypotheses are tempting because the normal infant behaves so naturally within its environment of evolutionary adaptedness, but there is no evidence that physically difficult labor or discomfort—or even cruelty or neglect in the first several weeks—limits the child's potential for future development unless tissue damage is sustained. In fact, the gravest congenital abnormalities requiring multiple surgical procedures and other painful methods of treatment ordinarily do not result in psychological maldevelopment. It is only later, when the child's psyche is organized by the quality and frequency of the caregiver's social responses, that we can speak of a truly psychological life in a child. Nevertheless, future research may reveal that certain early stimuli have epigenetic importance for optimal development later in life, and this possibility should be borne in mind in our handling of the youngest of infants (Stern, 1985).

We assume that "awareness" in neonates consists only of being comfortable or not and that infants differentiate only vaguely, if at all, between the outer and inner environments. The fixed-action patterns present at birth—rooting, sucking, postural adjustment, looking and listening, grasping and crying—stimulate the caregiver to provide what is needed to relieve discomfort. Although they seek to escape from unpleasant stimulation, the usual salient experience consists of repeated exposure, in a decidedly social context, to pleasurable and tension-relieving stimuli. (This "coming inside" of the external world, chiefly through the mouth in feeding but through other sensory modalities as well, has given rise to the concept of **orality** in psychoanalytic theory.)

The Role of the Father

The role of the father may be as important to the infant as that of the mother. If the mother is the primary caregiver, the father can be the first alternative caregiver. The relationship between fathers and infants is only now being examined closely, but it appears that fathers can serve as primary caregivers just as well as mothers. It is an advantage for infants if there is more than one attachment figure in the home, but the commonly held conviction that infants develop best in a home with both a father and a mother is based on convention and tradition rather than research data.

In the first weeks or months of life, infants begin to show characteristic styles of behavior that develop into consistent patterns. The constancy tends to persist until about 2 years of age, after which time traits of individual diversity start to appear. Caregivers react to the infant's style of behavior for better or worse according to their expectations and tolerance, and their responses tend to shape the child's behavior.

There is no question that "difficult babies" are a great trial to their caregivers, and this should be kept in mind in evaluating later behavior problems. The family's ability to provide a good emotional environment may be limited, and these deficiencies begin immediately to influence genomic potential so that a child's competence at age 2 or age 6 may fall short of its potential at birth (Sroufe, 1988).

Of all the characteristics of newborns that stimulate parental responses and affect what the child learns, the most striking is gender. Whether the infant is a girl or a boy elicits responses from the parents congruent with their hopes, fears, identifications, and preconceptions. These parental responses feed back into the child's developing self in a way that shapes the direction of the child's responses and, later, the child's feelings about himself or herself. Those who deal with newborns and infants often hear parents attribute qualities to their children that are not obvious to others. Boys, for example, are commonly seen by their fathers as tough, aggressive, and destined for success in sports, while girls are often described as sweet, shy, and in need of daddy's protection even though the two children may appear to an objective observer to be indistinguishable in behavior.

Aberrations of infant development that result from physical defects, extremes of constitutional style, etc, may be noted at or soon after birth. If dealt with skillfully by the caregiver, they may resolve, but such aberrations may persist despite ideal nurturing. If the caregiver continues to function without guilt, rage, or rejection and there is no further insult, the child will develop to the limits of its constitutional potential-which still may be defective. However, ideal nurturing in needy cases is not as common as might be wished. Caregivers are human and have their own problems stemming at times from their own suboptimal rearing. Considering the variations in environments, certain behavioral extremes of "deficiencies" may result even though not predetermined by any genomic predispositions. Such situations contribute to the diversity of humankind and, although unfortunate, cannot be considered pathological. An example would be a passive infant born to a very dependent woman with little formal education and low self-esteem. In the absence of contrary influences, it would be no surprise if this infant developed in a borderline retarded way, even though there were no indications of subnormal intellectual potential early in life.

Precursors of Attachment

Although from the start the infants orient themselves toward external signals emanating from human beings, they do not at first discriminate between one person and another but seem to be scanning for patterns and for things that move. Very young infants respond preferentially to soft, high-pitched voices and soothing, cooing sounds, and as early as the fourth week of life the infant will turn toward its primary caregiver's voice while ignoring others. The social smile becomes distinguishable from the reflex grimace between the fourth and eighth weeks. The infant's smile and its first gurgles and coos are powerful "social releasers" that elicit attention and affectionate behavior from the caregivers. As yet, however, the smile, vocalization, and general excitement at the appearance of a human face and the sound of a human voice are still fixed-action responses similar to the palmar grasp reflex.

The infant makes a ready and positive response to strangers up to about the 18th week. The infant's pleasure in these interactions is not simply related to anticipated relief of hunger or physical discomfort but is a **primary social behavioral system** provided by behaviors present at or soon after birth which mature and coalesce as the child associates the caregiver with gratifying experiences. The close child-caregiver bond provides protection and physical sustenance and is a necessary preparation for socialization in later life. What brings children and caregiving persons together for these protective and nurturing ends is **attachment behavior.** The appearance of the promiscuous social smile and the beginning of discrimination between the primary attachment figure and others signal the end of the prepsychological period of life.

THE PERIOD OF ATTACHMENT: THE INFANT AT 2–9 MONTHS

The Positive Phase of Attachment

During the third month, an infant recognizes the primary caregiver and soon begins to reserve its most

vivacious smiles and kicks for that person. Mothers will say, "He sees me now" or "She knows it's me." By 6 months, infants are alert, attentive to the environment, and eager to move out into it, and they grasp purposefully at whatever comes into view as long as they can see their own hands in the field. They try to sit up and to watch or follow anything that moves, as long as it does not approach too fast or make too much noise. They are especially eager to get at and stay close to mother, hold onto her, and climb on her. They lose awareness of objects out of sight and quickly lose interest, after a brief moment of perplexity, if a toy they have been playing with suddenly disappears under a blanket. By this time, they have begun to associate certain objects with activities that have provided gratification, such as holding a bottle.

Between 4 and 6½ months, most home-reared children narrow their attachment behavior to focus on the figure of their primary emotional caregiver and, to a lesser extent, the several other social respondents in the home, especially the father. Weakly attached infants are more likely to confine their social behavior to a single person. Social interaction with one or a few constant people is essential for formation of secure attachments. It is not known how much social interaction is necessary, and it probably varies. Between the fifth and seventh months, the tendency to focus on a particular figure is strongest, and when this attachment has been achieved, the tendency to seek other figures for attachment declines dramatically. This change is reminiscent of the critical periods for imprinting in animals. The sensitive phase within which attachment can be formed normally ends as early as the sixth month or as late as the eighth month. If the infant has not had consistent access to a figure on which to focus, the ability to form attachments seems to wane after about the 18th month, and thereafter it is extremely difficult to accomplish.

Investigations designed to determine whether multiple or changing caregivers might provide adequate infant care have not established conclusively that such arrangements would be suitable substitutes for the traditional main-caregiver/subsidiary-caregivers system that characterizes the human family unit. Data from natural experiments and from scientific projects are not comparable, and what constitutes a "good" outcome is difficult to agree upon. Most children reared in kibbutzim, communes, and other multiple-caregiver situations natural to the culture grow up to be indistinguishable, as a group, from the general population, but there is evidence that children reared primarily with peers rather than in traditional families have different—not necessarily deficient—personality structures.

While the complexity and richness of relations with attachment figures continue to grow, the endearing positive response to strangers, which is maximal at 14–18 weeks, gives way to sobering and staring at

18–24 weeks. This shift in attitude about strangers signals completion of the positive phase of attachment.

The Limiting Phase of Attachment

After 6 months, conditions for the development of attachment in home-reared children are complicated by the emergence of fear responses. As noted above, sobering and staring at strangers begin around the 18th week. Frank **fear of strangers** is manifest at variable times, beginning at about 26 weeks in home-reared infants, but is usually not well established until the eighth month. This response is fear of the stranger and not merely **separation anxiety,** because it occurs while infants are securely in the arms of their primary caregivers. It is important to note that these two types of behavior, although interrelated, are differentiable and may appear independently (either one before the other).

Separation anxiety, which prompts what has been described here as attachment behavior, is the sense of discomfort a child feels when being threatened by or experiencing an unpleasant separation from the attachment figure. Naturally, stranger fear and separation anxiety often function together; the child tries *to move away from* a frightening situation and *go toward* the person or place that offers protection and safety. Since fear of the stranger reinforces attachment behavior, it functions to enhance the already well-developed attachment drives, thus bringing to a close the positive phase of primary attachment. Thereafter, the infant may go to others and be friendly but will not develop the same emotional attachments accorded to his or her own emotional caregivers. This focus on the immediate family provides an apprenticeship in human relations that must be mastered before the child can move comfortably outside the family circle.

Screening for Attachment Adequacy

Since the most important achievement of the first year is a secure attachment to one or more caregivers, pediatricians and others caring for children must watch for normal development of that phenomenon or for its absence. Attachment behavior can be roughly assessed early in the first year primarily by noting the infant's response to the human face peering down. During the third and fourth month, the **social smile** is fully developed. Anyone can elicit such a smile in a well-attached baby of this age by approaching slowly and presenting one's face for inspection. Soft vocalizing helps. If the infant is well and not distracted, it will smile when the observer smiles. Although the infant may smile in response to other cues as well, the human face, smiling, nodding, and cooing, is the strongest stimulus. Absence of this characteristic response at this age warrants investigation for some physical or psychological abnormality.

Beginning in the seventh month, attachment to the primary caregiver can be easily tested in the clinic or elsewhere. The following is an example: As the pediatrician approaches the child and its mother, the child shows concern at the intrusion of a strange face. While safely on its mother's lap, a child not otherwise distressed will continue to smile broadly at her, reaching for her and playing with her hair— but will immediately become sober when looking at the pediatrician and will not return a smile but will turn back to the mother instead. This is the beginning of active discrimination between familiars and strangers that a fully attached infant will normally show. At 7 or 8 months, the child may cry when put on the examining table and protest vigorously when handled off the mother's lap. The child's distress at separation from the mother and the strange face of the examiner is an indication that the attachment system is in good order; it is not an occasion for disapproval or reproach of the child.

Cognitive Advances

At 6–9 months, when fear of strangers is developing, the first cognitively intentional acts are observed. In Piaget's charming phrase, the child learns to initiate "procedures calculated to make interesting spectacles last." Deliberate action begins. Since some kinds of behavior produce results, such as the noise of a rattle or the movement of a toy puppy pulled by a string, interest shifts from the action itself to its repeatable consequences. Still, the infant is inclined to equate the movement or gesture with the result, an essentially magical procedure.

THE INFANT AT 9–12 MONTHS

Physical & Cognitive Abilities

Near the end of the first year, the child can sit, crawl toward attractive objects and away from repugnant or fearsome ones, cruise at the rail, walk a few steps, fixate and track with the eyes, grasp with either hand, and convey what is grasped to the mouth. It has command over its motor systems, mental representations of familiar people and objects in the environment, and rudimentary devices for securing and retaining things and people that are wanted or needed. Objects now have an existence that survives loss of visual or tactile contact with them, so that the child may search for a toy that has somehow disappeared. If a ball is placed under a blanket where the child can see a bulge, it will reach under the blanket and retrieve the ball. However, if the ball is taken from under the first blanket and put under another one, even though the child sees this happen, it will not search at the second site. This illustrates Piaget's assertion that infants do not distinguish a "thing" from the motor action with which the "thing" is associated.

Attachment & Stranger Fear Responses

By 12 months, the infant is well attached to its primary caregiver and to others in the household to an equal or lesser extent. The ability to discriminate between people and the fear of strangers bind the child to the nuclear family and serve to protect the child from predators and other dangers. Sustained by the active social relationships formed, the young child is now equipped to venture into the world of experience beyond the caregiver's embrace. If the caregiver's own attachment to her mother was insecure, the chances are heightened that her own small children will experience difficulty in social relations (Main and Goldwyn, 1990).

Negative Effects of Overlong Separation

Since attachment is necessary for healthy physical and emotional development, and since separation is tolerable only in moderation, overlong separation in early life can be expected to have morbid consequences. Bowlby and coworkers have described how young, well-attached children respond to long separation from their parents without adequate substitutes- as happens, for example, when a child is left in a residential nursery because its mother has been hospitalized—with protest, despair, and detachment. The **protest phase** begins after about 3 days of separation, with crying, calling, and searching for the attachment figure. The child clamors for the attention of caretaking adults but knows they are only substitutes. Anger leads to ambivalence when the mother does return, so that the child may avert its face, reject the mother's offers of affectionate hugging, and cling to an attendant instead. In the **despair phase,** the child is still attached to the absent mother but communicates an air of hopelessness. Finally, if the separation continues, the child becomes **detached,** progressively more interested in the environment but more so in the material objects there than in people. If the mother returns before detachment occurs, the child may *appear* to be quite indifferent to her. This does not mean the child is not attached but that the security of that attachment has been dealt a blow. All this has put a great strain on the child's ability to trust the caregiving environment. If the primary caregiver responds to the child's apparent indifference by rejection, disastrous disaffection and estrangement may be the result.

Children placed for adoption can move from a foster home to the adoptive home with little difficulty until they are about 6 months of age; after that time, many children become visibly upset, and by the eighth month, all children show serious upset when moved from a foster home to the adoptive home—especially if the foster home was a socially stimulating one in which the child had developed strong affiliations. The distress is due to rupture of the attachment bond that begins to strengthen during the sixth month, and the sequence of protest, despair, and detachment occurs as just described. Some forms of such distress, especially protest and despair, continue to occur on long separations up to the third year or even later, regardless of the circumstances necessitating the separation and despite attention from multiple and changing nonattachment figures. The presence of a sibling, grandparent, or other secondary attachment figure can greatly reduce the stress of separation, and special attention by a trained substitute caregiver who does not rotate with others on a workshift schedule will minimize the potential damage.

Although many adults with moderate to severe emotional problems seem to have had insecure attachments in childhood (Dozier, 1990), this is not to say that there can be no repair or recovery if a child makes unsatisfactory primary attachments in infancy or must endure painful separations later. Initiation or resumption of affectionate care at any stage of development may reverse the process and limit developmental damage.

THE SECOND YEAR: MASTERY OF THE BODY

Physical and Social Advances

The child's second year is characterized by increasingly vigorous autonomous behavior but a corresponding ready distress upon unexpected separation from attachment figures. To be with someone who is familiar is of the utmost importance at this age. The fear of separation, however, is not the only fear experienced. Sudden sounds, the appearance of strange objects and unfamiliar people, and the rapid approach or looking presence of large objects initiate the fear response and stimulate attachment behavior. There is little indication that imagination or fantasy plays any part in the fear response; children are innately fearful of these things, and they learn to fear other things that have been associated with pain or frightening experiences, such as large animals or noisy machinery. They learn also to be aware of fear in their parents and siblings and express it as their own.

This year of life has been called the period of mastery of the body, since exploration of the child's own body, especially the erogenous sites, is a primary preoccupation. As new motor skills are acquired, the child takes great pleasure in using them, especially if the parents' praise and pleasure are forthcoming. Because motor development outruns the emergence of rationality and discretion, conflicts with what the parents consider appropriate behavior inevitably arise. When the child's demands are thwarted, frustration and rage may result, and the child sets out to test the limits of the parents' indulgence and tolerance. Since the child is small, the parents usually are successful in removal or restraint except in areas of physiological function where they cannot exert control—

eating, drinking, and excretion of urine and feces.

By the 18th month, the child is able to use spoons, cups, and other simple household items in appropriate ways. By age 2, small toys, cars, dolls, and playhouse furniture are beginning to be used in imaginative play.

At this point in life, both boys and girls are likely to have established an exuberant relationship with the world. Shyness with strangers lessens, and children resume the search for social relationships. This imposes new demands on the primary caregivers to keep up with their children and protect them from harm.

Parental Example & Intervention

During the child's second year, two major influences begin to exert their effect on behavior and personality: parental example (modeling) and parental intervention (positive and negative reinforcement). Even before this time, children are eager to imitate and identify with one or both parents; the peek-a-boo, patty-cake and baby-talk games of the first 6 months are common examples. Later, toddlers will delight in imitating complex parental behaviors based on observation without having grasped the purpose of the behavior. The cat is petted or its tail pulled, teddy bears punished or rewarded, and all manner of familiar adult behaviors are put into action. This propensity to imitate adults and to absorb their emotions reinforces the child's inclination to respond with fear, anxiety, or distress to the same stimuli that evoke these responses in the parents.

The shaping effect of parental intervention becomes more important as language becomes the chief means of interaction between parents and children. Although this influence may start to have some effect as early as the third month, it becomes maximal after age 1, when the child becomes able to divine the parents' intentions, "see through" their plans, and accurately assess their emotions. This awareness makes for conflict and the internalization of conflict. The child wants to do something, and the parents object. Their opposition is "internalized" as the child modifies its behavior in order to please them and avoid being discountenanced or punished. A common example is the absorption of the concept "No!" Toddlers often act as if "no" were still external. A child may reach for the television knobs and then, hand poised in the air, say "No!" firmly and pull away. Once internalized, the powerful concept of "No!" can be turned against the parents as the child realizes they can be opposed in some ways. The well-known oppositionism of this age group has been dubbed "the terrible twos."

During this period, toilet training depends partly on maturation of the nervous system. Bowel and bladder control is important to the extent the parents think it is. Overconcern about "accidents" focuses the child's attention on these physiological activities and confers an unwarranted importance on struggles between parent and child about matters over which neither has good control.

The child's interest in his or her body at this time emphasizes the parts that give pleasure and are under some kind of control. Excretory products are not repulsive at first. A little boy enjoys directing his stream of urine, and fecal play is a transient phenomenon in some children. A general tendency to "make a mess", is often noted, as are all physical activities that have some semblance of mastery of the environment. Since fine motor control is not yet achieved and judgment is immature, household items are at risk of destruction. Since this is also the time when the child has the power to expel or retain feces—and perhaps is engaged in a contest with the caregiver over who is to control that pleasurable activity—it has been called the anal sadistic stage in psychoanalytic descriptions of development.

Cognitive Advances

During the second year, the child can be observed studying situations and devising experiments in order to create new experiences. As new skills are acquired, they are perfected by repetition and practice. Consolidation by repetition is a recognized feature of mentation and shows that the function itself is a source of pleasure apart from any need to relieve boredom or tension or derive erotic pleasure. During this period, the child does with the body what it will later do with language, which eventually supersedes action as the chief means of dealing with the world and conforming to its social requirements. It is for this reason that Piaget calls the first 2 years of life the "sensorimotor" stage and considers it preintelligent (ie, prior to verbal conceptual thinking).

By about 16 months, as cognition matures, sensorimotor activity is slowly replaced by increasingly conceptual processes. Objects have acquired some permanency in memory and an existence independent from the actions with which they are associated. It is now common to imagine displacements of objects and logical to search for them in places where they might be lying hidden. Studies have shown that the primary caregiver is usually the first "object" to acquire such permanency in the child's mind and that children whose attachments are strong and positive are better able to develop mental images of other things.

The child's experiences in communicating with its parents serve as inner directives about which cognitive impulses can be freely entertained and which must be kept from consciousness because of their forbidden content. By this process, the "unconscious mind" begins to take form. Szurek (1969) argues that the parents' own unconscious sanctions are sensed by the child and received as authoritative along with their overt and conscious directives. As long as the parents are relatively free of conflict about their values, the child can tolerate rather strict "instructions'' about what may or may not be thought. The developmental processes are strong, however, and their force will sometimes be exerted against the parents' opposition.

Parents should tactfully help children gratify as many of their mental impulses as reasonably possible in the social and cultural context. When necessary frustration produces rage and tantrum behavior, children should be given a firm explanation of where, when, how, and with whom the sought-for gratification can be achieved rather than an angry or anxious negative or positive response. Parents should cultivate a habit of nonretaliatory acceptance of their children's anger but should not hesitate to use gentle physical restraint if the children try to hurt the parents or themselves.

THE CHILD AT AGE 2–4

Physical & Social Advances

The third and fourth years are those during which the expansion of mental life is most striking. There is an enormous increase in the ability to use words and symbols (pictures and gestures) and to combine them in new ways to enrich the inner life with fantasy and to explore and control the outside world. Although there is great variation in the age at which children master language, most children by age 2 have a speaking vocabulary of 100–300 words and are able to understand several hundred more. If their attachments are secure, they begin to spend less time with the parents and look outward for amusement, especially in the company of other children. **Parallel play** comes first, in which young children are observed playing ''together'' but not yet ''with each other.'' Between ages 2½ and 3, **associative play** evolves with elements of peer interaction and cooperation, and during the fourth year **cooperative play** with one other child is possible. It is not until the fifth year that cooperative play in a group becomes a regular feature of childhood behavior.

Fantasy

Fantasy play is the means by which children aged 2–4 master the world. In fantasy, they can manipulate, reverse, modify, and improve their lot in ways that are beyond their control in real life. After unpleasant or frightening incidents, the child can relive those experiences in fantasy and play and often revise and master them.

Sibling Rivalry

Age 2–4 is the time when a child is most likely to be presented with a baby brother or sister. Next to long separation from the primary attachment figure or other catastrophe in early life, the advent of a sibling is the most impressive psychological event in childhood, and its effects continue to be felt throughout life in attitudes about competitors and dependents. It provides a special opportunity for the development of important social skills but is also the nidus around which neurotic distortion may collect.

Most commonly, there is threatened or actual diversion of the mother's love and attention from the child who has enjoyed it undiluted for 2 or 3 years. The child may respond with babyish activity and demands for attention and may regress in behavior to an earlier stage of development. The parents' response to regression will determine whether adaptation with few residual effects will occur or whether it will remain a focus of anxious concern and bitterness for the child. Even the busiest new mother can find time to respond by allowing a bit of regression in her 2-year-old and to express her understanding of why it is happening. The birth of a sibling is a time when the father or other family adult not directly involved with the new baby should spend more time with the older child.

Transitional Objects

Many parents are annoyed when their children— even up to the school-age years—have some object they like to hold and carry about with them, usually a blanket, stuffed animal, or other article of soft material that they seek out in times of disappointment, fatigue, or pain. The psychodynamic explanation of this phenomenon remains a subject of debate (Winnicott, 1953), but there is no evidence that the practice has any pernicious effect so long as the child does not *prefer* the transitional object to the attachment figure.

Gender Identity

Children during the third and fourth years (if not earlier) discover the difference between boys and girls and have a natural curiosity about it. Starting in the second year, but mostly in the third and fourth, there is an increasing interest in bathroom matters and in the genitals and genital play, although this is usually forbidden by the adults in the family, who do not tolerate genital exhibitionism as they may have tolerated and encouraged other types of showing off. The restriction does not lead to conflict if the parents accept the impulse as natural but indicate that social tradition calls for privacy in these matters.

It is also at this age that awareness of being male or female occurs. How the parents act in their gender roles and what they demand from their sons and daughters determine how children internalize their gender.

Cognitive Advances

Age 2–4 is the time when children, having mastered the sensorimotor mechanisms of their bodies, begin to use symbols and syntax in dealing with the world. They ''reason'' by intuition rather than by logic. All things are judged by surface appearance and interpreted by post hoc reasoning. Children at this age are confused by causality, attributing effects to the loudest, most recent, or most impressive preceding event. For example, a 3½-year-old boy might assume that a thunderstorm has caused him to have a sore throat and that the doctor's examination cured it.

During this period, children maintain a relative egocentrism; they personalize their observations and experiences. Although many children show a spontaneous empathy for the distress of others even at as young an age as 1 year, they cannot be objective about why they feel that way, and they either do not comprehend at all or, at best, repeat without understanding what they are told.

THE CHILD AT AGE 4–6

Childhood Sexual Experience

During the years from age 4 to age 6, overt sexual behavior becomes differentiated from attachment behavior. Most adults cannot remember their own sexual preoccupations during this time, and many prefer to believe that children are "innocent" of such thoughts.

Whether this new, overtly sexual behavior constitutes the emergence of a new instinctual system or is an outgrowth of the old attachment system is still being debated. It is clear, however, that the forms taken by new sexual initiatives will be affected by what is acceptable in the family and will reflect parental attitudes, especially unconscious ones. Commonly, a father will be pleased by his daughter's coquettishly "feminine" behavior and will respond positively to it, and the mother responds in the same way to her son's "manly" behavior. Their positive responses to the sexual content of the children's behavior will be limited, however, so that in the long run, the child must endure disappointment. But the need for parental nonsexual love, attention, and direction—the attachment needs—continues for many years.

Sexual behavior adds a complex emotional dimension to the child's relationship with the parents. The child's understanding of this behavior is determined largely by the sophistication of its cognitive processes. Parental disapproval of sexual behavior by a small boy may arouse concern about potential harm to the penis, which he perceives as central to his sexual feelings. When he learns that females do not have penises, the immature little boy—and the little girl also—may wonder where the missing penis might be and how it came to be lost or hidden. Children of this age are not far removed from the phase of development when they dealt with the world only through their bodies, and they are greatly concerned about bodily integrity and any possible threats to it.

The little girl at age 2 or 3 may become concerned when she discovers she lacks a penis and may not be fully satisfied by reassurances that she has not lost hers, that she has something of equivalent value inside her body, and that she will someday be able to produce a baby. Despite the fear and doubts resulting from sexual thoughts and fantasies at this age, the child's self-respect still rests on how the parents behave toward her and how they behave toward each other. The mother's security as a female adult and the respect she receives from her husband is the daughter's best source of reassurance that she is a worthy and fully equal member of the family despite the absence of a penis. Although a girl of 4 or 5 can easily grasp the idea that she has *internal* organs of comparable value, for many youngsters at age 2 and 3, appearances are all-important even in the face of adult assurances otherwise. At this age, both boys and girls are very impressed with the penis. Later, when the mystery of procreation becomes comprehensible, both girls and boys are fascinated by that process. Some of the aggressive behavior boys direct toward girls—and their bragging and self-aggrandizing—can be traced to a wish that they could have the female's procreative abilities.

Boys at about age 4 focus a good deal of attention on the penis, and this leads naturally to use of the penis, especially when erect, as something to thrust against or into objects or people in a sensual or aggressive way. Girls commonly forget about this early interest in the penis.

The experience in Western culture is that between ages 4 and 6 years, both little boys and little girls go through a phase of immaturely perceived sexual love for the parent of the opposite sex, followed by the inevitable disappointment when it becomes clear that competition with the father (or mother) for exclusive possession of the other parent is a lost cause. The child must relinquish the parent as sex object without losing the parent's support and love and yet retain an interest in the opposite sex. How well the three parties handle the renunciation will determine to some extent the child's emotional stability and maturity in later life. If the parents are themselves free of conflicts about the child's sexual impulses and careful to avoid any semblance of participation in sexual behavior with the child, the child will eventually learn to select appropriate sexual objects outside the family. The result will be increased self-respect and even pride in having taken a step toward growing up.

The differences between sexual behavior in developing boys and girls may depend in part on the fact that, although the first love object for both is a woman, the boy must renounce the sexual elements of this love while preserving the possibility of such sexual love with another woman later. The girl does not have to experience this painful separation of loves so acutely, since her attachment to her mother can continue along with the development of her heterosexual interest in her father and other males.* It seems certain now that girls may achieve femininity without going through an acute phase of envying boys, although many girls go through a phase of wishing they had a penis (not necessarily wishing they were boys), and some girls experience a sense of deficiency about this, especially in families where boys are more highly valued by the parents. Girls may dress like boys and engage in activities traditionally associated more with boys than with girls, such as rough competitive play. Such behavior may be a repudiation of femininity. It is common in Western society for alternations of sex identification to continue for several years until a sense of self as female becomes established. Aside from those few who make this detour, girls who otherwise identify completely with their mothers and have no problems about accepting their own femininity may seek assertive goals much as boys do simply because of the physical mastery and competitive gratifications that can be achieved in that way. If the child's sexual feelings during this early period of sexual discovery and experimentation are accepted by the parents as natural and dealt with by means of simple explanations and reassurance, the child will turn its attentions to things in which success is possible while quietly continuing to explore sexuality when alone or in secrecy with other children.

If this period of life is disrupted by separation or by illness or injury of the child or parents or if there are covert seductions, sexualization of the child/parent relationship, reversals of the child/parent roles, vicarious encouragements of sibling sexual play, etc, anxiety will be experienced in the context of the child's sexual preoccupations and may leave psychic stains that will persist as dominant themes in psychological treatment later.

Guilt

The rudimentary moral sense developing in the child during this period engenders feelings of guilt that can be relieved by punishment and forgiveness. Guilt may arise over secret behavior or secret thoughts and fantasies. Provocative behavior toward the parents may be unconsciously calculated to elicit punishment for relief of guilt about sexual, hostile, or destructive fantasies of which the child feels the parents would disapprove. This inclination to punish oneself continues to some degree throughout life, in proportion to the dominance of an unconscious principle of wrongdoing and its deserved consequences ("an eye for an eye," etc).

The Role of Fantasy

One of the most remarkable human traits is the

---

*Controversy over the psychology of female sexual development has continued ever since Freud advanced his first tentative conclusions over 85 years ago. At present, opinion is widely diverse even among psychoanalysts.

capacity for fantasy and the use of words and symbols and directed memories to enhance fantasy. Children try to make sense out of experiences; they hypothesize, engage in research, and reach conclusions—as their elder counterparts must do also—on the basis of imperfect understanding, and attempt to control and change what they find unsatisfactory. When humans fail, they have recourse to imagination and verbal ratiocination where problems yield to magical solutions and defects can be relived as victories. All this is explicit in children's games, the stories they invent, and the fairy tales they love. Some of the fantasies of childhood survive in the unconscious and reappear in adult life in the form of dreams, in the free association of patients in psychiatric treatment, and in the waking lives of psychotic patients. The ability to fantasize increases as the cognitive skills gain sophistication. At each succeeding level of development, earlier conscious preoccupations are reworked. Through this process, some unconscious distortions, formed in childhood and resurfacing in psychotherapy, can be examined and corrected.

The Effects of Illness in Childhood

A child's reaction to illness or injury is conditioned by three factors: (1) the specifics of the disorder (severity, duration, signs and symptoms); (2) the stage of psychological development already achieved, and its stability; and (3) the response of parents and siblings. The most obvious reaction is regression, eg, clinging, whining, thumb-sucking, and bed-wetting in a child who has outgrown such "babyish" behavior. The younger child is most fearful of separation; an older preschooler may also fear mutilation (if surgery is necessary) or may perceive the illness as punishment for misdemeanors committed or contemplated.

Children also tend to take cues from their parents. If the parents are horrified, paralyzed with fear, disgusted, or angered by the child's misfortune, and if they withdraw, they will compound the psychological and physical damage. Psychological trauma can be minimized if the parents maintain a compassionate and supportive attitude and are especially attentive during the most stressful phase without being overindulgent.

Cognitive Advances

During the preschool years, the child's thinking is largely egocentric, as it was during the sensorimotor period. It is still impossible at this age to hold in mind both the concept of a thing in its entirety and the individuality of its parts. Appearance dominates judgment, so that something very long and thin may be considered "larger" than something with much more bulk but not so long. Most things are seen in terms of absolutes: best/worst, bad/good, etc. The 5-year-old is not adept at comparisons or basic mathematical concepts. When they are spread out in front of her, a little girl may know there are 10 pieces of candy. After they are lumped into a mound or put into a paper sack, she is no longer sure and must count them again.

Words are especially important in this very egocentric stage. Children are often deeply hurt by being called names, because words are perceived as concrete things and have a magical capacity to stand as accomplished facts, as if the name-caller were actually making them into the derogated thing.

Children of this age have only a vague concept of time. Today, yesterday, and tomorrow may be clear enough, but the child 4–5 years old has difficulty envisioning how long it will be from now until 2 or 3 days from now, and the distant past and recent past may be lumped together as "day before yesterday." A physical illness may be described as the result of some aspect of the child's personal experience, usually a single sensory experience. "How did you get sick?" "It was the night, at night," or "I played with John." Toward the end of this period, a grasp of impersonal causality begins to dawn and egocentrism weakens.

THE SCHOOL AGE YEARS: AGE 6–12

During the sixth or seventh year, most children have matured enough so that they can spend part of each day in some kind of educational experience and apart from their attachment figures. They have all the cognitive abilities and controls that are needed to conduct themselves well away from home. By this time, children have renounced incestuous love and have turned toward relationships with peers and interests in how the world works.

However, what may appear to be independent functioning at this age still depends on reliable adult continuity of care for its consolidation and continuance. Under conditions of social deprivation, when children of this age are left to their own devices, a premature and pathological spirit of independence and self-reliance may develop. Although perhaps permitting survival in abnormal circumstances such as war or mass disasters, too much independence too early prevents the full development of the individual.

Sexual Latency, or Moratorium

The disappearance of observable sexual behavior in most children in Western society at this age (and the disinclination of adults to acknowledge such behavior in children of any age) first suggested that this period was one of sexual latency and diminished sex drive. What seems more likely is that the energies formerly expended on sexual competition within the family are now turned outward (**sublimated**). Internally, eroticism continues in clandestine forms.

Despite frequent regression in the face of disap-

pointment and frustration, school-age children are resourceful in their own behalf and are beginning to be less rigid in their moral judgments. It is natural at this time to conform to the mores and "dress code" of schoolmates, and there is often also a general disillusionment—at least overtly—with the parental image. If the parents continue to offer loving support and guidance, the child will continue to identify with the general characteristics of the parent of the same sex. During elementary school years and adolescence, when issues of self-esteem are so important, the child needs the help of parents, older siblings, and teachers in gradually acquiring skills that call for patience and practice (Szurek, 1969).

During this period, there is an obvious voluntary separation of the sexes. Protestations of contempt by each group for the other may be an attempt to control uncomfortable interests in sexuality. Preference for playmates of the same sex appears to be a cultural phenomenon, since overt heterosexual behavior is evident and encouraged in some cultures during the preteen years.

Cognitive Advances

During this phase, maturation of the central nervous system and cumulative life experiences enable children to relate the parts of an object to its whole and to retain a concept of the whole while considering the parts. Children learn not only to conceive a course of events from the beginning to the end but also to understand it back from the end to the beginning. Piaget calls this **operational thought.** In the early (concrete) stage of operational thinking, the operations still depend on the child's perception of how things appear to be. Later, during adolescence, "formal" (abstract) thinking begins: thinking about thought.

In the concrete stage, children begin to understand systems of classification. For example, "nesting" is descriptive of all classes that are additive; each larger category sums up all of the previous parts. It is only now that they can understand the question, "Are there more birds or more crows in the world?" With this ability, children can conceptualize experiences individually and then organize them as parts of a larger whole. The change is from an inductive to a deductive way of understanding the world and from magical thinking to a more scientific approach. This knowledge precedes the ability to apply the knowledge very well or to put it into words—a 7-year-old has difficulty explaining *why* there are more birds than crows—and the new skills are used mostly in the service of the social and gratification aims characteristic of earlier phases of development, such as defeating others in competition or getting more treats.

Because the child at this age is better able to perceive cause and effect, there is a shift from categorical judgments learned by rote toward cognitive manipulation of rules and reasons. As the ability to understand and manipulate the environment increases, the environment becomes more stimulating, a better place to be. Cooperative play in groups occurs, since intrafamilial competitiveness can now be expressed through games and fantasies. As the child proceeds through the elementary school years, rules become more reasonable and ideas of punishment less strict. Right and wrong begin to lose their absolute qualities.

School

Going to school is the single most significant developmental event of childhood. When children leave their families and even their neighborhood groups to go to school for a significant part of most days, all of the deficiencies of social and behavioral interaction that have been tolerated or gone unnoticed in the home environment come to light. Although there are many causes of school difficulties and suboptimal achievement in class, the most prevalent ones are cultural or economic deprivation resulting in ego development inadequate to the task of schooling.

ADOLESCENCE

The task of describing the extraordinarily complex and variable normal adolescent experience is not undertaken here, but the following can act as an outline and summary of adolescent development.

Despite the time that has elapsed since Freud first began to write about it, the major developmental concerns of adolescence remain the same two he considered: (1) establishment of a firm individuality (a sense of self or ego identity) and (2) integration of the pubertal surge of sexual and aggressive impulses. Both of these, familiar from childhood, are the psychological concomitants of the physical developments of puberty: The maturing motor system of the body approaches adult strength and adeptness; the hormonal shift and spurt announce the capacity for fertilization; and the increase in neuronal complexity in the brain makes adult thinking and judgment possible. Social skills developed in relationships with family members, playmates, and others determine whether the transition to adulthood will be turbulent or smooth over a short or long course of time. Studies of other societies and of different social classes within Western society indicate vast differences in the degrees of difficulty experienced during this period.

Adolescence begins with the recognizable physical changes of puberty. The subsequent stages of psychological advance, regression and regrouping, partial fixation, and further advance are diverse and may occur simultaneously or in alternating fashion in any one young person. The end point of adolescence is defined by social rather than physical criteria and is the subject of much dispute between the generations.

Eventually, however, the press of physical maturation carries the young person out of adolescence and into adulthood.

For our purposes here, the end of adolescence is defined as that point in young life when the major social investiture for the given social class is complete—so that the obligations and privileges of adulthood are assumed. The duration of this process will be short or long in direct relation to local conditions of survival, ie, the need to augment the procreative, work, or fighting forces. In many societies it is quite short; in some classes of Western society, it is an extended period complicated by irresolution or enhanced by refinements of education, travel, pleasure-seeking activity, or volunteer service for others.

An Outline of Adolescence

Those who have studied and written about normal adolescence in North America commonly perceive three stages: early, middle, and late. Some add pre-adolescent and postadolescent (''youth'') phases, which helps to emphasize that this period is inextricable from what went before and what follows. In most instances, it is clear that in the year or so before the onset of puberty there begins a restless increase in motor and psychological needs typical of the same individual during ages 2–4. The young person is harder to get along with; the activities of the school years are no longer so satisfying; and parental control becomes difficult to sustain. A characteristic of this period is that children of both sexes turn away from their mothers, the boy to his ''gang'' and the girl to her circle of close friends. These changes intensify as physical development proceeds.

Early adolescence. Adolescence begins with the advent of pubertal change, when new ways of self-expression (sexual and social) and new skills emerge. These new interests are noticeable because people outside the family become the objects of further attachment. The relationships available within the family are no longer sufficient to gratify the new aspirations of a progressively more vigorous and sexual person. Early adolescents usually make an effort to contain their drives within the bounds of family life, and the result may severely test the parental relationship. If demands for growing space and sexual expression can be recognized and progressive emancipation allowed, the family will remain a source of support and guidance during these experimental sallies into a widening world.

Much has been written of the ''turbulence'' of adolescence in Western society. However, it is only when behavior is primarily antiself, antifamilial, or antisocial that one must suspect pathogenic forces at work, especially within the family. These potentially destructive forces sometimes lead young people to seek support and remedial experiences elsewhere. If a benevolent outside environment meets the need, the troubled youngster may be able to continue normal development and make a successful adult adjustment. More often, however, such conflicts lead to fixation at an immature stage, premature rupture of family relationships, or partial regression to earlier stages.

Despite the risks, most young people are irresistibly drawn toward the satisfactions and prerogatives older people seem to enjoy, especially in the area of sexual experience. Even in what is perceived to be a permissive modern society, young people continue to experience conflict over sexual impulses and their expression. Childhood fantasies about sexual anatomy and function may persist into these years in spite of free access to accurate information about sex and procreation.

In most socioeconomic classes, overt sexual behavior during early and middle adolescence is suppressed, deflected, or repressed, despite the exploitation of sexuality in our culture. Premature sexual experience is eluded through the escape channels of masturbation and verbalization with peers of the same sex and an exuberant family life.

Early adolescence is characterized by increased introspection and self-absorption, exciting but unspeakable new sensations (including masturbation to orgasm), and changes in physical proportions such that the body image established through the school years is destabilized. Since much of what is happening cannot even be discussed with the parents, young people at this age form intense personal relationships with one or two "best friends" of the same age and sex. Transient identification with adolescent or adult groups provides opportunities for young people to try various roles. The first contact with drugs usually occurs at this time—mostly marihuana and the inexpensive "uppers" and "downers." The influence of respected peers is of great importance in avoiding or pursuing destructive drug use. Constructive friendships, sexual fantasy, and growing pleasure in physical and intellectual activity are in most cases preferred alternatives to drug abuse or hazardous sexual escapades.

The attention of adolescents fluctuates back and forth from friend to self, to idealized heroes and back again to self. Bursts of activity alternate with almost interminable periods of passive absorption in music, reading, video games, and television. A wish to be different is paradoxically combined with a passionate insistence on sameness, so that having the same designer brand of jeans or jacket or the same earrings as their special friends becomes an urgent necessity. Adolescents seem to form a subculture—a world apart to which only the young can belong.

It was once assumed that a turbulent adolescence was essential to full development. However, research by Offer (1969) and others has demonstrated that only about one-fifth of normal adolescents have a stormy time; about the same proportion proceed smoothly to normal adulthood; and the remainder show turmoil and anxiety in surges, with spurts of development and periods of stress and stalled progress.

Middle adolescence. Eventually, after consolidation through relationships with peers has occurred and experience with fantasy loses its appeal, boys and girls become overtly interested in each other as the objects of sexual behavior, and middle adolescence holds sway. The boy has commonly focused until now on male identification models, whereas the girl has in most cases maintained an active interest in boys and in both male and female idols. Such interest is usually free of conscious sexual content. With the beginning of focused heterosexual interest, the preoccupation with intimate friendship, masturbation, and sexual play with members of the same sex are replaced by identifications with *groups* of people. The demanding, argumentative, dependent relationship with the father or (most often) mother often suddenly resolves. School clubs, athletics, and social activities of all kinds now provide opportunities to add a physical dimension to relationships with young people of the opposite sex. Access to cars, later hours, more money, and less adult supervision have the same effect.

During this period of increasing sexual expression, it continues to be obvious how private conversations with peers of the same sex protect against premature heterosexual activity. Excessive modesty (or its equivalent, nervous flirting) reflects the strength of the sexual impulses and the energy being expended on their suppression. Undoubtedly, some adolescents accelerate their development during this phase, while others, feeling hopelessly outclassed and frightened, falter and stop in some fixated state. Still a third group, inconsistently guided or ignored by their parents at earlier stages, take license for freedom and attempt by extreme behavior to provoke parents and other authority figures to set needed minimum limits.

In early mid adolescence, as the search for self-mastery and satisfying heterosexual relationships reaches its apex, we see all the forward, backward, and lateral movement that characterizes the adolescent in our society. The object of "first love" usually resembles in some way the parent of the opposite sex, or—if the conflict over renouncing the parent as a sexual goal was too intense—he or she may have diametrically opposite physical traits. The young person usually identifies with the parent of the same sex at this time, often in open imitation of dress and mannerisms. The boy becomes suddenly more integrated, genuinely manly, as compared with earlier strutting and posing. The girl becomes more womanly, as compared with her former vanities and affectations. This accomplishment marks the end of the middle adolescent period.

Late adolescence. In late adolescence, a consolidation of personality occurs, with relative stability and consonance of feelings and behavior. There is often a decrease in introspection and creative imagination characteristic of earlier adolescence. By the end of this period, one can recognize in young people's styles of behavior striking similarities to those they formerly repudiated in their parents. The admired and respected parental values have been made their own—for better or for worse—and in this way the generations are linked. The gender and libidinal struggles of mid adolescence yield center stage to the search for vocational choice and a satisfying position in the social group. Students who have done poorly in grades 8–11 suddenly, with the close of the major developmental press of the first two adolescent phases, may take up their studies with dedication and qualify for college.

For many young people in the middle and working classes, late adolescence means that school is finished and work and spousal choices are made or imminent. They pass immediately into adulthood. For others, late adolescence marks the beginning of long years of further schooling and professional training—a phase of adulthood beyond adolescence but short of the full investiture of adulthood. In this "youth" phase, some of the hallmarks of adolescent student status persist (Keniston, 1965).

Psychologically speaking, however, normal adolescence comes to a close in the college years (at about age 20) for those continuing in school. Adolescent-type conflicts may linger, but adolescence is over. A 24-year-old graduate student with identity diffusion or antisocial behavior, which might be normal for some 16-year-olds, is not a person with prolonged adolescence but an adult with problems.

Along with the maturing cognitive abilities, people in late adolescence usually become less preoccupied with themselves and more concerned with cultural values and ideologies. They become seriously interested in theology, ethics, or politics, but usually still in a tentative, reversible way, expecting that bad outcomes can be expunged, amnesty granted, and records sealed. Commitment to a "cause" may also represent some of the energy loosened from family ties and is an outlet for energies not yet invested in love and other ordinary adult preoccupations.

Cognitive Advances

During the elementary school-age years, problem-solving activity is mostly limited to actual situations in the real or fantasy world. At some time between ages 12 and 15—usually in the stage described here as early adolescence—some young people develop the ability to deal with abstractions, to think also about possibilities. Piaget calls this the **stage of formal operations** to emphasize that the form of the proposition is what is important, not the content, as the formulas of mathematics are different levels of abstraction. In formal-stage thinking, the individual extracts the key elements and then is able, through mental processes, to combine, reverse, and recombine them into possibilities that perhaps never were or

may never become actualized. This capacity contributes to the adolescent's propensity toward moral abstraction, grandiosity, idealism, and dedication to things that "could be but are not." Although Piaget described this development as the final stage in normal cognitive growth, it should be regarded as a special achievement rather than a universal expectation. As Dulit (1972) and others have demonstrated, only about one-third of adults function to a large extent in the formal stage; another third do so some of the time but have no need for it in their daily lives; and the rest seem never to achieve it at all. Although the capacity for formal thought is correlated with normal intelligence, it is not directly related to it. Failure to progress to the concrete stage from preoperational thinking is evidence of mental deficiency or disorder: a failure of development. This is not necessarily the case with failure to achieve the formal stage in adolescence. Most people move on from the concrete stage to learn workaday techniques for solving life's problems and have no practical use for the skills of the formal stage.

Attachment

The second decade of life is the time when people learn how to care for themselves in the world. The dependence on the primary attachment figures characteristic of the first decade—being cared for—gives way gradually to a measured independence. Physical and emotional separation from the parents occurs, sexual identity is consolidated, and sexual interest is directed toward peers. By the close of adolescence, love relationships reflect the quality of the old attachments, this time including tender and satisfying genital sexuality with an emotionally valued partner.

When this process is accomplished, usually early in the third decade, the young adult is prepared to care for others. The attachment cycle completes itself in the quality of care provided to a new generation. At this point, young adults can begin to return to their parents on a basis of equality. Old attachments continue to express themselves in attenuated form in letters, telephone calls, and visits, and attachment figures are sought out in times of sadness or adversity, giving structure and continuity to personal relationships over a lifetime.

ADULT DEVELOPMENT

At the beginning of this chapter, development was defined as lawful, qualitative change toward greater capacity for adapted living. It has been easy to see that the march through childhood and adolescence meets this formal definition of development, and these changes are so pronounced—and so rapid—that much space has been devoted to describing them. Despite the fact that the remainder of the life cycle is often three times as long as the 20 years or so it takes to reach adulthood, whether the changes that occur during the years of adult life remaining can be correctly deemed "development" is an unresolved question.

Freud thought that development was primarily a function of the first decade. However, most of the well-know theorists who have written about life span development, though having their roots in psychoanalysis, have disagreed with Freud on this point. Jung went against the flow and introduced the idea of life stages in 1933, including the concept of midlife crisis. Erikson was also a pioneer in maintaining that development proceeds throughout life, and, more recently, Vaillant, Gould, Levinson, and Colarusso and Nemiroff have made significant contributions. Central to these theories is the further evolution of **personal identity** or **self-concept.** The writers we have mentioned seek to describe how individuals come to think of themselves and how this identity changes and evolves over time (Whitbourne, 1986).

It seems reasonable—even self-evident—that the changes which occur over an adult's lifetime—love, career, marriage, children, retirement, proximity of death—must also force the achievement of developmental steps, just as the major changes of childhood do, but the scientific data supporting this idea are weak. In the remainder of this chapter, adulthood will be discussed in terms of how adults think (cognition), how they report on themselves (traits), and, finally, how Erikson sees the adult segment of the life cycle (the vicissitudes of identity).

Cognition in Adulthood

After achievement of the formal stage of intelligence in middle adolescence, there is evidence of a specific "postformal" stage that some people manage to develop. Many adults use a different logical path from the one characterized by Piaget, which is at once more complicated, relativistic, and context-specific. Research is proceeding on this issue and may some day explain why some well-functioning adults do not primarily use formal logic.

Beyond any shift of quality in adult cognition, there is also considerable controversy about whether there is significant decline in intelligence and other basic cognitive processes during adulthood—and, if so, when it first appears and in what processes. The answers to these questions have come in principal part from empirical research using batteries of cognitive tasks with large samples of healthy subjects.

It is generally conceded that from age 30 to 60 years, there is a variable decline in a variety of memory tasks, even when motivation and psychological factors are considered. There are multiple and conflicting hypotheses to account for this finding. It is agreed, however, that although ability to learn slows, persons of all ages can benefit from training.

In addition, depending on the measures used, there are contradictions in the data on intelligence. Using the Wechsler-Bellvue Intelligence Scales, a linear decline of up to 30 points has been demonstrated in the level of general intellectual functioning during the decades after age 30. Yet, as reflected in Thurstone's Primary Mental Abilities Test, intelligence appears to remain stable into the 50s, after which there is a progressive decline. The Raven Progressive Matrices, which test the subjects ability to apprehend relationships in puzzles, does not deteriorate with age, but it takes about twice as much time for a healthy 80-year-old to achieve the same score as a 20-year-old. Thus, no simple explanation seems to account for the observed change in cognitive functioning that occurs with aging (Salthouse, 1989). One promising new approach to investigation of the relationship of age and IQ is to correlate stability or decline in intelligence with general and specific health factors—conditions known to affect mental functioning.

What must be borne in mind is that any age differences in adult abilities described here are statistical, referring to whole groups or subgroups. Understanding any one person requires a knowledge of age-related factors for that person and the realization that anyone's current abilities are inextricably bound to the context of their life experience and their potential.

Traits in Adulthood

Trait psychology is a discipline that views personality as a collection of internal attitudes influencing thought, behavior, and self-representation. These attitudes can be measured by trait inventories that are atheoretical. The discipline has not been guided by any life span developmental theory but by empirical studies of how people behave and feel at any one point in their lives. Reliable cross-sectional research data have been produced showing many significant changes in traits, but no clear patterns have emerged (Haan et al, 1986). A summary of such research over the last 10 years shows—rather than characteristic development—an impressive degree of stability of traits over long intervals (Costa et al, 1986). It is true that most adults see themselves as stable in personality, but many report changes. A substantial subgroup of one study described themselves as changed, but when assessed longitudinally none of the five personality factors used in the inventory were consistently less stable (Costa and McCrae, 1988).

This tendency to stability in personality seems to contradict the idea that life span development occurs according to graded steps and in epigenetic progression. Nevertheless, prediction of the effect of illness or adversity is made easier by allowing the physician to draw data from how the person has dealt with such adversity in the past. Neugarten (1964) has offered one explanation for the lack of evidence that there is development in adulthood. She suggests that there is stability of socio-adaptational processes, as reflected in traits, and development in intrapsychic processes, as observed in psychoanalytic treatment or life span interviews.

Identity in Adult Life

The changes in attitudes and behavior that occur during life are so salient that the physician must have a framework for understanding the situation of any given patient. The concept of the life cycle is useful for appreciating expected changes. Erikson's model for understanding the stages of adult life is presented in Table 4–1 and discussed in the following paragraphs.

Erikson's Stage VI. Intimacy Versus Isolation: 20–30 Years

Continuing work by developmental theorists has underlined Erikson's premise that psychological change is continuous throughout life; adulthood cannot by understood just by projecting forward salient issues of childhood. Although each individual's life is unique, there are anticipated steps though perhaps unequal in outward impact or varying in chronological order.

Position of women. Most older developmental studies followed the time-honored tradition of studying men and extrapolating the results to women. Since the late 1970s, most students of the life span have included women. Currently, the issues are harder to define, because we are in a period of such rapid societal change. In less than a generation, the number of women holding jobs has more than doubled, mostly as a result of entry of married women into the work force. The chief impetus for this change is financial need, but the increased level of education achieved by women has not resulted in significantly higher economic status. For women, the issues of identity and autonomy may be only partially resolved when they enter the developmental phase of motherhood and then reenter the job market in later adult life. The stairstep pattern of developmental tasks is overlaid by more awareness of the biological timetable; choices about pregnancy can only be made during the fertile years. The impact of the range of choices—to marry or stay single; whether or not to have children; to stay at home or to combine career and family; to be gay or bisexual; to be a single parent or to raise children in a communal setting—will require careful study to be integrated with our current understanding of normal adult development.

Early adulthood is a period of abundant possibilities—biological, social, and otherwise—in which the individual must find some balance between settling down and moving forward. The task is to create a new life, apart from the parents but with a goal structure and openness to reattachment with new close ties.

Intimacy. Erikson writes, "It is only after a reasonable sense of identity has been established that real intimacy with the other sex—or, for that matter, with any other person or even oneself—is possible." This is the period of establishment of a stable love relationship in contrast to the more transitory ties of adolescence. The adult consolidation of the self as able to love helps in the resolution of earlier ambivalent relations with parental figures.

The fear of the commitment involved with intimacy can lead to a choice of isolation or of highly stereotyped interpersonal relations. It may seem safer to choose self-absorption than to seek an elusive closeness that seems potentially dangerous to one's own identity. There are other factors that interfere with intimacy. Young adulthood is a period of vigor and activity, with the establishment of a variety of different roles that are important in achieving identity and status.

When Freud was once asked what a normal person should be able to do, he replied simple, "To love and to work." In young adulthood, the balance of these—with love seen as the expansiveness of generosity as well as genital love and with work seen as a general productiveness that would not so preoccupy the individual that his or her capacity to be a loving, sexual being would be lost—may be a difficult goal to achieve.

The critical task of young adulthood, then, is the development of intimacy built on a strong sense of personal identity. The newly mature individual recognizes the essential loneliness of human existence and the vulnerability of closeness and yet chooses this special relatedness over protective self-absorption. The sense of self includes choices of vocation and life-style that are extensions of individual identity.

Such thoughts naturally lead to the next and major period of adulthood.

Erikson's Stage VII. Generativity Versus Self-Absorption or Stagnation: 30–65 Years

Generativity is primarily the interest in establishing and guiding the next generation, although this same impetus may be applied to other altruistic concerns or to creative activity. Attitudes toward one's own children seem to derive largely from the quality of one's own early parental ties. The birth of each child necessitates further adjustments and shifts in the marital relationship and family constellation. Family size has a direct bearing on the individualization of care for each child. Particular developmental periods in children may be harder for each parent to handle. There is a new sense of time. One woman put it like this: "It is as if there are two mirrors before me, each held at an angle. I see part of myself in my mother, who is growing old, and part of her in me. In the other mirror, I see part of myself in my daughter."

Possible life-styles. Many different possible life-styles are now open to most people. There may be a retreat from the demands of generativity to pseudointimacy, often with a pervasive sense of stagnation and interpersonal impoverishment; or the children may be clung to, since their departure will mean loss of identity. Perhaps as the cultural emphasis slowly shifts, a woman's sense of identity will be broader-based and not restricted to her reproductive function. For both parents, the maturation of children may provoke feelings of envy or unrealistic identification. The child's ultimate independence can leave the parent feeling rejected or deserted, a potential candidate for psychosomatic illness or depression.

Abandoning illusions. Mid life can be characterized as a period of surrendering illusions. Review of the road taken and reflection on the future make it clear that the world is no longer one of infinite possibilities. There are often discrepancies between what one had hoped to become and what one did become, uneasily expressed in the question, "Of what value is my life?" Preparation for the second half of life may be a time for perceiving creative new directions, with a sense of continuing growth and the interconnectedness of generations. It may also be a period of awareness of vague physiological changes, a growing sense of time limitation, with death no long an abstraction and time now measured in years left to live rather than time since birth. The neglected parts of the self urgently seek expression during a complex time when one may be responsible both for the care and education of the young and the care and retirement of the aged (Jung, 1933). Thus, the second developmental stage of adulthood is marked by a concern for the other two generations— a caring about the future rather than unsatisfying preoccupation with oneself.

The final stage of adulthood, with awareness of approaching death, is still the least well understood. It is taken up at length in Chapter 41.

Erikson's Stage VIII. Ego Integrity Versus Despair: 65 Years & Older

Biological aging. This is a period of biological decline. The process is perhaps best characterized by its tremendous individual variation, but there are some common experiences. Older people seeking medical care have many understandable concerns: What will be found? Will I still be seen as a worthwhile person? Will the advice seem merely palliative for one so close to the end of the race?

Erikson speaks of an ideal old age as the fruit of the seven earlier stages: a sense of integrity. "It means a different love of one's parents and an acceptance of the fact that one's life is one's own responsibility." It is a sense of history, of comradeship with the "ordering ways of distant times and different pursuits." A sense of integrity provides a successful solution to the fear of death as the end of an unfulfilled life. Older people may have a sense of pride in their past performances and in the achievements of their offspring or others whose lives they have influenced. They may show a sense of mellowness, a tolerance for self and others.

The goal to be sought in this final stage of life is a sense of wisdom and a readiness to accept the totality of the life cycle. This sense of adult integrity comes close to the earliest period of infantile trust. Erikson suggests that healthy children will not fear life if their elders have integrity enough not to fear death. Weisman (1972), in a study of the attitudes toward death of a large number of aging patients, comments that death is not always construed as a bitter blow of fate but may be welcomed as an appropriate and timely culmination of the events that make up a life. Death with open awareness may be more harmonious than death cloaked in a conspiracy of silence and depression.

The crisis of life ends with an echo of the original theme of basic trust, and the circle is complete. The patterns discussed here are but one way of representing the major pathways of growth and development in current Western civilization. Each stage bears the imprint of previous stages as well as the human ability to adapt. When life is viewed as a continuum of challenge and potential for growth, the perspective gained may help the individual deal with the developmental tasks of each period.

REFERENCES

Bowlby J: *Attachment,* 2nd ed. Vol 1 of: *Attachment and Loss.* Basic Books, 1983.

Bowlby J: The nature of the child's tie to his mother. Int J Psychoanal 1958;39:350.

Breger L: *From Instinct to Identity: The Development of Personality.* Prentice-Hall, 1974.

Colarusso C, Nemiroff R: *Adult Development: A New Dimension in Psychodynamic Theory and Practice.* Plenum, 1981.

Costa P Jr et al: Cross-sectional studies of personality: A national sample. Psychology Aging 1986;1:144.

Costa P Jr. McCrae R: Personality in adulthood: A six year longitudinal study of self-reports and spouse ratings on the NEO Personality Inventory. J Pers Soc Psychol 1988;54:853.

Dozier M: Attachment organization and treatment use for adults with serious psychopathological disorders. Dev Psychopathol 1990;2:47.

Dulit E: Adolescent thinking a la Piaget: The formal stage. J Youth Adolesc 1972;4:281.

Erikson E: *Childhood and Society,* 2nd ed. Norton, 1963.

Erikson E: *Identity and the Life Cycle.* Internat Univ Press, 1959.

Haan N, Millsap R, Hartka E: As time goes by: Changes and stability in personality over 50 years. Psychology Aging 1986;1:220.

Jung C: *Modern Man in Search of a Soul.* Harcourt Brace Jovanovich, 1933.

Keniston K: *The Uncommitted: Alienated Youth in American Society.* Harcourt Brace Jovanovich, 1965.

Lewis M, Volkmar F: *Clinical Aspects of Child and Adolescent Development.* Lea & Febiger, 1990.

Main M, Goldwyn R: Adult attachment classification system. In: *Behavior and the Development of Representational Models of Attachment.* Main M (editor). Cambridge Univ Press, 1990.

Metcalf A: Childhood from process to structure. In: *Hysterical Personality,* 2nd ed. Horowitz M (editor). Aronson. [In press.]

Neugarten B: *Personality in Middle and Late Life.* Atherton, 1964.

Offer D: *The Psychological World of the Teenager.* Basic Books, 1969.

Piaget J, Inhelder B: *The Psychology of the Child.* Basic Books, 1969.

Rutter M: Meyerian psychobiology, personality development and the role of life experiences. Am J Psychiatry 1986;143:9.

Salthouse T: Basic cognitive processes. In: *The Adult Years: Continuity and Change.* No. 5 in: *Masters Lecture Series.* Storandt M, VanderBos G (editors). American Psychological Association, 1989.

Sroufe LA, Cooper R: *Child Development: Its Nature and Course.* Knopf, 1988.

Sroufe LA: The role of infant-caregiver attachment in development. In: *Clinical Implications of Attachment.* Belsky J, Nezworski T (editors) Erlbaum, 1988.

Stern D: *The Interpersonal World of the Infant.* Basic Books, 1985.

Szurek S: The needs of adolescents for emotional health. In: *Modern Perspectives in Adolescent Psychiatry.* Howells J (editor). Oliver & Boyd, 1969.

Vaillant G: Theoretical hierarchy of adaptive ego mechanisms. Arch Gen Psychiatry 1971;24:107.

Whitbourne S: *Adult Development,* 2nd ed. Praeger, 1986.

Winnicott D: Transitional objects and transitional phenomena. Int J Psychoanal 1953;34:1.

The practice of psychiatry requires a working knowledge of brain structure and function as well as of individual psychology. Knowledge about psychodynamic concepts complements and strengthens the clinician's understanding of behavioral and intrapsychic changes associated with alterations in the structure and function of the central nervous system. In this chapter, a review of the gross anatomy of the brain is followed by descriptions of disorders of the central nervous system that illustrate the role of the brain in human behavior.

Until recently, psychiatric education has emphasized the diagnosis and management of schizophrenia, depression, and anxiety disorders. To a surprising extent, the study and management of memory disorders, aphasias, head trauma, epilepsies, and dementia syndromes have been neglected.

In evaluating and managing patients with brain lesions, several factors must be taken into account: Personalities, intellectual gifts, and cognitive processes prior to brain injury are highly individual; lesions that produce changes in behavior and cognition are themselves never exactly the same; and social support networks and the motivation to improve following brain damage vary tremendously. Nevertheless, many characteristics are shared by brain-injured patients, and a knowledge of common syndromes aids the clinician in developing an individualized approach. The psychiatrist who is unaware of neurobehavioral syndromes will miss those diagnoses, to the detriment of the patient's care. For example, altered behavior due to organic causes (eg, inattention or diminished language comprehension) may be mistakenly interpreted as a problem in psychodynamic motivation. The clinician must distinguish behavioral and cognitive changes due to brain lesions from psychological reactions due to the awareness of acquired deficits in mental and motor abilities. Since intact portions of the brain compensate for damaged portions, this task may be difficult.

GROSS ANATOMY OF THE BRAIN

An appreciation of neuroanatomy requires a knowledge of three different levels of the brain and the manner in which they are connected. MacLean (1969) used the term "triune" to describe three brains (Fig 5–1) essentially working as one: (1) a **neomammalian brain** (the neocortical mantle); (2) a **paleomammalian brain** (limbic or visceral brain); and (3) an ancient **reptilian brain** ("R complex"). These three levels will be discussed below under the headings of neocortical surface anatomy, limbic system anatomy, and brainstem anatomy.

Neocortical Surface Anatomy
(See Figs 5–2 and 5–3)

The adult human brain weighs about 1350 g and contains over 10 billion nerve cells. The surface of the four cerebral lobes (Fig 5–2) is irrigated by three major blood vessels: the anterior, middle, and posterior cerebral arteries. Major boundaries are formed by the **longitudinal cerebral fissure,** which separates the left from the right hemisphere at the midline;

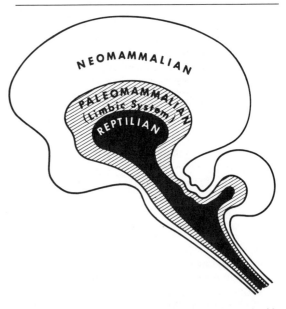

Figure 5–1. MacLean's "triune" brain. (Reproduced, with permission, from MacLean PD: The brain, empathy and medical education. J Nerv Ment Dis 1967;144:374. Copyright © 1967 by Williams & Wilkins.)

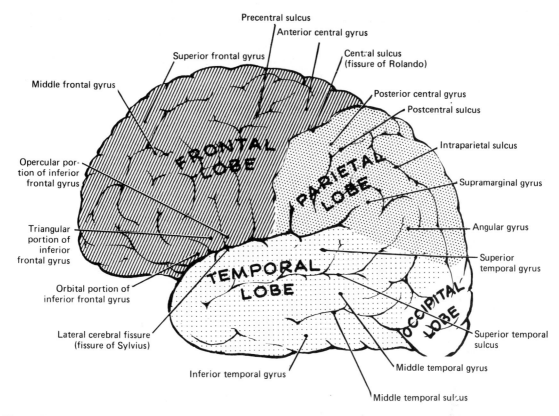

Figure 5–2. Lateral view of left cerebral hemisphere. (Reproduced, with permission, from Chusid JG: The brain. Chapter 3 in: *Correlative Neuroanatomy & Functional Neurology*, 19th ed. Lange, 1985.)

the central sulcus (fissure of Rolando), which separates the frontal from the parietal lobe; and the lateral cerebral sulcus (fissure of Sylvius), which forms the superior margin of the temporal lobe.

A. Organization of the Cortex: The cortex consists of motor, sensory, and association areas.

1. Motor cortex–The motor cortex lies anterior to the central sulcus and may be subdivided into motor, premotor, supplemental motor, and frontal eye field areas.

2. Sensory cortex–The primary sensory cortex consists of regions that receive projections from thalamic relay nuclei. (Note that olfactory stimuli have no thalamic relay stations.) **Auditory stimuli** activate the eighth cranial nerve, and the messages traverse brainstem pathways and are conveyed by auditory fibers from the medial geniculate body of the thalamus to Heschl's gyrus (the primary auditory cortex) in the superior temporal plane. Surrounding Heschl's gyrus is the auditory association cortex known as Wernicke's area, located in the posterior third of the superior temporal gyrus. **Visual input** is transmitted from the retina via the optic nerve and tract to reach the lateral geniculate body of the thalamus; the messages are then conveyed by fibers that sweep backward after a slight forward loop to reach the banks of the

calcarine fissure (the primary visual cortex) on the medial aspect of the occipital lobe. **Tactile input** is mediated by fibers arising in the trunk and limbs and traveling up the spinal cord and by fibers arising from the face; these fibers converge in the ventral basal complex of the thalamus and then are projected to the postcentral gyrus (the primary sensory projection cortex). Association fibers then pass to the superior parietal lobule.

3. Sensory association cortex–The sensory association cortex may be divided into unimodal, polymodal, and supramodal regions. The **unimodal association cortex** receives input exclusively from one sensory stimulus, whereas the **polymodal association cortex** receives input from more than one type of unimodal cortex. The **supramodal association cortex** performs a high-level integratory function. It receives no input from either the primary sensory or the unimodal association cortex; its only afferent source is the polymodal cortex.

B. Lobe Divisions: In addition to the functional division of the **frontal lobe** into motor, premotor, and prefrontal regions, three horizontal gyri—the superior, middle, and inferior frontal gyri—constitute major landmarks. In a similar fashion, the lateral aspect of the **temporal lobe** is also divided into supe-

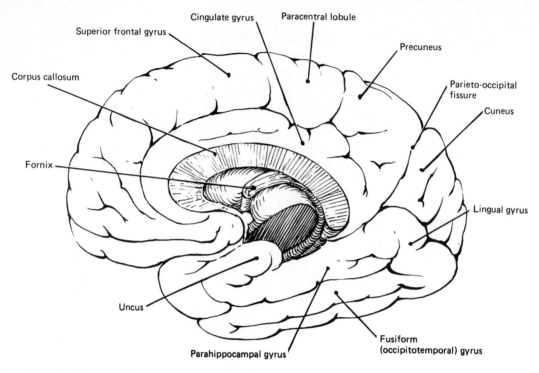

Figure 5–3. Medial view of right cerebral hemisphere. (Reproduced, with permission, from Chusid JG: The brain. Chapter 3 in:*Correlative Neuroanatomy & Functional Neurology*, 19th ed. Lange 1985.)

rior, middle, and inferior gyri. Major divisions of the **parietal lobe** are the postcentral gyrus, the superior parietal lobule, and the inferior parietal lobule. This last region, which consists exclusively of high-level (polymodal and supramodal) association cortex, is subdivided into supramarginal and angular gyri. The **occipital lobe,** also divided into superior and inferior gyri, contains the cuneus and lingual gyrus.

C. Sensory Cortex-Limbic System Connections: Through the sensory cortex-limbic system connections, the sensory information reflecting experience in the "outer world" is communicated to the "inner world" of emotions and drives, which are presumed to be governed by the limbic system.

Since the 1960s, it has been recognized that visual association fibers travel forward from the occipital region through the inferior and middle temporal gyri to reach the temporal pole. Fibers then sweep backward and medially to impinge on the amygdala, a component of the limbic system. The amygdala has been conceptualized as a gate, bridge, or way station between the sensory cortex and the hypothalamus.

D. Frontal Lobe-Limbic System Connections: Pathways that arise in the orbitomedial and dorsolateral prefrontal regions impinge on the hypothalamus and brainstem directly. Since these fiber systems are bidirectional, they offer a pathway whereby the frontal lobes not only can monitor but could also

actually modulate core brain or autonomic system activity.

Limbic System Anatomy

The term "limbic system" refers to a group of structures anatomically situated between the diencephalon and telencephalon. Functionally, these structures mediate transactions between the extracorporeal world (as elaborated in the sensory association cortex) and primitive internal or visceral drives and responses "represented" in the hypothalamus. To the extent that learning is a process whereby sensory experience achieves meaning or attains permanence in memory by being paired with the experience of pleasure or pain at the core brain or "visceral" level, all learning may be said to be mediated by the limbic system.

A. Limbic Circuits: Despite the fact that Willis in the 17th century and Broca in the 19th century used the term "limbic" to describe the ring of tissue on the medial surface of the hemispheres, it was not until 1937 that the notion of limbic circuitry had a major impact on psychiatry. In that year, Papez published "A Proposed Mechanism of Emotion," in which he suggested that a group of structures participated in transferring information from the hypothalamus to the cortex and back to the hypothalamus. Specifically, the Papez circuit (Fig 5–4) involves

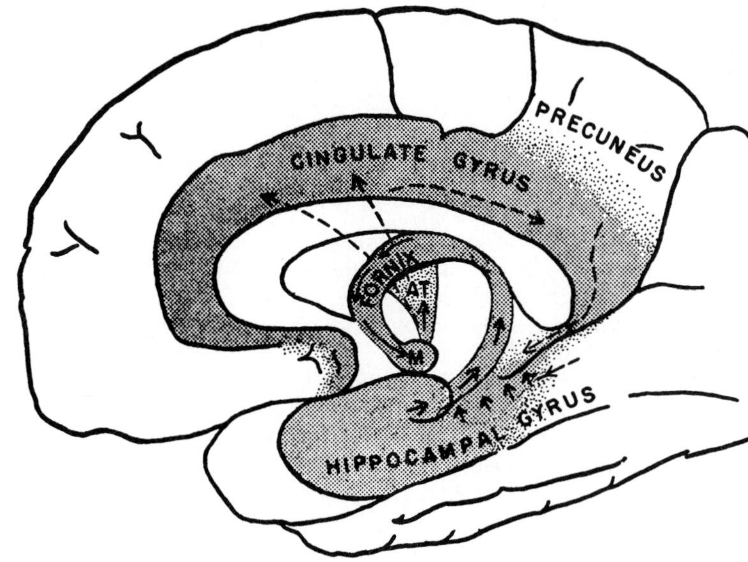

Figure 5–4. The Papez circuit, as described by MacLean. AT = anterior thalamus; M = mamillary bodies of the hypothalamus. (Reproduced, with permission of Elsevier Science Publishing Co., Inc., from MacLean PD: Psychosomatic disease and the "visceral brain." Psychosom Med 1949;11:340. Copyright © 1949 by The American Psychosomatic Society, Inc.)

the transfer of information from the hippocampus over the fornices to the mamillary bodies of the hypothalamus and then via the mamillothalamic tract to the anterior thalamus. From the anterior thalamus, fibers ascend through the anterior limb of the internal capsule to reach the cingulate gyrus, where they sweep posteriorly via the retrosplenial cortex to once again reach the hippocampus. Today the fornix is known to be a bidirectional pathway largely involving cholinergic pathways. It is believed to be part of an intrinsic or obligatory pathway involved in registering new information, and its role in emotional experience continues to be examined (Gray, 1983).

Eleven years after Papez published his now famous paper, Yakovlev (1948) suggested that in addition to the medial structures described by Papez, three lateral cortical regions (the orbitofrontal cortex, temporal pole, and insula) played an important role in motivation. Yakovlev also highlighted the strategic position of two subcortical structures that Papez had not included in his circuit, the amygdala and dorsomedial thalamus.

In 1952, MacLean explicitly linked the medial limbic circuit of Papez with the basolateral limbic circuit of Yakovlev, referring to them as the limbic system, or visceral brain. The following is a brief summary of the major limbic system connections: (1) Both circuits exert powerful downward and presumably regulatory effects on the brainstem. (2) Both circuits have intrinsic connections, and the Papez circuitry has been described as "reverberating." (3) The basolateral limbic circuit has particularly strong upward

connections to the sensory and frontal cortex, while the hippocampus (medial limbic circuit) receives sensory and frontal lobe input via multisynaptic pathways that converge on the entorhinal area before entering the hippocampus itself.

B. Limbic System-Neocortex Connections: Fibers arising from limbic structures in the medial temporal lobes travel to prefrontal regions by two distinct routes: a direct pathway via the uncinate fasciculus and an indirect pathway via the dorsomedial nucleus of the thalamus. Another example of limbic system-neocortex connections is the diffuse cholinergic projection system that arises from the nucleus basalis of Meynert in the basal forebrain and travels to widespread areas of the neocortex, as well as to the hippocampus and amygdala. Recent evidence suggests that degeneration of neurons in this limbic forebrain region may be responsible for the cholinergic deficit seen in Alzheimer's dementia.

Some Features of Brainstem Anatomy

Coursing through the brainstem is a dense network of interneurons known as the **reticular activating system.** From the reticular formation in the midbrain, fibers ascend both to the ventral forebrain and to the intralaminar and reticular nuclei of the thalamus. Thalamic fibers in turn project to diffuse areas of the cortex. Nauta (1958) coined the term **septo-hypo-thalamo-mesencephalic continuum** to describe a central core containing multiple neural tracts that connect (1) the septal region (the most anterior portion of the reticular activating system), (2) the hypothalamus, and (3) the midbrain. This continuum is roughly synonymous with MacLean's reptilian brain ("R complex") (Fig 5–1).

The **septal region** consists of a group of nuclei located beneath, in front of, and medial to the head of the caudate nucleus. In the 1960s, it was found that electrical stimulation of the septal region in both animals and humans resulted in a strong sensation of pleasure, and the septal area thus was labeled a "pleasure center" (see p 52).

The **hypothalamus** consists of multiple nuclei located behind and above the optic chiasm, beneath the thalamus, and above the pituitary. The hypothalamus forms the floor and part of the lateral wall of the third ventricle and has as its posterior border the mamillary bodies. The hypothalamus functions as an outflow pathway for autonomic discharge and plays a major role in regulation of pituitary function. It also contains regions central to the expression of drive states and appears to function as a homeostatic control device for maintenance of the internal milieu.

The **midbrain (mesencephalon),** a region of the upper brainstem, is of special importance to psychiatrists, since it is the site of origin of two major ascending **dopaminergic pathways.** Fibers arising from the substantia nigra and traveling to the neostriatum (caudate nucleus and putamen) form the **nigrostriatal pathway.** The **mesolimbic pathway** consists of fibers that arise from the ventral tegmental area of the midbrain and ascend to the frontal and limbic regions of the forebrain. (The antipsychotic effects of neuroleptic agents appear to be mediated by postsynaptic dopamine blockade in the mesolimbic pathways, while parkinsonian symptoms are produced by dopamine blockade at the level of the neostriatum.) Animal studies have implicated the mesolimbic dopaminergic pathway in the brain reward networks. There is evidence that the reinforcing properties of addicting drugs such as heroin and cocaine depend in part on activation of this system. In addition to these dopaminergic pathways, **noradrenergic pathways** and **serotonergic pathways** arise from the more posterior regions of the brainstem and, together with dopaminergic pathways, constitute the **medial forebrain bundle.**

In summary, the septo-hypothalamo-mesencephalic continuum has extensive intrinsic connections and exerts a powerful upward influence on the cortex via the ascending reticular network and the numerous pathways of the medial forebrain bundle. In addition, the continuum is itself subject to downward influences from the medial and basolateral limbic circuits.

ANATOMY & PHYSIOLOGY OF PAIN

Both perception of pain and response to pain vary greatly among individuals. These behaviors range from the reflex withdrawal of a burned finger from a hot stove to the experience of pain in a limb amputated long ago, and from the anesthesia of conversion disorders ("hysterical anesthesia") to the analgesia produced by placebos. Knowledge of the neuroanatomy and physiology of pain is critical to understanding behavior in response to pain. This brief discussion will focus on peripheral receptors and transmitters, spinal reflexes, a system for central transmission of pain, and a system for modulation of pain.

Pain Transmission Systems

Pain sensation is triggered by stimuli that are potentially damaging to tissue. Nociceptors ('pain'' receptors) in the periphery are probably free nerve endings. In peripheral nerve, the pain message is carried by two classes of small-diameter primary afferent fibers, the unmyelinated fibers and the myelinated fibers. Human peripheral nerve studies in which tungsten microelectrodes were used to stimulate single nerve fibers confirmed that pain is only elicited by activity in small-diameter myelinated and unmyelinated fibers. Although large-diameter fibers do not respond selectively to noxious stimuli, they are necessary for the "normal" quality of pain perception. When input from large-diameter primary afferent fibers is blocked, noxious stimuli produce an intense, qualitatively abnormal burning sensation. The activity in these large-diameter fibers is known to inhibit spinal pain transmission neurons, and this may account for the excessive response to noxious stimuli in subjects with large-fiber block.

The pain-transmitting primary afferent fibers bifurcate as they enter the spinal cord and run rostrally and caudally for several millimeters. They enter the gray matter and terminate in the dorsal horn, where they contact neurons of the projecting pain pathways such as the spinothalamic and spinoreticular tracts. The primary afferent fibers contact projection cells both directly and via small relay interneurons in the superficial layers of the dorsal horn. In addition to the primary afferent terminals, relay interneurons, and projection cells, the dorsal horn also contains inhibitory interneurons that function in pain modulation circuits (described below).

The present working knowledge of the central pathways transmitting pain is based on observations in the 1850s by Brown-Séquard, who demonstrated that "pain" involves crossed pathways in the spinal cord and that hemisection of the cord results in contralateral analgesia below the lesion. Gowers studied patients with discrete spinal lesions and reported in 1886 that the anterolateral column of the spinal cord was the important spinal pathway for pain. In 1911, Spiller, on the basis of studies of lesions in monkeys, encouraged the neurosurgeon Martin to cut the anterolateral column of the spinal cord in patients with severe pain, predicting that this would produce lasting pain relief. In fact, it did. Although the spinothalamic tract is in the anterolateral column, it is not clear that this tract is the only major pathway for pain sensation. Cutting the anterolateral quadrant of the cord also results in interruption of fibers that project to parts of the brainstem reticular formation, which in turn projects to the thalamus. This projection is called the spinoreticulothalamic pathway.

Phylogenetic development is accompanied by increasing size of the spinothalamic tract. To a certain extent, the spinoreticulothalamic tract also grows, and this pathway is phylogenetically the oldest. If we accept the hypothesis that subhuman animals feel pain, then we have to seriously consider the medial spinoreticulothalamic tract an important pathway of pain. Since lesions in the spinal cord and lower medulla must destroy *both* pathways, this does not resolve the question of which is the major pain pathway. In the rostral medulla, the direct spinothalamic fibers take a more lateral course, which is separate from the medial spinoreticular system. Although stimulation of either of these tracts produces pain, there is a qualitative difference in the experience the patients report. Stimulation of the lateral (direct) spinothalamic tract produces a sensation of *sharp* localized burning, numbness, or cold. Stimulation of the medial spinothalamic tract, presumably activating the spinoreticulothalamic system, produces a *severe* burning pain that evokes strong emotional responses (anxiety, fear).

In summary, there are at least two pain pathways: the lateral spinothalamic tract, which is more concerned with discrete, localized, acute pains, eg, pinprick; and the medial spinothalamic and spinoreticulothalamic pathway, which probably mediates more diffuse, chronic "clinical" types of pain. Cordotomy is an effective operation for pain relief probably because *both* pathways occupy the same region in the spinal cord and thus are simultaneously cut.

Cortical involvement in pain sensation is complex. The thalamic regions receiving fibers directly from the spinal cord project to somatosensory cortical areas in the parietal lobe. The connections of the other thalamic regions involved in pain sensation are more diffuse and may include cortical and subcortical limbic structures.

Central Pain Syndromes

Isolated lesions in the lateral spinothalamic tract in the brainstem result in pain in a high percentage of cases. A similar pain syndrome can be produced by lesions of the lateral spinothalamic tract in the thalamus (the pain of thalamic syndrome). These central pain syndromes may result from interruptions of the lateral (direct) spinothalamic tract while sparing the medial spinoreticulothalamic tract.

Pain Modulation Systems

There is good evidence to support the concept of a neural network that selectively inhibits pain trans-

mission. Stimulation of certain brainstem sites near the midbrain periaqueductal gray matter has been shown to produce analgesia in humans and laboratory animals. This modulating action is exerted at the level of the spinal cord dorsal horn. Stimulation of the periaqueductal gray matter inhibits spinal cord dorsal horn neurons that transmit pain. This action is mediated in part by a descending pathway that projects from the nucleus raphe magnus of the medulla to those regions of the dorsal horn where nociceptive projection cells are located.

The periaqueductal gray matter and the spinal cord dorsal horn contain high concentrations of opiate receptors, ie, membrane-bound proteins that stereospecifically bind opiate agonists (eg, morphine) and antagonists (eg, naloxone). Injecting small quantities of opiates at either site will produce analgesia. Furthermore, endogenous opioid peptides (endorphins) released by nerve cells can also produce analgesia by binding to opiate receptors. Examples of two such endorphins are leu-enkephalin and met-enkephalin. These enkephalins are found in very high concentration in the periaqueductal gray matter, nucleus raphe magnus, and spinal cord dorsal horn, and there is evidence that they are released in the presence of stress or pain and contribute to the action of the pain modulation system. Furthermore, there is evidence that morphine and other narcotic analgesics inhibit pain by activating cells in the periaqueductal gray matter and nucleus raphe magnus, which then project to and inhibit spinal cord pain transmission cells.

In addition to explaining how opiate analgesics relieve pain, knowledge of this pain modulation system has resulted in improved understanding of the variability of the pain experienced by different patients with similar tissue damage. One expression of this variability is the analgesic response of some patients to placebo. Placebo administration results in significant pain relief in about one-third of patients with severe pain (eg, postoperative or cancer pain). Recent studies have shown that this effect can be reduced by the opiate antagonist naloxone. This suggests that placebo analgesia results in part from activation of the endorphin-mediated analgesia system.

In summary, it is now clear that a full understanding of pain requires knowledge not only of the transmission system but of the modulation system as well. A more rational approach to the diagnosis and management of clinical pain problems can be expected to follow increased information about both systems.

EPILEPSY

Epilepsy and all seizure disorders illustrate the most basic relationship between the brain and behavior. These disorders result in intermittent paroxysmal dysfunction of the brain, which is manifested by synchronous high-voltage electrical discharges and by a variety of motor, sensory, and behavioral phenomena. Once called ''the sacred disease,'' epilepsy has served as a scientific model for understanding the role of the brain in human behavior.

Classification of Epilepsy

There have been many attempts to classify the epilepsies. Difficulties are encountered because a single underlying pathological process can produce various manifestations in different patients and because a variety of different processes (eg, tumor, infarct, vascular malformation) can result in clinically indistinguishable seizures. There are a variety of diseases whose sole manifestation is a seizure disorder. Each of these diseases has a somewhat different clinical and electroencephalographic manifestation. Thus, the epilepsies have two distinct aspects: First, epilepsy can be a general (nonspecific) response of the brain to a variety of metabolic and structural insults. Second, the epilepsies include a group of clinically distinct nervous system diseases.

Table 5–1 represents one clinically useful empirical classification scheme. The two major divisions are **primary epilepsies,** in which there is no known brain abnormality other than the clinical paroxysmal dysfunction; and **secondary epilepsies,** in which there is a known structural or metabolic abnormality of the brain.

Most (not all) primary epilepsies are generalized at onset—ie, there are electroencephalographic and clinical signs of widespread bilateral involvement of brain areas—with no preceding focal discharge. There is impairment of consciousness, and symmetric motor manifestations are seen. The **primary generalized epilepsies** usually appear before adolescence, are associated with normal intelligence, respond well to medical management, and may resolve, so that medication can be withdrawn. Seizures that are generalized at onset and have an obvious cause (eg, birth trauma, lipidoses) are termed **secondary generalized epilepsies** (previously called symptomatic epilepsies). If the underlying disease can be treated, the seizures will stop; if not, seizure control may be difficult or impossible.

Partial epilepsies are those in which the seizure discharge is limited to part of the brain, usually one hemisphere. If there is any impairment of consciousness during the seizure, it is referred to as a **complex partial seizure.** Partial seizures may spread and become generalized. They are then classified as secondary generalized epilepsy. Partial epilepsies are usually produced by structural lesions involving the limbic cortex, often the temporal lobe. Partial epilepsy includes temporal lobe or psychomotor seizures.

Complex partial seizures are of importance in psychiatry because the manifestations during seizures may resemble those seen in psychiatric illness. For example, visual and auditory hallucinations (including hearing voices) are not rare. Objects in the environ-

Table 5–1. Classification of epilepsies.*

Primary generalized epilepsies
Absence seizures:
  Classic absence seizures of childhood, with diffuse 3-Hz spike-and-wave complexes.
  Absence seizures of juvenile myoclonic epilepsy, characterized by staring and diffuse 3- to 6-Hz multi-spike-and-wave complexes during adolescence.
  Juvenile absence seizures with diffuse 8- to 12-Hz rhythms.
  Myoclonic absence seizures, with diffuse 3- to 6-Hz multi-spike-and-wave complexes.
  Myoclonic absence seizures, characterized by staring, fragmentary myoclonus, automatisms, and diffuse 12-Hz rhythms.
Myoclonic seizures:
  Myoclonic seizures of early childhood, with 3- to 6-Hz multi-spike-and-wave complexes without mental retardation (Doose's syndrome).
  Juvenile myoclonic seizures of Janz or benign myoclonic seizures of adolescence and late childhood, with diffuse 4- to 6-Hz multi-spike-and-wave complexes.
Clonic-tonic-clonic (grand mal) seizures.
Tonic-clonic (grand mal) seizures.
Partial epilepsies
Simple partial.
Complex partial:
  Simple partial at onset followed by impairment of consciousness and automatisms.
  Impairment of consciousness at onset:
    Motionless stare and impaired consciousness followed by automatisms (temporal lobe epilepsy).
    Complex motor automatisms at start of impaired consciousness (frontal lobe, somatosensory, or occipital lobe epilepsy).
    Drop attack with impaired consciousness and automatisms (temporal lobe syncope).
Secondary generalized epilepsies
Simple partial evolving to tonic-clonic (secondary tonic-clonic).
Infantile spasms (propulsive petit mal, infantile myoclonic encephalopathy with hypsarrhythmia, or West's syndrome).
Myoclonic astatic or atonic epilepsies (epileptic drop attacks of Lennox-Gastaut in children with mental retardation).
Progressive myoclonic epilepsies in adolescents and adults with dementia (myoclonic epilepsies of Lafora, Lundborg, Hartung, Hunt, or Kuf).
Unclassified epilepsies

*Modified from the classification of the International League Against Epilepsy and the World Health Organization.

ment may appear to shrink or move. Of particular interest are subjective changes such as a feeling of familiarity (déjà vu), of strangeness (jamais vu), or of unprovoked fear or anxiety. Other manifestations include automatisms such as lip smacking or chewing movements; more complex behavior including incoherent speech, driving, or walking may occur during the seizure, and the patient will have no memory of these acts. Strange smells, tastes, visceral sensations, or vertigo may occur and should raise the suspicion of complex partial seizures. In addition to these seizure phenomena, patients with complex partial seizures involving the temporal lobe may have an increased incidence of psychopathological manifestations between seizures. The two most frequent are aggressive behavior and a lasting schizophrenia-like illness that occurs after repeated seizures.

Newer monitoring techniques that simultaneously videotape the patient's behavior and electroencephalographic changes have permitted more accurate localization of the seizure focus. In cases of complex partial epilepsy that are refractory to anticonvulsant medication, excision of the seizure focus can lead to complete seizure control and some amelioration of the behavioral disturbance.

Mechanisms of Epilepsy

Partial epilepsies have been studied in a variety of animal species in which focal cortical lesions lead to paroxysmal discharge. In patients with partial epilepsy, the origin of the seizure can often be located between seizures by recording intermittent focal spikes on the electroencephalogram. In animals, such spikes can be produced by certain experimental focal cortical lesions. It is now clear that these surface spikes are generated by synchronous activity in cortical neurons. Intracellular recording has demonstrated that individual cortical neurons generate massive depolarizations that are synchronous with the spikes recorded at the cortical surface. These massive depolarizations are called paroxysmal depolarization shifts and are thought to represent a failure of normal synaptic inhibitory mechanisms. A variety of insults could produce this, including a reduction in the amount or efficacy of the inhibitory transmitter gamma-aminobutyric acid or an inadequate glial uptake of potassium.

In animals with induced focal cortical lesions, these intermittent focal spikes may increase in frequency until they produce a prolonged depolarization with continuous repetitive firing of cortical neurons. Under these circumstances, the seizure activity may spread to adjacent cortex or across the corpus callosum to become generalized.

Whether results in animal models are relevant to human partial epilepsy is uncertain; however, paroxysmal depolarization shifts have been recorded in human cortical tissue taken from a seizure focus.

DRIVES & DRIVE DISORDERS

At its most elemental level the human organism, like crawling life, has a mouth, digestive tract, and anus, a skin to keep intact, and appendages with which to acquire food. Existence, for all organisms, is a constant struggle to feed—a struggle to incorporate whatever other organisms they can fit into their mouths and press down their gullets without choking. . . If at the end of each person's life he were to be presented with the living spectacle of all that he had organismically incorporated in order to stay alive, he might well feel horrified

by the living energy he had ingested. The horizon of a gourmet, or even the average person, would be taken up with *hundreds* of chickens, flocks of lambs and sheep, a small herd of steers, sties full of pigs, and rivers of fish. The din alone would be deafening.

This quotation from Becker (1975) illustrates the pivotal role of drives—in this case, the drive to eat. Philosophers have long debated the meaning of universal and innate biological forces or drives manifested in all forms of life. Scientists have tried to translate these concepts into considerations of matter and energy, brain tissue and nerve transmission.

Freud's (1895) *Project for a Scientific Psychology* represented an attempt to consider how energy manifests itself and is transmitted in the brain and how objects in the external world begin to assume a particular charge or meaning for the observer. After hypothesizing the transfer of electrical energy (cathexis) from one neuron to another, Freud extended his model to include objects invested with or deprived of cathexis. For example, he spoke of infants as extending libidinal pseudopodia toward objects in the world.

While reflex behavior is fully *predictable*, other more complex forms of behavior exist that do not correlate as precisely with external stimulus conditions but are still far from voluntary. Students of behavior have invoked as hypothetical mechanisms the concept of motivational states that determine the intensity and direction of complex behaviors. Reflexes, drive behaviors, and fully voluntary behaviors thus seem to exist not as sharply demarcated features but along a continuum.

Theories of Drive

Various approaches to understanding drives can be seen in the work of ethologists, developmental psychologists, and anatomists.

A. Innate Capacities: Ethologists such as Lorenz and Tinbergen have made important discoveries about what they term "innate capacities." Turning away from the complexity of human behavior, ethologists have studied instinct or drive by working with animals such as fish, birds, and insects.

Tinbergen's work with the male stickleback fish is a good example of this approach. While the presence of male fish with bright red bellies during mating season provokes fighting or attack behavior in other males, it provokes approach or mating behavior in females. Colorless models resembling stickleback fish fail to elicit this behavior in either males or females. On the other hand, crude pieces of wood painted with a patch of red elicit only male approach. From this sort of work arose the notion of a "sign stimulus", or "releaser"—a particular configuration or feature embedded in a complex stimulus—that triggers instinctual behavior such as eating, mating, or attack. Since these stereotyped response behaviors occur in animals raised in total isolation, ethologists speak of them as operating through "innate releasing mechanisms."

The following is an example of the types of behavior arising from triggered innate release mechanisms: When parent thrushes alight on the nest of newborns and shake the nest, the mouths of the newborn chicks gape upward. A few days later, touching the side of the young thrush's mouth produces the same response. Shortly thereafter, the sight of the parent bird (or even of a human finger) elicits gaping behavior that is still vertically oriented. Still later, gaping behavior is directed toward the visual stimulus. Two distinct types of behavior are seen: (1) a response initially elicited and controlled by proximal (vestibular or tactile) stimuli and (2) a response gradually recruited by more distal stimuli such as visual stimuli.

B. Human Reflexes: Early reflex behaviors such as sucking, grasping, and turning the head toward a stimulus (eg, a nipple or a finger touching the infant's cheek) occur not only in awake infants but also in infants who are asleep or in coma. Sucking behavior also occurs in anencephalic infants. Although the extensor plantar response may persist for a year, most of these primitive reflexes disappear by the age of 4–6 months. However, they often reemerge in human adults with frontal lobe disorders (eg, tumor or advanced Alzheimer's dementia). Thus, these primitive behaviors appear to have been held in check by the frontal neocortex.

C. Anatomy of Specific Drive Behaviors:

1. Rage–In the 1890s, it was noted that cerebral decortication in dogs caused them to respond to trivial stimuli (pinching of the tail, being removed from the cage, or even having a fly land on the animal's nose) with disinhibited rage.

In the 1920s, Cannon studied adrenal medullary sympathetic discharge in decorticated cats and described their massive reaction to trivial stimuli (eg, touching the cat's back) as "sham rage," consisting of the following behavior: (1) pupils dilating and hair standing on end, (2) hissing and growling, (3) baring the teeth and fangs, and (4) arching the back and lashing the tail. In 1928, Bard pointed out that this entire sequence depended on the integrity of the posterior hypothalamus.

2. Eating–Feeding and eating have been studied in rather fine detail. Following initial observations that destructive lesions in the ventromedial hypothalamus resulted in hyperphagia and obesity, other reports began to document profound anorexia and weight loss following destruction of the lateral hypothalamus. Thus, there arose the concepts of a ventromedial "satiety center" and a lateral "feeding center," or "appetite center." Reports of stereotactic surgery of the hypothalamus in animals, along with a few dramatic case reports of humans with lesions in these areas, have supported these initial observations. However, several lines of inquiry—as shown in the examples below—suggest that it may be inappropriate to conceptualize hypothalamic areas as "centers" for eating or satiety.

Lesions in the hypothalamus interrupt ascending dopaminergic pathways of the medial forebrain bundle. Severing these fibers outside the hypothalamus also produces the diminished arousal and aphagia seen with lateral hypothalamic lesions. In fact, animals with lesions in the hypothalamus do not have an isolated or selective loss of interest in food. Rather, they appear to manifest syndromes of multimodal sensory inattention—ie, reduced responsiveness to visual, auditory, tactile, and olfactory stimuli presented to the side opposite the lesion.

Although animals with ventromedial hypothalamic lesions usually eat more food than animals without lesions, if the food is adulterated (eg, made bitter with quinine), they actually eat less than normal animals do. Thus, they seem to show an exaggerated response to both noxious and pleasant stimuli.

Animals starved prior to destruction of the lateral hypothalamus will eat and gain weight immediately after the lesion is produced—apparently in an attempt to bring their weight to a "set point."

These observations point to the difficulties in conceptualizing "centers" for activities as complex as eating.

A hierarchical network approach to eating behavior recognizes contributions to this behavior from three levels of control: (1) The hypothalamus, with its "hard-wired circuitry," regulates glucose levels, monitors fullness of the stomach (satiety versus hunger), and determines the "set point," ie, *how much to eat*. (2) The limbic system, in concert with the sensory systems, governs the selection of foods appropriate to appease the appetite, ie, *what to eat*. (3) The prefrontal regions are involved in decisions about table manners, ie, *when, where, and how to eat*.

Disturbances at each of these levels can be seen: (1) Tumors of the diencephalic region may disrupt carbohydrate metabolism and lead to hyperphagia, rage, and obesity. Patients with dysfunction of appetite regulation may even tear doors off refrigerators in order to satisfy the carbohydrate drive. This is termed "appropriate megaphagia," since the items ingested are not qualitatively different from what is normally eaten. (2) Patients with medial temporal lobe disorders (eg, Klüver-Bucy syndrome) may ingest items such as tea bags or cigarette butts. This "inappropriate hyperphagia" has been interpreted as reflecting sensory-limbic disconnection with consequent visual agnosia, manifested in this case by the inability to recognize and discriminate between the edible and inedible items. (3) Dementia or frontal lobotomy may lead to disruption of social behavior with loss of table manners.

3. Pleasure–Animal experiments begun in the 1960s have shed light on the neural substrates for "pleasure." After electrodes were implanted in certain regions of the medial forebrain bundle, the animal could press a bar to receive an electric current to the brain (pleasure stimulus). Animals were observed to press the bar repeatedly—even to the point of neglecting water and food or to the point of exhaustion—and to cross an electric grid to receive further pleasure stimulation. It is now clear that a major component of the brain pathway for reinforcement is the mesolimbic dopaminergic projection from the ventral tegmental area of the midbrain to the nucleus accumbens, located near the septal area. This same pathway contributes to the rewarding effects of food, fluids, and certain drugs of abuse.

Modulation of Drives

Drives depend on neural circuits whose developmental maturation is vulnerable to chemical and structural insults. Structurally intact circuits are themselves subject to modification and modulation by numerous forces. Examples of factors that shape and modulate the circuitry from which drives arise include the following:

A. Genetics: Individuals with Down's syndrome (trisomy 21) appear to have a biological disinclination to violent behavior.

B. Circadian Rhythms: Cortisol secretion, motor activity, and body temperature are all subject to 24-hour cycles. A pathway from the retina to the supraoptic nucleus of the hypothalamus plays a major role in adjustment to changes in the light-dark cycle.

C. Hormones: Castration and antiandrogens are used to treat sex offenders in Europe. The human brain itself may have a "sexual identity": A region of the anterior hypothalamus (preoptic nucleus) has been termed "dimorphic" in rats, since its gross anatomy is shaped by exposure to circulating estrogens. Alpha-fetoprotein produced by the fetal liver protects the developing human fetal brain of both sexes from masculinization by circulating maternal estrogens. The third or fourth month of human gestation appears to be a critical period" for the development of sexuality.

Drive Disorders

Psychiatrists and neurologists seldom see isolated drive disorders. Constellations of drive disorders, however, are seen frequently in the context of neuropsychiatric disorders. The following are examples of human drive disorders:

A. Anorexia Nervosa: This disorder is characterized by loss of 25% of baseline ideal weight; altered body perception and fear of obesity; amenorrhea; lanugo; hypotension; bradycardia; and peculiar behavior associated with eating and weight control, such as hoarding food, abusing laxatives, binge eating (bulimia), and vomiting. Anorexia occurs more frequently in females than in males (20:1) and is most common in the age group-from 15 to 25 years. The role of psychodynamic factors in this disorder is unclear. Behavioral regimens (eg, confinement to bed

until satisfactory weight gain occurs) in conjunction with psychotherapy appear to be the only successful approach to treatment (see Chapter 28).

B. Kleine-Levin Syndrome: Episodic hypersomnia (up to 20 hours) alternates with hyperphagia, gorging of food, and hypersexuality (masturbation and aggressive sexual behavior) in this syndrome in adolescent boys. Patients are amnesic for these episodes, which recur at intervals of 3–6 months, last 1–3 weeks, and remit spontaneously.

C. Depression: Major depression is associated with the following neurovegetative signs:

1. Sleep—The amount of sleep is classically diminished in depression. Early morning awakening and rumination are prominent manifestations, but prolonged sleep with frequent arousals can also characterize major affective disorders. Hypersomnia is well recognized in "atypical depressions."

2. Eating—Anorexia with weight loss is common, but overeating is often seen in "atypical depressions."

3. Sex drive—Diminished interest in sex is often seen as one manifestation of anhedonia (inability to find pleasure in events that previously afforded enjoyment).

4. Motor activity—Psychomotor retardation is common in depression.

D. Mania: Diminished need for sleep, hyperactivity, pressure of speech, and hypersexuality are common in manic states.

E. Klüver-Bucy Syndrome: Manifestations include placidity (tameness), visual agnosia, lack of sexual inhibitions, and a tendency to place objects in the mouth.

F. Complex partial Seizures: Hyposexuality and increased preoccupation with abstract intellectual interests (eg, philosophy, religion, and morals) are seen in patients with complex partial seizures. It is as if these intellectual interests had preempted biological drives.

G. Wernicke-Korsakoff Syndrome: Korsakoff's amnestic syndrome is preceded by the characteristic triad of Wernicke's encephalopathy, ie, confusion, ataxia, and eye movement disorders (nystagmus or ophthalmoplegia). As part of Korsakoff's syndrome, one may see profound apathy in which neither sex nor alcohol interests the patient. Korsakoff's syndrome is a useful model for a drive disorder, with lesions distributed in strategic midline structures: (1) mamillary bodies in the posterior hypothalamus (part of Papez circuit); (2) the periaqueductal region (from the third to fourth ventricles), with lesions interrupting the ascending fibers of the medial forebrain bundle and the reticular activating system; and (3) the dorsomedial nucleus of the thalamus, which is a crucial bridge between multiple limbic regions and the frontal lobes.

SLEEP & SLEEP DISORDERS

Sleep has many of the attributes of a drive. Sleep deprivation leads to an increased "urge" to sleep and to extended periods of sleep immediately following the deprivation. After several days of sleep deprivation, a confusional state may occur with disordered attention, emotional lability, reduced memory, delusions, and even hallucinations. The physiological function of sleep is unknown.

Physiology of Sleep

Most animals experience a daily cycle of changes in levels of alertness and arousal as well as sleep and waking. Sleep was originally thought to be a passive process (ie, essentially a functional deafferentation), based on observations of animals falling into continual sleep or coma if the forebrain is deafferented by transection of the brainstem at the mesencephalic level. However, the observation that lesions of the pons just in front of the trigeminal nerve cause animals to be hyperalert and sleep much less than normal indicates that normal sleep is an active process that requires activity of neurons in the brainstem. In fact, neurophysiological studies have demonstrated that nerve cells in the pontine reticular formation begin to discharge minutes prior to the onset of certain stages of sleep.

The sleep cycle consists of several distinct stages defined by the appearance of certain wave patterns on the electroencephalogram. The time required to pass through the complete sequence of sleep stages is about 90 minutes, and the cycle is repeated 3–5 times each night. There are two distinct states of sleep: **slow-wave sleep** and **rapid eye movement (REM) sleep.**

Slow-wave sleep—also called non-rapid eye movement (NREM) sleep—is divided into four stages (Fig 5–5): Stage 1 is characterized by an electroencephalogram in which the alpha rhythm has disappeared and the electroencephalographic background consists of low-voltage fast activity. In stages 2–4, the electroencephalogram becomes more synchronized (lower frequency, higher amplitude) and the subject more difficult to arouse. The longest and deepest period of slow-wave sleep each night is the first period of stage 3 and 4 sleep, usually within 2 hours after falling asleep. During this period, subjects are aroused with great difficulty and frequently demonstrate a transient confusional state. Stage 4 sleep, the deepest stage of slow-wave sleep, resembles hibernation in that blood pressure, pulse, respiratory rate, and body temperature all drop and the brain oxygen consumption is very low. It is not known where in the brain slow-wave sleep is initiated, but its electrical manifestations can still be observed in cortex that is disconnected from the brainstem.

After the initial slow-wave sleep stages, the electroencephalographic pattern usually shifts abruptly to the desynchronized (higher frequency, lower amplitude) pattern seen in stage 1 sleep. Despite some similarity with the "waking" electroencephalographic pattern it is difficult to waken subjects in this stage of sleep. This is sometimes referred to as

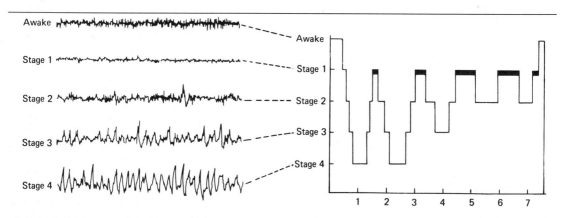

Figure 5–5. Left: Electroencephalographic recordings during different stages of wakefulness and sleep. Each line represents 30 seconds. The top recording of low-voltage fast activity is that of an awake brain. The next four tracings represent successively deeper stages of NREM (slow-wave) sleep, characterized by lower-frequency, higher-amplitude waves. **Right:** A typical night's pattern of sleep staging in a young adult. The time spent in REM sleep is represented by a dark bar. The first REM period is usually short (5–10 minutes), but periods tend to lengthen in successive cycles. Conversely, stages 3 and 4 dominate the NREM periods in the first third of the night, but they are often completely absent later. (Reproduced, with permission, from Kelly DD: Physiology of sleep and dreaming. Chapter 40 in: *Principles of Neural Science.* Kandel ER, Schwartz JH [editors]. Elsevier, 1981. Copyright © 1981 by Elsevier Science Publishing Co., Inc.)

"paradoxic sleep." One of the most striking features of this stage is intermittent rapid eye movements. Because of these eye movements, this stage is termed rapid eye movement (REM) sleep. During REM sleep, there is also a striking loss of limb muscle tone, which resembles paralysis. In normal subjects, REM sleep only occurs after a preceding period of deeper (stages 2–4) sleep. Studies indicate that dreaming occurs mainly during REM sleep. More than 80% of subjects aroused during REM sleep report vivid and colorful visual imagery. Subjects aroused 10 minutes after the REM period has terminated seldom report complete dream imagery. Since subjects usually have several REM episodes each night, they probably have several dreams, although they rarely remember more than one. If REM sleep is selectively blocked by wakening the subject at the beginning of REM sleep, a specific "REM debt" builds up, and the subject does not feel adequately rested. REM sleep is apparently triggered by neurons in the dorsolateral midbrain and pontine reticular formation.

Sleep Disorders*

Several of the drive disorders described previously are characterized by abnormalities of sleep. Hypersomnia is a key feature of the Kleine-Levin syndrome, and disorders of sleep are seen frequently in patients with depression and mania. Insomnia (ie, trouble falling asleep, waking up during the night, or awakening too early without a rested feeling) is one of the most common complaints in general medical practice and occurs in about 30% of the normal population.

A. Insomnia: Insomnia is usually considered to be sleep deprivation or a marked change in the perceived sleep pattern. Factors contributing to insomnia include (1) situational problems such as transient stress, job pressures, and marital discord; (2) aging; (3) medical disorders that inevitably include pain and physical discomfort; (4) drug-related episodes, including withdrawal from alcohol or sedatives; and (5) psychological conditions, particularly the major mental illnesses such as schizophrenia and affective disorders.

Schizophrenic patients vary markedly in the degree of sleep disturbance they endure. In acute episodes, the disruption is severe, even to the point of total insomnia. The chronic schizophrenic or the patient in remission often has no complaints, and an electroencephalographic pattern is not remarkably abnormal.

Sleep disturbance is one of the most common symptoms of affective disorders. Some patients with bipolar disorder sleep more when they are depressed and less when they are manic, but there is much variation. Primary depressions usually show sleep continuity disturbances, shortened REM stage latency, more

REM sleep at the beginning of the night than in early morning hours, and a marked reduction in sleep stages 3 and 4. In the manic phase, REM sleep is decreased, but there are varying reports on slow-wave sleep. In both unipolar and bipolar disorders, patients in the depressed phase usually have a decreased total sleep time. The incidence of excess sleep in depression is low—about 8%. There is no correlation of particular types of depression with specific types of sleep problems.

B. Hypersomnia: Hypersomnia is seen in narcolepsy, Kleine-Levin syndrome, and sleep apnea.

1. Narcolepsy–This sleep disturbance usually occurs before age 40 and includes one or more of the following four conditions: sleep attacks, cataplexy, sleep paralysis, and hallucinations. **Sleep attacks** are sudden, reversible, short (lasting about 15 minutes) episodes occurring during any type of activity. Electroencephalographic recordings usually show a direct progression to REM sleep. The patient awakens refreshed, and there may be a refractory period of 1–5 hours before another attack occurs. **Cataplexy** is a sudden loss of muscle tone, with effects ranging from weakness of specific small muscle groups to general muscle weakness that causes the person to slump to the floor, unable to move. Cataplexy is often initiated by an emotional outburst (laughing, crying, anger) and lasts from several seconds to 30 minutes. **Sleep paralysis** involves acquisition of flaccid muscle tone with full consciousness, either during awakening or while falling asleep. There is usually intense fear, which is occasionally accompanied by auditory hallucinations. The attack is terminated by touching or calling the patient. **Hypnagogic hallucinations,** either visual or auditory, may precede sleep or occur during the sleep attack. If the hallucinations occur during awakening, they are called **hypnopompic hallucinations.** The occurrence of the symptoms of the narcoleptic tetrad are as follows: sleep attacks, almost 100%; sleep attacks and cataplexy, about 70%; sleep paralysis alone, about 5%.

2. Kleine-Levin syndrome–Hypersomnic attacks may last up to 20 hours and occur infrequently (3–4 times per year). There is confusion upon awakening. This syndrome is a separate entity from narcolepsy.

3. Sleep apnea–Apneic episodes occur in both REM and NREM sleep. Noisy, stertorous snoring and hypersomnolence the next day are common. Intellectual and personality changes include decreased attention span, decreased memory, and hyperirritability. There are two types of sleep apnea: **central apnea,** in which there is a cessation of respiratory movement with loss of airflow; and **obstructive apnea,** in which there is persistent respiratory effort but upper airway blockage.

C. Stage 4 Sleep Disorders: The most common of these disorders is enuresis, which is usually seen with variable nightly occurrence in children. While

---

* This section is contributed by James J. Brophy, MD.

it often seems that the wetting occurred during dream sleep, it is actually seen most frequently in stage 4 sleep, with some preponderance in the first third of the night. **Somnambulism** also is reported mostly in children, usually during stage 3 and 4 sleep. **Pavor nocturnus** (night terrors) usually occurs in young children, predominantly in stage 4 sleep. As in somnambulism, amnesia for the episode occurs.

SYNDROMES OF DENIAL, NEGLECT, & INATTENTION

The parietal lobe receives and integrates tactile, visual, and auditory information. As it has grown through evolution, it has (1) pushed the motor area anteriorly, (2) pushed the visual cortex backward and downward, and (3) led to the development of an operculum (flap) composed of temporal, parietal, and frontal cortex.

The right parietal lobe region and the prefrontal region have been referred to as "silent areas," since lesions in these regions may not produce gross disturbances of motor or sensory function. On the other hand, it is definitely not the case that the surgeon can remove these areas with impunity.

Assessment of Parietal Lobe Disorders

Several factors complicate assessment of parietal lobe disorders. Patients with lesions of the left parietal lobe frequently have receptive aphasia and, therefore, may be unable to understand the examiner's statements and questions. Patients with lesions of the right parietal lobe have problems sustaining and directing attention and may be only marginally cooperative. Since patients with parietal lobe disorders may be either unaware of their deficits or unable to communicate with the examiner, the history obtained from friends and family becomes invaluable.

During the mental status examination, extreme care must be taken to avoid overlooking any of the following: (1) language problems (see Language Disorders, below); (2) problems with the distribution of attention; (3) visual, spatial, or constructional deficits (see Apraxia and the Callosal Syndromes, below); (4) body image distortions; (5) tactile problems; (6) motility disturbances; and (7) other neuropsychiatric disturbances.

Denial of, Neglect of, & Inattention to Illness

In 1914, Babinski coined the term anosognosia to denote neglect of left hemiplegia following right cerebral infarction. He observed that his patients either were unaware of or seemed to ignore their deficits. His first patient was a woman who, despite an otherwise excellent recovery, never once over a period of years complained of or even alluded to her hemiple-

gia. When asked to move her arm, she behaved as if the examiner were talking to someone else. A second patient not only failed to move her paralyzed arm when asked to do so but would sometimes say, "There, it's done" without having moved at all. Babinski noted that each of these patients had left-sided weakness with sensory deficits in the affected limb. He speculated that anosognosia might be peculiar to patients with lesions of the right hemisphere. It is important to note that "denial of illness" is a somewhat clumsy translation of Babinski's original term, since it implies that patients have some level of awareness of their deficit but either repress or suppress this knowledge. Because most cases of anosognosia occur in association with right parietal lobe disorders and because neglect or inattention can also be produced in animals by surgically manipulating the parietal lobes, it seems unlikely that psychodynamic factors play a primary causative role in most neglect syndromes.

Right hemispheric lesions in at least five different areas can each produce striking neglect syndromes both in animals and in humans. These areas include the inferior parietal lobule, the prefrontal convexity, the cingulate gyrus, the thalamus, and the hypothalamus. It has been postulated that each of these areas is part of an anatomic loop connecting cortical, limbic, and reticular structures. Lesions at any level of this loop might thus produce attentional deficits. It is of particular interest that structures in the left parietal lobe play a role in the distribution of attention to objects and events in the right hemispace, while homologous structures in the right parietal lobe appear to play a role in the distribution of attention not only to the contralateral but also to the ipsilateral hemispace.

Body Image Distortions

Patients with lesions of the parietal lobe may deny the existence of a paralyzed limb or may admit its existence but repudiate ownership, claiming that it belongs to someone else. One male patient with left hemiplegia constantly lay on his right side, protesting that he had a paralyzed brother beside him. He explained that because this situation was offensive to him, he preferred to turn his back on his brother. On one occasion, without being aware that he was being observed, the patient was overheard addressing his brother: "How are you?" "Do you want a cigarette?" In another case, a physician observed a male patient searching under the bed for his left arm, which he felt was missing. A patient whose limb is paralyzed secondary to parietal lobe disorder may adopt a facetious or condescending attitude toward the compromised limb, referring to it as a "piece of meat" or "dumb slob" or giving the offending body part a pet name. (Critchley [1979] used the term "misoplegia" to describe a violent dislike for the paralyzed limb.)

Tactile Sensory Disturbances

Patients with parietal lobe disorders may have tactile sensory disturbances despite the absence of gross sensory deficits. Their response to a tactile stimulus may be delayed, or they may have a distorted perception of the stimulus. Patients may experience **tactile (haptic) hallucinations,** such as the hallucination of a three-dimensional object in the hand or of a "phantom limb." Persistence of tactile experience or displacement of sensory experiences from one side of the body to the other may also occur. More commonly, however, careful examination discloses striking deficits in the synthesis, interpretation, and differentiation of primitive sensory experiences. **Astereognosis** (tactile agnosia) refers to the inability to recognize a three-dimensional object by palpation. Disorders of tactile discrimination are not limited to the appreciation of shape and may occur with reference to texture **(hylognosis),** size **(macro-** or **microstereognosis),** or pattern **(graphanesthesia).** Finally, impaired ability to recognize the posture of an extremity **(statagnosia)** tends to be associated with bizarre subjective experiences and may play a major role in determining a patient's mental attitude toward the disability.

Motility Disturbances

Patients with parietal lobe disorders manifest greater unilateral incapacity than would be expected on the basis of their motor weakness. Unilateral diminution in spontaneous movements and wasting of the hand muscles and shoulder girdle muscles suggest the importance of intact sensory pathways to motor activity and to the maintenance of muscle mass.

LANGUAGE DISORDERS

Aphasia usually suggests pathological changes in the left hemisphere. Aphasic patients with posterior lesions may present with acutely disorganized and incoherent speech that is sometimes mistaken for schizophrenic "word salad," while patients with anterior lesions are often noted to be severely depressed, frustrated, or irritable. Aphasia-like disorders may be induced by medications; lithium toxicity, for instance, may produce **dysnomia** (word-finding difficulty). Management of patients with organic brain disease and especially those with language disorders requires an appreciation of both the functional deficits and preserved skills of the patient. Without assessing a patient's ability to comprehend, name, repeat, read, or write, the clinician's ability to help either the patient or the patient's family is severely limited.

Language Versus Speech Disorders

Although combinations of speech and language disorders may be seen, it is important to distinguish these two types of disorders. **Dysarthrias** (disorders of speech) are due to pathological changes in the neuromuscular apparatus responsible for the mechanical production of speech. Dysarthria may be seen either with lower brainstem lesions affecting the cranial nerves subserving motor speech outflow or with disruption of corticobulbar fibers traveling from the cortex to the brainstem. In speech disorders, articulation is characterized as spastic, flaccid, ataxic, or hypo- or hyperkinetic. In contrast, **aphasias** (disorders of language) are due to disruption of the neural machinery responsible for the reception, processing, and production of language-dependent ideas. Aphasic patients demonstrate abnormalities not only in spoken but also in written communication.

Language Circuitry of the Left Hemisphere

Since the 1860s—based on the work of Pierre Paul Broca, a French surgeon and anthropologist—it has been known that the vast majority of language disorders occur following damage to the left hemisphere. Ninety-seven percent of right-handers have left hemispheric dominance for **propositional language** (the ability to use semantics and syntax to convey an idea or proposition). Ten percent of the population are left-handed, and over two-thirds of left-handed individuals have left hemispheric dominance for language skills.

The language circuitry of the left hemisphere (Fig 5–6) involves regions of the temporal, parietal, and frontal cortex surrounding the lateral cerebral (sylvian) fissure. Damage to the perisylvian* region produces major aphasic syndromes whose features depend on the size, extent, and location of the lesion. Auditory fibers travel from the medial geniculate body of the thalamus to Heschl's gyrus in the superior temporal plane. Surrounding Heschl's gyrus is the auditory association cortex known as **Wernicke's area.** From Wernicke's area, fibers sweep backward and upward in the arcuate fasciculus, traveling through the inferior parietal lobule to reach the foot of the third (inferior) frontal gyrus. This frontal region, known as **Broca's area,** can be thought of as motor association cortex. As an extension of premotor cortex, it serves as an auditory encoder that generates articulatory programs for the region of the motor cortex subserving the mouth, tongue, and larynx.

Since the entire perisylvian area is supplied by the middle cerebral artery, varieties of aphasia reflect which branch or branches of this artery are occluded.

Aphasias Due to Lesions in the Perisylvian Area (Table 5–2)

The three major aphasias discussed below all result from pathological changes in the perisylvian area of

---

* By "perisylvian" is meant the area surrounding the lateral sulcus, also known as the sylvian fissure or sulcus.

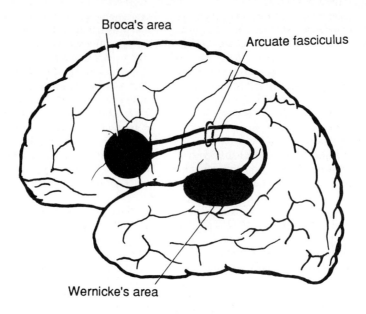

Figure 5–6. Perisylvian language circuitry.

the left hemisphere, and all three are characterized by inability to repeat spoken language. Patients with **Wernicke's aphasia** cannot repeat because they are unable to decode auditory messages. Those with **Broca's aphasia** fail to repeat because they cannot encode messages that have been understood. Patients with **conduction aphasia** cannot repeat because they are unable to transfer information from an intact auditory decoding apparatus to an intact auditory encoding apparatus. If the entire perisylvian area is destroyed, patients lose both spontaneous speech and auditory comprehension. These unfortunate individuals, whose lesions lie either in the internal carotid artery itself or near the organ of the middle cerebral artery, are said to have global aphasia.

A. Broca's Aphasia: Broca's aphasia ("motor" aphasia) is characterized by poor articulation and severe impairment of verbal fluency (the ability to produce spontaneous, effortless speech) and is often accompanied by paralysis of the right face and arm. Comprehension is relatively unimpaired, and following recovery, patients often report that they knew precisely what they wanted to say but were unable to say it.

Table 5–2. Classification of aphasic syndromes.

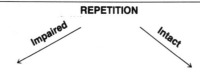

	REPETITION	
Impaired ↙		↘ Intact

Perisylvian Syndromes			Nonperisylvian Syndromes
	Fluency	**Comprehension**	
1. Broca's aphasia	−	+	1. Anomic aphasias
2. Wernicke's aphasia	+	−	2. Transcortical aphasias
3. Conduction aphasia	+	+	Motor
4. Global aphasia	−	−	Sensory
			Mixed ("isolation of the speech area")
			3. Subcortical aphasias
			Basal ganglia/internal capsule
			Thalamus
			Marie's quadrilateral space

Because the speech of these patients consists mainly of noun and adjective phrases or clichés, with omission of connecting words such as conjunctions and prepositions, it is often described as "telegraphic" and "agrammatical." Despite severe impairment in fluency, patients are sometimes capable of serial speech such as counting or reciting. Cursing and singing may also be preserved. Patients with Broca's aphasia tend to be angry, depressed, and frustrated. Surprisingly, however, suicide attempts in this population are extremely rare.

B. Wernicke's Aphasia: Wernicke's aphasia often occurs in the absence of motor impairment. Speech is fluent and effortless but devoid of meaning, and comprehension is grossly impaired. Lesions producing this "fluent" aphasia are located in or near Wernicke's area. Since the auditory association cortex functions as an auditory decoder or phonetic analyzer for spoken language, destruction of this area leads to inability to extract meaning from spoken language.

The affective behavior of patients with Wernicke's aphasia ranges from euphoric indifference to paranoid agitation. Management is complicated by the patients' lack of insight into their illness, and rehabilitation therapy cannot be initiated until they become aware of their deficits. Individuals with Wernicke's aphasia are at risk for suicide at two points in the course of their illness: (1) following sudden onset of a comprehension deficit, when their lack of insight and misinterpretation of others' actions may lead to chaotic paranoid behavior; and (2) as they begin to become aware of their impairment.

C. Conduction Aphasia: In conduction aphasia, spontaneous speech and comprehension are both preserved, but the patient has almost complete inability to repeat spoken language. This condition results from lesions that spare both Broca's area and Wernicke's area while disrupting the fibers of the arcuate fasciculus that connect these two regions.

Aphasias Due to Lesions Affecting Nonperisylvian Language Areas

The following language disorders result from lesions in the nonperisylvian area of the left hemisphere. Patients with these disorders are able to repeat spoken language.

A. Anomic Aphasias: Anomic aphasias are characterized by severe impairment of word-finding ability. (As a general rule, all aphasias are accompanied by some difficulty with word finding.) Patients with anterior lesions appear to have problems with word **production,** while patients with posterior lesions have difficulty either with **selection** of the correct word or with **access** to their "central word lexicon." The most severe anomic aphasia is that associated with lesions in the region of the dominant inferior parietal lobule. Damage to either the angular or supramarginal

gyrus can produce anomia of such severity that patients not only fail to benefit from phonemic or semantic cues but may also be unable to recognize the name of a common item when presented with a list containing the word.

Word-finding difficulty may occur in the absence of a structural lesion, eg, with physical exhaustion, dehydration, fever, or metabolic encephalopathy. Thus, care should be taken to differentiate true anomic aphasia from transient language disorders that merely reflect physiological disequilibrium.

B. Transcortical Aphasias: These aphasias are characterized by impairment of either fluency or comprehension, depending on whether the lesion is anterior or posterior. The aphasias are termed transcortical because they typically result from infarctions at the border zone between the middle cerebral artery and either the anterior or the posterior cerebral artery.

C. Subcortical Aphasias: The third group of language disorders in which repetition is preserved is referred to as the subcortical aphasias. Three types have been described: The anterior type results from vascular disorders in the basal ganglia or anterior limb of the internal capsule. The posterior type results from vascular disorders in the thalamus. Both of these are characterized by an initial period of mutism. While the first evolves into transcortical *motor* aphasia, the second evolves into a transcortical *sensory* aphasia with prominent paraphasias. The third type of subcortical aphasia arises from pathological changes in the area known as Marie's quadrilateral space, and in this type, initial mutism persists as global aphasia. The importance of the subcortical aphasias is 2-fold. First, they demonstrate that language circuitry is not limited to neocortex, Second, the subcortical syndromes may represent an exception to the general rule that word-finding difficulty accompanies all aphasic disorders.

Disturbances of Prosody

The "expressive" ability to modulate pitch, melody, and rhythm to impart emotional coloring (prosody) to one's own speech and the receptive ability to detect prosody in the speech of others are important "nonpropositional" aspects of language. Patients with Broca's aphasia, Parkinson's disease, and moderately advanced dementia have difficulty with the inflection, rhythm, and melody of their speech. Recent evidence suggests that patients with damage to the right frontal region homologous to Broca's area may lose the ability to impart prosody to their speech, while patients with posterior right hemispheric lesions in areas homologous to Wernicke's area may lose the ability to decode or perceive affective coloring in the speech of others. Although a prosody and dysprosody are only now beginning to be studied, the possibility of dissociations between felt inner emotion and affective expression is clearly of significance to psychiatrists, since it confounds the diagnosis of depression in patients with organic brain disease and may also represent an under-recognized complication of neuroleptic drug administration.

APRAXIA & THE CALLOSAL SYNDROMES

The term "apraxia" has been used in a confusingly large number of ways. In fact, many clinicians still use the term to denote disorders of movement they are unable or unwilling to characterize in some other way. The clinician who accepts another's diagnosis of apraxia without personally examining the patient adopts the ambiguity and uncertainty of the previous examiner. Thus, clinicians are advised to ask the previous examiner to specify what has been observed and then to examine the patient personally.

Constructional Apraxia

The term "constructional apraxia" is a somewhat awkward means of denoting difficulty with "constructions," eg, copying a simple drawing or reproducing a pattern. Constructional ability may be assessed in several ways (see Chapter 11). Since the earliest reports of constructional difficulty appeared, debate has continued about whether the deficit reflects (1) a perceptual problem with the spatial aspects of visual and tactile experience or (2) a motor disorder of programming complex movements in space. It now seems that the right and left hemispheres make separate and distinct contributions to performing complex constructional tasks. The right hemisphere appears to play a largely perceptual role, while the left hemisphere is instrumental at the executive or planning level of motor constructions. Thus, differences in constructional deficits are based on whether lesions are right-sided or left-sided.

Patients with right-sided lesions draw energetically and often add extra strokes. Their productions tend to be scattered and fragmented; boundaries are not observed, and virtually all aspects of spatial relations appear to be lost. These patients may also have difficulty dressing themselves and show hemispatial neglect (for the left side of space).

Patients with left-sided lesions draw slowly and seem to benefit from having a model to copy (this does not help patients with right-sided lesions). Their drawings tend to be somewhat more coherent but are simplified and lack inner detail. The coexistence of language disturbances and elements of Gerstmann's syndrome—alexia, agraphia, right-left confusion, and finger agnosia—may be seen.

Apraxia for Dressing

Difficulty in orienting articles of clothing with reference to the body can be seen in patients with dementia or right parietal lobe disorders but is probably most common in confusional states.

Apraxia of Gait

Patients with expanding frontal lobe lesions or lesions in the region of the supplemental motor area and patients with normal-pressure hydrocephalus may have great difficulty in initiating gait. Because they look as if their feet are glued to the floor, they are sometimes said to have a "magnetic gait." Patients with apraxia of gait are unable to use their limbs properly despite unimpaired strength and intact sensation. Their deficits are not limited to walking and appear to reflect a diffuse problem with the initiation of movements in the lower extremities. These patients may, for example, be unable to perform on command such acts as kicking an imaginary ball or drawing a circle with their feet while lying supine.

Apraxia of Speech

Apraxia of speech is a communication disorder intermediate between true aphasia and dysarthria. It is characterized by prolongation and segregation of syllables. Apraxia of speech, along with dysarthria, is often a component of Broca's aphasia. Apraxic "groping for articulatory postures" lends a plaintive quality to patients with Broca's aphasia. For the speech pathologist, however, it suggests that a particular therapeutic strategy (melodic intonation therapy) may be helpful

Ideational Apraxia

Ideational apraxia denotes disturbance in the planning of a complex gesture or act even though each of its component parts can be executed singly without difficulty. The problem is one of the sequencing and integration of motor behavior over time.

Ideomotor Apraxia

Ideomotor apraxia denotes a disconnection syndrome wherein certain skilled movements cannot be performed in response to verbal commands, although they can be performed spontaneously. Behavioral neurologists in the USA use the term ideomotor apraxia only if the following criteria can be met: (1) Motor systems are intact, ie, no paralysis, paresis, slowing of movements, incoordination, or other movement disorder; (2) there is no sensory loss in the limbs; and (3) the disorder is not the result of inattention, lack of cooperation, poor comprehension, or intellectual deterioration.

Ideomotor apraxia is caused by interruption of the pathways between the perisylvian area involved with language and the motor association areas involved with voluntary (willed) behavior. A review of these pathways may be helpful. When one is asked to perform a particular act with the right hand, comprehension and performance involve the circuitry from Wernicke's area via the arcuate fasciculus to Broca's area and thence to the left motor cortex. If one is asked to perform the same act with the left hand, the command must be relayed from Wernicke's area in the dominant hemisphere to the right motor cortex. Two possible pathways might be imagined: (1) from Wernicke's area in the left hemisphere via the posterior commissure to the Wernicke's area homolog in the right hemisphere, and then to the right motor cortex; or (2) from Wernicke's area via the arcuate fasciculus to Broca's area, from Broca's area via the anterior corpus callosum to the Broca area homolog in the right hemisphere, and then to the right motor cortex). Since there is no clinical evidence that patients with lesions of the posterior corpus callosum (infarction of the posterior cerebral artery) have difficulty using the left hand to follow complex commands, the anterior route appears to be the actual pathway.

Apraxia may occur with damage to the pathway from Wernicke's area to the right motor cortex at any of three sites: (1) If the anterior portion of the corpus callosum is damaged (due to commissurotomy or infarction of the territory irrigated by the anterior cerebral artery), the pathway from Wernicke's area to Broca's area and then to the left motor cortex is intact, and patients can perform tasks on command with the right hand. However, since the left hemisphere cannot communicate with the right hemisphere homolog of Broca's area, these patients are unable to carry out commands with their left hand despite fully intact strength, coordination, and sensation in the left hand. (2) Lesions producing Broca's aphasia are usually large enough to produce paralysis of the right arm. Even though comprehension is intact, the patient is unable to perform the task with the paralyzed limb. Since the command cannot travel from the left hemisphere to the right motor cortex, the patient will also be unable to use the left hand. (3) Apraxia can result from left middle cerebral artery infarctions that spare Broca's and Wernicke's areas as well as the pathways that cross the corpus callosum but disrupt fibers traveling from Wernicke's area to Broca's area (ie, as in conduction aphasia).

Since left middle cerebral artery infarctions are not rare, one might expect ideomotor apraxia to be common. In fact, it is infrequently reported. There appear to be several reasons for this: (1) Apraxia may be a transient phenomenon that disappears as edema diminishes or as alternative pathways are recruited. (2) Patients themselves are usually unaware of ideomotor apraxia, since they can perform volitional acts spontaneously. (3) Patients with apraxia are sometimes considered to be simply confused or to have comprehension problems. (4) Those testing for apraxia may fail to utilize strict criteria.

It is important to remember that one of the criteria for apraxia is intact comprehension. Comprehension can be tested in aphasic patients (1) by asking them questions of graded difficulty that require head nodding, head shaking, or yes and no responses; and (2) by asking them to perform movements involving use of the axial muscles (movements that can be executed with extrapyramidal motor systems whose origins appear to arise from diffuse areas of the cortex) or eye movements. Intact comprehension is demonstrated if the patient can perform these tasks.

Callosal Syndromes

The corpus callosum, composed of 200 million fibers, is the largest of several nerve fiber bundles connecting the hemispheres. Three other telencephalic interhemispheric pathways are the anterior commissure, hippocampal commissure, and massa intermedia. In addition, there are two midbrain commissures: the posterior and habenular commissures.

When surgical section of the corpus callosum was first performed in patients with intractable convulsions, behavior did not appear to be affected by the procedure. Large-scale studies in the 1940s led researchers to comment jokingly that the corpus callosum served only to transmit seizures from one hemisphere to the other or to keep the hemispheres from collapsing onto themselves. After Sperry's pioneering work on animals whose interhemispheric pathways had been surgically sectioned, Geschwind et al (1962) were able to document symptoms of callosal syndrome in a patient whose corpus callosum had been severed to control seizures. Since that time, a uniform clinical picture has been described in patients whose corpus callosum has been surgically transected or damaged by disease. These patients behave as if their two hemispheres were functioning autonomously. For example, the patient may open a drawer with one hand and immediately close it with the other or may button a shirt with the left hand and then unbutton it with the right hand (the "alien hand syndrome"). From observations that patients who wrote in a normal fashion with the right hand were unable to write with the left and were unable to name (although they could demonstrate recognition of) pictures of items that had been seen exclusively by the right hemisphere, researchers have gained insight into hemispheric specialization. Particularly important was the recognition that even though the right hemisphere was essentially mute, it was still able to process things in complicated ways. Geschwind's research on disconnection syndromes in animals and humans, published in 1965, has become a cornerstone of behavioral neurology in the USA. Even though the apraxias were not the first disorders of higher cortical dysfunction to be conceptualized as disconnection syndromes, they have served as a prototype for the study of mind-brain relations.

MEMORY DISORDERS

Korsakoff's (Amnestic) Syndrome

Wernicke's encephalopathy constitutes the acute phase of two distinct disorders—Wernicke's syndrome and Korsakoff's syndrome—both of which are caused by thiamine deficiency. Confusion, ataxia, and eye signs (nystagmus or ophthalmoplegia) comprise the traditional triad of symptoms in patients with Wernicke's encephalopathy. Because these patients are profoundly inattentive, it is inappropriate to characterize them as having a memory disorder (see Chapters 11 and 17). In the chronic stages of thiamine deficiency, however, apathy and memory disorder are the two most salient features. The hallmark and sine qua non of Korsakoff's syndrome is a dissociation between immediate recall and recent recall (the latter sometimes referred to as recent memory or short-term memory). In addition to significant problems registering new information, these patients demonstrate long-term memory problems (retrograde amnesia). One can think of this long-term memory deficit as a reflection of the difficulty these patients had registering new information at earlier times (anterograde amnesia). Thus, the extent of retrograde amnesia probably reflects the period of time over which the patient has suffered anterograde amnesia.

Unless formal testing of memory is performed routinely (see Chapter 11), the memory deficits associated with thiamine deficiency are easily mixed, since these patients often converse in what appears to be a normal or even glib fashion. Moreover, their performance on tests of intellectual functioning is not significantly impaired by their amnestic state. Confabulation (the filling-in of memory blanks with what may appear to be fanciful information) is not an invariable part of the syndrome but tends to occur in the earlier stages and during recovery. While confabulation has been construed as intentional misleading of the examiner, it is probably best viewed as an attempt by the patient either to make sense of the world or to cooperate with the examiner despite depleted information stores.

Since lesions in Korsakoff's syndrome are localized to specific anatomic sites, the syndrome provides a model for the study of amnesia and brain localization. Petechial hemorrhagic lesions stretch from the third to the fourth ventricle in the midline along the cerebral aqueduct. Lesions in the mamillary bodies and in the dorsomedial nucleus of the thalamus are also predictable findings. While the periventricular lesions lie in the ascending reticular network, lesions in the mamillary bodies lie in the medial limbic circuit described by Papez. The dorsomedial thalamus is a prominent way station for fibers passing from medial limbic structures such as the amygdala to the prefrontal cortex.

Alcoholic Memory Blackouts

In contrast to Korsakoff's syndrome, in which both the anatomy and pathophysiology are reasonably well understood, alcoholic blackouts represent a common occurrence whose pathogenesis is poorly understood. Two types of blackouts have been described: en bloc and fragmentary.

The onset of **en bloc blackouts** is abrupt, and the duration is from minutes to days. During blackouts, patients are incapable of registering new information and may ask the same question or tell the same story repeatedly. Despite their anterograde amnesia, these patients may have unimpaired ability to move about, drive an automobile, and perform routine tasks. The hallmark of the en bloc blackout is that forgetting is complete and memory cannot be recovered for a period of time despite attempts to "jog the memory" with cues, hypnosis, or amobarbital interviews.

Fragmentary blackouts are more common than en bloc blackouts. Patients with fragmentary blackouts have "spotty" recall for events that happened during the blackout and sometimes report that events happened "as in a dream" or "a picture out of focus." During recovery, islands of recall seem to coalesce, and retrieval of information is facilitated by "jogging the memory." Casual observers cannot distinguish behavior of patients during alcoholic blackouts from their behavior during mild states of inebriation.

Transient Global Amnesia

The typical picture of transient global amnesia is that of a 50- or 60-year-old man who experiences a sudden onset of confusion with loss of ability to learn new information. Attacks last hours to days, and during this period patients tend (in contrast to patients having an alcoholic blackout) to be agitated and aware of their problem. They may, for example, repeatedly ask questions such as "Where am I?" or "What is happening?" An attack rarely (if ever) occurs more than once in any individual. Seizure activity, vasospasm, and occlusive transient ischemia of medial temporal lobe structures have been suggested as possible causes of transient global amnesia.

Traumatic Amnesia

Following nontrivial head injury, memory problems are common. Traumatic amnesia refers to loss of memory both for a period of time preceding the head injury (retrograde amnesia) and for events following the injury (posttraumatic [anterograde] amnesia). Posttraumatic amnesia prevents the patient from registering new information. For example, a hospitalized patient may recognize visitors and talk with them but the next day have no recollection of the visit. In general, posttraumatic amnesia lasts minutes to hours following return of consciousness; if it exceeds 24 hours, the patient usually has sustained severe and permanent neurological deficits such as those associated with prolonged coma. Termination of posttraumatic amnesia tends to be abrupt and often occurs after a period of sleep or following some emotionally meaningful event such as the visit of a close friend. Because the extent of retrograde amnesia immediately following injury may initially encompass years of the patient's life but later shrinks to a minute or less in all but the severest cases of head injury, the term "shrinking retrograde amnesia" is appropriate. Phenomenological studies of traumatic amnesia reveal that shrinkage of retrograde amnesia follows and depends on resolution of the anterograde amnestic deficit. Following head injury or confusional states, a remarkable phenomenon known as "reduplicative paramnesia" involving bizarre distortions of memory is sometimes observed. For example, a patient with paramnesia who is asked, "Where are you?" may admit being in a hospital but insist that the hospital itself is across the street from his or her home or that the hospital room is even in a wing of the home.

Amnesia Following Seizures

Following major motor seizures, patients are invariably amnestic for the seizure itself as well as for a variable period after the seizure. In general, the same is true of complex partial seizures, although some patients have such seizures during which they remain conscious. During the confusional period that follows seizures, patients may respond to gentle attempts to assist them with agitation or aggression but will later be amnestic for this period of abnormal behavior. Continuous absence ('petit mal') is a rare condition in which patients lose touch with the environment for prolonged periods and thus are amnestic for events.

Acute Confusion

Although acute confusion of toxic, metabolic, or infectious origin is not considered a true amnestic state, patients with acute confusion may be unable to register new information over prolonged periods. If examined following resolution of their confusion, they may appear "amnestic" for the confusional period. Toxic states for which a person has no recall can occur with phencyclidine (PCP) abuse. This drug is a known "dissociative/amnestic" agent, and a person under its influence may commit crimes of violence for which he or she later has no recall.

Memory Impairment

Memory impairment unaccompanied by other evidence of intellectual deterioration is termed an amnestic syndrome. Early problems with memory become increasingly more severe in presenile and senile dementia of the Alzheimer type. The term "benign senescent forgetfulness" has been used to designate the almost universal memory problems that occur with increasing frequency in the seventh, eighth, and ninth decades. This "benign" variant of forgetfulness is in all likelihood related to the memory deficits seen in dementia syndromes, differing only in degree of impairment.

Patients with moderately advanced dementia are usually unaware of their memory dysfunction and therefore not concerned about it. Depressed patients with complaints of cognitive deficits (depressive pseudodementia) are preoccupied with what they take to be memory deterioration and may seek help for this complaint. Thus, even though some patients in the earliest stages of dementia may be aware of and upset by their memory problems, patients who present with complaints of memory problems are more likely to have an affective illness.

Differential Diagnosis of Organic & Functional Amnestic Disorders

Among the nonorganic (psychogenic) memory disorders are the following: dissociative episode (fugue state), feigned amnesia (malingering), factitious amnesia (a variant of Ganser's syndrome), and conditions in which thought processes are disrupted by intrusive thoughts or images (major affective illness, schizophrenia, posttraumatic stress disorder). Although the latter are psychiatric conditions, their "biological" features suggest that the term "psychogenic" is used here in a somewhat strained sense.

In differentiating organic from functional amnestic disorders, the clinician should consider the following factors: age; medical history (especially history of neurological disorders); psychiatric history; the presence or absence of psychosocial precipitants (in what environment or under what circumstances the amnestic episodes occur); affective behavior during the episode; the patient's desire for recovery; what type of information is forgotten (loss of personal identity implies functional illness); evidence that the patient is registering some types of information while selectively ignoring others; the patient's response to cuing techniques (eg, hypnosis, use of amobarbital); and where the patient is when memory function is recovered.

FRONTAL LOBE SYNDROMES

Understanding the behavioral manifestations of frontal lobe disease requires a knowledge of frontal lobe functions and of frontal connections to the rest of the central nervous system.

Frontal Lobe Connections

A. Sensory Input: Sensory input to the prefrontal region does not arise from primary sensory regions but rather from the high-level (polymodal and supramodal) association cortices of the temporal, parietal, and occipital lobes. Sensory information presented to the frontal lobes is therefore already highly processed. Input to the frontal convexities from the inferior parietal lobule serves as one example of such highly processed sensory input.

B. Motor Output: The frontal lobe cortex contains four motor areas: (1) the motor strip containing giant pyramidal (Betz) cells, (2) the premotor region, (3) the frontal eye fields, and (4) the supplemental motor area. The frontal cortex, along with much of the neocortex, projects to the basal ganglia. Projections to the head of the caudate nucleus (which are not bidirectional) are particularly prominent. The importance of these frontostriatal ("psychomotor") pathways is suggested by the fact that the head of the caudate nucleus also receives limbic system input from such regions as the hippocampus and the amygdala. Thus, the basal ganglia can be seen as a point of convergence for frontal lobe and limbic system information.

C. Limbic System Input: As mentioned in the earlier discussion of limbic system anatomy in this chapter, there are numerous links between prefrontal and limbic areas. These may conveniently be subdivided into three categories: (1) direct pathways from the medial temporal lobe structures to frontal cortex via the uncinate fasciculus; (2) indirect fibers connecting frontal and limbic system regions via the dorsomedial nucleus of the thalamus; and (3) indirect fibers passing from the hippocampus to prefrontal regions via the cingulate gyrus.

D. Septo-Hypothalamo-Mesencephalic Continuum Input: There are direct pathways from the dorsolateral convexities and orbitomedial portions of the prefrontal area to the septo-hypothalamo-mesencephalic continuum.

Behavioral Changes in Frontal Lobe Syndromes

Behavioral changes following frontal lobe damage may be grouped into three broad categories: personality, intellect, and motor function disturbances.

A. Personality Disturbances: The case of Phineas P. Gage, a 25-year-old construction foreman working on a railroad bed in Vermont, is perhaps the most famous example of personality disturbance associated with frontal lobe syndromes. According to the case report of Harlow (1868), Gage was using a tamping iron to pack blasting powder into a hole when the powder exploded. The explosion drove the tamping iron through his face and out the top of his skull, transacting his frontal lobes. After the accident, he became, in the words of his physician, ". . . fitful, irreverent, indulging at times in the grossest profanity (which was not previously his custom), manifesting but little deference to his fellows, impatient of restraint or advice when it conflicts with his desires, at times pertinaciously obstinate yet capricious and vacillating, devising many plans for future operation which are no sooner arranged than they are abandoned in turn for others appearing more feasible. . . . His mind was radically changed, so that his friends and acquaintances said he was no longer Gage."

Studies of individuals who suffered penetrating head injuries during World War I showed personality disturbances of two distinct types. Individuals with orbitomedial disorders appeared puerile, disinhibited, and euphoric ("pseudopsychopathic"). Those with brain injury limited to the dorsolateral convexities appeared apathetic and indifferent ("pseudode-

pressed"). Since patients rarely have lesions limited to either of these regions, it is more common to see admixtures of these two personality types. Geschwind has described these patients with irritability, apathy, and euphoria as manifesting "the impossible triad of frontal lobe pathology."

B. Intellectual Disturbances: Characterization of intellectual deficits following frontal lobe damage has been a vexing problem. In the late 1940s (10 years after psychosurgery had come into use), essentially no neuropsychological changes had been consistently noted in postsurgical patients even though psychologists searched diligently for intellectual deterioration in these patients. Failure to correlate intellectual deficits with prefrontal lobe damage called into question the established view that the frontal lobes were the highest seat of human intelligence and suggested that they might even be superfluous structures, since they could apparently be removed with relative impunity. Since that time, the consequences of frontal lobe damage have been somewhat clarified, largely as a result of the work of Luria, a Russian neurologist and neuropsychologist (see Luria, 1980). After seeing thousands of patients personally, Luria concluded that the frontal lobes have four functions: (1) generating plans for action; (2) programming the components, or subroutines, of actions; (3) monitoring ongoing activity with reference both to the goal and to environmental shifts; and (4) correcting the course of activity already in progress.

Obviously, the frontal lobes do not act independently. They depend on high-level sensory input from the temporal, parietal, and occipital lobes. Patients with frontal lobe damage may have the following problems: (1) difficulty suppressing irrelevant associations, or intrusions; (2) inability to anticipate the consequences of their actions, ie, physical damage to property, self, or others and emotional consequences for self and others; (3) inability to formulate an approach to complex problems that extend over time; (4) remarkable dissociation of speech from action (eg, a patient told to "squeeze a ball when the light goes on" may say "I must squeeze the ball" when he or she sees the light but will fail to carry out the action); and (5) difficulty understanding metaphors, similes, and parables (the "inability to assume the abstract attitude" described by Goldstein in the 1940s as the hallmark of organic disease).

Patients with frontal lobe damage have been said to manifest "frontal amnesia." In actuality, these patients do not have amnestic problems similar to those of patients with Korsakoff's psychosis. However, they are sometimes unable to hold in conscious awareness the various pieces of information required for a specific action. It has been speculated that these individuals fail to generate mnemonic associations; thus, their forgetting may reflect not so much a retrieval blockade as a disinclination to remember or a failure to generate "limbic tags" for events.

Intelligence tests do not appear to measure well the type of deficits seen following frontal lobe damage. The Wisconsin Card-Sorting Test (in which patients are asked to infer from the examiner's responses whether they are shifting cards by the appropriate criterion) and various maze-learning tasks have proved helpful in neuropsychological assessment of frontal lobe damage. Tests that measure the ability to sustain, shift, or direct attention might be expected to be most sensitive to frontal lobe lesions.

C. Motor Function Disturbances: The motor changes following frontal lobe damage may include the appearance of primitive reflexes such as grasping, sucking, and snouting reflexes. However, in many patients with significant prefrontal lobe damage (eg, lobotomized psychiatric patients), these reflexes cannot be elicited. The grasp reflex is most frequently observed in patients over age 60, but its presence does not correlate well either with gross brain damage or with intellectual deterioration.

Disturbances associated with difficulty in overcoming motor inertia are seen in patients with frontal lobe damage. These include apraxia of gait, characterized by difficulty initiating gait; decreased "ocular palpation of the environment," which may contribute to the patient's tendency to make judgments on the basis of incomplete information; and palilalia, characterized by repetition of the last elements of an utterance (either the entire last word or the last syllable). Difficulty "changing sets" has long been recognized as a problem following frontal lobe damage. Patients asked to draw a series of geometric shapes such as a circle, triangle, and square may perseverate the production of one of these three elements. Luria has recommended the use of a simple bedside test in which patients are asked to perform a 3-step command—striking the top of a table with the edge of an open hand ("cut"), then striking the table with a closed fist ("pound"), and finally striking the table with an open palm ("slap")—as one index of frontal lobe function.

Many of these problems with inertia and perseveration resemble symptoms that arise from disorders of the basal ganglia. Since there are strong frontostriatal connections, it becomes difficult and even somewhat meaningless to attempt to separate frontal (cortical) from striatal (subcortical) symptoms.

MOVEMENT DISORDERS

Although virtually all neurological diseases have psychological correlates, the movement disorders serve as striking prototypes of neuropsychiatric disorders. The connections between neurology and psychiatry are particularly strong in Parkinson's disease, Huntington's disease, tardive dyskinesia, Gilles de la Tourette's syndrome, and Wilson's disease. Therefore, each of these disorders will be considered here.

Parkinson's Disease & Other Extrapyramidal Motor Disorders

A. Pathological Physiology: Tremor, muscular rigidity, and bradykinesia (the parkinsonian triad) are due to pathological changes in the posterior portion of the septo-hypothalamo-mesencephalic continuum—specifically, in the substantia nigra of the midbrain This darkly pigmented area lies at the junction between the cerebral peduncles and the tegmentum of the midbrain. Dorsal and medial to the substantia nigra lies the ventral tegmental area of Tsai, which is the origin of the mesolimbic dopaminergic pathways projecting to the limbic and frontal cortices. Destruction of the dopaminergic neurons in the substantia nigra leads to a decrease in the dopamine content of the neostriatum (caudate nucleus and putamen) and alters the cholinergic-dopaminergic balance. This imbalance of acetylcholine and dopamine may be treated with either dopamine agonists or anticholinergic drugs.

B. Dementia in Parkinson's Disease: For many years, it was thought that intellectual deterioration was not an intrinsic feature of Parkinson's disease, It now appears that parkinsonian patients are at high risk (10 times that of age-matched controls) of developing dementia. The incidence of neuropathological changes of the Alzheimer type is higher in patients with Parkinson's disease than in age-matched controls. Because so many symptoms of dementia in parkinsonian patients seem to involve a *slowing* of both mentation and motor activity, it has been suggested that the basal ganglia may play an important role in cognitive activity. Since dopaminergic pathways that ascend from the ventral tegmental region of the midbrain also travel to the frontal lobe cortex, damage to these mesolimbic and mesofrontal pathways may play a role in the dementia of Parkinson's disease.

C. Drug-Induced Parkinsonism: Drug-induced parkinsonism may occur within 5–30 days after starting neuroleptic treatment. Although the parkinsonian triad of symptoms is present, the severity of symptoms in drug-induced parkinsonism differs from that in Parkinson's disease in that bradykinesia is often the most prominent feature, muscular rigidity is less pronounced, and tremor may be insignificant.

Acute **dystonia,** if present, usually appears in the first 5 days of neuroleptic treatment and is very painful. Dystonic reactions may be seen in the eyes, neck, tongue, jaw, or trunk and are frequently misdiagnosed as hysteria, malingering, or seizures. A drug such as benztropine mesylate, diphenhydramine, or diazepam should be administered intravenously. If dystonic reactions recur or persist, a neuroleptic agent or lower potency such as thioridazine or chlorpromazine may be indicated. Serum calcium levels should be measured to rule out hypocalcemia.

Akathisia, an inner sense of restlessness that may or may not be accompanied by gross motor restlessness, may occur 5–60 days after initiating treatment with dopamine blockers. Antihistamines and propranolol are more efficacious than purely atropinic substances in treating akathisia.

"**Rabbit syndrome,**" a fine perioral tremor, may appear months after starting an antipsychotic agent. It is frequently misdiagnosed as tardive dyskinesia but is actually a parkinsonian phenomenon that responds to treatment with anticholinergic agents.

Huntington's Disease

Movement disorder and dementia are the two major features of Huntington's disease. The age at onset of this autosomal dominant disorder ranges roughly from 25 to 50 years, with peak onset in the fourth decade. Recent work on localization of the gene for Huntington's disease raises hope that early detection and possibly even treatment may be forthcoming. It is impossible to distinguish tardive dyskinesia from Huntington's disease, except on the basis of a family history of Huntington's disease.

Although patients may present with either motor or psychiatric symptoms, the former are more likely to bring the patient to medical attention. Initially, patients may fidget, twitch, grimace, and speak in a slurred fashion. As the disorder progresses, movements become conspicuously clumsy, of greater amplitude, and assume a bizarre and grotesque quality.

Personality disorder, thought or affective disorder, and dementia may occur. Violence and hypersexuality (often of a bizarre nature) are among the striking behavioral abnormalities that Huntington noted:

In patients with Huntington's disease, atrophy of the caudate nucleus leads to ballooning of the lateral ventricles, which can be seen on CT scan in the late stages of illness. Metabolic changes in the head of the caudate nucleus can be demonstrated early with positron emission tomography.

Since the mean life expectancy of patients with Huntington's disease is 16 years following diagnosis, it is important to realize that symptomatic relief is available. The movement disorder, the agitation, and the violent behavior described above can be treated with dopamine blockers such as haloperidol. For disturbances of affective behavior, which may reflect either depression due to a biochemical imbalance or reactive depression, treatment with lithium or tricyclic antidepressants should be considered.

Tardive Dyskinesia

In 1956, two years after approval of chlorpromazine as an antipsychotic agent, the first cases of persistent abnormal movements following discontinuation of the drug were reported.

A. Pharmacological Factors Affecting Onset and Treatment: Tardive dyskinesia is a late-onset disorder that occurs months to years after initiation of treatment with dopaminergic blocking agents. Suggested mechanisms for a functional dopaminergic ex-

cess have included (1) increased circulating blood levels of dopamine, (2) increased dopamine release by dopaminergic neurons, and (3) increased responsiveness to dopamine at the postsynaptic receptor sites. The precise pharmacological basis remains unclear. In all likelihood, tardive dyskinesia involves an imbalance of neurotransmitters (eg, dopamine, acetylcholine, and gamma-aminobutyric acid) and perhaps neuropeptides such as cholecystokinin and somatostatin as well.

Discontinuing dopamine-blocking agents is desirable but may not always be possible if psychosis is poorly controlled. Temporary worsening of the movement disorder is to be expected following cessation of administration of these agents. Drug holidays (weeks or months) are indicated to determine whether patients continue to require antipsychotic medications.

Increasing the dose of dopamine-blocking agents is not suitable treatment for tardive dyskinesia, since it will only mask the symptoms while pathophysiological changes continue.

If patients are being treated with anticholinergic agents such as tricyclic antidepressants or with antihistamines, discontinuing these agents may produce dramatic alleviation of the movement disorder.

Although lecithin and choline have been used for treatment of dyskinesia, these agents do not appear efficacious. Lecithin causes a fishy odor, and choline must be given in massive doses.

B. Types of Tardive Dyskinesia: Patients may present with one or more of the types of tardive dyskinesia described below. Older patients tend to have the buccolingual-masticatory and orofacial syndromes, whereas adolescents and young adults are more likely to develop choreiform movements primarily of the extremities.

1. Buccolingual-masticatory dyskinesia–The movements for this type include twisting, turning, protruding, and smacking the tongue and lips.

2. Orofacial dyskinesia–This form is characterized by facial tics, grimacing, and blinking.

3. Axial dyskinesia–Truncal movements such as shoulder shrugging, lordotic posturing, and pelvic thrusting may all be seen in patients with axial dyskinesia.

4. Appendicular chorea–Choreiform movements of the fingers, hands, arms, or legs have a rapid, dancelike quality. Since these choreiform movements are usually accompanied by some degree of athetosis (slow, writhing movements), the term choreoathetosis is often employed. Ballistic movements, eg, a throwing movement of the arm, are occasionally seen.

C. Differential Diagnosis: It is impossible to distinguish tardive dyskinesia from Huntington's disease clinically. This leads to a particular problem: If a patient with a psychotic behavioral disturbance is treated with antipsychotic agents and years later develops a movement disorder, the clinician seeing the patient for the first time is likely to attribute the movement disorder to prior neuroleptic drug treatment. Thus, Huntington's disease can be masked unless a family history is determined.

Gilles de la Tourette's Syndrome

This syndrome is characterized by chronic multiple motor and vocal tics. The age at onset is 2–15 years. Motor tics frequently consist of sniffing, snorting, or blinking; vocal tics consist of clicks, grunts, barks, coughs, or yelps. Coprolalia (the compulsive uttering of obscenities) is said to occur eventually in 60% of cases. Although mental and mood changes are not an intrinsic part of the syndrome, suicide may occur secondary to profound social disruption produced by the disorder. Tourette's disease may exist for many years before the diagnosis is made. The cause and pathogenesis are unknown, but administration of central nervous system stimulants such as methylphenidate may precipitate the disorder. Dopamine-blocking neuroleptic agents usually afford some symptomatic relief (see also Chapter 32).

Wilson's Disease (Hepatolenticular Degeneration)

Wilson's disease is an autosomal recessive disorder in which copper is deposited in the liver and lenticular nucleus (putamen and globus pallidus) of the basal ganglia. The defect in copper metabolism consists of diminished levels of ceruloplasmin, which may be documented by serum assay. The neurological manifestations of the disease reflect progressive extrapyramidal dysfunction accompanied by deterioration of personality (eg, irritability, depression, psychosis) and intellect. Early signs include tremor, bradykinesia, dysarthria, and dysphagia. Eventually, the patient develops a characteristic picture—a "vacuous smile," great difficulty chewing and swallowing, constant drooling, and a coarse "wing-flapping" tremor when the arms are outstretched. Deposition of copper in the cornea (Kayser-Fleischer ring) may be seen with a slit lamp in advanced stages. Treatment consists of reduction in dietary copper, use of sulfurated potash to prevent absorption of copper, and administration of the copper-chelating agent penicillamine.

Family members should be screened once the diagnosis is made.

REFERENCES

Babinski MJ: [No title.] Rev Neurol (Paris) 1918;34:365.

Babinski MJ: Contribution à létude des troubles mentaux dans l'hémiplégie organique (anosognosie). Rev Neurol (Paris) 1914;27:175.

Bard P. A diencephalic mechanism for the expression of rage with special reference to the sympathetic nervous system. Am J Physiol 1928,84:490.

Becker E: *Escape From Evil*. Free Press, 1975.

Benson DF: *Aphasia, Alexia and Agraphia*. Churchill Livingstone, 1979.

Benson DF: *Psychiatric Aspects of Neurologic Disease*. Vol 2. Grune & Stratton, 1982.

Broca P: Anatomie comparée des circonvolutions cérébrales: Le grand lobe limbique et la scissure limbique dans la série des mammifères. Rev Anthropol [Series 2] 1878;1:385.

Broca P: Perte de la parole: Ramollissement chronique et déstruction partielle du lobe antérieur gauche du cerveau. Paris Bull Soc Anthropol 1861;2:219.

Brodal A: *Neurological Anatomy*, 3rd ed. Oxford Univ Press, 1981.

Brophy JJ: Psychiatric disorders. Chapter 18 in: *Current Medical Diagnosis & Treatment 1991*. Schroeder SA et al (editors). Lange, 1991.

Critchley M: Misoplegia, or hatred of hemiplegia. In: *The Divine Banquet of the Brain*. Raven Press, 1979.

Critchley M: *The Parietal Lobes*. Hafner, 1953.

Freud S: Project for a scientific psychology (1895). In: *Standard Edition of the Complete Psychological Works of Sigmund Freud*. Vol. 1. Hogarth Press, 1966.

Geschwind N: The apraxias: Neural mechanisms of disorders of learned movements. Am Sci 1975;63: 188.

Geschwind N: Disconnexion syndromes in animals and man. (2 parts.) Brain 1965;88:237, 585.

Geschwind N, Kaplan E: A human cerebral disconnection syndrome. Neurology 1962,12:675.

Goldstein K: The effects of brain damage on personality. Psychiatry 1962;15:245.

Gray JA: *The Neuropsychology of Anxiety*. Oxford Univ Press, 1982.

Harlow JM: Recovery from the passage of an iron bar through the head. Mass Med Soc Publications 1868;2:329.

Lorenz K: *The Foundations of Ethology*. Springer, 1981.

Luria AR: *Higher Cortical Functions in Man*, 2nd ed. Basic Books, 1980.

MacLean PD: The brain, empathy and medical education. J Nerv Ment Dis 1967;144:374.

MacLean PD: Some psychiatric implications of physiological studies on the frontotemporal portion of the limbic system (visceral brain). Electroencephalogr Clin Neurophysiol 1952;4:407.

MacLean PD: *A Triune Concept of Brain and Behavior*. Univ Toronto Press, 1969.

Marsden CD, Fahn S: *Movement Disorders*. Butterworths, 1981.

Mountcastle VB: *Medical Physiology*, 14th ed. Mosby, 1980.

Mueller J: Neuroanatomic correlates of emotion. Chapter 10 in: *Emotions in Health and Illness*. Temoshok L, Van Dyke C, Zegans LS (editors). Grune & Stratton, 1983.

Nauta WJH: Hippocampal projections and related neural pathways to the midbrain in the cat. Brain 1958;81:319.

Papez JW: A proposed mechanism of emotion. Arch Neurot Psychiatry 1937;38:725.

Pfaf DW: *The Physiologic Mechanisms of Motivation.* Springer, 1982.

Plum F, Posner J: *The Diagnosis of Stupor and Coma,* 2nd ed. Davis, 1972.

Sperry R: Some effects of disconnecting the cerebral hemispheres. Science 1982;217:1223.

Willis T: *Cerebri Anatome.* Martzer and Alleftry (London), 1664.

Yakovlev PI: Motility, behavior and the brain: Organization and neural coordinates of behavior. J Nerv Ment Dis 1948; 107:313.

Neurobehavioral Chemistry & Physiology

6

Jack A. Grebb, MD, Victor I. Reus, MD, & Nelson B. Freimer, MD

Modern psychiatry seeks to correlate the vast amount of new research in basic neurosciences with observations of normal and abnormal human behavior. Research has focused on the identification of specific neurochemical pathways in the brain, the classification of receptor subtypes for each neurotransmitter, and the continued elucidation of the physiology and behavioral role of the neuroactive peptides (eg, endogenous opioids).

The virtual explosion of information in the basic neurosciences has resulted from the expanded application of existing research tools as well as new technological advances. Positron emission tomography is particularly useful because it permits in vivo determination and measurement of metabolic and neurochemical processes in human brain. Early studies focused on mapping brain metabolism with 2-deoxyglucose. Recently, scanning techniques have been adapted to the study of neurotransmitters and their receptors. For example, the functional activity of dopamine receptors has been visualized using binding with labeled spiperone, a neuroleptic agent with presumed high affinity for D_2 receptors. Additional in vivo imaging techniques (eg, topographic magnetic resonance spectroscopy) promise similar focal metabolic assessment with considerably less invasive risk to the patient. Psychiatrists must now be familiar with at least the basic concepts of these techniques in order to fully understand and critically evaluate much of the recent literature.

TRANSMISSION OF NERVE IMPULSES IN THE CENTRAL NERVOUS SYSTEM

The most important fundamental unit of transmission of nerve impulses in the central nervous system is the synapse, which is a specialized area of contact between nerve cells that enables interneuronal communication to occur. There are three types of synapses. First and most important, there are **chemical synapses,** which use a chemical messenger that is released by the presynaptic neuron when it is stimulated. Once in the synaptic cleft, this chemical can act on receptors located either on presynaptic cell

membranes (autoreceptors) or on postsynaptic cell membranes. The effects of this receptor interaction may be either stimulatory or inhibitory; however, in the central nervous system, it is the combined effects of multiple inputs to a single neuron that determine its actual functioning. Second, there exist **electrical synapses,** whose role remains poorly understood. Third, there are **conjoint synapses** that operate via both chemical and electrical transmission of nerve impulses. In addition to facilitating synaptic communication, nonsynaptic areas of neuronal membranes may contain receptors for chemical signals floating freely in the brain extracellular fluid. Neurons may be further affected by changes in pH, electrolyte concentrations, and other chemical constituents of the surrounding extracellular fluid and cerebrospinal fluid. For example, cerebrospinal fluid prostaglandins and especially calcium have major regulatory functions in transmission of nerve impulses.

Chemical transmission has been the focus of most of the recent research in neurobehavioral sciences, and three general categories of neuroregulators have been described: neurotransmitters, neuromodulators, and neurohormones. Although the differentiation of these messengers is clear in theory, they often have overlapping roles in vivo. **Neurotransmitters** are the "classical" chemical signals. They are released into the synaptic cleft quickly (1–2 ms) by the presynaptic neuron when it is stimulated. They then bind to receptors on either the postsynaptic or presynaptic cell membranes. The physiology and chemistry of neuromodulators are not yet clearly understood. It is known, however, that **neuromodulators** also bind specifically to receptors, although their function is to modify the response of the receptor to the neurotransmitter by tempering or adjusting transfer of the message rather than to actually transmit the message. Neuromodulators may be released by presynaptic nerve cells and may exercise their effects on a single synapse. It is also possible that neuromodulators may come from nonneuronal tissue and be distributed in cerebrospinal or extracellular fluid, thereby affecting large numbers of neurons. In addition, it appears that neuromodulators have a longer duration of effect (perhaps minutes) than do neurotransmitters. The distinguishing feature of **neurohormones** is their release by nerve cells directly into the systemic circulation rather than into the synaptic cleft, extracellular fluid, or cerebrospinal fluid. Neurohormones may then be transported throughout the body to affect peripheral organs as well as the central nervous system.

Discovery of the **coexistence of neuroregulators**—the presence of more than one neuroregulator (neurotransmitter, neuromodulator, or neurohormone) with a single neuron—is one of the most important recent developments in neuroscience. It now appears that many neurons in the central nervous system demonstrate coexistence. The number of coexisting neuroregulators released upon stimulation apparently varies; however, the basic physiology of these coexisting neuroregulators is largely unknown. Coexistence has significant implications for understanding regulatory mechanisms in normal and disease states. It is possible, for example, that a nerve cell might contain both a neurotransmitter and a neuromodulator. If the neuromodulator decreases the response of the postsynaptic neuron to the neurotransmitter and if an apparent overactivity of the neurotransmitter is noted in disease states, the cause may be an excess of neurotransmitter, a deficiency of neuromodulator, or both.

Steps in Synaptic Transmission

The first three steps in synaptic transmission are the synthesis, transport, and storage of the chemical messenger. The actual release of the chemical messenger usually involves a calcium-dependent process that causes a synaptic vesicle containing the neuroregulator to fuse with the postsynaptic membrane and release its contents through exocytosis.

The principal site of action of neuroregulators is the synapse. Synapses are not only axodendritic but also axoaxonic, axosomatic, and dendrodendritic. Synaptic receptors are complexes of one or more proteins floating in the lipid portion of the nerve cell membrane. Current knowledge suggests that synaptic receptors may have as many as three basic components: a recognition site, a modulator, and an effector. Each component and its corresponding functions may be represented by one or more proteins existing in a common area of the membrane and interacting when the receptor is stimulated.

The **recognition site** of the receptor exists on the external membrane and is responsible for the specificity of receptor response by preferentially binding only certain neuroregulators. The modulator component may exist as a separate protein that connects the activated recognition site to the effector. The **modulator protein** may itself have binding sites located on the external membrane, where neuromodulators or neurohormones bind to modulate receptor function. For example, a neuromodulator may bind to a modulator protein and change the latter's conformation. This change in conformation may affect the conformation of receptor proteins and inhibit binding of the neurotransmitter.

The **effector protein** is usually either a nucleotide cyclase or an ion channel. The effector protein is often adenylyl cyclase, which catalyzes the conversion of adenosine triphosphate to cyclic adenosine 3′,5-monophosphate, which is often called the "second messenger" because it links extracellular chemical messengers and the physiological response. The cyclic adenosine 3′,5-monophosphate can then activate cytoplasmic enzymes, phosphorylate membrane proteins, induce synthesis of messenger RNA, or affect microtubular assembly at the cellular level. An ion channel (the other common type of effector protein), when activated, changes its conformation to increase or decrease passage of specific ions into the neuron.

Termination of neuroregulator activity may occur through three mechanisms. First, the neuroregulator or products of its degradation may be brought back into the neuron through active, energy-dependent reuptake. Second, the neuroregulator may be degraded by enzymes either extraneuronally or intraneuronally. Third, the released neuroregulator may diffuse away from the postsynaptic cell into the brain extracellular fluid.

It is necessary to think of the steps in synaptic transmission as a dynamic flow, with change in one step affecting all other steps. Most drugs currently used in psychiatry initially exert their specific action on a single component of the synaptic receptor; however, the specific acute change may have complex effects on other components, and acute effects may differ markedly from chronic effects once the central nervous system has attained a state of equilibrium with the drug.

Regulation of Synaptic Transmission

Because recent research about the biology of behavioral disorders has centered on abnormalities of the regulation of chemical transmission, it is critical to understand the normal regulation of this process. The amount of neuroregulator that is synthesized may be controlled by varying the amount of necessary precursors and by altering the activity of the synthetic enzymes for specific neuroregulators, particularly enzymes controlling rate-limiting steps. The transport and storage of neuroregulators are also subject to regulation by changes in microtubule, microfilament, and vesicle assembly and function at the cellular level.

The actual release and action of neuroregulators have received most of the emphasis in research on regulatory processes. Presynaptic inhibition may occur through a variety of mechanisms; eg, with repeated stimulation, a presynaptic neuron eventually releases smaller amounts of neuroregulator. Presynaptic neurons with autoreceptors may respond to the released neuroregulators to decrease (or possibly increase) synthesis and release of neuroregulators. The amount of neuroregulator released may also be reduced either by an independent inhibitory presynaptic neuron with an axoaxonic connection or by an inhibitory presynaptic neuron stimulated by a collateral fiber of the presynaptic neuron itself. Postsynaptic inhibition may be either direct or indirect. Direct inhibition occurs when an inhibitory postsynaptic potential is generated in the cell by an inhibitory neurotransmitter. Indirect inhibition occurs during the refractory period after the development of an action potential in a postsynaptic cell.

The sensitivity of the receptor is also subject to regulation, and the concepts of supersensitivity and subsensitivity are widely accepted. **Sensitivity** denotes the degree of neuronal response to a particular agonist. Changes in sensitivity may occur through a change in the absolute number of available receptors or through a change in the actual function of the receptor complex. The modulation of receptor sensitivity is thought to be involved in the development of tolerance and dependence. In **tolerance,** the chronic administration of a drug results in the need for an increasing amount of the drug to achieve the same effects originally produced by a smaller amount. In **dependence,** a state of homeostasis occurs in an organism as a result of the presence of an active drug in the system. If the drug is stopped, the system is no long in homeostasis, and withdrawal phenomena occur.

The proteins of the receptor complex exist in the fluid matrix of the bilayer lipid membrane, which itself is a site of regulation of neuronal homeostasis and activity. There is an increasing awareness that localized areas of the membrane may rapidly become more or less fluid (viscous), primarily as a function of phospholipid methylation. Such changes in membrane viscosity may hypothetically affect the function of receptors in various ways. For example, a more viscous membrane might force more receptor recognition sites out into the synapse, thereby increasing sensitivity. Conversely, a more fluid membrane might allow the various proteins of the receptor complex to become more widely separated and result in decreased sensitivity.

A new concept in neuroregulation is **chronobiology** (study of the effect of time on living systems), based on the observation that most biological systems in the central nervous system—including neuroregulator production, neuroendocrine function, receptor sensitivity, and behavioral attributes such as rest and activity—follow a regular temporal cycle in their occurrence. **Circadian rhythms** are variations in biological activity occurring during the course of a day (ie, 24 hours). Other important rhythms occur at the same time each month or each year. Rhythms may be regulated either by endogenous mechanisms or by exogenous (environmental) cycles (eg, the light-dark cycle of day and night or the varying daylight hours at different times of year). The various rhythms in normal controls are said to be synchronous. In disease states these rhythms may become asynchronous, and daily patterns of sleep or appetite may be disrupted.

The biological basis of the pacemaker for circadian rhythms in humans is poorly understood, though the suprachiasmatic nucleus and pineal gland are thought to play important roles. Circadian rhythms have many implications for neurobehavioral physiology. The time of measurement of any central nervous system function must be noted, since activity may vary dramatically during the course of a day. Furthermore, the concept of biological rhythm implies that the response of the central nervous system to environmental stimulation and to drugs changes over a period of time. Some have postulated that asynchronous biological rhythms contribute to some mental illnesses, eg, abnormalities in sleep rhythms and in diurnal mood variations as well as the tendency for recurrence and seasonal occurrence of depression. In support of this hypothesis, antidepressant agents have been shown to affect circadian rhythms, and these effects may be the mechanisms of the drugs' therapeutic actions in some patients.

Recent study of the role of ion complexes in regulating cell function is important in psychopharmacology and in understanding the mechanisms of pathological behavior. The calcium messenger system is the focus of particularly intense investigation. Calcium ions (Ca^{2+}), acting as both extracellular and intracellular messengers, regulate neurotransmitter and hormone secretion. Gross changes in extracellular Ca^{2+} concentration have been implicated in mood state changes in patients with bipolar affective disorder. It is likely, however, that disequilibration of the tightly controlled system regulating intracellular Ca^{2+} concentration is of greater significance. A complicated pump system maintains a large Ca^{2+} concentration differential across the cell membrane by regulating Ca^{2+} entry into the cell. The process depends upon control of the activity of specific Ca^{2+}-binding proteins, with calmodulin probably the most important in brain. Stimulation of the Ca^{2+}-binding system by hormones, neurotransmitters, or depolarization results in alteration of intracellular Ca^{2+} concentration through either intracellular Ca^{2+} release or opening of membrane Ca^{2+} channels. Small changes in Ca^{2+} flux can result in significant disequilibrium; whether such disequilibrium results in behavioral change is unclear. However, evidence for mood-stabilizing effects of Ca^{2+} antagonists active at voltage-dependent Ca^{2+} channels suggests that depolarization abnormalities may be important. These agents do not seem to block Ca^{2+} channels directly; they act by binding to nearby receptors.

There appear to be marked variation and heterogeneity in the concentration of Ca^{2+} antagonist receptors in brain. The functional significance of such variation is still unclear; however, mood-stabilizing effects have been described for different classes of Ca^{2+}-blocking agents with varying receptor specificities.

NEUROTRANSMITTERS

The three classes of neurotransmitter substances are the monoamines (biogenic amines), amino acids, and peptides. The monoamines include the catecholamines (dopamine, norepinephrine, epinephrine), an indoleamine (serotonin), a quaternary amine (acetylcholine), and an ethylamine (histamine). (See Table 6–1 for a summary of major precursors, enzymes, and metabolites of these substances.)

Neurotransmitter Research

The synthesis and metabolism of individual neurotransmitters are discussed below for two reasons. First, many of the synthetic enzymes as well as the products of metabolism serve as markers in research for the presence and activity of these neurotransmitter systems. Second, both synthesis and metabolism may be affected by drugs. It is unlikely that individual pathways specifically related to complex behaviors will be found; however, it may be that small groups of major pathways will be shown to be essential for proper expression of certain emotions or behaviors.

One focus of investigation is receptor subtypes for specific neurotransmitters. It seems that for most neurotransmitters, there is more than one type of receptor that will respond specifically to that neurotransmitter. These different receptor types vary in their sensitivities, structural characteristics, and responses to the neurotransmitter. Research is therefore being directed toward the development of drugs that affect specific receptor subtypes but not others. Ideally, new drugs will affect the receptors involved with the abnormal behavior and not cause the adverse effects associated with some currently used drugs.

Research in most neurotransmitter systems also includes neurotransmitter challenge tests. **Challenge tests** involve in vivo testing of the biological state of a specific neurotransmitter or neuroendocrine system by means of baseline measurement of a biological or behavioral variable, followed by the administration of a specific biologically active agent affecting a neuroregulator system. The effects on the original variable are then measured over time. For example, it has been thought that some depressed patients might have abnormally sensitive receptors for acetylcholine. Physostigmine is a potent inhibitor of acetylcholinesterase, which is the major mechanism of termination of acetylcholine neurotransmission. Challenge testing in this case would involve measurement of baseline mood and pupillary size, administration of physostigmine, and assessment of its effects on those measurements.

It now appears that neurotransmitter synthesis and release are partially controlled by the concentration of their precursors in dietary intake. High-carbohydrate, low-protein meals elevate brain tryptophan levels and accelerate serotonin synthesis. Brain concentrations of tyrosine and its catecholamine products may be elevated by consumption of protein and, as shown in preliminary studies, by consumption of the artificial sweetener aspartame. The behavioral effects of caffeine appear to depend upon its regulation of release of adenosine, a nucleic acid that may have neuroregulatory properties.

Dopamine

Dopamine is synthesized through a number of enzymatic steps from the amino acid tyrosine. The rate-limiting enzyme is tyrosine hydroxylase, which requires pteridine cofactor for activity. The principal degradative path is through the action of monoamine oxidase to 3,4-dihydroxyphenylacetic acid and then through catechol-O-methyltransferase to homovanillic acid, the major metabolite of dopamine. It has been demonstrated that there are two types of monoamine oxidases (MAO-A and MAO-B) in the central nervous system that differ in their substrate affinity, with MAO-B more selectively metabolizing dopamine and MAO-A more selectively metabolizing norepinephrine and serotonin.

The importance of MAO in dopamine metabolism has been highlighted by serendipitous observations of the effects of 1-methyl-4-phenyl-1,2,3,6-tetrahy-

Table 6–1. Monoamine neurotransmitters and related compounds.

Neurotransmitter	Principal Synthetic Enzymes	Primary Precursors	Primary Brain Metabolites
Dopamine	Tyrosine hydroxylase*	Tyrosine L-Dopa	Homovanillic acid
Norepinephrine	Tyrosine hydroxylase* Dopamine β-hydroxylase	Tyrosine L-Dopa	Methoxyhydroxyphenylglycol
Epinephrine	Tyrosine hydroxylase* Dopamine β-hydroxylase Phenylethanolamine-N-methyltransferase	Tyrosine L-Dopa	Methoxyhydroxyphenylglycol
Serotonin	Tryptophan hydroxylase*	Tryptophan	5-Hydroxyindoleacetic acid
Acetylcholine	Choline acetyltransferase*	Choline	No specific metabolite
Histamine	Histidine decarboxylase*	Histidine	No specific metabolite

*Rate-limiting enzyme, or enzyme associated with rate-limiting step in synthesis.

dropyridine (MPTP), a central nervous system toxin. An epidemic of parkinsonism among users of a synthetic heroin containing MPTP suggested a model for studying dopamine depletion in the substantia nigra. It is now known that the dopamine-depleting effects of MPTP depend upon its conversion to 1-methyl-4-phenylpyridinium iodide (MPP^+), a reaction that is catalyzed by MAO-B and blocked by MAO-B-selective inhibitors. These findings have led to the hypothesis that parkinsonian syndromes may result from environmental toxins that aggravate the diminution in dopaminergic function associated with aging.

Together with norepinephrine, dopamine regulates motivational arousal and the reward-reinforcement system; however, these functions have not been localized to a specific pathway. Dopamine is also thought to be involved in temperature regulation, which may be relevant in neuroleptic malignant syndrome, a disorder associated with administration of some antipsychotics (eg, phenothiazines). (See Chapters 17 and 32.)

A. Dopaminergic Pathways: There are five recognized dopaminergic neuronal pathways in the central nervous system.

1. The nigrostriatal pathway has cell bodies of dopaminergic neurons in the substantia nigra. These neurons project to the caudate nucleus and putamen of the corpus striatum. Normally, this pathway is involved in the initiation and coordination of muscle movement. Dopamine shares a dynamic balance with acetylcholine in this pathway. It is thought that there is a dopamine excess and an acetylcholine deficiency in Huntington's chorea and Gilles de la Tourette's syndrome. The reverse imbalance exists in Parkinson's disease. An excess of both dopamine and acetylcholine may possibly lead to idiopathic orofacial dyskinesia (Meige's dystonia, or Brueghel's syndrome). This pathway is involved in neuroleptic-induced extrapyramidal syndromes and probably in the development of tardive dyskinesia as well (see Chapter 5).

2. In the mesolimbic-mesocortical pathway, cell bodies of dopaminergic neurons exist in an area medial and superior to the substantia nigra. These neurons project to the limbic system and neocortex. This pathway is thought to be involved in the control of normal emotions and behaviors and is conceivably the site of pathological changes in schizophrenia and other psychotic illnesses.

3. The tuberoinfundibular (tuberohypophyseal, hypothalamic-hypophyseal) pathway has cell bodies of dopaminergic neurons in the arcuate nuclei and periventricular area; these neurons project to the median eminence of the hypothalamus and to the posterior pituitary. This pathway regulates release of prolactin from the pituitary. Dopamine itself is thought to act as a prolactin-inhibiting hormone.

4. The medullary periventricular pathway has cell bodies of dopaminergic neurons in the motor nucleus of the vagus nerve and the nucleus tractus solitarii. The projections are not well defined, but this group of cells is thought to be involved in the control of food intake and perhaps in the physiological derangements causing eating disorders (see Chapters 5 and 28).

5. A group of incertohypothalamic neurons project from the dorsal and posterior hypothalamus to the dorsal anterior hypothalamus and the lateral septal nuclei. The role of these neurons is unknown.

B. Dopaminergic Receptors: Three types of dopamine receptors have been characterized. The existence of D_1 and D_2 receptors has been firmly established; the existence of D_3, D_4, and D_5 receptors remains controversial.

1. D_1 receptors are located on postsynaptic cells and activate dopamine-sensitive adenylyl cyclase. They are essentially absent in the tuberoinfundibular pathway.

2. D_2 receptors are located on postsynaptic cells and either do not affect or may actually inhibit dopamine-sensitive adenylyl cyclase. Guanosine triphosphate further regulates the effects produced by stimulating these receptors. This is the only type of dopamine receptor in the pituitary.

C. Dopamine Hypothesis of Schizophrenia: (See also Chapter 20.) The dopamine hypothesis of schizophrenia proposes that hyperactivity of the dopamine system (possibly the D_2 receptors in the mesolimbic-mesocortical pathway) may exercise a causative role in schizophrenia. The major support for this hypothesis is that the clinical potency of the neuroleptics is well correlated with their ability to block D_2 receptors. Postmortem examination of the brains of schizophrenic patients has revealed an increased number of D_2 binding sites; however, this may be partially attributed to the effects of neuroleptic medication. There appear to be some schizophrenic patients with low monoamine oxidase activity, which would reduce the rate of degradation of dopamine. There may also be a subgroup of people with low dopamine β-hydroxylase activity. This enzyme converts dopamine to norepinephrine; therefore, low dopamine β-hydroxylase causes a relative dopamine excess and norepinephrine deficiency. Since the various aspects of this hypothesis are still the focus of current research, it is more important to understand the concepts of dopamine regulation than it is to comprehend any of the currently hypothesized specific dysfunctions.

There is an increasing awareness of the role dopamine plays in the affective disorders. The hypothesis is that dopamine levels are low in depressed patients, particularly those with significant motor retardation. Conversely, dopamine levels are thought to be high in mania and may be particularly important in the shift from depression to mania. The biological correlates at the time of major clinical change in patients (eg, shift from depression to mania or from nonpsychotic to psychotic states) are of major interest for researchers. Dopamine challenge tests with measurement of growth hormone or prolactin response are being used to assess the functional status of a patient's dopaminergic system.

D. Neuroleptics: (See also Chapters 20 and 32.) Neuroleptics are the major drugs used to treat psychotic conditions, including schizophrenia. The antipsychotic effects of neuroleptics may not become apparent for 3 weeks, whereas their dopamine receptor-blocking effects occur immediately. Many neuroleptics also significantly block alpha-adrenergic, serotonergic, histaminergic, and cholinergic receptors; therefore, not all of the actions of neuroleptics can be directly ascribed to their immediate dopamine-blocking effects.

The major adverse side effects associated with neuroleptics are parkinsonism-like symptoms and the potential development of tardive dyskinesia. The traditional explanation of this disorder is that chronic dopamine blockade by neuroleptics causes the equivalent of denervation and postsynaptic dopamine hypersensitivity. Although this theory may explain withdrawal dyskinesias, more recent research indicates that presynaptic oversecretion of dopamine coupled with noradrenergic hyperactivity is the cause of tardive dyskinesia in at least some patients with this disorder. This theory fits in with the observation that the most effective drugs for tardive dyskinesia involve beta-adrenergic blockers and gamma-aminobutyric acid-containing drugs, which may decrease dopamine activity. The use of cholinergic drugs to help correct a hypothesized dopamine-acetylcholine imbalance has not been of much clinical benefit. Also, recent reports have noted that in some patients with bipolar affective disorders who have been treated with neuroleptics, tardive dyskinesia is active during depression and absent during mania. This observation supports the hypothesis of dopamine overactivity in mania.

Norepinephrine & Epinephrine

Norepinephrine shares the synthetic pathway of dopamine. Dopamine is converted to norepinephrine by dopamine β-hydroxylase, a copper-containing enzyme. Norepinephrine is metabolized by monoamine oxidase (more selectively by MAO-A) and catechol-O-methyltransferase to methoxyhydroxyphenylglycol. Epinephrine is currently considered to play only a minor role in central nervous system function. It is produced when phenylethanolamine-N-methyltransferase converts norepinephrine to epinephrine. The noradrenergic pathways are thought to play a role in regulation of mood, learning, memory, reinforcement, anxiety, and the sleep-wakefulness cycle. Beta receptors—specifically, those located in the hippocampus and septal nuclei—seem to be involved in the sensation of anxiety. Alpha receptors may regulate the initiation of feeding, and beta receptors may participate in the induction of satiety.

A. Noradrenergic Pathways: There are two large groups of noradrenergic neurons:

1. The locus ceruleus in the upper pons is the site of most noradrenergic neurons. These neurons project to the cerebral cortex, hypothalamic and thalamic nuclei, and limbic system.

2. The lateral tegmental neurons are loosely scattered within the lateral ventral tegmental fields and may be an important source of noradrenergic fibers to the basal forebrain, hypothalamus, and amygdala.

B. Adrenergic Pathways: Epinephrine-containing neurons are intermingled with the noradrenergic neurons of the lateral tegmental area and are found also in the dorsal medulla. They are believed to project to the locus ceruleus, mesencephalon, and hypothalamus. Epinephrine-containing neurons in the nucleus tractus solitarii may play a role in the control of blood pressure.

C. Noradrenergic Receptors: There are at least five types of noradrenergic receptors:

1. Alpha$_1$ receptors are postsynaptic and do not activate adenylyl cyclase when stimulated.

2. Most α_2 receptors are presynaptic, activate adenylyl cyclase when stimulated, and are more sensitive to alpha-adrenergic agonists than are postsynaptic adrenergic receptors. They function to reduce norepinephrine synthesis in the presynaptic neuron. Some α_2 receptors are postsynaptic.

3. Beta$_1$ receptors are postsynaptic and may be presynaptic. They activate adenylyl cyclase when stimulated.

4. Beta$_2$ receptors are postsynaptic and activate adenylyl cyclase when stimulated. There is some evidence for presynaptic β_2 receptors that function to increase presynaptic function. Both types of beta receptors predominate at the ends of the locus ceruleus tracts, and there may be beta regulation of α_2 receptors in the mammalian central nervous system.

D. Monoamine Hypothesis of Affective Illness: (See Chapter 22.) The monoamine hypothesis of affective illness states that a functional underactivity of norepinephrine or serotonin may cause depression and that increased activity in the noradrenergic and serotonergic pathways may result in mania. The basis for this hypothesis rose from two major observations. First, researchers noted that reserpine not only depleted central stores of catecholamines and indoleamines but also inhibited their storage. It also caused depression. Second, antidepressant drugs (see Chapter 32) either blocked reuptake of catecholamines and serotonin or effectively blocked their degradation. The major problem with this hypothesis and the supporting evidence is that although the acute changes associated with antidepressant drug therapy seem to increase noradrenergic and serotonergic activity, the chronic changes are significantly different. Studies of patients undergoing chronic (1–3 weeks) treatment with antidepressant drugs have indicated the following changes: decreased postsynaptic β receptor and presynaptic α_2 receptor sensitivity or activity; increased α_1 receptor sensitivity; and increased norepinephrine release (possibly due to decreased α_2 receptor sensitivity). These studies seem to support a different hypothesis—namely, that noradrenergic overactivity is involved in depression and that treatment with antidepressant drugs reduces overall noradrenergic activity. Research on the monoamine hypothesis of affective illness continues.

Recent models of mood disorders have highlighted the importance of disequilibrium of the noradrenergic system. There is evidence to support the following criteria for disequilibrium: impairment of feedback control, erratic basal output, disruption of normal circadian rhythms, decreased selectivity in response to environmental stimuli, and restoration of efficient regulation by mood-stabilizing drugs. The postsynaptic α_2 receptor system, which normally provides negative feedback inhibition to norepinephrine release, appears to be desensitized in some depressed patients. A singular change has been hypothesized in patients with panic disorder. Yohimbine, a selective α_2 receptor antagonist, for example, reproduces panic symptoms in susceptible individuals.

Investigators have pursued two additional lines of study in their research into the role of the noradrenergic pathway in depression. First, it has been noted that urinary excretion of methoxyhydroxyphenylglycol in depressed patients follows two patterns. Patients with low urinary methoxyhydroxyphenylglycol levels have a norepinephrine deficiency, whereas those with normal or high levels may not. Second, noradrenergic challenge tests with clonidine (a specific α_2 agonist) or amphetamine followed by measurement of their effects on the neuroendocrine system have been used to assess central noradrenergic function. These challenge tests may enable clinicians to differentiate subtypes of depressed patients on a biological basis and may eventually have implications for treatment.

Although much research in schizophrenia has focused on the role of dopamine, there is evidence to support overactivity of norepinephrine as a causative factor in some schizophrenic patients. Both clonidine and propranolol (a beta-adrenergic blocker) have been successful in the treatment of a few psychotic patients.

E. Drugs Commonly Used in Affective Disorders: (See Chapters 22 and 32.) Many commonly used psychotropic drugs have major effects on the adrenergic system. The tricyclic antidepressants and the monoamine oxidase inhibitors have strong noradrenergic effects as well as a broad range of action s affecting the serotonergic, cholinergic (mostly muscarinic), and histaminergic ($H_1 \gg H_2$) systems. The antiadrenergic antihypertensive drug clonidine has been used to treat opiate withdrawal. Presumably, clonidine binds to presynaptic α_2 receptors and reduces the amount of norepinephrine synthesized and released during the withdrawal period. The beta-adrenergic blocking drugs, of which propranolol is the best known, either are nonselective in their blockade

effects or have some selectivity for β_1 blockade. No specific blockers of β_2 receptors are in clinical use. Lithium inhibits stress-induced release of norepinephrine as well as norepinephrine reuptake. Chronic lithium treatment may decrease beta receptor function and increase alpha receptor function. The major adverse adrenergic side effects of monoamine oxidase inhibitors and tricyclic antidepressants are mediated primarily by α_1 receptors and consist of postural hypotension, dizziness, and reflex tachycardia. Tyramine-induced hypertensive crises in patients taking drugs also inhibit liver and intestinal monoamine oxidase activity. A surge of adrenergic activity occurs when tyramine-rich foods such as cheese, beer, or wine are consumed.

Serotonin

Serotonin is synthesized through a number of enzymatic steps from the amino acid tryptophan. The first enzyme in this pathway is tryptophan hydroxylase, which requires oxygen and pteridine cofactor for activity. The concentration of tryptophan is a primary regulatory factor. Serotonin is metabolized by monoamine oxidase (preferentially by MAO-A) to 5-hydroxyindoleacetic acid (5-HIAA). It is not known how much cerebrospinal fluid 5-HIAA is derived from the spinal cord and how much comes from brain. Serotonin is thought to play a role in circadian rhythms, the perception of pain, the sleep-wakefulness cycle, and mood. It is also involved in control of feeding, motor activity, and temperature. It affects the prolactin, cortisol, growth hormone, and possibly the β-endorphin neuroendocrine systems.

A. Serotonergic Pathways: Serotonergic neurons are concentrated in the area of the median and the dorsal raphe nuclei, caudal locus ceruleus, area postrema, and interpeduncular area. Both the medial and dorsal neurons project to the thalamus, hypothalamus, and basal ganglia. The medial neurons also project to the amygdala, piriform cortex, and cerebral cortex. Descending fibers from this group of serotonergic neurons innervate the spinal cord, modulate the sensitivity to pain input, and therefore probably play a key role in mediating the analgesic actions of morphine and related opioid compounds. Antidepressants that affect the serotonergic system have been widely used clinically to control chronic pain.

B. Serotonergic Receptors: Three classes of serotonergic receptors have been identified. S_1 receptors incorporating three different subtypes preferentially bind serotonin, require guanosine triphosphate for activity, and activate adenylyl cyclase. S_2 receptors, also containing three subtypes, preferentially bind spiperone (a neuroleptic not available for clinical use in the USA), do not require guanosine triphosphate for activity, and do not activate adenylyl cyclase. S_3 receptors, the subtypes of which remain to be identified, show moderate affinity for agonists such as serotonin and high affinity for novel selective antagonists such as zacopride. Currently, a number of pharmacological agents specific to one or more of these receptor subtypes are being investigated for possible efficacy in the treatment of anxiety, depression, obsessive-compulsive disorder, and obesity.

C. Role of Serotonin in Affective Illness and Schizophrenia: (See Chapter 22.) Traditional psychiatric theory has claimed that low serotonin levels are associated with depression and high serotonin levels with mania. Some depressed patients have been shown to have decreased levels of 5-HIAA in cerebrospinal fluid, and these patients seem to show greater anxiety and to be at greater risk for suicide than other patients. The "permissive serotonin hypothesis" states that low levels of serotonin "permit" low levels of catecholamines to cause depression, whereas high levels induce mania. Somewhat in conflict with these theories is the observation that chronic treatment with antidepressant drugs reduces the number of S_2 receptors, which might imply an overactivity of serotonin in at least some types of depression.

The transmethylation hypothesis of schizophrenia postulates that metabolic errors in the serotonergic system might produce psychotomimetic indoleamine derivatives. Major support for this hypothesis has come from research into the actions and effects of LSD, which has extraordinarily specific effects on the serotonin system as a receptor blocker and as a partial agonist even though it affects both the serotonergic and dopaminergic pathways.

D. Psychotropic Drugs: Most traditional antidepressant drugs increase serotonergic function through blockade of reuptake. Several recently developed agents (fluoxetine, sertraline) are highly specific in this regard. Others, such as buspirone, an S_{1A} agonist, have differing selectivity. Loading with L-tryptophan (a precursor of serotonin) has been shown to increase central nervous system levels of serotonin; this amino acid has been used both as a hypnotic and as an adjuvant chemotherapeutic agent for antidepressant treatment. At the onset of therapy, lithium likewise increases serotonin levels; however, after 2–3 weeks, lithium appears to reduce stimulant-induced release of serotonin.

Acetylcholine

Acetylcholine is synthesized from choline and acetyl-CoA by the enzyme choline acetyltransferase. Acetylcholine is rapidly metabolized in the synaptic cleft by acetylcholinesterase. About half of the choline produced by this degradation is taken back into the presynaptic neuron. Acetylcholine synthesis is regulated mostly by the availability of choline and somewhat by the feedback of acetylcholine in the choline acetyltransferase enzyme.

In the normal central nervous system, the cholinergic neurons are thought to modulate arousal, rapid eye movement sleep, pain perception, learning, memory, and thirst. Perhaps the most significant role of the cholinergic system in disease occurs in Alzheimer's dementia. A specific destruction of the neurons of the nucleus basalis of Meynert has been observed in at least a subgroup of patients with this disorder. (See Chapters 7 and 17.) Dementia in general is associated with a decrease in acetylcholine concentrations in the temporal neocortex, hippocampus, and amygdala. Attempts to facilitate cholinergic function with increased amounts of choline precursors such as lecithin in the diet have been disappointing, although this approach may prove useful in a subgroup of patients with dementia.

A. Cholinergic Pathways: Cholinergic neurons are found in the corpus striatum, nucleus accumbens septi, motor cortex, and thalamus. A large ascending system of cholinergic neurons originates in the reticular formation and projects to the hypothalamus, thalamus, hippocampus, and neocortex. A specific concentration of cholinergic cells in the nucleus basalis of Meynert projects to the cerebral cortex.

B. Cholinergic Receptors: Cholinergic receptors are subdivided into muscarinic and nicotinic types. Many psychotropic drugs, including tricyclic antidepressants, monoamine oxidase inhibitors, and neuroleptics, lead to the common anticholinergic adverse side effects of blurred vision, dry mouth, sinus tachycardia, constipation, and urinary retention. Nicotinic receptors are much less common than muscarinic receptors in the central nervous system; however, they do exist and are responsible for the stimulating effects of tobacco. A third type of presynaptic cholinergic receptor may also exist.

C. Role of Acetylcholine in Affective Illness: There is an increasing appreciation of the possible role of acetylcholine in the genesis of affective disorders. A homeostatic balance of acetylcholine with norepinephrine has been hypothesized. Depression is thought to be associated with cholinergic overactivity and mania with adrenergic overactivity. It has been suggested that the shortened interval between initial onset of sleep and onset of rapid eye movement sleep seen in depression may reflect cholinergic hypersensitivity in the central nervous system; furthermore, response to early correction of this disturbance with antidepressant therapy may predict the eventual therapeutic outcome. It has been further suggested that the derangement of the cortisol axis seen in depression is also due in part to cholinergic overactivity in the central nervous system. Cholinergic challenge tests with cholinomimetic agents may prove to be useful markers of cholinergic function in the central nervous system.

D. Psychotropic Drugs: Drugs with anticholinergic activity (benztropine, trihexyphenidyl) are frequently used to treat neuroleptic-induced extrapyramidal symptoms. (See Chapter 32.) They function by decreasing the dopamine-acetylcholine imbalance caused by dopamine blockade. Although they are usually effective in this role, there is contrary epidemiological evidence that use of anticholinergic drugs increases the likelihood of tardive dyskinesia; therefore, these drugs should be used with caution.

Histamine

Histamine is synthesized from histidine by the enzyme histidine decarboxylase.

A. Histaminergic Pathways: Histamine is found in the highest concentrations in the hypothalamus and is believed to be a neurotransmitter in projections to the cerebral cortex, thalamus, corpus striatum, nucleus accumbens septi, and hippocampus.

B. Histaminergic Receptors: There are two types of histaminergic receptors: H_1 and H_2. H_1 receptors are therapeutically blocked by antihistamine medications used to control allergic symptoms. H_1 blockade may lead to sedation, weight gain, and hypotension. H_2 receptors activate adenylyl cyclase and are found in the neocortex and hippocampus.

C. Psychotropic Drugs: Cyproheptadine is a potent H_2 antagonist that also has complex effects on the dopamine, acetylcholine, serotonin, and norepinephrine pathways. It has been used successfully in the treatment of Cushing's disease and anorexia nervosa. Doxepin, a tricyclic antidepressant, is a potent blocker of H_1 and H_2 receptors, being about six times more powerful than cimetidine as an H_2 blocker and about 1000 times more powerful than diphenhydramine as an H_1 blocker.

Amino Acids (Including Gamma-Aminobutyric Acid)

Gamma-aminobutyric acid (GABA) is an inhibitory amino acid neurotransmitter present in 60% of synapses in the human central nervous system. Other possible inhibitory amino acid neurotransmitters include glycine, taurine, and β-alanine. Glutamic acid appears to act as an excitatory amino acid neurotransmitter at many sites in the human central nervous system. Other probable excitatory amino acid neurotransmitters include aspartic acid, cysteic acid, and homocysteic acid. A variety of excitatory amino acid receptor subtypes have recently been identified showing specific sensitivity to such agonists as rainic acid, quisquilic acid, and N-methyl-D-aspartate. Neurotoxicity resulting from abnormalities in excitatory amino acid regulation have been implicated in a host of neurological and psychiatric degenerative diseases. Elucidation of the action of amino acid neurotransmitters is complicated by the fact that they play common metabolic roles as well as perform neurotransmitter functions. Neurons containing GABA appear to affect anxiety, emotions, and the control of eating. Disease or derangement of the neuronal system containing GABA may lead to disorders in these functions as well as to overt seizure disorders.

GABA is synthesized from glutamic acid by the enzyme glutamic acid decarboxylase and is metabolized eventually to succinic acid by GABA transaminase. Both of these enzymes require pyridoxal phosphate as a cofactor for activity.

A. GABA-Containing Neuronal Pathways: GABA is widely distributed in inhibitory interneurons but is concentrated in the substantia nigra, globus pallidus, hypothalamus, and cerebellar and cerebral cortices. It is the neurotransmitter for the cerebellar Purkinje cells, which project to the vestibular and cerebellar nuclei. There is also a tract of cells containing GABA running from the corpus striatum to the substantia nigra that may interact in a complex relationship with the endogenous opioid system.

B. GABA Receptors: There are probably at least two different types of GABA receptors in the central nervous system; however, they have not yet been well differentiated.

C. Psychotropic Drugs: The receptor at which benzodiazepines work exists as a recognition site on the GABA receptor, independent of the primary agonist recognition site. Molecular cloning studies have shown that these protein structures, along with recognition sites for barbiturates and ethanol, are directly linked to a chloride channel, which in turn regulates cell membrane permeability. Both anxiolytic and anxiogenic endogenous ligands for the benzodiazepine binding site have been identified.

PSYCHOENDOCRINOLOGY

Psychoendocrinology (more specifically, psychoneuroendocrinology) is a subspecialty of endocrinology that takes into account the fundamental relationships between central nervous system biology, behavior, and the endocrine system. The classical chemical messengers of the endocrine system are the hormones, which are chemical signals released into the systemic circulation that may exert either local effects close to their site of release or effects far distant in the body. The three major structural classes of hormones are the steroids, peptides, and amino acids. It is the peptide class that has attracted the most interest in psychoendocrinology.

As mentioned above, the peptides coexist with the biogenic amines in presynaptic terminals—ie, are cotransmitters—and are apparently released along with the biogenic amines when the neurons containing them are stimulated. Table 6–2 contains a list of some currently known coexisting biogenic amines (specifically, monoamines) and peptide neuroregulators. Until recently, it was thought that only one neuroregulator existed in any one type of cell. Given the importance of the biogenic amines in both normal and abnormal human behavior, the relationship between the two classes of compounds is thought to be important, although it is not completely understood at this

Table 6–2. Examples of monoamines and peptides that are found in the same neurons.

Monoamines	Coexisting Peptides
Dopamine	Cholecystokinin Enkephalins
Norepinephrine	Enkephalins Neurotensin Somatostatin
Serotonin	Substance P Thyrotropin-releasing hormone
Acetylcholine	Enkephalins Vasoactive intestinal peptide
Epinephrine	Enkephalins

time. There is evidence that peptides not only act as neuromodulators and neurohormones at distant sites but also may have local effects similar to those of classical neurotransmitters. Many of these peptides (eg, corticotropin-releasing factor, adrenocorticotropic hormone) are also involved in regulation of the traditional hormonal axes (eg, the cortisol axis).

An important quality distinguishing peptides from classical neurotransmitters is their polymorphism; there are now known to be at least nine endogenous opiates and five forms of cholecystokinin, each of which may be localized to different neurons. The identification and isolation of new peptides have been revolutionized by DNA technology. Molecular cloning has permitted the exact sequencing of a number of peptides and their precursors. Through examination of precursor sequences predicted by cloned mRNA, it is now possible to postulate the existence of previously undetected peptides. Such sequencing techniques are likely to identify and localize enzymes required for the formation of peptides from precursors, as well as for the inactivation of peptides. This information will help clarify the functional significance of specific peptide systems.

The synthesis of neuropeptides involves transcription of DNA in the cell nucleus to form RNA, which through the process of translation, guides the production of proteins in cytoplasm. Both of these steps are under multiple regulatory controls. The product of translation is a precursor protein that is metabolized into active components by peptidases. This system allows many peptides to be derived from a single gene product and involves yet another step that can be regulated. The peptides are transported, stored, and released in a manner basically similar to that described for conventional neurotransmitters.

It is hypothesized that in contrast to monoamines and amino acids, peptide neuroregulators can act at sites more distant from their site of release; can affect neuronal function over a longer period of time; can

modulate rather than directly transmit messages; and can coordinate complex behaviors rather than simply activate single cells. The action of the peptides is terminated by the action of peptidases.

The basic role of neuroendocrine systems and the peptides in particular in mental disorders is still largely unknown; however, abnormalities in these systems have been identified in some mental disorders. These abnormalities of regulation may represent markers of dysfunction or may themselves be directly responsible for pathophysiological changes.

Central Nervous System-Hypothalamic-Anterior Pituitary Axis

The basic organization of the central nervous system-hypothalamic-anterior pituitary axis involves input from the limbic system and cortex to the hypothalamus, which in turn releases releasing and inhibitory factors affecting the pituitary. The pituitary releases trophic hormones that may stimulate the peripheral glands to release hormones. All of the released products have the potential to provide feedback regulation to previous components of the axis. Although the following sections discuss the hypothalamic factors and pituitary trophic hormones under the heading of the final hormone of their systems, many of the substances have been found to exist elsewhere than in the hypothalamus, and many may have direct effects unrelated to their hormonal action.

A. Cortisol: The regulatory controls in the levels of cortisol are corticotropin-releasing hormone and adrenocorticotropic hormone. A diurnal variation in adrenocorticotropic hormone and cortisol occurs in humans, with peak cortisol levels occurring around 6–7 AM. Hypercortisolism (Cushing's syndrome) may cause depression, mania, confusion, and psychosis. Apathy, fatigue, and depression are common symptoms in hypocortisolism (Addison's disease). The entire axis is important in the physiological response to stress and may be involved in the control of mood and behavior. In addition to its direct hormonal actions, cortisol also induces protein synthesis and modulates production of synthetic enzymes in the central nervous system. Both corticotropin-releasing hormone and adrenocorticotropic hormone have been shown to exist in the central nervous system outside the hypothalamus. Extrahypothalamic adrenocorticotropic hormone is found in the brain stem, thalamus, and limbic system, where it may play a modulating role in attention, memory, and learning. High cortisol levels with loss of the usual diurnal variation in levels have been reported mainly in patients with depression but may also be found in some patients with mania, obsessive compulsive disorders, schizoaffective disorders, or eating disorders. The role of extrahypothalamic corticotropin-releasing hormone is not known.

There is a good deal of interest in the possible

direct effect on behavior of corticotropin-releasing hormone. When administered centrally in animals, it causes behavioral effects similar to those observed in animal models of anxiety and depression. A subgroup of depressed patients has also demonstrated an attenuated adrenocorticotropic hormone response to corticotropin-releasing hormone stimulation. This response contrasts with that of control subjects and with the adrenocorticotropic hormone hyperresponsivity of most patients with Cushing's disease.

B. Gonadal Regulatory Steroids: The peptides involved in the regulation of production of estrogens, progesterone, and androgens are gonadotropin-releasing hormone, luteinizing hormone, and follicle-stimulating hormone. The primary role of the gonadal regulatory system is regulation of gonadal function and control of gonadal steroid hormone production, with specific reference to puberty, the menstrual cycle, and menopause. Disturbances in regulation are undoubtedly involved in premenstrual tension syndrome.

Gonadotropin-releasing hormone is structurally similar to thyrotropin-releasing hormone and exists chiefly in the hypothalamus but is also found in the amygdala and midbrain. There is evidence that gonadotropin-releasing hormone functions as a neuromodulator and that it has both inhibitory and excitatory effects on postsynaptic cells. Its primary effect is presumably on sexual behavior; however, it may also be involved in the general control of alertness and anxiety as well as in early development of the central nervous system.

Anorexia nervosa is characterized by pathological changes in the gonadal regulatory system—specifically, by reversion to prepubertal patterns of secretion of the hormones of this system, with low levels of gonadotropin-releasing hormone and no circadian or monthly variation in hormone levels.

There is evidence that estrogens have an antidepressant effect in some women, and antiandrogens have been reported to be of use in the treatment of male sexual offenders. The observation that many serious mental illnesses have their onset at puberty may be related to the dramatic changes in the gonadal regulatory system that occur at that time.

C. Thyroid: The peptides involved in the regulation of triiodothyronine (T_3) and thyroxine (T_4) production are thyrotropin-releasing hormone and thyrotropin. The thyroid regulatory system is known to play a critical role in central nervous system development, as shown by the profound neurological and other abnormalities seen in perinatal hypothyroid states. In adults, gross hyperthyroidism may cause anxiety, restlessness, and irritability. "Apathetic" hyperthyroidism, characterized by depression and withdrawal, may also occur, especially in geriatric patients. Hypothyroid states are characterized by depression, cognitive impairment, confusion, and psy-

chosis. Thyrotropin-releasing hormone is widely distributed outside the hypothalamus in the cerebral cortex, brain stem, spinal cord, periventricular area, amygdala, and basal ganglia. Thyrotropin-releasing hormone is released from neurons upon stimulation (and therefore has neurotransmitter-like properties). It generally has an inhibitory effect on postsynaptic cells. It is thought that thyrotropin-releasing hormone is involved in the regulation of mood and behavior in addition to and independently of its traditional endocrine role.

A blunted thyrotropin response to infusions of thyrotropin-releasing hormone has been noted in about one-third of patients with major depression (see Chapter 22), and abnormal augmented responses have been observed in a number of all depressed women. The latter finding is frequently associated with increased antithyroid antibody titers. Triiodothyronine as a supplement to tricyclic antidepressant has been shown to accelerate response to antidepressants in some individuals, particularly women. Supplementing tricyclic antidepressant therapy with triiodothyronine also has been effective in treating depressed patients who have failed to respond to tricyclic antidepressants alone (see Chapter 32). These effects may be related to the observation that the regulatory peptides and hormones of the thyroid system are able to regulate the number of available central nervous system beta-adrenergic receptors. It should be noted that many patients with acute psychiatric illness have transient elevations of thyroid hormone levels at the time of admission to the hospital, although the interpretation of this finding is unclear.

D. Growth Hormone: The peptides regulating the release of growth hormone are growth hormone-releasing factor and somatostatin (growth hormone-inhibiting factor). Gross disorders of growth hormone regulation result in acromegaly or dwarfism. Release of growth hormone increases with exercise and stress. The growth hormone response to growth hormone-releasing factors is altered in depression, as is the normal sleep-associated release pattern. Somatostatin is found in high concentrations outside the hypothalamus, especially in the cerebral cortex and amygdala, but it is also found in the brain stem, basal ganglia, and hippocampus. It has been demonstrated that somatostatin is released from neurons upon stimulation and serves as a potential neurotransmitter or neuromodulator; it may also have an inhibitory effect on postsynaptic neurons. The behavioral effect of somatostatin is to decrease activity and increase sedation. A significant alteration in somatostatin regulation may account for many of the neuroendocrine changes noted in major depressive illness, and the role of somatostatin as a possible neuromodulator of acetylcholine may be important in the mechanism of Alzheimer's disease.

E. Prolactin: The controls regulating the release of prolactin are prolactin-inhibiting hormone, prolactin-releasing hormone, and GABA. Prolactin bears certain structural similarities to growth hormone. It is found in increased levels during sleep, exercise, pregnancy, and nursing. Neuroleptics cause a marked increase in circulating prolactin, because they block the tuberoinfundibular receptors for dopamine, which may function physiologically as prolactin-inhibiting hormone. Hyperactivity of the prolactin regulatory system may lead to lethargy, irritability, and increased thirst.

F. Melanocyte-Stimulating Hormone: The regulatory peptides for melanocyte-stimulating hormone are melanocyte-stimulating hormone release-inhibiting hormone and melanocyte-releasing hormone. Little is known about the role of these substances in the central nervous system; however, melanocyte-stimulating hormone may be involved in learning and memory, and there have been a few reports that melanocyte-stimulating hormone and melanocyte-stimulating hormone-inhibiting hormone have an antidepressant effect.

Central Nervous System-Hypothalamic-Posterior Pituitary Axis: Vasopressin & Oxytocin

Vasopressin (antidiuretic hormone) and oxytocin are both synthesized in the supraoptic nuclei and paraventricular nuclei of the hypothalamus. These nuclei send projections to the posterior pituitary, whence the hormones are released into the circulation. The two hormones are derived from two different precursors. These two precursors also produce the two specific neurophysins, or carrier proteins. These carrier proteins may also have independent effects on the central nervous system. The paraventricular nuclei also project to the amygdala, locus ceruleus, thalamus, nucleus tractus solitarii, hippocampus, and septal nuclei.

Neurons containing vasopressin project to the anterior pituitary and into the cerebrospinal fluid through cells ending in the third ventricle. Release of vasopressin is increased by pain, stress, exercise, morphine, nicotine, and barbiturates and is decreased by alcohol. Vasopressin is thought to play a role in attention, memory, and learning and may also have an antidepressant effect. Inappropriate secretion of vasopressin can be induced by various psychopharmacological agents but—for unclear reasons—can also occur spontaneously in psychiatric patients. A number of specific agonists and antagonists of vasopressin have recently been developed, and their use in experimental animal models will help clarify the role of vasopressin in the central nervous system.

Oxytocin has been shown to be released by neurons and may function as a neurotransmitter; it appears to have an inhibitory effect on postsynaptic cells. Recent research has implicated oxytocin in the initiation and maintenance of maternal behavior, social bonding, and sexual receptivity.

Central Nervous System-Pineal Gland Axis: Melatonin

Melatonin is synthesized from serotonin in the pineal gland by the action of serotonin-N-acetylase and 5-hydroxyindole-O-methyltransferase. The pineal gland also contains many other peptides, including vasopressin and luteinizing hormone-releasing hormone. The major regulator of melatonin synthesis is the light-dark cycle, with synthesis being increased during darkness. Regular fluctuations in the production of melatonin occur even without light-dark cues but create a longer cycle. The pineal gland is thought to be regulated by a major beta-adrenergic mechanism, and propranolol decreases melatonin synthesis. Melatonin itself seems central to the regulation of circadian rhythms and sexual maturation.

Other Central Nervous System Peptides

A. Endogenous Opioids: The endogenous opioids consist of a large number of naturally occurring morphine-like compounds. The two major enkephalins are met-enkephalin and leu-enkephalin. The enkephalins are found in high concentrations in the brain stem, amygdala, cerebral cortex, corpus striatum, thalamus, and periaqueductal gray regions.

The α-, β-, and γ-endorphins are derived from a large, nonopioid precursor protein. Beta-endorphin is found in high concentrations in the pituitary, anterior hypothalamus, septal region, and periaqueductal gray regions.

Mu receptors bind morphine preferentially and may be involved in the mediation of the analgesic effects of the endogenous opioid system. Delta receptors bind enkephalins preferentially and may be the opioid receptors primarily affecting behavior and seizure threshold. Kappa receptors bind dynorphan preferentially. They are located deep in the cerebral cortex and are thought to influence sensory integration. This function is manifested clinically by sedation and analgesia. Other types of receptors include σ and ϵ; however, these have not yet been clearly characterized.

Beta-endorphin release is increased by stress, and the general role of the endogenous opioids would appear to include regulation of pain, anxiety, and memory. Other likely effects include regulation of sexual activity, feeding, temperature, and blood pressure. A variety of endogenous opioid abnormalities have been reported in schizophrenia, affective illnesses, and eating disorders. Treatment of mental disorders with both opioid agonists and antagonists (eg, naloxone) has thus far yielded conflicting results.

B. Substance P: Substance P may be the principal neurotransmitter for the primary afferent sensory fibers from the dorsal root ganglion to the substantia gelatinosa of the spinal cord. Substance P is found in particularly high concentrations in the hypothalamus, median eminence, and basal ganglia; it is also found in the brain stem, amygdala, hippocampus, and cerebral cortex. It has been demonstrated that substance P is released from neurons upon stimulation and serves as a possible neurotransmitter. It often has an excitatory effect on postsynaptic cells. Substance P appears to modulate pain perception and possible motor control. Levels of substance P have been reported to be markedly reduced in patients with Huntington's chorea.

C. Cholecystokinin: Cholecystokinin has also been shown to be released from central nervous system neurons and may therefore be a neurotransmitter. It is found in high concentrations in the hippocampus and cerebral cortex as well as in the brain stem, basal ganglia, hypothalamus, and amygdala. It is thought that cholecystokinin may partially mediate the sensation of satiety, and its coexistence with dopamine in the nucleus accumbens septi argues for a prominent role in the pathophysiology of schizophrenia.

D. Vasoactive Intestinal Peptide: Vasoactive intestinal peptide is structurally similar to glucagon and is released from central nervous system neurons upon stimulation (thereby indicating a possible role as a neurotransmitter). It is found in especially high concentrations in the hippocampus and the cerebral cortex, where it appears to be organized within single cortical columns. It is also found in the brain stem, basal ganglia, hypothalamus, and amygdala. The role of vasoactive intestinal peptide is not known.

E. Angiotensin II: Angiotensinogen is converted by renin into angiotensins II and III. Although angiotensin II has received the most attention, all three compounds may be active in the central nervous system as neuroregulators. Angiotensin II is concentrated in the periventricular region; its major behavioral effect thus far discovered appears to be stimulation of water drinking, although angiotensin-converting enzyme inhibitors have been reported to have antidepressant properties.

F. Neurotensin: Neurotensin may be an excitatory regulator and is found in the highest concentrations in the hypothalamus and substantia nigra as well as in the nucleus accumbens septi, septal area, spinal cord, brain stem, interneurons of the substantia gelatinosa, and the motor trigeminal nucleus. It has been thought to regulate pain, sensitivity, arousal, and body temperature as well as to regulate the inhibitory modulation of dopaminergic activity.

FUTURE DIRECTIONS

Three new areas of research in biological psychiatry and the related basic neurosciences are psychoimmunology (properly psychoneuroimmunology), developmental psychobiology, and molecular genetic neuroscience.

Psychoimmunology is analogous to psychoendocrinology in that it expands the study of immunology to include the relationships between central nervous system biology, behavior, and the immune system. In reference to the biopsychosocial model of disease, two lines of research demonstrate how environmental influences may affect immune function. First, animal models have demonstrated that environmental stress may affect the immune system and the immune function may, in fact, be a conditioned response. Second, it is known in clinical medicine that both the onset and course of illnesses involving the immune system (eg, rheumatoid arthritis, systemic lupus erythematosus, and cancer) may be altered by psychosocial "stresses (see chapter 3)."

The immune system is reciprocally linked with the nervous and endocrine systems, centrally and peripherally. In animal studies, hypothalamic and limbic system lesions may either impair or amplify suppressor T cell activity. In addition, various peptide and catecholamine receptors are found on the surface of circulating lymphocytes.

Although glucocorticoids were thought to suppress immune function, it is now apparent that they can either amplify or depress immune response under different physiological conditions. Various immune products, eg, thymosin (the thymic hormone) or lymphokines, influence the secretion of corticotropin-releasing hormone and adrenocorticotropic hormone or may independently affect behavioral function. Preliminary evidence indicates that lymphocyte receptors for glucocorticoids and catecholamines are altered in subsets of depressed patients. The plethora of opiate receptors on lymphocytes suggests an additional mechanism for hormone-immune system interactions. Studies of stress response may elucidate these interactions; acute exposure to stressors tends to suppress humoral immunity, whereas repeated exposure often leads to enhanced antibody response.

The linked evolution of the nervous, endocrine, and immune systems may be thought of in terms of a progressive sophistication in the process of distinguishing "self" from "nonself" in complex organisms. Aberrations in the recognition of self and nonself are thought to be the basis of autoimmune disease; an increasing number of diseases with behavioral manifestations are now known or suspected to be of autoimmune origin, including Graves' disease, Hashimoto's thyroiditis, multiple sclerosis, lupus erythematosus, and myasthenia gravis.

Developmental psychobiology is the study of the influence of the external environment on the development, maintenance, and natural degeneration of the central nervous system. It is a common misconception that brain development is unaffected by the environment until puberty, after which functioning then slowly degenerates with age. Experiments in which animals were exposed to environmental stresses, specific patterns of learning, dietary changes, and varying degrees of sensory input have clearly demonstrated that such fundamental central nervous system properties as receptor number, cell division and migration, branching of dendrites, formation of synapses, and protein synthesis may all be affected by environmental factors. Recognition of these forces has resulted in increased research in behavioral teratology and has led to evidence that any significant environmental stimulus (eg, drugs; psychological or physical stress) occurring during a critical period of neural develop-ment may have subtle but permanent effects on neural regulation and behavior.

Workers in **molecular genetic neuroscience** are exploring central nervous system function and dysfunction through the application of molecular genetic principles. The importance of protein synthesis in central nervous system development and function is already clear, and modern techniques in genetic research make it conceivable that genetic markers and genetic manipulations may become critical in the understanding of the molecular basis of mental disorders.

REFERENCES

Andreasen NC: Brain imaging: Applications in psychiatry. Science 1989;239:1381.

Bain J: Hormones and sexual aggression in the male. Integrative Psychiatry 1987;5:82.

Baraban JM, Worley PF, Snyder SH: Second messenger systems and psychoactive drug action: Focus on the phosphoinositide system and lithium. Am J Psychiatry 1989;146:1251.

Baxter LR et al: Reduction of prefrontal cortex glucose metabolism common to three types of depression. Arch Gen Psychiatry 1989;46:243.

Berridge MJ: Inositol trisphosphate, calcium, lithium, and cell signaling. JAMA 1989;262:1834.

Black I et al. Biochemistry of information storage in the nervous system. Science 1987;236:1263.

Cooper J, Bloom F, Roth R: *The Biochemical Basis of Neuropharmacology,* 5th ed. Oxford Univ Press, 1986.

Coppen AJ, Doogan DP: Serotonin and its place in the pathogenesis of depression. J Clin Psychiatry 1988; 48(Suppl No. 8):4.

Dunn AJ: Psychoneuroimmunology for the psychoneuroendocrinologist: A review of animal studies of nervous system-immune system interactions. Psychoneuroendocrinol 1989;14:251.

Frost JJ: Imaging neuronal biochemistry by emission computer tomography: Focus on neuroreceptors. Trends Pharmacol Sci 1987;7: 490.

Gold PW, Rubinow DR: Neuropeptide function in affective illness: Corticotropin-releasing hormone and somatostatin as model system. In: *Psychopharmacology: The Third Generation of Progress.* Meltzer HY (editor). Raven Press, 1987.

Gonzalez-Heydrich J, Peroutka SJ: Serotonin receptor and reuptake sites: Pharmacologic significance. J Clin Psychiatry 1990;51(Suppl No. 4):5.

Halbreich U (editor): *Hormones and Depression.* Raven Press, 1987. Koob GF, Bloom FE: Cellular and molecular mechanisms of drug dependence. Science 1988;242:715.

Lipinski JF et al: Adrenoreceptors and the pharmacology of affective illness: A unifying theory. Life Sciences 1987;40:1947.

Lynch DR, Snyder SH: Neuropeptides: Multiple molecular forms, metabolic pathways, and receptors. Annu Rev Biochem 1986;55:773.

Miles A, Philbrick D: Melatonin and psychiatry. Biol Psychiatry 1988;23:405.

Nemeroff CB: The interaction of neurotensin with dopaminergic pathways in the central nervous system: Basic neurobiology and implications for the pathogenesis and treatment of schizophrenia. Psychoneuroendocrinology 1986;11:15.

Nicoll RA: The coupling of neurotransmitter receptors to ion channels in the brain. Science 1988;241:545.

Olney JW: Excitatory amino acids and neuropsychiatric disorders. Biol Psychiatry 1989;26:505.

Richelson E: Synaptic pharmacology of antidepressants: An update. McLean Hosp J 1988:13:67.

Schwartz JH, Costa E: Neuropeptide synthesis and function. Annu Rev Neurosci 1986;9:277.

Shepard G. *The Synaptic Organization of the Brain,* 3rd ed. Oxford Univ Press, 1990.

Snyder SH: Drug and neurotransmitter receptors. JAMA 1989;261:3126.

Snyder SH: Neuronal receptors. Annu Rev Physiol 1986; 48:461.

Stacher G: Effects of cholecystokinin and caerulein on human eating behavior and pain sensation: A review. Psychoneuroendocrinol 1986;11:39.

Stein M, Miller AH, Trestman RL: Depression, the immune system, and health and illness. Arch Gen Psychiatry 1991;48:171.

Swerdlow NR, Koob GF: Dopamine, schizophrenia, mania and depression. Toward a unified hypothesis of corticostriatopallidothalamic function. Behav Brain Sci 1987;10:197.

Zorumski CF, Isenberg KE: Insights into the structure and function of GABA-benzodiazepine receptors: Ion channels and psychiatry. Am J Psychiatry 1991;148:162.

Social & Cultural Aspects of Health, Illness, & Treatment

7

Gerard J. Hunt, PhD

This chapter will discuss how a number of social factors influence (1) the etiology and course of illness, (2) the decision to seek treatment and the kind of treatment sought, (3) the treatment itself, and (4) the patient's response to treatment and its outcome. The social factors that will be considered include age, sex, race, socioeconomic status, marital status, family situation, ethnicity, and cultural beliefs. The following case illustrates how social factors interact with biological and psychological aspects of people's lives to produce specific outcomes.

Illustrative Case

Ms G is a 57-year-old white middle-class woman who presents herself in the emergency room at 11:00 AM after a fall in her home at 3:00 AM. She reports that she got up to go to the bathroom and instead of turning left to go down the hall, she walked straight ahead in the dark and fell down a half a flight of stairs, hitting her head and knocking herself unconscious. She had lived in this house for 14 years and had walked in the dark to the bathroom at night many times.

Her husband, who accompanies her, reports that he heard her fall and when he arrived she had regained consciousness, but lost consciousness twice as he attempted to help her back up the stairs to bed. He called 911, and Ms G was examined by the paramedics but refused hospitalization.

The following morning, she continued to be dizzy and somewhat nauseated and, at the urging of her physician, who was contacted by her husband, went to the emergency room. Over the next 8 hours, vital signs were taken every half-hour, blood work was done, Ms G was x-rayed for possible spinal injury, and a CT scan of the head was performed. Her husband remained with her the entire time she was in the emergency department.

Although all tests proved negative, she was admitted overnight for observation, and in the morning the attending neurologist making rounds agreed with the resident's preliminary diagnosis of "postconcussive syndrome." She was released and returned home.

Comment: A household fall that could have resulted in tragedy fortunately ended without major sequelae.

However, some salient questions remain unanswered. Why did Ms G fall in the first place? Why did she fall on this particular night? What was going on in her life at the time of the accident, and how likely is it that Ms G will have another accident or serious illness?

And who has the responsibility for asking these questions? The emergency room physician? The neurology resident who saw Ms G in the emergency room? The attending neurologist? The internist who was called by her husband? If you were one of these physicians, what questions would you ask Ms G? What hypotheses about her fall would you start with?

SOCIAL FACTORS & THE BIOPSYCHOSOCIAL MODEL

It is difficult to deal with social factors apart from biological and psychological ones. Could Ms G have had a transient disruption in brain functioning that caused a momentary disorientation as she walked to the bathroom? Could she have been under some psychological stress that influenced her central nervous system responses? Could that stress have been caused by interpersonal problems with her husband or other members of her family? Could all of these factors be operating at the same time? Interacting with each other to produce the fall?

While we are not certain of the answers to these questions, evidence is accumulating that the biological, psychological, and social factors in people's lives interact with one another to influence every aspect of the phenomena of health and illness, the treatment of illness, and the response to treatment.

THE INFLUENCE OF SOCIAL FACTORS ON THE ETIOLOGY & COURSE OF ILLNESS

1. AGE, SEX, RACE, SOCIOECONOMIC STATUS, & ETHNICITY

Age

Persons in different age groups are at risk for different medical problems. Congenital abnormalities and prematurity contribute to most infant deaths during their first year. Many of these are related to maternal risk factors during pregnancy such as poor nutrition, smoking, the use of alcohol and other drugs, pregnancy after age 38, and lack of prenatal care. (Hingson et al, 1981). Young persons die mostly from accidents (primarily automobile accidents) and suicide. People over the age of 65 suffer predominantly from chronic illness such as arthritis, hypertension, and heart disease.

Life expectancy for all Americans has been increasing over the past 100 years. In 1900, a person born in the USA could expect to live to age 47, compared to almost 75 years at present. This improvement—and the decline in the infant mortality rate from 16% in 1900 to less than 3% at present—can be attributed to a number of social factors, including improvements in the standard of living for all Americans and the improved quality and more abundant quantity of available health care services (Cohen-Cole, 1990).

Sex

American women live longer than men. In 1984, the average life expectancy for white women was 79 years compared to 72 years for white men. Nonwhite women live to be about 74 years on average; nonwhite men to about 66 years (Cockerham, 1986).

The differences in longevity between males and females appears to be an interaction of physiological, psychological, and social processes. Prenatal and neonatal death rates for males are higher than for females, indicating a physiological vulnerability. Males typically die in greater numbers from accidents and under violent circumstances and, until recently, may have experienced greater cultural pressure to succeed, with the stress that accompanies such a mandate (Cockerham, 1986).

There are also differences in the kinds of mental illness suffered by men and women. The Epidemiologic Catchment Area Study (Regier et al, 1988) report that women tend to suffer from anxiety and depressive disorders while men are more prone to substance abuse disorders. The total prevalence of mental illness seems to be about the same in men and women, though women are more likely than men to seek help for it (Cohen-Cole, 1990).

Race

Racial differences in the causes and course of different illnesses clearly exist in the United States. Black infants have twice the mortality rate of white infants (2% versus 1%). Since there is no racial difference in mortality until the immediate postnatal period, it appears that the difference in the rate is caused mostly by social inequality.

Black persons are especially prone to hypertension, which accounts for deaths of black males between the ages of 25 and 44 years—15 times the rate reported for white males. The death rate from the consequences of hypertension in black women is 17 times that in white women. Contributing factors to these differences include a combination of genetic factors, dietary habits, and access to health facilities (Cockerham, 1986).

Social Class

Social class is a composite measure of income, education, and occupation. In the USA, social class is a major factor in the development and course of many illness. In general, the lower one's social class, the more vulnerable one is to illness and death. Increased life expectancy is correlated with high social class for all age groups, and persons of lower socioeconomic status have been shown to be more susceptible to illnesses such as hypertension, arthritis, upper respiratory infections, speech difficulties, and eye diseases (Cohen-Cole, 1990).

Mental illnesses are also strongly associated with social class, with the highest rates of mental illness consistently being found among the lowest classes (Dohrenwend and Dohrenwend, 1974; Leighton et al, 1963; Srole et al, 1962).

Two especially prevalent illnesses do not follow the general rule that the lower the social class, the higher the illness and mortality. Coronary artery disease has been shown to be higher among middle-class and upper-class men, and breast cancer appears to be higher among middle-class and upper-class women.

Ethnicity

Susceptibility to disease varies among ethnic groups in the United States. High rates of alcoholism have been reported for persons of Irish and Scandinavian descent and for Native Americans, low rates for persons of Asian background. Jews suffer more from Tay-Sachs disease and a variety of other metabolic diseases than the general population, and black Americans from hypertension and from sickle cell disease. More will be said later in this discussion about the important role of ethnicity in health, illness, and the treatment of illness.

This information is valuable to a physician since, when a patient arrives for treatment, the major social categories into which the patient falls provides clues to the kinds of disease that might be present. Even if a "typical" disease is not found for a particular patient, knowing the potential vulnerabilities of that patient prompts the doctor to educate the patient in preventive measures—especially the benefits of early detection of disease.

2. THE EFFECT OF FAMILY ON THE DEVELOPMENT & COURSE OF ILLNESS

Family life influences the development and course of illness in at least three ways. First, a family's life-style strongly defines a person's patterns of eating, drinking, and use of tobacco, alcohol, and other drugs. Attitudes toward body size, cleanliness, and preventive health measures are learned at an early age and reinforced within the family context. If all members of a family are overweight or if all smoke or abuse alcohol, the chances increase that new members will incorporate these behaviors.

Second, a family can influence the health and illness of its members by its patterns of interaction. Family therapy interventions into the ways in which family members interact have been shown to improve treatment outcomes for children with "brittle" diabetes, asthma, and anorexia nervosa (Minuchin, 1975) and also to prevent exacerbations of schizophrenia (Falloon et al, 1982).

Third, a family may act as a buffer against certain kinds of illnesses. In a study in Israel, Medalie et al (1973) found that men who reported the fewest family problems developed angina pectoris at about one-third the rate of those who reported the most family problems. Medalie and Goldbourt (1976) also reported that the wife's love and support lowered the risk of angina even when other high-risk factors were present. Brown and Harris (1978) found that women most vulnerable to depression were those who lacked intimate relationships (among other factors).

The mechanisms by which family interaction assists in lowering its members' vulnerability to illness are not completely clear. However, there is a good deal of evidence that the presence of various social supports has a positive influence on psychological states and general measures of morbidity as well as compliance with treatment regimens (Broadhead et al, 1989). Conversely, there is evidence that psychosocial stress, especially in the absence of social supports, contributes to both physical and psychological illness (Doherty and Baird, 1983; Dohrenwend, 1975; Goldberg and Breznitz, 1982).

THE INFLUENCE OF SOCIAL FACTORS ON THE DECISION TO SEEK TREATMENT & THE TYPE OF TREATMENT SOUGHT

Because physicians and patients experience sickness differently, it is helpful to maintain a distinction between "disease" and "illness." Disease can be defined as a malfunctioning of the organism (Cohen-Cole, 1990). It is disease that is usually identified by the physician, whereas illness is a morbid subjective state experienced by the patient. What a patient does about this subjective state has been called **illness behavior** (Kleinman et al, 1978). Clearly, there can be disease without illness, as in the case of hypertension, which causes no symptoms; and illness without disease, as when a patient complains of not feeling well and the physician can find no organic malfunction.

This distinction is important when considering what people do when they experience illness. Age, sex, and socioeconomic class all influence a person's reactions to symptoms of illness. The leading cause of death for men between 30 and 60 years of age is myocardial infarction. (DiMatteo and Friedman, 1982). However, what people do when they experience chest pain varies. Although 56% arrive at the hospital within 4 hours after the occurrence of symptoms, 16% arrive more than 14 hours after they have noticed chest pain. Problems with transportation account for only about 10% of these cases; it is likely that psychosocial factors are involved in the decision about when to go to the hospital (Cohen-Cole, 1990).

Older people seek help less readily than younger ones, and older women are especially slow in seeking help for chest pain, probably because they are less likely than men to believe that their symptoms are connected with heart disease.

Lower-class persons are also slower to seek treatment than their upper class counterparts. Financial problems and difficulties with transportation may account for some of these variations. It should be noted that Medicaid and Medicare have reduced financial obstacles to medical care for the elderly, the disabled, and the poor to some extent, and physician visits now appear to be more equal across social class lines (Cohen-Cole 1990).

Mental Illness

As with physical illness, social factors play an important role in a person's decision to seek treatment for mental or emotional illness. Mechanic (1980) has outlined five such elements: (1) whether or not normal activities and the performance of social roles are disrupted by the symptoms; (2) how sophisticated the evaluator is about psychiatric matters; (3) whether or not the symptoms can be ignored or normalized; (4) subcultural norms regarding irrational or inappropriate behavior; and (5) the perceived embarrassment or stigma caused by the symptoms and potential treatment (eg, hospitalization).

Some people seek help for emotional and mental illnesses on their own, while others must be manipulated or even coerced into treatment by family and friends. The more bizarre and disruptive the symptoms, the more likely it is that the person will seek care or be forced to accept it (Clausen and Huffine, 1975).

Social variables seem to exert their strongest influence on *where* rather than *whether* a person seeks help for an emotional illness (Cockerham, 1986). Several studies have shown that a "lay referral network" has often been instrumental in guiding people to professional help for medical as well as emotional problems. This network is composed of small groups of friends who have received help for the kind of problem the person is facing (Kadushin, 1969; Horwitz, 1978).

THE INFLUENCE OF SOCIAL FACTORS ON TREATMENT & ITS OUTCOME

Virtually all forms of medical care are rendered in an interaction between two or more people. Thus, an understanding of how social factors influence medical care is essential to successful treatment outcomes. Indeed, understanding is only part of the doctor's task. In order to provide effective treatment, physicians must develop the skills necessary to generate healing exchanges between themselves and their patients.

So far, evidence from both the popular press and the professional literature indicates that problems exist in this area. Patients want two things from their doctors: (1) technical competence and (2) an indication of caring (Hingson, 1981). Regarding the first, patients insist that the physician make an accurate diagnosis and implement or recommend an effective treatment regimen. Studies have shown that an important reason patients leave physicians is failure to carry out these operations. (Mechanic, 1968).

However, these same studies have also indicated that patients require more of their physicians than technical competence. Patients want to know that the physician is interested in them and their ideas and beliefs about the illness. It is here that problems arise. One study indicated that on average, physicians interrupted their patients within the first 18 seconds of the interview, leaving the patients feeling that they did not get to tell their story and that the physician did not understand their most important problems. (Beckman and Frankel, 1984)

Noncompliance with medical advice has been documented to vary between 15% and 93%, with an average of about one-third (Mumford, 1981). Some of this failure to comply with physicians' recommendations is the result of faulty communication between physicians and patients in the social exchange between them. Indeed, training to improve physicians' motivational and educational skills has produced improved patient outcomes (Cohen-Cole and Bird, 1986).

With this as background, the next section examines how the interactions between physicians and patients have been conceptualized. The more physicians appreciate the social context of the patient's life, the better able they will be to understand their patients'

world view, including their attitudes toward and beliefs about their illnesses. If this understanding is communicated to patients, they will feel that the physician is interested in them and cares about them as persons and not just "subjects" or "cases."

1. PATIENT & PHYSICIAN ROLES: COMPLEMENTARY OR CONFLICTING?

Parsons (1951) has outlined the general norms that govern being sick in this society. Essentially, two "expectations" and two "privileges" accompany this "sick role." Sick people are expected to be motivated to get well and to seek competent help for the problem. In return, they are not held responsible for their illness and are exempted from their customary social duties and responsibilities.

For the physician, Parsons similarly notes two privileges and five obligations. The privileges include (1) access to physical and emotional intimacy with the patient and (2) professional dominance. Obligations include (1) acting for the welfare of the patient, (2) being guided by standards of ethical professional behavior, (3) applying professional skills and knowledge as competently as possible, (4) being objective and emotionally detached, and (5) engaging in professional self-regulation.

Extending Parsons's thinking, Szasz and Hollander (1956) outlined three models within which they believed physicians and patients might interact: (1) activity-passivity, (2) guidance-cooperation, and (3) mutual participation. Acting within the first model, the doctor does something to the patient, who usually is a passive recipient. This is illustrated clinically by emergency medical illness or acute trauma. In the second type of interaction, the physician tells the patient what to do and the patient cooperates by doing it. The treatment of acute illness is an example of this type of interaction. In the third instance, the physician helps patients to help themselves—each is a partner in the effort to get well. Rehabilitation of the patient with chronic disabilities is the applicable clinical situation.

While these models provide a beginning in conceptualizing the interaction between physicians and patients, they have been criticized for not fully exploring the complexity of the encounter and for attributing too much power and control to the doctor. Parsons sees the imbalance in the relationship to be caused by the difference in competencies between physicians and patients. In matters of health, physicians are acknowledged to have more learning and technical expertise than patients. Furthermore, when one is ill, an emotional dependency may arise that might place the patient in a subordinate role vis-à-vis the doctor. Thus, Parsons argued for "professional dominance" in the physician-patient encounter.

While the above may be an accurate description

of the relationship between physician and patient in acute and emergency care conditions, it might not apply quite so readily in chronic care situations. In the latter cases, the patient may indeed know more about his or her condition than the physician and may actually be more adept at handling it. Under these conditions, the physician may become a *consultant* to the patient, seeking to add knowledge and expertise to what the patient has already acquired.

Critics have also pointed out that these models fail to deal with physician-patient interactions where patients do not define themselves as ill (eg, alcoholism, some forms of mental illness, hypertension) or are ambivalent about the motivation to get well. Under these circumstances, the relationship between the doctor and the patient may be strained. However, competent medical care, which includes interest in and caring about the patient, is still required. For example, an athlete with chronic musculoskeletal impairments may know more than the physican about what warm-up exercises to perform, what activities will exacerbate pain and limitation of motion, and when to rest, but may need consultation on the effects of an intercurrent illness or a medication on the musculoskeletal system.

Perhaps the most important criticism of the Parsons model for the physician is that it assumes too much complementarity. It sees physicians and patients operating in the same ways toward the same ends and ignores important differences that may exist between them. While more will be said in the next section regarding the influences of cultural beliefs on health, illness, and treatment, it can be noted here that in the physician-patient encounter at least three sets of cultural beliefs are always exerting an influence: (1) the physician's personal values and beliefs, (2) those of the patient, and (3) the values and beliefs of the institution of medicine as currently practiced in the local social context. Each of these sets of perspectives influences the interaction between the patient and the doctor, and most of the time they are unspoken.

What beliefs might Ms G have been operating under when she first refused to be taken to the hospital by the paramedics? Were these different from her husband's? What personal beliefs did the physician have about household falls when he called Ms G? What might have been his medical beliefs? How much complementarity or difference might there have been between these views?

2. ROLE OF THE FAMILY IN TREATMENT

The role of a family member is highlighted in the case of Ms G. It appears that Mr G's beliefs about household falls and blows to the head that cause unconsciousness were not such as to convince her to seek treatment. However, when her physician called and urged her to go the emergency room, she did so. The interaction of the physician and the husband helped Ms G to obtain care.

The role of the family can be seen by the physician from two perspectives. First, family members can be an important therapeutic ally of the physician. Second, family members themselves may need assistance as a consequence of the disease, disability, or death of one of their members. These two viewpoints can be examined for acute, chronic, and terminal illnesses.

The Family & Acute Illness

Family members are a rich source of information for the physician regarding any acute or emergent problem. What are the circumstances under which the problem arises? Why did the problem arise at the present time? Has it ever occurred before? What were the circumstances then? What has been done in the past by the patient, the family, or other doctors to treat this problem? Answers to these questions can be of great use to the physician, especially when the patient is unable or unwilling to respond.

The family can also be useful to the physician in providing information about cultural behaviors that support the health of its members or contribute to their developing illness. Depending upon the problem confronting the physician, questions about diet, use and abuse of alcohol, use of tobacco, and views about dangerous lifestyles or behaviors may be helpful.

Families may need assistance from the physician in dealing with the acute illness of one of its members. For example, information about such things as diet and activity—especially sexual activity—may be helpful to the family of a patient recovering from a myocardial infarction. Information regarding the potential dangers of specific dietary patterns or social activities (heavy drinking, riding a motorcycle without a helmet) may be necessary.

The physician may also wish to ask the family about the effect on them of the patient's illness. One trauma surgeon was surprised to see the devastating effect of the injury on the family of a young man he was treating for a broken leg. To the surgeon, the problem was minor compared with his usual fare. To the family, it meant shattered dreams. Their son was a local track star, and his success meant a lot to them. They deeply appreciated the surgeon's empathy and counsel at that time.

The Family & Chronic Illness

A member with a chronic illness or disease or physical disability changes the structure of a family and the process of its interactions. Special dietary and other environmental considerations must be provided for those with diabetes, asthma, or hypertension. Even greater accommodations must be made for the member with paraplegia or quadriplegia or for those with chronic mental illness such as schizophrenia. Families often wish to know as much as possible about the illness and how they can help their loved one. Often of greater importance is what they can do to help prevent a recurrence of the illness once it has been brought under control.

However, the role of the family as medical ally is not always an easy one. While it may be of great use to the doctor to have a dedicated family member at home helping to take care of a chronically ill patient, that responsibility often represents a great burden to the family member and can distort the normal structure and functioning of a family in ways that are detrimental to its members. The physician with a chronically ill patient must take care to see that this does not happen. By determining the extent of the burden carried by a family member or members and developing alternatives, if possible, the physician can ensure that each member will be able to develop and function in as normal a manner as possible.

A second way in which the doctor can assist family members of chronically ill patients is by assuring them that they are not the cause of the patient's illness or disability nor the agent of its recurrence. Families often carry great guilt and—with certain chronic illnesses—shame concerning their role in the patient's illness. For these reasons, explanations of the etiology of the illness can help family members greatly.

Third, in some families, the chronic illness of one of its members can serve a function or can actually be an organizing principle. For example, a child's asthma can deflect conflict between the husband and wife, or a mother's alcoholism can create cross-generational alliances between a father and his daughter in which she becomes a surrogate wife to him and surrogate mother to her younger siblings. Under these circumstances, the physician can be of great help to the family by referring them to a family therapist so that a more normal structure and individual functioning can be reestablished (see Chapter 37).

The Family & Terminal Illness

Again, when a patient is dying, family members can both be of help and be in need of help themselves. Providing physical and psychological comfort to the dying patient is a role physicians and families must share. Helping a patient prepare to die by attending to practical details such as making a will and important "goodbyes" is another responsibility that family can fulfill. Arrangements can be made between the family, the physician, and the patient regarding "heroic measures" to prolong life and when to allow death to come without intervention. These are sensitive issues, and compassion, openness, and tact are required from the physician if the doctor is to work closely with the family as an ally.

Family members' grief may be expressed in a variety of ways. Granting permission to experience whatever feelings might be present and providing a safe context for their expression may be one way in which

a doctor can help a family deal with the its loss (Epperson, 1977).

The loss of any member of the immediate family unbalances the delicate structure of family relations, and assistance may be necessary from the physician and other medical staff in helping them to reorganize in new ways.

In the beginning of this section, it was suggested that one of the privileges of the physician was access to both physical and psychological intimacy with patients. Many physicians may be more skilled at physical interventions than with psychological ones. However, the latter can be as helpful to patients as the former, and, while they do require skill, they are within the reach of most physicians.

THE INFLUENCE OF CULTURE

The most powerful social influence on human behavior is the culture in which the individual lives, works, procreates, and dies. Culture can be viewed as the aggregate of all beliefs, customs, language, history, and technological achievements of a people. Culture influences not only directly observable behavior but also the values and beliefs that govern that behavior. It provides us with notions of what is right and wrong and gives meaning to our actions.

All societies have as part of their culture a medical system that assists its people in dealing with the universal experience of disease and death. These systems contain a theory explaining the causes of illness as well as techniques for its diagnosis and treatment. Some of these medical systems are closely connected to the culture's system of religious beliefs, and some, such as those in the United States, are not (Brown and Ballard, 1990). As Kleinman et al (1978) have noted, we learn appropriate ways of being ill and what to do about it.

As noted above, the transaction between the physician and the patient is influenced by (1) the personal culture of the physician, (2) the personal culture and subculture of the patient, and (3) the culture of the institution of medicine itself.

1. THE INFLUENCE OF CULTURE ON PHYSICIANS

Medicine exists as a part of a wider culture and as such is influenced by the values and beliefs of that social context. What is defined as a disease and what should be done about it are factors influenced by culture. Payer (1988) provides examples of this in noting that patients in Great Britain are only about one-sixth as likely to have coronary bypass surgery as their American cousins and only about half as likely to have an x-ray for any reason. French physicians commonly prescribe lactobacillus from yogurt culture along with antibiotics to counteract stomach upsets from those medicines, a practice that is not routine in other western societies.

Culture influences the definition of psychological health, illness, and treatment as well. The *DSM-III-R (Diagnostic and Statistical Manual of Mental Disorders–Revised)* and the *ICD-9* (manual of the *International Statistical Classification of Diseases, Injuries, and Causes of Death*) each contains both verifiable signs and symptoms as well as subjective, culture-based judgments about what is normal and abnormal behavior and what are appropriate methods of treatment.

Science itself is not exempt from the influence of culture, since it exists as part of a wider context. What is important to study, what will be supported by government agencies as well as by citizens, and how the results will be received (on the front page or "buried" in obscure journals) are all culturally determined.

Since antiquity, healers have known and utilized the powerful effects of patients' beliefs in helping them to recover from illness. With the advent of Hippocratic medicine, this "placebo effect" emerged as a major adjunct to the physician's arsenal. Currently, it is seen as a powerful ally as physicians realize that what they and their patients believe about a medicine or a form of treatment can greatly influence the effectiveness of that remedy (Frank, 1975).

2. INFLUENCE OF CULTURE ON PATIENTS

Kleinman et al (1978) have increased our understanding of the influence of culture on transactions between physicians and patients by examining the "explanatory model" patients bring to the interaction. Patients do not arrive with a blank slate concerning medical care, nor do their beliefs and values necessarily correspond to those of the treating physician. Rather, patients arrive with their own model, which may contain an etiological explanation of why they got sick in the first place; how this illness is likely to affect them; what course it might take and what should be done about it.

With this in mind, the physician can consider that for every difference in social characteristic (age, sex, social class, ethnicity), there may be a corresponding difference in beliefs and values between doctor and patient. Thus, if Ms G, a white, middle-class woman in her 50s, is being treated by an emergency room physician who is black, male, and in his 30s, there might well be differences between them even with regard to the seriousness and treatment of a fall!

How is the physician to determine and deal with these differences? Kleinman et al (1978) have provided us with the following questions that can be incorporated into the medical interview.

1. What do you think has caused your problem?
2. Why do you think it started when it did?
3. What do you think your sickness does to you?
4. How severe is your sickness? Will it last a long or a short time?
5. What kind of treatment do you think you should receive?
6. What are the most important results you hope to receive from this treatment?
7. What are the chief problems your sickness has caused you?
8. What do you fear most about your sickness?

These questions can be of great help to the physician in seeking to determine how the patient views his or her illness. However, at least two problems may arise in their use. First, physicians may feel awkward in asking the patient what is wrong and what should be done about it. The physician may feel—and the patient may agree—that under the cultural norms of this society, *the physician is supposed to determine what is wrong and what to about it*. This problem can be handled by prefacing the questions with a comment: "I have my ideas about what your problem is and what to do about it, and I am aware that sometimes patients have their own ideas about their illnesses, and I was wondering about what you were thinking." Friendly overtures of this nature let the patient know that the physician is interested in how they view the problem and may contribute to their perceiving the physician as someone who cares about them.

The second problem in eliciting the patient's model is that it may be different from the physician's. Where there are no direct conflicts between the two in terms of treatment, the patient's model can be respectfully accepted by the physician. Elements of the patient's model can often be incorporated into the physician's treatment regimen, thereby strengthening it.

However, sometimes the patient's and physician's models are in violent disagreement about important treatment issues. Patients may want or expect a form of treatment that the physician deems harmful or useless, or the patient may regard what the physician is recommending as useless or in conflict with important cultural beliefs. **Negotiation** is an important tool to be utilized here, and in many cases **time** can be the element that must be negotiated. Would the patient be willing to try the physician's prescription for a specified period of time, and then, if the desired results are not forthcoming, switch to the patient's remedy? Would the patient prefer to try his or her own prescription first and then, after a specified period of time, the physician's?

Again, negotiating these issues requires some skill and a small investment of time. However, eliciting the patient's model allows physicians to determine whether or not their patients' cultural beliefs are in harmony with their own. If done with sensitivity and respect, this should improve compliance among patients.

The above discussion is intended to assist physicians in dealing with individual patients. Is there general information available that the practitioner can use as guidelines in determining the differences that may exist between patients and doctors? The answer is yes, with an important caution about stereotypical thinking.

ETHNICITY & STEREOTYPING

Avoid Stereotyping

Can the physician use what is known about similarities between peoples without falling into the trap of assuming that each patient will be like every other patient from the same racial or ethnic group? Blacks may be quite different from whites about certain specific variables, but it is dangerous to assume that any given patient must share the characteristics of his or her racial group.

If the physician can avoid the temptation to stereotype the patient, information about different racial and ethnic groups may be useful as guidelines for diagnosis and treatment. Some of this information is presented below.

Berlin and Fowkes (1983) have suggested guidelines for treating patients from different cultures. They offer the mnemonic *LEARN,* in which the physicians first *l*istens to the patient's view of the problem— his or her explanatory model. Next, the doctor may *e*xplain his or her own perception of the problem and then *a*cknowledge and discuss any differences that might exist. The physician may *r*ecommend treatment and finally *n*egotiate an agreement.

Black Americans

Blacks constitute the largest ethnic minority group in the United States, comprising approximately 12% of the population. Blacks have higher incidences of hypertension and stroke than whites and thus have a higher mortality rate in different age classifications. They are also much more likely to die from trauma and violence.

Blacks constitute a very heterogeneous group, however, and any generalizations about their family structure, health beliefs, and attitudes toward health and illness are bound to suffer from stereotyping and racial bias. It is important for the physician to realize that what is often seen as the result of the racial characteristics of blacks (sometimes attributed to biological factors) may be instead a product of social class and the disadvantaged position most blacks have experienced in the United States.

While research has indicated that most blacks utilize orthodox biomedicine almost entirely for their health care, it is important to note that some blacks believe in both natural and unnatural causes of illness, with the latter (''rootwork'') requiring the power of religious practitioners. Furthermore, ethnographic studies of blacks in different geographic areas have revealed specific beliefs about health and illness. These findings indicate that physicians should utilize the questions listed above in an effort to elicit their black patients' explanatory models (Brown and Ballard, 1990).

Hispanic Americans

Spanish-speaking people from Puerto Rico, Mexico, and Cuba as well as those from other countries in Central and South America and the Caribbean constitute what is referred to as the Hispanic population in the United States. While this group is extremely diverse, some commonalities have been noted. Among these are difficulties in communicating in English, which is associated with economic disadvantages and problems in health care utilization. Problems associated with migration and with ethnic discrimination in jobs and education have also been part of the heritage of these groups in the United States (Brown and Ballard, 1990).

Overall norms and beliefs include placing a high value on the extended family as well as idealized concepts of what constitutes manliness and feminine virtue. Many groups have both natural and folk beliefs regarding health, illness, and treatment, and folk healers are utilized in many communities along with orthodox medical practitioners.

One of the mostly widely known alternative systems of cultural beliefs is the hot/cold theory of disease held by some Puerto Ricans (Harwood, 1971, 1981). In this system, foods, illness, and treatments are classified as either hot or cold. Illness is seen as either an excess or shortage of hot or cold humors. For example, arthritis, upset stomach, and respiratory infections are seen as cold *(frío)* conditions, while diarrhea, skin eruptions, and ulcers are thought of as hot *(caliente)*. The treatment of these illnesses requires rebalancing the body by supplying a remedy of the opposite character. However, problems can arise when physicians unfamiliar with this theory prescribe a hot remedy to treat a hot disease. This will violate the cultural beliefs of the patient, and noncompliance may result. Harwood (1981) presents a solution in the ''principle of neutralization'' in which the balance sought can be obtained by taking the hot remedy with a cold medium. For example, a pill which is regarded as ''hot'' can be ingested with a cool drink.

Other Ethnic Americans

Asian Americans, people from the Middle East, and Native Americans constitute other heterogeneous ethnic groups within our society. Each has culturally derived beliefs about health, illness, and its treatment that influence the way they view illness and what they do about it. Sensitive and respectful inquiry by the physician may reveal beliefs and values that can be utilized in the overall care of the patient. However, members of some groups may be reticent to share their views even with the most open and compassionate practitioner who is not of their background. Under these circumstances, when the outcome of treatment is involved, the use of indigenous consultants may be appropriate. The use of native persons may also be helpful when problems of language arise.

REFERENCES

Beckman HB, Frankel RM: The effect of physician behavior on the collection of data. Ann Intern Med 1984;101:692.?R Berlin EO, Fowkes WC: A teaching framework for cross-cultural health care. West J Med 1983;139:130.

Broadhead WE et al: Functional versus structural social support and health care utilization in a family medicine outpatient practice. Med Care 1989;27:221.

Brown GW, Harris T: *Social Origins of Depression: A Study of Psychiatric Disorder In Women.* Free Press, 1978.

Brown PJ, Ballard B: Culture, ethnicity and behavior and the practice of medicine. In: *Human Behavior: An Introduction for Medical Students.* Stoudemire A (editor). Lippincott, 1990.

Clausen JA, Huffine CL: Sociocultural and social/psychological factors affecting social responses to mental disorder. J Health Soc Behav 1975;16:405.

Cockerham WC: *Medical Sociology,* 3rd ed. Prentice-Hall, 1986.

Cohen-Cole SA: The biopsychosocial model in medical practice. In: *Human Behavior: An Introduction for Medical Students.* Stoudemire A (editor). Lippincott, 1990.

Cohen-Cole SA, Bird J: Interviewing the cardiac patient. III. A practical guide to educate patients and to promote cooperation with treatment. Qual Life Cardiovasc Care 1986;3:101.

Dimatteo MR, Friedman HS: *Social Psychology and Medicine.* Oelgeschlager, Gunn & Hain, 1982.

Doherty WJ, Baird MA: *Family Therapy and Family Medicine.* Guilford, 1983.

Dohrenwend BP, Dohrenwend BS: Social and cultural influences on psychopathology. Ann Rev Psychol 1974; 25:417

Dohrenwend BP: Sociocultural and social-psychological factors in the genesis of mental disorders. J Health Soc Behav 1975;16:365.

Epperson MM: Families in sudden crisis: Process and intervention in a critical care center. Soc Work Health Care 1977;2:265.

Falloon IRH et al: Family management in the prevention of exacerbations of schizophrenia. New England J Med 1982;306:1437.

Frank JD: The faith that heals. Johns Hopkins Med J 1975;137:127.

Goldberg L, Breznitz S: *Handbook of Stress.* Free Press, 1982.

Harwood A: *Ethnicity and Medical Care.* Harvard Univ Press, 1981.

Harwood A: The hot-cold theory of disease: Implications for the treatment of Puerto Rican patients. JAMA 1971;216:1153.

Hingson R et al: *In Sickness and In Health: Social Dimensions of Medical Care.* Mosby, 1981.

Horwitz A: Family, kin and friend networks in psychiatric help-seeking. Soc Sci Med 1978;12:297.

Kadushin C: *Why People Go to Psychiatrists.* Atherton, 1969.

Kleinman A et al: Culture, illness and care: Clinical lessons from anthropologic and cross-cultural research. Ann Intern Med 1978;88:251.

Leighton A et al: *The Character of Danger.* Basic Books, 1963.

Mechanic D: *Medical Sociology.* Free Press, 1968.

Mechanic D: *Mental Health & Social Policy.* Prentice-Hall, 1980.

Medalie JH, Goldbourt U: Angina pectoris among 10,000 men: II. Psychosocial and other risk factors as evidenced in a multivariate analysis of a 5-year incidence study. Am J Med 1976;60:910.

Medalie JH et al: Angina pectoris among 10,000 men: Five-year incidence and univariate analysis. Am J Med 1973;55:583.

Minuchin S et al: A conceptual model of psychosomatic illness in children: Family organization and family therapy. Arch Gen Psychiatry 1975;32:1031.

Mumford E: The responses of patients to medical advice. In: *Understanding Human Behavior in Health & Illness.* Simons RC (editor). Williams & Wilkins, 1985.

Payer L: *Medicine and Culture.* Holt, 1988.

Parsons T: *The Social System.* Free Press, 1951.

Regier DA et al: One month prevalence of mental disorders in the United States. Arch Gen Psychiatry 1988:45:977.

Srole L et al: *Mental Health in the Metropolis: The Midtown Manhattan Study.* McGraw-Hill, 1962.

Szasz T, Hollander M: A contribution to the philosophy of medicine: The basic models of the doctor-patient relationship. AMA Arch Intern Med 1956;97:585.

8

Psychopathology: Diagnosis & Psychosocial Formulation

Howard H. Goldman, MD, PhD, & Steven A. Foreman, MD

Psychopathology is the study of mental disorder and abnormal thoughts, feelings, and behavior. Clinical psychiatry is thus concerned with two related processes: (1) diagnosing mental disorder and (2) assessing psychiatric factors in health and illness. The former is a specialized domain, defined by concern for particular disorders (eg, schizophrenia, depression). The latter is a generic process common in evaluating all patients regardless of diagnosis and may extend beyond the traditional boundaries of medicine to include assessment of ''problems in living'' and normal human behavior. Clinical psychiatry shares this two-dimensional approach with other medical specialties. Cardiologists, for example, are concerned not only with diagnosing cardiac disease but also with assessing cardiovascular function in all patients. Although they share important similarities in the objectives of patient assessment, psychiatry and other medical specialties have some important differences as well.

The basic processes of diagnosis are quite similar in the various branches of clinical medicine. The clinician observes patterns of signs and symptoms characteristic of a syndrome or specific disorder and decides on a name, or diagnosis. The diagnostic label implies that *this* patient's pattern of signs and symptoms is similar to the pattern observed in other patients with the same diagnosis. The pattern of signs and symptoms may have the same cause (etiology) or may develop in the same way (pathogenesis) or may be associated with the same abnormalities (pathology). The diagnostician observes the patient and tries to answer two questions: (1) Does the patient have frank . . . [mental, cardiac, etc] disease? (2) Does the patient have signs or symptoms of . . . [mental, cardiac, etc] dysfunction that suggest the onset of disease or suggest that the patient's clinical status would be compromised or deteriorate under stress such as an intercurrent illness, surgery, or death of a loved one? The clinician may also look for evidence of special skills or strengths or signs of abundant health that may enable the patient to adapt well to a particular situation or stress.

For most purposes of clinical assessment, it is sufficient to say that there *is* or *is not* evidence of disease.

In some cases, however, the diagnostician may want to speculate about the circumstances (tolerance limits) under which the patient can be expected to function within ''normal limits.'' In clinical psychiatry, the diagnostician first determines whether mental disorder is present or absent (**diagnosis**) and then goes on to assess the patient's mental function, behavior, social circumstances, and personality—a process called **psychosocial formulation.** Each patient is described uniquely, and the description is expanded to include personal information useful in patient care. To conclude only that a patient's psychiatric status is ''within normal limits'' generally is unsatisfactory. Psychodynamic formulation is one type of psychosocial formulation based on psychoanalytic theories of mental function and dysfunction. It is the most common formulation encountered in clinical psychiatry and is discussed later in this chapter.

There is a growing body of knowledge about the significance of behavior, emotion, personality, social circumstances, life-style, and stressful life events on health and illness. Clinical evaluation is incomplete without an assessment of these factors (psychosocial formulation). Unlike the diagnostic process, which tells us how one patient is similar to others, the process of psychosocial formulation tells us how each patient is unique. It attempts to explain why a patient presents at a particular time with a specific set of complaints. For example, a man with hemoptysis who waited 2 months before seeking treatment presented with vague complaints of chest pain. The physician found the chest pain to be benign, and hemoptysis proved to be the clue to malignant disease. Questioning the patient revealed that he presented with complaints on the anniversary of his child's death following cardiac surgery; and because his mother had died of lung cancer, he had denied the significance of the cough out of fear. The psychosocial formulation made on each patient can help the physician understand the patient's psychological defenses and personality, so that an individualized approach to treatment can be planned.

How can the physician help the patient understand the illness and cooperate in making informed decisions about treatment? What psychosocial factors will affect compliance with treatment? What are the patient's social and family resources in coping with the illness? Is special assistance needed at times of stress? The process of psychosocial formulation parallels the diagnostic process both in medicine and in psychiatry. Its goal is to enable the therapist to understand each patient individually.

THE BIOPSYCHOSOCIAL MODEL

Current thinking in clinical psychiatry holds that no *single* or "unitary" theory of psychopathology is adequate to explain all that needs to be explained about mental disorders. Instead, psychiatry has embraced a biopsychosocial model, recommended by George Engel and others before him, that attempts to integrate three perspectives into a comprehensive view of human behavior in health and illness. Drawing upon biomedical, psychological, and social theories of psychopathology, the biopsychosocial model permits us to distinguish the two major patient assessment processes in clinical psychiatry and, for that matter, in general medicine: (1) diagnosis and (2) individual psychosocial formulation. In the absence of a widely accepted theory of psychopathology to explain the pathogenesis of mental disorder, diagnosis becomes a process of categorizing signs and symptoms that occur together in recognizable patterns. This descriptive (phenomenological) process seeks to define disease entities carefully enough so that similarities of underlying pathogenesis or etiology can be discerned.

Criteria for inclusion or exclusion from a diagnostic category consist of verifiable signs and symptoms with a specified duration and intensity and a common natural history, prognosis, and response to treatment. Once a diagnosis has been made and the patient placed in a particular diagnostic category, the process of individual psychosocial assessment can begin. As noted in the introductory paragraphs, whether the diagnosis is psychiatric or somatic, individual psychosocial assessment is essential for evaluating patients comprehensively. As Francis Scott Smyth, former Dean of the School of Medicine, University of California (San Francisco), once noted, "To know what kind of a person has a disease is as essential as to know what kind of disease a patient has" (Smyth, 1962:499).

For the present at least, the search for a unitary theory of psychopathology can be said to have intellectual appeal but no urgent utility. We do not need a theory linking diagnosis and pathogenesis in order to arrive at a correct diagnosis, a realistic individual psychosocial assessment, and an effective plan of treatment. It is not essential to associate psychological development or personality in a causal relationship with a diagnosis of depression, schizophrenia, or ulcerative colitis. As a practical matter, it is sufficient

to diagnose mental illness in a biomedical mode and to assess our patients individually in a psychosocial mode. The diagnostic process enables us to select a known category of dysfunction or disorder that fits the patient's symptoms and signs—ie, to define how the patient is similar to other patients. The more difficult process of psychosocial assessment helps us to understand the meaning and expression of this disorder in a unique individual.

CLINICAL USE OF THE BIOPSYCHOSOCIAL MODEL

Ordinary People was a popular novel and successful movie in which Conrad Jarrett, the young protagonist, is portrayed as being depressed. The character will serve as a clinical example to illustrate two important points: (1) the utility of the biopsychosocial model to guide clinical assessment and (2) the benefit of both diagnosis and psychosocial (in this case, "psychodynamic") formulation for patient evaluation and treatment. We have selected this example because the young man has a disorder—a major depressive episode—that may be explained and treated both biomedically and psychosocially. The case demonstrates the need to diagnose a disorder for its biomedical benefits and to formulate the individual psychodynamics for its psychosocial benefits. Occasionally, patients can be treated successfully from only one perspective. Generally, a biopsychosocial perspective encouraging both diagnosis and formulation is optimal.

Conrad Jarrett was hospitalized and treated with electroconvulsive therapy after a suicide attempt following an extended period of depressed mood with guilt feelings marked by self-reproach, hopelessness, and thoughts of death. He was socially withdrawn and seemed to have lost all sense of pleasure. He also experienced difficulty sleeping, agitation, and poor appetite. He had nightmares in which he reexperienced a boating accident that cost his older brother his life. With the help of a psychiatrist, he eventually came to realize that his guilt over having survived the accident might explain his depression.

Conrad had always resented his brother and felt he was neglected by his mother, who favored the dead brother. He suspected that some part of him wanted the brother to die and that he did not try hard enough to rescue the drowning boy. The feelings left him despondent and angry. The suicide attempt represented an unconscious wish both to be punished and to punish his mother.

It is useful to examine these events from both a biomedical-diagnostic and a psychosocial perspective. Our understanding of Conrad and our approach to his treatment will be influenced by both points of view: He is suffering from a major depressive episode, characterized by depressed mood and a pattern of behavior including withdrawal from pleasurable activities, guilt and self-reproach, hopelessness, and suicidal thoughts. He is also suffering from a sleep and appetite disturbance. Such an illness usually responds to biomedical treatments such as antidepressant medication or electroconvulsive therapy. The psychodynamic formulation, developed during psychotherapy, provides an individualized understanding of the psychosocial forces contributing to this patient's depression. The formulation helps us understand the unique presentation of this young man undergoing a major depressive episode.

As is often the case in practice, we do not know whether the biomedical-diagnostic or the psychosocial perspective contributes more to our understanding of the cause and pathogenetic mechanism of Conrad's illness. We do not know if some still unidentified constitutional predisposition must be present for major depressive disorder to occur. We do not know if the physiological findings (such as abnormalities in dexamethasone suppression or a depletion of catecholamines in the brain) are the cause of the depressive episode or the result of psychodynamics. We do know that not all patients with major depressive episodes have the same psychodynamic formulation and that not all individuals with the same personality structure and similar life experiences suffer major depressive episodes.

Since we have agreed not to seek unitary explanations for this and other types of mental disorder, we need not restrict ourselves to any one therapeutic resource. Controlled clinical trials have demonstrated that electroconvulsive treatment of antidepressant medication is usually necessary for optimal control of depressive symptoms in major depressive episodes and that psychotherapy (especially focused on social adaptation) is indicated for maximal recovery of social function. Insight psychotherapy is intellectually satisfying for some patients and may help prevent the painful repetition of depressive episodes by enabling patients to recognize their mixed feelings toward loved ones, even after the death of loved ones or their loss through divorce, separation, etc. Medication has also been shown to prevent recurrences of depressive symptoms, even without psychodynamic understanding of the disorder.

Continuing research may someday clarify the connection between the psychodynamics of depression and the psychobiology of major depressive episodes. Meanwhile, a dual perspective—biomedical and psychosocial, diagnostic and individualized—is essential to comprehensive patient care.

DIAGNOSIS & PSYCHOPATHOLOGY

Diagnosis in psychiatry is a complex and challenging process even though it may require less experience than psychodynamic or psychosocial formulation. Diagnosis serves several purposes, some of which benefit the patient, while others benefit the provider of care, the patient's family, or society. We diagnose mental disorders in an attempt to communicate more reliably and effectively with one another about a certain class of problems. A diagnosis is a type of "shorthand" for defining an individual's problems in a way that will be recognized by patients, doctors, and society. In addition, the act of diagnosis confers the "sick role" on the patient, granting exemption from certain responsibilities as well as giving permission to engage in certain types of behavior and to expect certain types of behavior from others.

A diagnosis also implies a degree of understanding of a pattern of illness, suggesting a specific treatment and an expected outcome, or prognosis. Establishing a diagnosis may also make the physician or other care provider feel better about dealing with the uncertainties of illness, human suffering, and death. Sometimes the process of diagnosis is all the physician can offer, but it should be offered even so. The danger that a psychiatric diagnosis may function as a social label or stigma is a risk that must be accepted. The benefits of specific treatment may depend on specificity and precision in diagnosis. Leprosy, syphilis, lung cancer, tuberculosis, and mania are all stigmatizing diagnoses. Failure to make the diagnosis could deprive a patient both of specific treatment and of the general supportive care called for in such cases.

Precision in diagnosis is important also for research. If we are to understand illness, we must be able to describe it reliably enough to achieve a degree of homogeneity in a study population and perhaps in that way discover a common cause of a pattern of illness or dysfunction. Communication, research, and treatment are three important reasons why phenomenological descriptions and classification into specific disorders are important even without a full understanding of underlying causes and pathophysiological mechanisms.

Diagnosis involves three processes that will be discussed in turn in the following sections. The diagnostician begins by organizing a set of **symptoms and signs** elicited from the history and from the physical and mental status examinations. These observations are then grouped into **syndromes.** Further specification produces diagnoses of **mental disorders.** Mental disorders are characterized by deviations from a socially defined norm in thoughts, perceptions, mood, and behavior that impair social functioning. As noted above, psychopathology is the study of these deviations, the symptoms and signs of mental disorders, and their etiology and pathogenesis.

Symptoms are subjective complaints; signs are objective evidence of a pathological state. A symptom could be a headache, a fear, or a report of auditory hallucinations; a sign may be nystagmus, tachycardia, or loosening of associations. Symptoms frequently occur in characteristic clusters called syndromes. A syndrome is a set of symptoms and signs that occur together in a recognizable pattern.

A disorder is more specific than a syndrome. A disorder is also a set of symptoms and signs but with a specified course of the illness, premorbid history, and pattern of familial occurrence. It is assumed that every disorder has a specific pathogenesis, although the pathogenesis may be unclear. The same syndrome can occur in many different disorders or diseases. In psychiatry, the term "disorder" is occasionally distinguished from "disease." A disease is even more specific than a disorder in that a known cause and a specific pathogenesis are implied. Table 8–1 describes the various levels of diagnostic conceptualization.

The goal of medicine is to understand pathological processes so they can be prevented or treated effectively. Most medical treatment is symptomatic or syndromic in nature. We would prefer to base all treatment on an etiological diagnosis, as we do with antibiotic drugs or vitamin therapy for specific infectious diseases or vitamin deficiencies, but in most cases we treat symptoms (pain), signs (fever, inflammation), or syndromes (congestive heart failure, hypercortisolism [Cushing's syndrome], dementia, depression). Therapy differs with the level of diagnostic specificity. For example, fever can be treated with aspirin, but it is important to know whether the fever is part of a syndrome along with productive cough that might respond to antibiotic therapy, in contrast to a syndrome of fever, joint pain, and rash, which might suggest a different therapy,

A syndrome consisting of fever and productive cough, without more, might represent a bacterial or fungal disorder. Further historical details, physical examination, x-ray studies, and laboratory procedures will help make the distinction, If the sputum cultures grow *Streptococcus pneumoniae* and the chest x-ray shows a patchy density in the right lower lobe, we can make the diagnosis of a specific disease: pneumococcal pneumonia. For the patient with this diagnosis, specific antibiotic treatment is indicated.

In psychiatric disorders the pathological features are rarely shown on x-ray films. No bacillus or enzymatic defect has been shown to cause schizophrenia or bipolar affective disorder. For this reason, we rarely speak of **diseases** with known causes and pathophysiological mechanisms. Instead, we speak of **disorders** we think represent particular underlying but as yet unknown disease processes. In some cases, the disorders are little more than **syndromes**—clusters of observable symptoms and signs.

The third edition of *Diagnostic and Statistical Manual of Mental Disorders (DSM-III)* together with its revision *(DSM-III-R),* now the standard diagnostic text in psychiatry, attempts to formalize the nomencla-

Table 8–1. Levels of diagnostic conceptualization.[1]

Level	Definition	*DSM-III-R* Examples
Sign	An objective manifestation of a pathologic condition. Signs are objectively observed by an examiner and not reported subjectively by the patient.	Catatonia, as in schizophrenia, catatonic type.
Symptom	A subjective manifestation of a pathologic condition. Correctly refers to subjective complaints by the patient; however, often used to include the concept of "sign" as well.	Phobia, as in phobic disorder.
Dysfunction	General term for difficult or abnormal function. Can be synonymous with sign or symptom.	Functional vaginismus (could also be sign or symptom).
State	General term for the current status of a patient's signs and symptoms.	Psychosis, as in atypical psychosis.
Trait	General term for an enduring characteristic of an individual, presumably one that distinguishes him or her from other individuals.	Paranoid personality traits.
Syndrome	A group of signs and symptoms that occur together in a recognizable pattern.	Dementia or any of the organic brain syndromes.
Disorder	Similar to a syndrome but implying more certainty regarding the discreteness of the condition as well as the possibility that it *may* represent a single disease.	Bipolar affective disorder.
Disease	A syndrome with a known cause or pathophysiologic process.	Alcohol hallucinosis.

[1] Courtesy of Jack E. Grebb, MD.

ture by organizing psychopathology into a series of disorders. In most instances, *DSM-III* makes no assumptions about the causes or the pathophysiological mechanism underlying the disorders. It recognizes limitations to our understanding of psychopathology. *DSM-III* defines disorders by means of **inclusion and exclusion criteria.** The criteria consist chiefly of the clinical manifestations (symptoms and signs) along with a statement about duration of the pathological state, the course of illness, the premorbid history, impairment of function, and whether the patient meets the criteria for a different disorder. For further details on psychopathology and psychiatric diagnosis, the reader is referred to Chapter 16 for a discussion of the DSM-III-R and to the Glossary of Psychiatric Signs and Symptoms in the Appendix to this book.

REFERENCES

Campbell RJ: *Psychiatric Dictionary,* 5th ed. Oxford Univ Press, 1981.

Diagnostic and Statistical Manual of Mental Disorders (DSM-III), 3rd ed. American Psychiatric Association, 1980.

Diagnostic and Statistical Manual of Mental Disorders (DSM-III-R), 3rd ed, revised. American Psychiatric Association, 1987.

Engel G: The need for a new medical model: A challenge for biomedicine. Science 1977;196: 129.

Guest J: *Ordinary People.* Viking, 1976.

Medical Essays. Houghton Mifflin, 1895.

Smyth FS: The place of the humanities and social sciences in the education of physicians. J Med Educ 1962;37:495.

Spitzer RL, Skodol AE, Gibbon M: *Psychopathology: A Case Book.* McGraw-Hill, 1983.

Section II. Psychiatric Assessment

Introduction to Clinical Assessment: The Mayor of Wino Park

9

Howard H. Goldman, MD, PhD

Wino Park is an unoccupied rectangle of land "south of Market" in San Francisco, open on two sides, which has been somewhat crudely developed as a temporary haven for a shifting population of about 50 men and a few older women who lounge there out of the wind during the day and are allowed to sleep in metal shelters at night if they have no better bed to go to. The police leave them alone if they stay quiet. There have been a few assaults and small-change robberies in Wino Park but no murders, no rapes, no drug dealing that anyone knows of.

John Francis ("Red") Kimball, self-appointed Mayor of Wino Park, whose full story is told in more detail in Chapter 15, has lived in the park for 4 or 5 months. After a night in jail, he is now in restraints in a police ambulance on his way to Memorial Hospital Emergency. As the ambulance backs to the unloading dock he shouts and struggles, complains loudly of brutal treatment, threatens legal action, invokes retribution by powerful "friends downtown." With professional skill and no hard feelings, the attendants transfer the Mayor from the ambulance litter to a hospital gurney, strap him down, exchange paperwork and a few words of explanation with hospital intake personnel, and depart along a beam of revolving blue light in a crackle of radio code words.

In the reception area the Mayor alternately scowls and cajoles. He wants a cigarette. He wants to be liked and knows he won't be, a trashy Irish drunk in a bored, intolerant time and place, a burden on the taxpayers, uncared for, welcome nowhere, all but homeless. He was married once but drank too much, was impotent, hit his wife, and lost her to California's smoothly functioning no-fault marital dissolution system. He lived for a while in a hotel in the Tenderloin district where the night manager agreed to receive and hold monthly SSDI checks by arrangement with adult protective services workers. The Mayor now lives in Wino Park as his life slowly worsens. He drinks only wine, and not a lot of that by skid row standards—"up to 2 quarts a day" in Chapter 15. When not somnolent with drink he postures and harangues his fellows in the Park, turning away scorn with knowing glances. In occasional bursts of resolve he holds "news conferences" at downtown crosswalks, speaking right into nonexistent microphones, raising an arm to take questions from the less favored correspondents in the back rows, fielding tough questions with quotable quips, expounding plans to extend ever grander services to his threadbare constituency if only the supervisors had the guts, the vision. Now there is talk of closing Wino Park. Nothing is so fierce as the functionary's loyalty to his function. The Mayor gets wild sometimes thinking about it.

•　　•　　•

The Mayor has been to Memorial before, but he's worse this time. His assaults are more than bluster, and he gets three injections of diazepam that night. When he wakes he is nervy, somehow jaunty, sexually aggressive with the nurses. He is assigned to a senior medical student not yet at ease with psychiatric patients whose job it is to deal with the Mayor until a decision can be made about what to do with him. Dealing with him means first of all recording vital signs and starting some tests for the Mayor's bulging file. With help from a technician, blood is drawn and sent for analysis. A urine sample is taken, a stool sample. There is much vulgar comment and protest. The student has an ophthalmoscope and would like to use it. It's his favorite instrument but not an easy one to use. You have to get close, and this patient smells. You have to focus, and this patient jerks around. He stands uncertainly with it in his hand, wondering what to do, for all the world like a television reporter with a field mike. Tomorrow is

Father's Day and he hasn't sent a card. Why is this rumball "mayor" standing there as if he wants something? Without thinking he asks the most interesting question the Mayor has ever heard:

"Mr Kimball, what brings you to the hospital at this time?"

.　　.　　.

THE MAYOR GRANTS AN INTERVIEW*

"I'm the Mayor of Wino Park. They talk about closing me down. That's how I started drinking more and got real bad, turning yellow, blacking out. Next thing I know, I'm staring you in the face, like old times, we're buddies from way back, I remember last night, everything. You were scared, I could tell. I was a mess, right? But I walked in under my own steam, right? The Mayor don't need help. I see double, did you know that? I have pains in my belly, too.

"I wasn't always like this. They didn't elect me Mayor for nothing. I have the gift. Sometimes I talk

---

* The Mayor's account here varies somewhat from the facts developed in Chapter 15.

too much, give away my secrets. Like that cop, moving me along. I wasn't causing nobody any trouble. I was doing God's own work. It's my secret fate to help people, I whispered that to the cop. I shouldn't have touched him, you can't touch cops these days, they overreact, like my old man, *He just couldn't stop hitting me! Sure I talked back to him! The way he yelled at Ma, then he was sorry. She couldn't have kids after me, something was wrong, she didn't come home with me from the hospital they said.* [Long pause.] He died in one of these places. God damn him. [Starting to cry.] God damn him."

.　　.　　.

INTRODUCTION TO CLINICAL ASSESSMENT

This was the first of many interviews with the Mayor. He stayed at the hospital for 3 weeks, undergoing extensive diagnostic evaluation, beginning treatment, and continuing in monitored rehabilitation after discharge. His evaluation included daily interviews, examinations and tests, and a personality assessment. These subjects are discussed in Chapters 10–14. Chapter 15 consists of the details of the assessment procedure and its results, presented in one commonly used case study format.

The Psychiatric Interview

10

David E. Reiser, MD

Patient interviewing is a core skill in medicine. Despite technical advances, the bedrock of diagnosis and treatment continues to be communication. The doctor and patient must talk. Both, but especially the doctor, must also know how to listen. No diagnostic test or apparatus can ever replace the human bond that forms the basis of medical practice, the doctor-patient relationship. The primary tool the physician utilizes to cement that relationship is a skillful and sensitive interview.

SIMILARITIES BETWEEN THE PSYCHIATRIC INTERVIEW & THE GENERAL MEDICAL INTERVIEW

The goal of all communication between doctor and patient is to facilitate **diagnosis and treatment** and further the aims of the **working alliance** between doctor and patient. Because of this, the psychiatric interview is similar in many ways to the general medical interview. It is useful to review the similarities before underscoring important differences.

Diagnosis

Diagnosis and individualized assessment (formulation) are major goals of medical interviewing. An accurate diagnosis is at the heart of every evaluation, and the diagnosis becomes the benchmark against which treatment success or failure is subsequently measured. This may seem obvious. What is not always appreciated, however, is the relationship between effective interviewing and accurate diagnosis.

Many patients withhold important medical information, fearing that it is too trivial or perhaps embarrassing to bring up. This is most apt to occur if the physician appears busy or impatient. For example, a modest girl in her teens presents to her family practitioner with complaints of fatigue. She has only recently entered puberty and is bashful about her sexuality. A brusque and hurried interview that focuses too quickly on a checklist of her symptoms may fail to elicit a symptom that embarrasses her—she has frequent urges to urinate. To the physician, this information is vital to a possible diagnosis of diabetes. To the patient, however, it is embarrassing, and it will be disclosed only in an atmosphere of openness and trust.

The interview also determines *what* is diagnosed.

In a hurried, narrowly focused interview, for example, a physician might be able to elicit symptoms of congestive heart failure in a 60-year-old man. This information will do little good, however, if the physician notices nothing about the temperament and coping style of the patient. A skilled interviewer might go on to learn that for the past year this patient has been despondent over the death of his wife. Since her death, in fact, he has been noncompliant in the matter of taking medications, including digitalis. He says, ''They gave my wife drugs toward the end, and that's what killed her.'' Bringing out these fears and attitudes is just as critical as eliciting a 10-day history of severe orthopnea.

Thus, good interviewing is essential both in establishing an accurate diagnosis and in gaining insight into the personality and coping style of the patient.

Treatment

Effective interviewing is also essential for effective treatment. For example, a physician makes a diagnosis of pneumococcal pneumonia in a 78-year-old widow living in a hotel for pensioners. He prescribes oral ampicillin; his receptionist schedules a return visit; and he considers his job done. Five days later, he learns that the patient has been admitted to the hospital in severe respiratory distress. What the physician failed to appreciate was the presence of Alzheimer's disease (discussed in Chapters 5 and 17). Not only had the patient failed to take her medication—she had never had the prescription filled, forgetting all about it as soon as she left the physician's office.

Studies of patient compliance show that only 50–70% of patients comply with the therapeutic regimens prescribed by their physicians (Davis, 1966). Distrust, unexpressed anxiety, and confusion about physicians' instructions are the common reasons for noncompliance. *Most instances of noncompliance, in fact, seem to stem from breakdowns in the doctor-patient relationship.* Doctors think they communicate clearly to their patients, and patients think they understand what their physicians tell them—yet serious breakdowns in communication still occur.

The interview can be therapeutic in its own right. The prospect of help, the experience of being understood, and the impact of new insight offered by a trusted and respected physician all can have a therapeutic effect.

Effective interviewing must include, at a minimum, creation of an atmosphere conducive to a patient's expression of questions and concerns, opportunities for appropriate patient education, and meaningful follow-up. The doctor who walks out the door saying, "Call me if you have any questions," has not done enough. Patient education pamphlets, videotapes, and reprints can all be helpful. Yet there seems to be no substitute for an effective doctor-patient relationship, with the interview being the agent that cements it.

The Working Alliance

No treatment protocol is maximally effective if a good doctor-patient relationship has not been established. Regardless of our biotechnical skills, success depends to a great extent on the patient's compliance and trust. The working alliance can be defined as an agreement between physician and patient, based on mutual rapport and trust, to undertake treatment *together*. Steps in that process may entail discomfort and risk; they are deemed worth the risk when both believe that such steps may improve the patient's condition. In some treatments, this working alliance may simply be assumed. In others, it must not be taken for granted. A physician prescribing penicillin for streptococcal sore throat is not apt to read the patient every paragraph of a pharmacology textbook concerning adverse drug reactions. At the other extreme, in the realm of "heroic medicine," there are dramatic instances of high technology being applied to medical conditions once thought to be unmanageable by any means. In such cases, patients may have to be given detailed information about all potential risks of treatment, and the working alliance obviously entails much communication between physician and patient regarding numerous critical details. Between such extremes lie most of medicine's daily challenges. In almost all cases, however, a physician's success with patients depends on the ability to establish an alliance based on trust and to communicate the necessary facts effectively.

As the foregoing is intended to suggest, there are many similarities between the psychiatric interview and the medical interview. This deserves emphasis, for the psychiatric interview is too often set apart in the clinician's mind as something abstract and specialized, based on knowledge and principles that need to be grasped only by psychiatrists. But as Harry Stack Sullivan (1962) has said, "Man is more simply human than otherwise." Psychiatric patients are not so different from other patients: Something has gone wrong, and they are seeking help. But like most patients, they are ambivalent about help, wanting it yet fearful of what might lie in the future–knowing that they need an expert to intervene yet unhappy with the realization that they cannot handle the problem themselves.

DIFFERENCES BETWEEN THE PSYCHIATRIC INTERVIEW & THE GENERAL MEDICAL INTERVIEW

The psychiatric interview differs from the medical interview in that the psychiatric patient must communicate personal concerns about disturbed mental functioning through language that can only be formed as a process of mentation. Depending on the psychiatric condition, this problem can be great or small; but in all cases, special tact and sensitivity are required of the psychiatric interviewer.

Diagnosis

The impediments to diagnosis posed by a psychiatric condition can vary considerably. A patient with a nonpsychotic disorder characterized by anxiety or depression may be able to communicate with no greater difficulty than any other patient. Many psychiatric conditions, however, affect the patient's ability to communicate and comprehend what is going on, as shown in the following examples:

(1) A patient suffering from a psychotic disorder such as paranoid schizophrenia may be experiencing a flood of derogatory and frightening auditory hallucinations at the time of the interview. He may be convinced that someone is plotting to poison him and steal all of his possessions. The physician who walks into the room, extends a hand, and begins with a friendly introduction may be in for a rude surprise. Instead of smiling back obligingly, the patient may back into a corner, raise his fists in front of him, and say, "You're not coming near me with that poison!" (2) A manic patient may rush about the examination area uttering profanities, hardly able or willing to heed the doctor's reassurances. She may be busy testing all of the water faucets in the emergency area, convinced she has a magic formula for converting tap water into liquid uranium.

(3) A demented patient may be outwardly cooperative. He will sit compliantly, nod when asked if he understands, and smile affably. Unfortunately, he thinks it is 1924 and is firmly convinced that the doctor interviewing him is his high school football coach.

(4) A sociopathic patient may give a heart-wrenching story about the anguish of narcolepsy, leading the physician to miss the twinkle in her eyes as she asks for a prescription for 100 amphetamine tablets, "just like my doctor gives me back home."

The psychiatric interview may require multiple evaluations over time. A patient suffering from a psychiatric disorder, especially in its acute stage, may not be able to tolerate a detailed, lengthy interview at the first meeting. A depressed patient may be too despondent and withdrawn to be helpful at this stage of the illness as a detailed informant. A manic patient may be more interested in reeling off profit projections from her latest scheme to establish a nationwide chain of boutiques than in reporting that she stopped taking her lithium. A paranoid patient may eye the clinician suspiciously, convinced that there are microphones strapped to his body. In all such cases, the clinician must be prepared to terminate the interview and resume it later when the patient's condition improves. Nothing is gained by attempting to force patients to endure the interviewing process beyond a comfortable limit.

The more acutely impaired a psychiatric patient is, the more the science of observation becomes critical. The science of observation will be elucidated further in the next section. It will suffice here to note that words are not the only source of information during an interview. Communication in a variety of other modes—including facial expressions and body language—conveys the underlying mood. If a clinician walks into the examining room and finds a disheveled, tense young man with clenched fists darting fearful glances around the room, the clinician has observed a great deal though the patient has not yet said anything.

The psychiatric interviewer must be prepared to seek out ancillary sources of data. People are usually part of a social network. Important members of this network will often be present in the emergency or acute care setting with the patient—friends, employers, spouses, ex-spouses, etc. When such people come with the patient to the acute care setting, it is usually worthwhile to spend some time talking with them, always with the patient's knowledge. Even when no one comes in with the patient, it is often good practice to seek such people out later for the help they can give as informants. Stresses in a relationship often underlie psychiatric decompensation. The collateral information from people who know the patient is often invaluable.

Similarly, the physician should search old medical records, call prior treating physicians, and seek out other potential sources of data (school, military, employment records, etc) that may help in understanding the patient now. The patient's confidentiality, dignity, and trust must always be respected, but data obtained from collateral sources may be critical for effective diagnosis.

Treatment

There was a time when little other than communication was available to a psychiatrist for treating patients. Antipsychotic drugs, effective antidepressants, and benzodiazepines are quite recent developments. The future holds prospects for effective somatic and pharmacological treatments, but communication will not doubt continue to play a central role.

The Working Alliance

Psychiatric patients, like many medical patients, are ambivalent about needing professional help. Even though they want help with problems they are unable to solve, they may feel humiliated and defeated by the mere fact of needing assistance. Wanting to change patterns of behavior, they nevertheless fear giving up familiar ways of coping. Patients who have great hopes for the results of treatment may also have great fear of failure. Cultural proscriptions and taboos about psychiatry and the "stigma" of psychiatric treatment reinforce such attitudes. A patient with a diseased heart or kidney usually does not feel shame to the same degree a patient with alcoholism or psychosis does. For these reasons, the interviewer must be sensitive to the importance of empathy, respect, and trust in order to develop a good working alliance with the patient. Regardless of what patients say or how they behave, the interviewer should assume that seeking psychiatric help is a distressing and conflict-laden event for all patients.

THE SCIENCE OF OBSERVATION

Illustrative Case

A group of medical students and their preceptor went to interview a 79-year-old woman in the orthopedics unit. She was in a semiprivate room and had a visitor, a woman in her mid 40s. Flowers, cards, and a framed photograph on the bedside table—of a handsome man in his late 50s wearing clothes styled in the late 1950s—showed that the patient was not alone in the world. She was in good spirits, with a hip that was only sprained and not more seriously injured. She asked her visitor to return another time—happy, she said, "to have some young people to talk to."

The preceptor was then unexpectedly called away to an emergency and urged the students to proceed with the interview for at most 20 minutes.

Later, the preceptor offered to anticipate the students' impressions of the old woman though he had been with her less than a minute before he was called away. The students were astonished at how much he had been able to observe in that time: that she was a widow, because she wore a wedding band and the picture would have been more recent—or there would have been none—if her husband were still alive; that she had grown children and maintained close ties with them, because a greeting to "the kids" (her grandchildren?) had gone with the visitor, who said, "Goodbye, Mom," and because the patient related so well to the young medical students; and that she belonged to several clubs and social groups, because there were so many flowers and cards—some with a great many signatures—in the room.

Most students think of the interview chiefly as something that they *do, perform,* and *conduct.* This is true, of course, but the interview is also a time to *observe, perceive,* and *take in.* The first concept of the interview is active and intrusive; the second is passive and receptive. In fact, the interview involves both, but most physicians err in the direction of being too active. One of the essential skills of observation is staying quiet so the patient can talk and so things can happen that need to be noted.

There are two phases to the observation component of the interview: active vigilance, and what Freud (1912) called even-hovering attention.

Active vigilance is most appropriate during the first few minutes of the interaction. The "first few" minutes begin right away, as soon as the therapist and patient see each other, and not when they have settled down, with names exchanged and notes taken, so that the interview can formally "start." In the illustrative case above, the phase of active vigilance began the instant the group walked to the patient's bedside. During this phase of the interview, the student should take in as much as possible, actively and aggressively processing data that come in through all of the senses. How does the patient first greet the interviewer? Does he or she offer a hand or sit passively? Does the patient make eye contact? Is the handclasp firm and warm, or is it cold and clammy? Are there any books on the bed or table? What is the patient wearing? What are the first jokes and casual banter uttered by the patient? Are there any unusual sounds or smells in the room?

When the interview formally begins, the phase of active vigilance continues for the first few minutes of the dialogue. The student should make an effort to remember *everything* the patient says. What was the *very first* thing the patient said? What was the accompanying emotional tone? The following illustrate the importance of the patient's initial remarks:

(1) "Whatever it is they're accusing me of, I didn't do it!" one patient "joked" at the start of an interview. It turned out that this man had been riddled with guilt since the suicide of his son 2 years previously. That is when his health began to fail.

(2) "I wouldn't have nothin' to offer anyhow! Go away and leave me alone!" This patient turned out to be deeply tormented and embittered by her children's recent decision to place her in a nursing home.

After the phase of active vigilance, the student should shift to **even-hovering attention.** Students will discover, especially if they have been vigilant in the first few minutes of the interaction, that they can remember the rest of the interview without resorting to detailed notes. Note taking is in fact discouraged except in order to jot down a few key facts, since a student with head lowered over a notepad is not looking at the patient and paying attention.

After the first few minutes, simply adopt a relaxed and receptive stance. *Listen!* Allow whatever the patient is saying to come into your mind freely. Allow yourself also to attend the thoughts, ideas, and random associations that you yourself are having while the patient is talking. There will be time for more focused and directive interviewing later.

Many students have conceptual difficulties that interfere with observation. One involves finding a balance between skeptical inquiry and jumping to conclusions. Another is an almost universal tendency to attribute what transpires in an interview to how well the interview was conducted. In the illustrative case, although most of the students were impressed by the preceptor's acumen, a few of them were angered by it and even felt the preceptor had jumped to conclusions. This does happen, and students are right to be cautious. Any conclusions drawn from limited data should be regarded as hypotheses, not certainties, and physicians should not hesitate to modify or expand their ideas about patients' problems as more data become available. At the same time, they should give the science of observation the benefit of the doubt before dismissing all hunches that can be extracted from small pieces of observable data. To be nonjudgmental and resist premature appraisal is laudable, but physicians cannot afford to ignore the clinical data the initial interaction so often provides.

The converse of this is that physicians should never assume that the data a patient provides are always perceived by them and the patient in the same way. Just as some interviewers ignore small yet important facts, others erroneously assume that they understand what the patient means even when the patient speaks in ambiguous terms. Patients talk about "not being myself lately" or being "out of sorts," "without get-up-and-go." The clinician should never assume that these and similar phrases are automatically clear. "Not being myself" could mean "I've been sexually impotent," or it could mean "I cry all night, and I've just bought a gun to kill myself with." It never hurts to ask, "What do you mean when you say you are not yourself?" "Out of sorts in what way, specifically?" "What do you mean by get-up-and-go?" The clarifying responses the patient then provides may startle the physician, who thought the patient meant something else entirely.

Regarding the student's second concern—that he or she is always responsible for how an interview goes—only experience will teach that the interview is less influenced by what the examiner does than by the temperament and mood of the patient. It is primarily patients who shape the interview—and they do so with the same coping styles, wishes, fears, and conflicts with which they shape (or fail to shape) their lives. This is precisely why the interview provides such valuable data: It *replicates* the coping pattern and difficulties of the patient.

Students are always eager to learn how to correct what they did wrong and to understand what they could have done to make an interview go better. Interviewing technique is important, and students are right to ask for constructive criticism. But they must also sooner or later understand that how an interview goes usually says more about the patient than about the student. To assert this principle is not to deny responsibility for contemplating one;s own limitations but to recognize an important diagnostic principle of psychiatry.

CONTENT & PROCESS

Illustrative Case

A 51-year-old construction foreman was being evaluated on a neuropsychiatry unit for symptoms of forgetfulness. He had had only a sixth-grade education but was highly regarded on the job and boasted of being a "self-made man." A medical student was conducting the initial evaluation interview. In responding to a question about the family, the patient began to speak derisively about his son, whom he had sent to college but who was now staying at home, collecting unemployment insurance, and playing a guitar and dreaming of riches on the rock scene. "He may have a college degree, but there's things I know that only life can teach!"

The medical student listened attentively and respectfully. Then he said, "It sounds like your son doesn't always respect what you know, what experience has taught you."

"That's right!"

The medical student then made an important intuitive connection. "I'm probably about the same age as your son," he said. "I hope I don't come across as a know-it-all with you. I'm a student—I told you that. Be sure to let me know if I'm not understanding something."

"No, doc, you're doing all right. You're all right."

All interpersonal communication has both a content and a process (Reiser and Schroder, 1980). Everyone is accustomed to focusing on the **content** of communication, but it is often the **process** that communicates what is most important. Music offers a good analogy: The content forms the basic notes of communication, while process comprises the rhythm, timing, chord structure, and harmony. Content is the literal *what* that is being said; process is the timing and flow, the all-important *way* in which something is said.

While there is process communication in all interactions, its importance obviously varies. If one is asking a store clerk how much something costs, the process is hardly important unless local custom encourages bargaining. In the doctor-patient interaction, however, process is always important. Regardless of what the problem is, the patient will always have concerns about the doctor. "Can this person help me?" "Does he care about me?" "Does she find my problem disgusting?" 'Trivial?" "Has he ever seen anyone with my problem before?" The foreman in the illustrative case had an important concern: Would the young "doctor" treat him with understanding and respect?

While the specifics may vary, the concerns are universal, and addressing them sympathetically will help establish a good working alliance. Because patients can rarely express these concerns directly, they almost always do so through process, though they are not always aware of it.

Mastering and understanding the process level of communication is an exacting skill that takes time and experience to acquire. The interviewer can usually detect the process level of a patient's communications by asking three questions: (1) What is the patient telling me about his or her concerns *right now?* (2) What is the patient telling me about his or her feelings *right now?* (3) What is the patient telling me about his or her feelings concerning what is going on between us *right now?*

This is how the student understood his patient's concerns in the illustrative case. *Right now,* the patient was saying he was concerned about whether the young student would patronize him. *Right now,* he was saying that he wanted to be treated with respect even though he was not an educated man.

Attention to process often answers another key question in the psychiatric interview: *Why now?* A 46-year-old man with a 20-year history of manic-depressive illness comes to the emergency room markedly depressed. *Why now?* A young college senior develops a delusion that he is part of an international scheme. *Why now?*

What has been going on in the patient's life? The answer is always critical. More often than not, it will be found in the process of a patient's communication more than in the content. In the case of one very depressed man, for example, the process level of his communication dwelt extensively on themes of rejection and loss. He even told a sad joke about a man who was a cuckold. This process unfolded while the patient ostensibly disclosed only content. "I've been married 15 years to a good woman." This prompted the interviewer to inquire further about the patient's marriage and enabled him to learn that the patient suspected his wife had started an affair. This was the *why now?* for this patient's illness.

Finally, the concept of process is closely related to the phenomenon of **transference,** discussed in Chapter 33. In the psychiatric relationship, the intense feelings a patient has toward his or her therapist may be critical. Success in psychotherapy often depends on the skillful handling of these feelings. In certain forms of therapy, such as psychoanalysis and psychoanalytically oriented psychotherapy (see Chapter 33), an understanding of the patient's transference actually becomes an integral part of the process of treatment itself. With few exceptions, the nature and extent of the transference will also be communicated in process.

THE "A.R.T." OF INTERVIEWING

Every psychiatric interview may be conceptualized as having three phases: *A*ssessment, *R*anking, and *T*ransition (Reiser and Schroder, 1980).

Assessment

The assessment phase of the interview is the maximally open-ended, nondirective phase of the interaction. The setting should be a quiet and private place where doctor and patient can talk in an unhurried manner. Both should be seated and able to interact in normal tones at about the same eye level. If such a setting is not available, an empathic interview can go a long way toward overcoming the disadvantages of noise and lack of privacy. In all cases, the interviewer should try to ensure the best setting possible under the circumstances.

The interviewer should introduce and identify himself or herself, clearly explain the purpose of the meeting with the patient, and then invite the patient to begin in as open-ended a manner as possible. Some interviewers use a standard phrase, eg, "What sort of troubles have you been having?" Or, "Tell me about the problem that brings you here." Some simply begin with a look of interest and an inviting gesture of the hand.

There are several reasons why it is important to start in an open-ended manner. First, an invitation to talk tells the patient, "You're important to me. I am interested in everything about you. Everything that concerns you is potentially of concern to me." Communicating this attitude is always important in medicine but is even more so when working with patients who have problems that damage their sense of self-worth and their ability to trust others. Second, the clinician can often discern subtle but important clues to disturbances in thought processes. In response to the open-ended beginning of the interview, does the patient proceed to tell his or her story in a logical, goal-directed manner? Or does the patient ramble in a loose and incoherent way about seemingly unrelated concerns? Or does the patient start to cry and seem unable to articulate any story at all? Is there inappropriate laughter? Is there a rush of language amounting to pressure of speech? These and similar incongruities of affect and cognitive disturbances (see Chapter 11) can be readily diagnosed if the interviewer is appropriately nondirective. If the examiner too quickly launches into a content-intensive, checklist style of interviewing, such data may be missed. A third reason for beginning in an open-ended manner is perhaps the most important of all. The physician may be wrong in assuming he or she knows what is most important in the patient's presentation. If a patient entering an emergency room appeared belligerent and paranoid and expressed fears of gangland revenge, the physician may have initially assumed that the person was suffering from a psychosis of the paranoid type, probably schizophrenia. Yet this conclusion would have to be reassessed if, in the course of an open-ended interview, the patient began to talk about his activities as a drug dealer and his recent heavy use of cocaine.

During the assessment phase, the patient will raise concerns, describe symptoms, and offer other clues the clinician will wish to investigate further. These will range from the patient's medical and past psychiatric history to family relations and vocational and financial difficulties. After a time—usually 3–10 minutes—the clinician will be ready to begin the second phase of the interview process.

Ranking

During the ranking phase of the interview, the physician makes decisions about the order in which different areas of inquiry should be examined. During the 3- to 10-minute assessment phase, the patient may introduce a half-dozen areas of interest worth pursuing. What comes first? It is common practice to proceed first with the medical history, especially the present illness, but this is seldom necessary (except of course in true emergencies) and may be ill-advised. It is best to postpone the medical history if it is suspected that the patient has apprehensions about the doctor-patient relationship itself. These concerns are usually expressed in process (as in the illustrative case described above). When these concerns are significant, they need to be dealt with before other data are obtained. Thus, the physician might rank a given patient's problems as follows: (1) concerns about whether I will understand that he is afraid to come to the hospital, (2) a 3-week history of depression and suicidal ideation, (3) breakup of marriage, and (4) loss of job after 20 years. The physician might then proceed by saying, "Before we talk further about your depression, Mr Smith, do I get the feeling you're afraid I'll insist you be hospitalized tonight?" Within each ranked area, the examiner should proceed from an open-ended, nondirective style to progressively more focused and defined inquiry. Thus, the physician might say, "Tell me more about this feeling of hopelessness." After the patient has attempted to do so, the clinician's inquiry would become progressively more directive: "Have you lost any weight over the past few weeks?". . . "How many pounds would you say you've lost?" etc. Finally, questions that require the most specific type of responses may be asked: "Would you say you've lost a couple of pounds or 10 pounds in the last 2 weeks?" A good rule in ranking is to let the patient's priorities control whenever possible. The physician may be eager to elicit data concerning sleeplessness and euphoria or a 20-year drinking history. The patient may be much more troubled by concerns about being hospitalized or perhaps by something else altogether—something concerning the family or changes in employment or health.

Transition

Assessment and ranking are complex clinical skills that develop gradually as experience and knowledge increase; transitions are fairly easy from the first day. A transition consists of telling the patient when and why the subject of the interview is being changed. After the assessment phase, for example, the clinician may say, ''It sounds like you're very concerned about the effect your drinking is having on your wife. But right now I'd like to hear more about why you think you want to end it all.'' In this instance, the clinician has properly given assessment of suicidal ideation a very high priority. The clinician ranked this consideration first after listening to many of the patient's concerns and then made a transition by telling the patient exactly what the focus of attention was and why.

Transitions may also be used to return to a more open-ended interview, after a specific line of inquiry has run its course. After a careful review of systems, the clinician might say, ''Now that I've gotten the basics I need concerning your medical history, perhaps we could return to something you mentioned earlier—that your grandmother was hospitalized once for a psychiatric problem and things didn't go well. Could you tell me more about that?''

The line of questioning is usually clear in the clinician's mind, but the patient cannot be expected to understand what the clinician is up to. Great care must be taken to avoid confusion in changing the topic of inquiry.

"A.R.T." Sequence

Although assessment, ranking, and transition have been presented here in that sequence, all three actually go on simultaneously. For example, during a review of systems, the clinician may come upon a new fact that should be assessed more thoroughly then and there, indicating a need to return to the assessment phase of the interview. As the doctor-patient relationship proceeds, new facts are always emerging that require reassessment and ranking.

SPECIFIC INTERVIEWING TECHNIQUES

The foundation of good psychiatric interviewing—indeed all medical interviewing—is a working alliance between doctor and patient in a spirit of growing mutual trust. No amount of skill in technique can compensate for basic defects in this alliance. Conversely, a patient will usually forgive the doctor any number of mistakes if basic trust is there. The most potent single interviewing technique, therefore, is **empathy,** an appreciation of what the patient is going through. It is far more important than any special technique, more meaningful to the patient than anything learned from this or any other book. With that

understood, the remainder of this chapter can be given over to comments about ''tricks of the trade'' of interviewing adapted from Reiser and Rosen (1984).*

(1) Pay attention to the patient's comfort. Too often, students see patients in crowded institutional settings where their dignity, privacy, and comfort are neglected. Doctors converge around the bedside in large groups and literally ''talk down'' to the supine patient. Introductions are mumbled or omitted altogether. Perhaps some of this is inevitable, but the psychiatric interviewer should be more meticulous in such matters. A quiet and private setting should be found if possible. Doctor and patient should both be comfortable and able to interact at eye level. Perhaps this sort of courtesy should not be called a technique at all. But its benefits for the patient and the interviewing process are so frequently overlooked that it must be underscored.

(2) Remember the basics. As emphasized in previous sections, *understanding* the patient is more important than rigid adherence to classic technique. Nevertheless, a few of the standard interviewing rules and nostrums are helpful. (a) Don't ask two questions at the same time. (''Have you ever been bothered by voices or odd beliefs?'') (b) An open-ended question is usually preferable to a closed-ended one. (c) Don't ask questions calling for negative answers. (''You haven't had any experience with 'voices,' have you?'') (d) Avoid being judgmental. (''Have you had any disgusting or obscene thoughts?'') (e) Make liberal use of facilitating remarks. (''I see. . . . Tell me more. . . . How was that for you?. . . Go on. . . .'') (f) Ask for clarification. (''Can you explain what you meant by that? I'm not sure I exactly followed that.'')

(3) Don't be afraid to be yourself. The student should not try to imitate a portrait of Freud in a double-breasted suit. If a patient tells a joke and the joke is funny, go ahead and laugh. If the patient wants to know something about you—where you come from, whether you are married and have children—go ahead and answer. It is an unfortunate myth that the doctor-patient relationship should be totally unilateral, with the patient telling all and the doctor nothing. In an unselfconscious way, always respecting the patient's dignity, you should feel free to tell who you are, both in the facts you disclose and the attitude you convey. There are times when it is appropriate—indeed indicated—to touch a patient on his or her hand or shoulder. That may be perceived as ''phony'' if you are naturally reserved, and so you may not be able to bring it off. If that is the case, don't force it. But you should never be afraid to reach out and be human. Physical contact is a potent ''drug'' which—like any drug—may have major side effects.

---

* Adapted and reproduced with permission of the copyright holder, University Park Press.

It takes experience to know when to touch as well as when not to. Still, too much has been written about the psychiatrist as iceberg—silent, cold, unbending. Remember also that a patient can be "touched" in many ways. An empathic expression of understanding or a sincere look of concern on your face can often touch a patient more deeply than your hand on his or her shoulder. Be yourself. When you communicate, whether through words or by laying on your hands, be guided by your answer to the question, "Am I doing this for my patient?"

(4) Encourage the expression of feelings. Some patients are under strong cultural proscriptions against public displays of affect, especially grief and rage. Physicians may have the same attitude, and if so may believe that if a patient starts to cry, for example, something must have gone wrong with the interview. Most psychiatric patients are in emotional states they feel they cannot express—usually rage and sorrow. Almost without exception, they should be encouraged to let these feelings come out. ("There are tears in your eyes. His death has left you *very* sad, hasn't it?") The only case in which encouraging expression of affect is contraindicated is when a patient is in danger of total loss of control, signaled by escalating behavior—a louder and louder voice, tenser body habitus, etc. In such circumstances, the interviewer should demand that affect be controlled.

(5) Consider the patient in developmental terms. As this textbook makes clear, growth and development do not cease at age 21. It is often useful to consider the patient's stage of development. Might this depressed 50-year-old woman be suffering from "empty nest syndrome" (depression because the children have all left home)? Might this agitated psychotic young man be struggling with emotional conflicts related to sexual intimacy and separation from his family? A developmental perspective can assist the interviewer in understanding the patient's concerns, especially if the patient and interviewer are of widely disparate ages.

(6) Remember that the patient is more scared than you are. A young man is nervous about meeting you and about the implications of having a psychiatric disturbance. Will you read his mind? Will you find him unlikable? Is he on a course leading to incurable insanity? Or do you find his problems laughably trivial, not worthy of serious attention or compassion? Inexperienced clinicians are often apprehensive in approaching a psychiatric patient but not nearly so apprehensive as the patient usually is, and knowing this may enable you to be of help sooner than otherwise.

(7) Tell the patient what you think he or she is feeling. Imagine that you yourself are suffering from a psychiatric disorder—eg, that you have developed severe phobic symptoms. You have become afraid to travel by air, then by car, and now are afraid even to leave your home on foot. Which of the following would seem more empathic to you? "Can you describe your reaction to these events?" or "You must feel like a prisoner! How painful for you!" Some clinicians argue against what may seem like putting words in a patient's mouth. That is a pitfall to be avoided, but the risk is exaggerated. If you are occasionally wrong about what a patient is feeling, the patient will tell you so. If you are consistently wrong, something has prevented you from forming an empathic bond with that patient. If you are not sure you know what the patient is feeling, it is easy enough to ask, "What is this like for you?" or "How was that for you?" in order to elicit a report of the patient's affective experience. Clinicians miss a good opportunity to interact therapeutically when they do know how the patient is feeling but fail to communicate their insight to the patient.

(8) When an interview bogs down, try repeating the patient's last words. This technique was first popularized by the psychologist Carl Rogers (1951), who felt it was maximally nondirective and encouraged patients to proceed in the direction they preferred. Overreliance on this technique, however, is counterproductive. All psychiatric interviews have a purpose, which is not restricted to letting a patient go wherever he or she wants. The interview should follow the patient's lead, but sometimes the physician must be directive. Repeating the patient's last words is a technique that can be effective and should be used when needed. Encouraging nods of the head or supportive murmurs can accomplish the same thing. Periods of silence should be permitted also.

(9) Go ahead and ask the "unaskable." If you are in touch with your own feelings as well as those of your patient, you may realize that a patient is very scared, angry, or depressed. It may even occur to you that the patient is thinking of committing suicide. Fortunately, most do not, but even if a patient does not act on suicidal thoughts, he or she may feel terribly isolated and alone. Many patients think about death but feel they cannot tell anyone. A similar burden is imposed by other intense affects patients dread sharing. If you think that a patient might be suicidal, ask the question, tactfully and respectfully. It is impossible to put such an idea into a patient's head, which is what interviewers sometimes fear; but it is quite possible and very dangerous to ignore a patient's nonverbal signals. Most people who attempt suicide have seen a physician recently, often without indicating their intent, and many go on to use medications prescribed by the physician in the attempt. Thus, in the case of suicide, clinicians must always ask the "unaskable."

The same principle applies to many other areas—if you suspect alcoholism, drug abuse, child battering, or some other socially "delicate" problem, you must not be afraid to inquire. Occasionally you may give offense, but less often than one might think. Special note should be made of the subject of sexuality. Despite our "liberated" times, it is surprising how often interviewers overlook inquiring about sexual concerns. Sex is part of being human and is frequently affected by illness, especially psychiatric illness. Usually, however, the physician must inquire firmly and directly if he or she hopes to be of any help in this aspect of the patient's welfare. Ultimately, it is not just suicide and sex but all taboos to which the admonition ask! applies: fear of death, mutilation, sexual dysfunction, madness, suicide. A patient will let you know if you should back off. More often, the patient will open up with an outpouring of gratitude and relief.

(10) Learn to be quiet. When patients come to a point in their story where they are about to disclose something uncomfortable, they will often fall silent. Silence can be socially awkward, but as a psychiatric interviewer you must learn to take advantage of it. When a patient falls silent, be silent too. The pressure does build, and it may seem awkward for a time, but the patient usually goes on to tell the interviewer what is really bothering him or her. Most interviewers would do well to listen more and talk less. If silence becomes unduly protracted, it may be useful to say something neutral—"Go ahead. . . . Yes, go on. . . . I'm listening"—to relieve awkwardness and encourage the patient to continue.

(11) Pay attention to body language. Body language is one of many ways in which patients try to communicate. This subject has received considerable attention in both medical and lay publications, perhaps more than it deserves. Yet body language is an important way in which both patients and doctors express themselves. And unlike the tongue, the body seldom lies.

Body language can be particularly revealing at the beginning of the interview. Observe how patients position themselves and move. Watch how they sit or stand, seek or avoid eye contact, etc. Body language is a reliable form of communication that everyone uses. The trick, as with other observational skills, lies in being *conscious* of what is observed.

(12) Start broadly and then focus in. As the above discussion of the *"A.R.T."* of interviewing makes clear, it is rarely necessary to focus narrowly on any agenda at the outset of an interview. Allow the patient at least 3–10 minutes for assessment, the most open-ended phase of the interview. Books about interviewing list many techniques for staying broadly focused or narrowing in. They speak of open-ended versus closed-ended questions, of compound versus simple sentences, of facilitating responses, etc. While such labeling may be useful for some students, most do not find this kind of analysis helpful. Instead, as in cinematography, the interviewer should think of technique as involving a gradual focusing in, from wide-angle distance shots to narrow-angle close-ups. The interviewer's responses during the assessment phase are broadly focused wide-angle responses consisting of empathic silences, repeating the patient's last words, identifying the patient's affect ("That must have made you very sad!"), requesting clarification, etc. As the interviewer begins to focus in, questions become more directed: "Tell me more about this depression, Mr Jones." Or, "You mentioned that you and your wife have been fighting. Tell me more about what's going on there." As the camera angle narrows progressively, the questions naturally become more constricting: "How long have you been feeling that life was hopeless?" "How many pounds have you lost?" Now the emphasis is on specific data, chronology of symptoms and their nature and severity, their relations to other symptoms, etc. At this stage, the interviewer inquires about symptoms and signs directly related to the diagnostic criteria for specific mental disorders. Finally, the interviewer may focus in on the most narrowly directed question of all– those that can only be answered yes or no: "Have you ever had blackouts?" "Have you found yourself thinking that everyone is against you?"

SUMMARY

The 12 interviewing techniques discussed above, coupled with an understanding of the content/process distinction and the *"A.R.T."* of interviewing, should enable the psychiatric interviewer to obtain a meaningful story from the patient. The interviewer should always remember, however, that technique is invariable secondary to the human dimension of interviewing—above all, establishing empathy, respect, and trust.

REFERENCES

Balint M: *The Doctor, His Patient, and the Illness.* Internat Univ Press, 1972.

Davis M: Variations in patients' compliance with doctors' orders: Analysis of congruence between survey responses and results of empirical investigations. J Med Educ 1966;41:1037.

Freud S: Recommendations to physicians practicing psychoanalysis (1912). In: *Standard Edition of the Complete Psychological Works of Sigmund Freud.* Vol 12. Hogarth Press, 1958.

MacKinnon RA, Michels R: *The Psychiatric Interview in Clinical Practice.* Saunders, 1971.

Reiser DE, Rosen DH: *Medicine as a Human Experience.* University Park Press, 1984.

Reiser DE, Schroder AK: *Patient Interviewing: The Human Dimension.* Williams & Wilkins, 1980.

Rogers CL: *Client-Centered Therapy.* Houghton Mifflin, 1951.

Sullivan HS. *Schizophrenia as a Human Process.* Norton, 1962.

The Mental Status Examination

11

Jonathan Mueller, MD, Ralph J. Kiernan, PhD, & J.W. Langston, MD

The mental status examination is an instrument the clinician uses to assess a patient's orientation, attention, feeling states, speech, thought patterns, and specific cognitive skills. Like a lens or filter, it allows the clinician to perceive details and patterns whose nature might otherwise be only vaguely delineated. This examination, along with a careful history, physical examination, and laboratory examination, provides the foundation for psychiatric diagnosis and clinical assessment. Table 11–1 lists the major elements of the mental status examination organized in hierarchical format.

As Hughlings Jackson pointed out, functions most recently evolved (phylogenetically and ontogenetically) are the most vulnerable to disruption. Psychiatrists study disruption of thoughts, feelings, and behaviors that emerge from the organic functioning of the brain: The hierarchical structure of the mental status examination reflects the fact that higher cortical functions, such as abstract thought, may be distorted or disrupted by pathological processes at many levels. It is obvious that one cannot test a stuporous patient's appreciation of abstract similarities, but it is often forgotten that other factors also constrain assessment of thought processes. For example, a patient who is unable to attend because of fever or metabolic disturbance cannot make new memories, although the neuronal substrate for "memory making" may be structurally intact. Among the factors that affect the interpretation and conduct of the mental status examination are disturbances of attention, vigilance, or concentration; emotional turmoil; perceptual disturbances (impaired vision or hearing); and receptive or expressive language disorders. A patient unwilling to cooperate with the examination will neither reveal intact functions nor disclose deficits. Failure to recognize limitations at any of these levels will lead to errors both in diagnostic formulation and in determination of appropriate treatment.

Table 11–1. Organizing the mental status examination (hierarchical format).

1. Presentation.
2. Motor behavior and affect.
3. Cognitive status.
4. Thought.
5. Mood.

Although the mental status examination will be presented here as a separate part of the clinical examination (chief complaint, history of present illness, past medical, psychiatric, and social history, etc), it must be emphasized that the mental status examination is not simply an encapsulated or isolated part of the evaluation. Information noted throughout the interview will later be reported in the mental status examination, and information gained during formal mental status testing may prompt the physician to reevaluate the medical history or to seek confirmation of details by returning to specific items later in the examination. When a patient has a memory disorder, for example, the clinician should suspect omissions and inconsistencies in the history and investigate other sources if needed.

Physicians do not always have multiple opportunities to evaluate patients and may be called on for urgent decisions about a patient's capacity for self-care, potential for violence, suicidal risk, or hold on reality. Especially in emergency room and consultation/liaison settings, there is a premium on prompt assessment. To maximize the yield of the mental status examination, the clinician must be ever mindful of the privileged nature of the relationship with the patient and of the impact specific questions may have on the patient. Initially, the examiner should explain the purpose of the mental status examination, indicating that it is part of every complete patient evaluation. It may help reduce the patient's anxiety and avoid offending the patient to add, "You may find some of the questions very easy and some quite difficult to answer." The clinician must be able to note subtle behavioral clues (a change in voice tone, averted gaze, a tear, a swallow, a sigh, or hesitancy to discuss a particular matter) without losing track of material that must be covered in order to complete the examination. Although the examiner should have a structured scheme for covering all aspects of the mental status examination, a "shopping list" approach is not appropriate. Nevertheless, certain complaints, signs, or symptoms do require that a mental checklist be consulted. For example, if a patient experiences hallucinations, it is essential to obtain a detailed description of the phenomenon. (1) Are hallucinations auditory, visual, tactile, olfactory, or gustatory? (2) Are they elementary (simple points or lines) or complex (formed figures)? (3) Do visual hallucinations occur only in one part of the visual field? (4) Are they disturbing or comforting? (5) Is the hallucinating patient commanded to perform certain acts (eg, do things harmful to self or others), and if so can the commands be resisted? (6) Do the hallucinations seem to emanate from a particular source?

GENERAL FORMAT OF THE MENTAL STATUS EXAMINATION

The goal of the mental status examination is to assess—both qualitatively and quantitatively—a range of mental functions at a specific time. A clear record of the data provides a baseline for future examinations. Quantification of elements of the mental status examination enables the clinician to assess deterioration or improvement in specific functions over time.

Assessment of cognitive strengths and weaknesses traditionally has been done by psychologists. Physicians who wish to benefit from precise measurement of cognitive function must either master the psychological literature on the subject or learn to make their own assessments. Quantitative assessment of higher cortical functions (cognitive status examination) is a process that is essential for proper diagnosis and management of organic mental disorders. Specifically, attention, language, constructional ability, recent memory, calculation, and reasoning abilities such as appreciation of similarities and practical judgment can all be assessed in a graded fashion.

One practical way to characterize cognitive dysfunction is to systematically probe areas of intellectual functioning with **screening** questions difficult enough that a right answer implies an adequate level of function in that area and renders further testing of that area unnecessary. If the patient fails the screening item, the examiner presents a very easy question followed by a series of increasingly difficult ones (the **metric**). This ''screen/metric'' approach provides a graded quantitative measure of the degree of functional impairment in specific areas. Such an approach is rapid and efficient, since time is not wasted examining areas in which the patient has obvious strengths.

Several standardized brief mental status examinations serve as cognitive screening devices but are insensitive to important aspects of mental status. Textbooks often provide very detailed ''laundry list'' approaches to mental status examinations that may exhaust both patient and examiner when used rigidly and in their entirety. Such mental status examination formats are rarely presented hierarchically and do not provide quantifiable results. The following approach to the standardized and quantified mental status examination is recommended for routine use in single or serial assessments. Although its organization differs from that of standard examinations in current use, it contains the same elements. A detailed outline of this mental status examination is provided in Table 11–2. Many of the terms are defined in the Glossary of Psychiatric Signs and Symptoms or elsewhere in the text.

PRESENTATION

Level of Consciousness

Fluctuations in degree of alertness should be documented as precisely as possible. (For example, ''Pa-

Table 11–2. Detailed elements of the mental status examination (hierarchical format).

1. **Presentation:**
   Level of consciousness: coma to alert wakefulness (Glasgow Coma Scale; see Table 18–2).
   General appearance: body habitus; hygiene; cosmesis; dress.
   Attitude: degree of cooperation and effort.
2. **Motor behavior and affect:**
   Motor behavior: akinesia; involuntary movements; mannerisms.
   Affect: facial expression; gestures; speech characteristics; pressure, volume, prosody.
3. **Cognitive status:**
   Attention:
      Attention span: digit span; number of trials required to learn 4 words.
      Concentration and vigilance: serial subtraction; letter cancellation tasks; months of year backwards.
   Orientation: for personal identity; place; time.
   Language:
      Fluency: spontaneous speech; description of picture.
      Comprehension: of spoken or written language; performing commands of graded complexity; response to "yes/no" questions; pointing to named or described items.
      Repetition: sentences of graded difficulty; isolated words; letters; numbers.
      Naming: objects and parts of objects to visual confrontation (or on tactile presentation).
      Reading: aloud vs for comprehension; paragraph; sentence; words; letters; numbers.
      Writing: written description of picture; write name and address; write from dictation; copy a written phrase, word, or letter.
      Spelling: words of graded difficulty.
   Memory:
      Verbal memory: 4 unrelated words recalled after 5 minutes; recall of short story or paired words.
      Visual memory: reproduction of figures; recall of where examiner hides object.
   Constructional ability: reproducing figures from memory; copying figures; constructing blocks or token designs.
   Calculations: addition, subtraction, multiplication, and division.
   Reasoning:
      Practical judgment.
      Abstraction: similarities and proverb interpretation.
4. **Thought:**
   Process: coherence; goal directedness; logicality.
   Content: hallucinations; delusions; preoccupations; suicidal or homicidal ideation.
   Insight: nature of illness and awareness of factors that affect the course of the illness.
5. **Mood:**
   Relation to affect and congruence with thought content.

tient yawning and drowsy but responds to verbal encouragement with cooperation that never lasts more than 20 seconds.'') Level of consciousness can be described along a continuum from coma to full alertness. **Coma** is a state in which neither verbal nor motor responses can be elicited by noxious stimuli. (In moderate to light coma, motor reflexes may be elicited but not psychological responses.) **Stupor** is a state in which vigorous and repeated stimulation is required to rouse the patient. **Somnolence** and **lethargy** are less obtunded states in which drowsy, inactive, and indifferent patients respond to stimulation in delayed or incomplete fashion. **Drowsiness** is a sleeplike state from which the patient cannot be roused fully by minor stimuli. **Alert wakefulness** is a state in which responses to auditory, tactile, or visual stimuli are prompt and appropriate.

The Glasgow Coma Scale (Table 11–3) developed by Teasdale and Jennett (1974) is a graded approach to assessment of impaired consciousness on the basis of eye opening and verbal and motor responses to various stimuli. The scale ranges from 3 for deep coma to 14 for alert wakefulness. It has demonstrated great value for assessing and predicting degree of recovery.

General Appearance

The examiner notes clothing, personal hygiene, and any use of cosmetics, documenting details of fastidiousness or inattention (eg, ''a 3-day growth of beard with food spilled on his nightshirt''). Is the patient robust in appearance? Does he or she appear physically ill, with signs of alcoholism (eg, palmar erythema, facial flushing, spider angiomas) or endocrine disease (eg, cushingoid)? Special attention is paid to idiosyncrasies of appearance. These details should be recorded carefully enough so that a third party would be able to recognize the patient from the description without having seen the patient.

Attitude

Is the patient cooperative, evasive, arrogant, bemused, or apathetic? The patient's attitude toward the examiner and the examination situation determines to a large extent how much and what kind of information will be derived.

MOTOR BEHAVIOR & AFFECT

Motor Behavior

Are the patient's movements rapid, abrupt, clumsy, graceful, or totally absent? Is the level of motor activity fairly constant, or do abrupt periods of fitful hyperactivity alternate with apathetic withdrawal? If the patient displays unusual responses, how are they provoked? Are movements coherent and goal-directed, or do they have no discernible purpose? Are there bizarre repetitive stereotyped movements? Does behavior include nail biting (anxiety), tapping the feet (anxiety or akathisia), or sticking out the tongue and licking the lips repetitively (buccolingual-masticatory syndrome of tardive dyskinesia)?

If the patient is mute, does he or she consistently avoid the examiner's gaze, closing eyes tightly and resisting efforts to lift the lids (catatonic negativism or malingering)? Do the patient's movements repeat those of the examiner (echopraxia)? Will the patient's limbs remain in unnatural positions if placed there (called catalepsy, or ''waxy flexibility'')? Is a mute patient able to write if handed a pencil or to nod yes or no in response to certain questions (indicating either aphemia or hysterical mutism)? Is there any change in behavior depending upon whether the examiner discusses nonpersonal events rather than more personal issues such as the health of either the patient or the patient's immediate family?

Affect

''Affect'' may be considered the observable correlate of emotion, ie, the outer manifestation of inner states. It may be characterized as bright, sluggish, voluble, expansive, anguished, tearful, etc. The examiner pays particular attention to the range, intensity, lability, and appropriateness of affective behavior.

Affect has three components: facial expression, gestures, and speech. Although speech and language are often described together, there is a rationale for considering the flow, volume, pressure, rhythm, and intonation of speech as kinetic phenomena apart from language. The emotional coloring (prosody) of speech may be impaired in major depression, in dysfunction

Table 11–3. Glasgow Coma Scale.

	Coma Scale
Eyes open (E)	
Spontaneously	4
To speech	3
To pain	2
None	1
Best motor response (M)	
Obeys commands	5
Localizes pain	4
Flexion to pain	3
Extension to pain	2
None	1
Best verbal response (V)	
Oriented	5
Confused	4
Inappropriate words	3
Incomprehensible sounds	2
None	1

Summed Glasglow Coma Scale = E + M + V.
Range: From 3 for deep coma to 14 for alert wakefulness.

of the basal ganglia, in Broca's aphasia ("motor" aphasia), or secondary to damage of the right cerebral hemisphere (see Chapter 5).

The term "witzelsucht" refers to a facetious jocularity sometimes observed in association with frontal lobe lesions.

"Blunted" affect is grossly diminished in range of emotional expression.

Explosions of tears or anger ("catastrophic reactions") can occur in organically impaired individuals confronted with tasks once simple but now difficult or impossible to perform.

COGNITIVE STATUS

Arguments can be made for assessing the patient's cognition at either the outset or the conclusion of the mental status examination. The authors believe that a structured assessment of the patient's cognitive status is best performed immediately after the clinician has noted the patient's initial presentation, motor behavior, and affect, before an attempt is made to assess thought and mood. Impairments in cognitive ability may masquerade as either thought disorder (aphasia may appear as "concreteness of thought") or mood disturbance (an amnestic patient given the diagnosis of cancer 2 days previously may make no spontaneous mention of this and may therefore appear to deny or be indifferent to the diagnosis).

Attention

Is the patient so preoccupied or easily distracted that cooperation with the examiner is impossible? Is there a visual field cut, inattention to a visual hemifield in the absence of a field cut, or neglect of one side of the body?

A. Immediate Recall: Immediate recall refers to the retention of small amounts of information for up to 30 seconds. Material "in" immediate recall requires further processing before it can enter more permanent memory stores.

Proper assessment of attention is of great importance, since it may have implications for further evaluation and treatment. In the presence of an attentional deficit, the examiner must be wary of drawing inferences from further testing of higher cortical functions. Since inattention is a hallmark of acute confusional state, its presence should prompt a search for remediable (toxic, metabolic, or infectious) medical problems. However, inattention may also be seen in nonorganic mental disorders such as brief psychotic reaction and posttraumatic stress disorders. As a general rule, digit span (see below) is preserved in the early stages of dementia, and it is not until cortical degeneration is well advanced that one finds impaired attention.

Attention span may be assessed by having the patient repeat a list of words or a digit sequence presented at the rate of one digit per second. It is important that the digits not be grouped (by rhythmic clusters or intonation) and that they be somewhat random (eg, not all odd or all even). This should be practiced, since it is difficult to present a string of digits in this fashion without clustering. Intact repetition of six digits forward rules out major attentional disturbance. Inability to repeat at least five digits is considered abnormal.

Patients who fail the initial screening task of six-digit repetition are presented with a metric: digit sequences of increasing length, beginning with three-digit numbers. The examiner discontinues this task only after the patient has missed twice at a given level (eg, two mistakes at the five-digit level).

B. Concentration and Vigilance: The ability to sustain attention over a longer period may be referred to as "concentration" or "vigilance." Serial 7s (see p 115) or repetition backward of a digit sequence or the months of the year (or days of the week) may be used to assess concentration. Psychiatric disorders such as anxiety, depression, and schizophrenia may impair vigilance without disrupting digit repetition.

Orientation

Orientation is assessed with reference to person, place, and time. Orientation to **person** (ability to give one's own name when asked to do so) reflects "overlearned" information and is seldom if ever lost in organic brain disease. Failure to give one's own name occurs in hysterical dissociation and most often reflects negativism, confusion, distraction, hearing impairment, or receptive language disorder.

Orientation to **place** can be tested with reference to country, state, county, city, type of building, name of building, location of building, and location in the building. A patient may know he or she is in a hospital but not know the city or state.

Orientation to **time** may be tested with reference to year, season, month, day of week, and date. Because time changes more frequently than location, it is more vulnerable to disruption and thus is the most sensitive index of disorientation. (One cannot, however, use time of day as a screen for orientation to time, since patients may know or guess the time of day from numerous cues but have no idea of the month or year.)

Language

Failure to assess language in a systematic fashion is a shortcoming of many mental status examinations and can lead to diagnostic confusion. Word-finding difficulty (anomia), for example, may be mistakenly thought to reflect a disorder of memory or judgment. Aphasia (see Chapter 5) is a language disorder often mistakenly attributed to confusion, dementia, hysteria, or psychosis.

Language proficiency is assessed by testing four parameters: fluency, comprehension, repetition, and naming. (Reading and writing will not be discussed here.)

A. Fluency: Fluency refers to the ability to produce sentences of normal length, rhythm, and melody. It is commonly assessed by listening to the patient's spontaneous speech. Is speech hesitant, stammering, or inarticulate? Are words mumbled or spoken too softly to be heard? Is the volume constant, or does it decrease toward the end of the sentence? Does the patient use bizarre syntax resulting in nonsense? What is the range of vocabulary? Is speech "empty," consisting of few substantive words and frequent circumlocutions? (The function or some particular attribute of an item may be offered as a substitute for its name—eg, "the thing that holds it on your shirt," rather than "the clip of the pen.") Patients may become adept at masking word-finding difficulty by skirting certain issues or using unobtrusive circumlocutions.

A helpful method for assessing fluency is to have the patient describe what he or she observes in a picture. Although this is not truly spontaneous speech, there are distinct advantages to presenting each patient with a uniform speech stimulus. The examiner quickly learns to note neglect of details and to recognize subtle word-finding difficulties. Upon completion of the patient's description, the examiner can return to specific details of the picture that have been omitted or incorrectly described. Verbatim recording of a patient's description of the picture is essential. Special attention is paid to paraphasic errors, which consist of distortions involving either individual letters ("brain clumor") or whole words (eg, "stick" for pencil). Speech is described for clinical purposes in an all-or-nothing fashion as either "fluent" or "nonfluent."

B. Comprehension: Just as intact auditory perception is essential for optimal interactions between geriatric patients and friends or hospital staff, language comprehension is also crucial. Since repetition and comprehension may be "dissociated" in language disorders that spare the perisylvian speech areas (see Chapter 5), it is dangerous to infer intact comprehension from a patient's ability to repeat what is said. Thus, any tendency by the patient to consistently echo or repeat should actually raise a question of comprehension deficit. It is as if these patients are trying to "run the tape by" one more time in order to extract from it as much information as possible.

There are many ways to assess comprehension at the bedside. The patient can be asked to point to objects the examiner names or whose function is described. This method is limited by objects that are at hand and by the examiner's skill in abstract description of common objects. Another approach is to present questions that can be answered yes or no. If this is done, the examiner must ask at least six questions, since the patient has a 50–50 chance of answering any one question correctly. (It should also be noted that some aphasic patients are unable to say yes or no even when they know the answer.)

A graded screening and metric approach to testing comprehension that has proved useful is as follows:

The screening item consists of obeying a 3-step command. At least five objects are placed in front of the patient, who is told to "turn over the paper, hand me the pen, and point to your nose." A patient who fails this task is asked to perform the metric, which consists of three one-step commands, two two-step commands, and one three-step command. Success in performing each of the one-step commands rules out major apraxic problems. (See Chapter 5 for discussion of ideomotor apraxia.)

The metric is performed (for example) as follows:

One-step commands: (1) Pick up the pen. (2) Point to the floor. (3) Hand me the keys.

Two-step commands: (1) Point to the pen and pick up the keys. (2) Hand me the paper and point to the coin.

Three-step command: Point to the keys, hand me the pen, and pick up the coin.

A surprising number of patients are unable to perform a three-step command despite intact cooperation, attention, and auditory acuity. Careful documentation of inability to comprehend and comply with complex requests (ie, subclinical language disorder) is of great value to the nursing staff and others who manage the patient on the ward. Documentation of such deficits minimizes the risk that these patients will be wrongfully considered negativistic or uncooperative.

C. Repetition: Sentences that are short and contain high-frequency ("everyday") words are the easiest to repeat. Longer sentences that contain low-frequency words or short grammatical function words with no objective referents ("from," "and") are more difficult to repeat. An appropriate screening sentence for repetition might be "The beginning movement revealed the composer's intention," The patient who fails this is given a series of phrases or sentences of graded difficulty as the metric: "Out the window." "He swam across the lake." "The winding road led to the village." "He left the latch open." "The honeycomb drew a swarm of bees." "No ifs, ands, or buts." Because the bizarre speech of patients with Wernicke's aphasia is fluent, the physician may incorrectly conclude that these patients are psychotic or in a confusional state. Demonstration of paraphasic errors on repetition tasks provides elegant proof of primary language dysfunction. Repetition is impaired in all of the major perisylvian aphasic syndromes.

D. Naming: Naming parts of an object (eg, "tentacle") is even more difficult than naming the object itself ("octopus"). Thus, an appropriate screening question turns out to be naming a pen and its parts on visual confrontation: cap or cover, point or nib, and clip. (The patient who can name a pen and its parts has intact naming ability and does not have aphasia.)

Although an individual who names items correctly does not have aphasia, not every patient who manifests naming difficulties has aphasia. Otherwise healthy individuals who are physically exhausted or sleep-deprived often manifest dysnomia, Dysnomia may be an early nonspecific sign of generalized cerebral dysfunction secondary to metabolic disturbance. Aphasic dysnomia may occur as an isolated and dramatic deficit with localized left hemispheric lesions, or it may exist as part of a larger aphasic syndrome.

Unless naming is carefully assessed, the clinician runs the risk of mistaking word-finding difficulty for "thought blocking," amnesia, or impaired judgment. Accordingly, language is assessed prior to memory.

Memory

A. Verbal Memory: A general impression of the patient's memory can be gained from the way in which he or she presents the history. Is there internal consistency, or are there gaps and contradictions? Does the patient remember the physician's name from a past encounter, or does the patient confabulate, claiming to have met an individual whom he or she has never seen before? Is there a period for which the patient has poor recall? If so, is the patient unable to recall either personal or general information from that period (organic amnesia), or is there selective inability to recall personally relevant information (psychogenic amnesia)?

1. Recent memory–Ability to recall events of the past minutes or days reflects recent memory. (Orientation to place and time also actually reflects memory.) Recent memory is assessed clinically by asking the patient to learn new information. This is commonly done by presenting four unrelated words. The patient is told that he or she will be asked for these words later in the examination. The examiner must be certain the patient can repeat all four words before going on with other parts of the examination, which constitute "interference material." (The number of trials required to learn four words is another measure of attention.) Failure to make sure that the patient can repeat all four words invalidates any conclusions about recent memory as a specific ability area—the patient may simply not have been attending to the task, and apparent failure to recall may really reflect initial failure to register material.

For each word a patient is unable to recall after 5 or 10 minutes, a category prompt (eg, "a color" or "an animal") is given. If the patient is still unable to recall the word, a list of three or four words— one of which is the test word—is presented. Points may be assigned on the basis of whether a word is recalled on command (3 points), following a prompt (2 points), or recognized from a list (1 point). Five to 10 minutes after a depressed patient or a severely amnestic alcoholic has been given four words to learn, neither may be able to recall any of the words when asked to do so. The depressed patient, however, will usually respond to category prompts or recognize the words from lists, whereas an alcoholic patient with Korsakoff's syndrome may not even recall having been given a list of words to learn. The examiner who simply records "none of four words recalled at 5 minutes for both of these patients fails to distinguish two very different situations. Moreover, a maximum 12-point scoring system (four items, each rated 0–3) allows the clinician to monitor improvement or deterioration of memory following administration of agents such as thiamine, digitalis and diuretics, or tricyclic antidepressants. Clinicians who ask patients what they had for breakfast should verify the answer by asking the nursing staff also. It is worth repeating that the distinction between attentional and amnestic deficits is crucial. *The diagnosis of amnestic syndrome cannot be made in the presence of an attentional deficit.*

2. Remote memory–Ability to recall the events of weeks or years ago is difficult to assess clinically, since the examiner seldom knows enough about the patient to ask pertinent or verifiable questions. Unless the examiner is prepared to seek corroboration (such as what schools the patient actually attended or the dates of military service), there is no point in asking such questions. Questions about past presidents, dates of wars, and events that affect everyone (such as President Kennedy's assassination) are helpful, but evaluation of responses remains problematic, since failure to recall may reflect increasing forgetfulness (as in senile dementia) or a period of time during which the patient was unable to lay down memories. With resolution of memory problems (eg, following traumatic amnesia secondary to head injury, or in response to thiamine treatment of Wernicke-Korsakoff syndrome), older memories tend to return before more recent ones (Ribot's law).

B. Visual Memory: Patients may be asked to reproduce designs or report details of pictures after delays of seconds or minutes. Alteratively, the examiner may ask the patient to remember a series of items (eg, clock, window, chair) or where the examiner places or hides an item such as a dollar bill (eg, behind a picture).

Constructional Ability

While testing of constructional ability is frequently omitted from the routine mental status examination, it may be helpful in the detection of organic brain disease. Patients may be asked to copy drawings, manipulate blocks, or reconstruct a figure using tokens. Before the examiner draws conclusions about a patient's constructional ability, it is essential to assess visual acuity, motor functions (strength, praxis, and coordination), and tactile sensation.

As a screening test for constructional ability, the

patient is instructed to study two figures for 10 seconds and is then asked to reproduce them from memory. Successful completion of the screen requires intact immediate visual recall as well as significant visual-spatial ability.

Individuals who fail the screen are asked either to copy a series of increasingly difficult figures.

Calculations

The patient's education and professional background should be considered before calculating ability is tested. The traditional "serial 7s" task, in which the patient is asked to "subtract 7 from 100 and then continue, subtracting 7 from each answer," is a difficult task for many high school graduates (ie, over two-thirds are unable to get into the 50s without an error in less than 30 seconds). In addition to calculating ability, the task requires sustained concentration and is easily disrupted by anxiety; for this reason, difficulty with serial 7s should not be taken as evidence of dyscalculia. Simple addition, subtraction, and multiplication often assess rote learning (a type of remote recall) rather than calculating. Thus, an appropriate assessment of calculations involves tasks that fall somewhere between the two examples. Some patients find it simpler to address problems in daily life, such as making change from a purchase, rather than solving formal math problems. As a screening device, the question "How much is 5×13?" is appropriate. Examples of metric items are shown below.

How much is $5 + 3$?
How much is $15 + 7$?
How much is $39 \div 3$?
How much is $31 - 8$?

Reasoning

Cognition can be subdivided into two areas: practical judgment and abstraction (similarities and proverb interpretation).

A. Practical Judgment: Assessing practical judgment is especially important in the evaluation of thought disorders, character disorders, or dementia. This area is difficult to appraise because many judgment questions can be answered "correctly" by the aid of simple memory (remembering what one's parents or teachers said should be done in a given situation). Practical judgment also reflects the patient's social and financial background. (A prosperous physician who loses his wallet in the airport in Denver, Colorado, might call home to have money wired to him, whereas an adolescent runaway might turn to Traveler's Aid, go to a local church, or try to hitchhike.)

1. Screening question–The patient is asked, "What would you do if you were stranded in the airport in Denver, Colorado, with only a dollar in your pocket?" Acceptable answers are calling a friend or family member to wire money and going to Travel-er's Aid. If the patient claims to know people in the Denver area, the examiner should say, "For the purposes of this question, imagine you are in an airport far away from anyone you know." If the patient suggests using credit cards, the examiner should say, "For the purposes of this question, imagine you do not have credit cards." Patients should be asked to explain their answers further when vague or partially correct answers are given.

2. Metric–The patient is asked the following series of questions. A score of 2 points is given for a fully correct answer, 1 point for a partially correct or vague answer, and no points for an incorrect answer. Examples of 2-point, 1-point, and 0-point answers for each item are given below.

a. What would you do if you woke up at 1 minute before 8:00 AM and remembered an appointment downtown at 8:00 AM? *Answers:* 2 points—call the person; 1 point—dress as quickly as I can and rush downtown; 1 point (vague)—cancel the appointment; 0 points—go back to bed.

b. What would you do if while walking beside a lake you saw a 2-year-old child playing alone at the end of a pier? *Answers:* 2 points—remove the child from the pier and look for the parents; 1 point—tell the child to get away from the water; 1 point (vague)—make sure the child is not harmed; 0 points–yell for help; look for a lifeguard; go for help.

c. What would you do if you came home and found a broken pipe was flooding the kitchen? *Answers:* 2 points—shut off the main water valve; 1 point—call the plumber; 1 point (vague)–stop the water; 0 points—mop up the mess.

B. Abstraction: (Similarities and proverb interpretation.)

1. Similarities–Ability to appreciate the commonality between two objects is tested as part of the Wechsler Adult Intelligence Scale. Low native intelligence, psychosis, distraction, or dementia may produce impairment in abstracting ability.

a. Screening question–The patient is told, "I am going to ask you how some things are alike." A specific example is then given: "For example, a hat and a coat are alike because they are both clothing." As a screening item, the patient is asked, "In what way are painting and music alike?" Only the abstract responses "art" or "forms of art" are passing. Less specific abstract responses, such as both are "artistic" or "created," are not passing answers.

b. Metric–The patient is told, "I have some other pairs of items. Again, I want you to tell me how they are alike. In what way are a rose and a tulip alike?" Each item is similarly introduced. The first time a patient responds with a difference between the items, that response is recorded and the patient is told, "That is how they are different. I want you to tell me how they are alike." Regardless of whether the patient goes on to give a good answer, no credit is given. Subsequent "difference" responses are not corrected or credited with points.

(1) Rose-tulip: 2 points—flowers; 1 point—grow, have petals, need water, smell nice; 0 points—pretty, same color, fresh, outdoors.

(2) Bicycle-train: 2 points—vehicles, means of transportation; 1 point—ride them, wheels, toys; 0 points—go fast, have tracks.

(3) Watch-ruler: 2 points—measuring instruments; 1 point—have numbers, tell how much; 0 points—are useful, have many parts.

(4) Corkscrew-hammer: 2 points—tools; 1 point—used by humans, made of metal, do work; 0 points—cut into things; are strong.

2. Proverb interpretation–Another means of assessing a patient's capacity to abstract is to ask for the patient's interpretation of a proverb. Proverbs such as "There's no use crying over spilled milk" and "The grass is always greener on the other side of the street" are easier than "People who live in glass houses shouldn't throw stones" or "Every cloud has a silver lining." Proverb interpretation is strongly influenced by culture, educational level, and socioeconomic class.

THOUGHT

Assessment of thought may be divided into several areas: process, content, cognitive functions (abstraction and judgment), fund of knowledge, and insight. Each will be discussed briefly.

Thought Process

Process of thought is assessed by noting coherence of speech and reflects the way in which mental associations are made. Thought process may be described as concrete, tangential (getting off the track of the subject and failing to return), circumstantial (digressive but able to return to the subject), perseverative (sticking to a single thought, phrase, or word), loose (absence of logical thought progression), or incoherent. Thought blocking" refers to sudden cessation of thought or speech. It may occur in schizophrenia, and lesser degrees are seen in anxiety states such as obsessive compulsive disorders. In rare instances, thought process may be so disrupted that the examiner has little or no idea of the content of a patient's thought.

Thought Content

In assessing the content of a patient's thought, the examiner notes preoccupations, ambitions, phobias, and perceptual disturbances (such as illusions and hallucinations). Patients may be asked, "Do you have the feeling that you control your own thoughts?" On careful questioning, patients may admit that they believe thoughts are inserted into or withdrawn from

their minds or broadcast to others, or that their thoughts are controlled by outside forces.

Specific fears or beliefs should not be taken at face value, but their origins should be explored. A statement such as "I don't want to go out of my house," for example, may have widely different meanings. A patient with a right parietal lobe tumor may no longer be able to find the way home after walking to a nearby store. One suffering from a major depressive disorder may feel too tired to go for a walk or may have lost all interest in former sources of pleasure. A schizophrenic patient may fear being overtaken by enemies and tortured. Yet another individual may fear open streets or becoming trapped in a crowd.

Patients who deny specific delusions may still claim to have a special relationship with God. It is often helpful to ask patients, "How do you think others feel about you?" (admired, shunned, unappreciated, etc).

Although visual and olfactory hallucinations may occur in "functional" psychoses such as schizophrenia or mania, they tend to occur more frequently in association with organic disease. Patients should be asked to describe how vivid and frequent their hallucinations are, in what circumstances they occur (on falling asleep or waking), and whether they are pleasant, comforting, or terrifying. They should be asked to identify the source of the hallucination (whether it originates within the patient or is projected from some outer source). If hallucinations consist of commands, patients should be asked whether they are able to resist the commands. Patients who are asked if they have special bodily feelings may respond that they feel dead or unreal inside.

Insight

The patient's degree of understanding of his or her medical or psychological problems is a measure of insight. The patient may be asked, "How do you understand your problems?" or "What has been most helpful to you in dealing with this problem in the past?" Although insight and understanding are often essential to working with patients, some patients are able to acquire insight only after their behavior has changed. It is always important to look for cognitive, perceptual, or informational explanations of "poor insight" before imputing to patients psychodynamic defenses against insight.

MOOD

Since patients with word-finding difficulty or memory disturbances may be unable to describe or recall their mood over the past few days or weeks, interpreting a patient's subjective report of mood requires knowledge of language skills and memory function.

It is for this reason that mood is not assessed or described until cognition has been assessed.

The term "mood" denotes a persisting subjective state of feeling tone as reported by the patient. If the patient does not volunteer a description of his or her mood, the examiner may ask, "How are you feeling inside?" or "What are your spirits like?" Mood may be characterized (for example) as blue, despondent, anxious, fearful, bored, exuberant, irritable, or restless.

Are there dissociations between affect and reported mood? Does the patient with immobile facies say that he or she feels nothing inside or report that he or she feels sad but cannot cry? Does the facial expression of a schizophrenic patient who describes inner feelings of fear or emptiness reflect this, or does he or she wear a "silly" smile while describing inner turmoil? Patients with pseudobulbar palsy (due to disruption of fibers connecting frontal motor cortex with brainstem nuclei subserving emotional expression) may report episodes of laughing or crying uncontrollably, breaking into laughter when they feel blackly depressed, or crying when amused.

MENTAL STATUS & INTELLIGENCE

Mental status examination and intelligence testing are often combined. Elements of the mental status examination are tested in formal tests of intelligence. Abnormalities in mental status (eg, attention or memory) clearly affect ability to complete tests of intelligence (see Chapter 13 for a detailed discussion of tests of intelligence). Conversely, some rough measures of intelligence, especially fund of knowledge, often are included in mental status examinations. Our formal examination format does not include measurement of fund of knowledge, but it is briefly described here for the sake of completeness.

The patient's **fund of knowledge** may be assessed by asking questions about a wide range of subjects (politics, literature, art, history, geography, etc). In addition to reflecting educational level, the questioning may also help evaluate recent and remote memory. Although intelligence often manifests itself in a wide range of interests, some individuals with superior intelligence actually have very restricted interests. Vocabulary (noted under speech) represents a particular example of fund of knowledge and correlates highly with intelligence.

REFERENCES

Benson DF: *Aphasia, Alexia and Agraphia.* Churchill Livingstone, 1979.

Cummings JL: *Clinical Neuropsychiatry.* Grune & Stratton, 1985.

Diagnosis and psychiatry. Chapter 12 in: *Comprehensive Textbook of Psychiatry/IV,* 4th ed. Kaplan HI, Freedman AE, Sadock BJ (editors). Williams & Wilkins, 1985.

Hinsie LE, Campbell RJ: *Psychiatric Dictionary,* 4th ed. Oxford Univ Press, 1970.

Kiernan RJ, Langston WJ, Mueller J: The neurobehavioral mental status examination. Presented at the American Psychological Association Meetings, October, 1983.

Taylor J (editor): *Selected Writings of John Hughlings Jackson.* Basic Books, 1958.

Teasdale G, Jennett B: Assessment of coma and impaired consciousness: A practical scale. Lancet 1974;2:81.

Van Dyke C, Mueller J, Kiernan RJ: The case for psychiatrists as authorities on cognition. Psychosomatics 1987;28:87.

Walsh KW: *Neuropsychology.* Churchill Livingstone, 1977.

12

Physical Examination & Laboratory Evaluation

Jonathan Mueller, MD

The ability to perform a physical examination is, like any other skill, acquired and maintained by frequent practice. Many psychiatrists who have completed their training—and particularly those who have exclusively outpatient practices—do not perform physical examinations. This is unfortunate, since internists and other specialists often perform abbreviated neurological examinations despite neuropsychiatric symptoms. As the role of the neurosciences and other branches of medicine becomes increasingly important in the practice of modern psychiatry, the psychiatrist's ability to perform relevant examinations should become a central concern of psychiatric education. Since the purpose of the physical examination is to confirm or refute hypotheses that have been formulated on the basis of the patient's history and a review of systems, these areas will be considered first.

MEDICAL HISTORY & REVIEW OF SYSTEMS

Medical History

Detailed attention to the medical history reassures patients that they are being seen by a physician who recognizes the interplay between physical and mental distress. As an expression of concern for the patient's reactions to and feelings about illness, history taking serves to initiate a working alliance between patient and therapist. The medical history obtained from a psychiatric patient may provide clues to the actual cause of changes in mental status and inevitably sheds light on the patient's biological limitations—limitations of what existential psychotherapists term the patient's "being in the world."

The earliest events that influence central nervous system development are experienced in utero. These may include physical assaults and deprivation endured by the mother during pregnancy and maternal addiction to substances such as alcohol, heroin, nicotine, or other psychoactive drugs. Patients are often unaware of major prenatal events. Thus, documentation from previous medical records and history obtained from siblings, parents, or other relatives may be crucial.

Early childhood illnesses may be significant either because of enduring effects on major organ systems or because of suspicions they raise about immunological compromise. **Major medical illnesses** in a child or other members of the family may result in prolonged separation of the child from the parents or a significant decrease in time spent with and interest shown in a developing child's accomplishments or difficulties.

Surgical procedures, regardless of the age at which they are performed, have special importance as events during which control of the body is relinquished to a team of professionals. Hip fracture in an elderly patient may precipitate a series of physical and psychological events culminating in loss of autonomy. Any major surgical procedure exposes the patient to risks of hypotension and anesthesia. "She has never been the same since her operation" is a frequent observation made by friends and family of elderly patients. All current medications and dosage schedules should be listed, along with past and present use of alcohol and other substances.

Special attention should be devoted to documenting the occurrence of **neurological disturbances.** Seizures, head trauma, blackouts, loss of consciousness, and language or memory problems all have great bearing on psychiatric assessment. Likewise, **endocrine disturbances** in patients with diabetes, thyroid or parathyroid disease, or hyper- or hypofunction of the adrenal glands can present as psychiatric illness.

Review of Systems

The following list is not exhaustive but provides examples of physical dysfunction with major implications for psychiatric assessment and management.

A. Nervous System and Sensory Organs: Complaints of headache may arise from a wide range of causes, including stress, migraine, hypoxia, brain tumor, subarachnoid hemorrhage, and meningitis. Since diplopia very rarely represents a conversion phenomenon, complaints of double vision should always trigger a search for disorders of neurological origin, such as Wernicke's encephalopathy, multiple sclerosis, or diabetic cranial nerve palsy. Visual hallucinations or illusions may arise from structural damage to any part of the visual system, eg, from lesions of the retina, the optic nerve, tract, visual radiations, or the occipital cortex. Hallucinations confined to one visual hemifield or one visual quadrant always suggest structural damage from disease or injury. Older patients should be asked about changes in hearing or vision, since correction of these deficits (hearing aid or glasses) can improve patient's ability to care for themselves and lead independent social lives. Loss of hearing may lead to paranoid ideation.

B. Cardiovascular System: Recurrent anxiety may reflect cardiac arrhythmia (especially paroxysmal atrial tachycardia), angina, or mitral valve prolapse. Worsening of congestive heart failure with attendant drowsiness or hypoxemia may be easily mistaken for depression. Any history of angina, arrhythmia, or myocardial infarction should be noted. Heart disease may impose significant limitations on the patient's life-style, and cardiac medications may have psychoactive effects.

C. Respiratory System: Episodic shortness of breath or hyperventilation may occur secondary to panic attacks or may be seen in the context of general anxiety disorders. Conditions such as chronic obstructive pulmonary disease, congestive heart failure, pulmonary embolism, and pneumonia must always be excluded when anxiety is assessed.

D. Gastrointestinal System: Vague recurrent abdominal symptoms may be seen in patients with somatoform disorders (eg, conversion disorder and somatization disorder), but abdominal distress due to organic causes (eg, regional enteritis, ulcerative colitis, and porphyria) may be accompanied by prominent psychological distress. Anorexia is a vegetative sign of depression, but loss of appetite may also arise from numerous organic causes, particularly cancer. Hyperphagia with weight gain may be a sign of diabetes mellitus (eating habits reflect rapidly changing blood glucose levels) or may occur in atypical cases of depression or rare cases of ventromedial hypothalamic disorders. Diarrhea may be due to irritable bowel syndrome or a malabsorption syndrome. Diarrhea accompanied by nausea, polyuria, and polydipsia may be a sign of lithium toxicity. Hypomotility or atony of the bowel, on the other hand, may be caused by use of psychiatric medications with anticholinergic properties (eg, tricyclic antidepressants, low-potency neuroleptics, and antiparkinsonism medications).

E. Genitourinary System: Frequency of urination is a cardinal symptom of diabetes mellitus but may also reflect anxiety states, use of diuretics, or lithium toxicity. Inability to initiate urination should suggest anticholinergic toxicity in patients taking psychiatric medications and is a major concern in elderly men with prostatic hypertrophy. Episodes of incontinence, if accompanied by loss of consciousness, suggest either vasovagal phenomena or seizures. Spinal cord lesions (eg, secondary to trauma or multiple sclerosis) above the S1–2 level can produce a spastic bladder. The triad of dementia, ataxia, and incontinence in an elderly individual should raise the question

of normal-pressure hydrocephalus—a potentially reversible condition.

PHYSICAL EXAMINATION

The patient's general appearance tells the clinician a great deal about the severity and acuteness or chronicity of the illness. Failure to note subtle or obvious signs of physical illness may lead to prolonged, costly, and unnecessary or inappropriate treatment. Detection of a physical sign, on the other hand, may afford the physician unexpected leverage in treating an illness that was initially thought to be psychiatric. It is the rule rather than the exception that medical illnesses have behavioral manifestations and emotional consequences. In addition, some somatic illnesses present with psychiatric symptoms.

Vital Signs

It is essential to record vital signs early in therapy with psychiatric patients—if possible before medications are started or before they are changed. Orthostatic measurements (with the patient lying supine and then standing) of pulse and blood pressure are particularly valuable.

A. Pulse: Tachycardia may reflect anxiety, pain, or ingestion of adrenergic agonists or anticholinergic substances. Furthermore, some arrhythmias (especially paroxysmal atrial tachycardia) produce marked anxiety. Bradycardia is common in patients with anorexia nervosa. Return of the pulse rate to the normal range in these patients is one means of monitoring protein ingestion.

B. Blood Pressure: Hypertension has multiple medical causes and places the patient at significant risk of cerebrovascular and cardiovascular accidents as well as renal complications. Situational stress may elevate blood pressure on a transient or chronic basis. Concurrent ingestion of monoamine oxidase inhibitors and wines or cheeses containing tyramine may lead to dangerous episodes of hypertension. Some antihypertensive drugs can produce episodes of major depression and may also cause impotence. In addition, psychotropic medications may produce postural hypotension via peripheral blockade of alpha-adrenergic receptors.

C. Temperature: Hypothermia is a potentially dangerous complication of antipsychotic medications in the elderly. Hyperpyrexia may reflect infection anywhere in the body (including the central nervous system), atropine poisoning, toxicity due to dopamine-blocking agents ('neuroleptic malignant syndrome'), or the hypermetabolic state of delirium tremens.

D. Respiratory Rate: While hyperventilation may arise in the context of stress disorders, anxiety states, or panic attacks, it may also reflect metabolic acidosis with a compensatory respiratory drive. Central respiratory drive may be diminished by barbiturates, benzodiazepines, alcohol, or brainstem compression or lesions.

Head

Evidence of head trauma such as skull deformities or scars should be noted. Patients may be amnestic for the actual event if the trauma was associated with loss of consciousness. An increase in cranial circumference or an unusual cranial shape suggests congenital abnormalities or developing hydrocephalus.

A. Face and Mouth: Hyper- or hypotelorism (wide- or narrow-set eyes) may suggest congenital central nervous system abnormalities. Adenoma sebaceum (multiple papules over the bridge of the nose and cheeks) occurs in tuberous sclerosis. A "port wine" stain over the second division of the fifth cranial nerve suggests Sturge-Weber syndrome. A "butterfly" rash over the nose and cheeks suggests the possibility of systemic lupus erythematosus. A round or moon-shaped face may reflect idiopathic Cushing's disease or ingestion of corticosteroids. Hair loss from the lateral eyebrows occurs in syphilis, leprosy, and hypothyroidism. A sore, raw tongue reflects vitamin deficiency; a large tongue, hypothyroidism; and greenish discoloration of the tongue, brominism. Repetitive tongue movements are common in edentulous patients but may also be seen in patients with involuntary buccal, lingual, and masticatory movements (tardive dyskinesia), which may occur as a late complication of neuroleptic drug use. Regular tremor of the lips (an early parkinsonian complication of dopamine-blocking drugs) has been termed the "rabbit syndrome." Lack of facial expression may be a symptom of schizophrenia, major affective disorder, dementia, or idiopathic Parkinson's disease or may reflect drug-induced akinesia.

B. Eyes: Dilated pupils may reflect stress, anticholinergic toxicity, or hyperadrenergic states secondary to amphetamine abuse. Constricted pupils suggest ingestion of a narcotic, but brainstem lesions at the pontine level may also cause pinpoint pupils. Herniation of the uncus (a structure on the medial aspect of the temporal lobe) secondary to increased intracranial pressure compresses the pupilloconstrictor fibers of the third cranial nerve, causing the ipsilateral pupil to become fixed and dilated. Extraocular muscles may be affected in Wernicke's encephalopathy, in progressive supranuclear palsy, or following ingestion of phencyclidine, phenytoin, or barbiturates. Copper-colored rings at the limbus of the iris (Kayser-Fleischer rings) are a hallmark of Wilson's disease.

Neck

Thyroid enlargement or tenderness is significant, since symptoms of both hyper- and hypothyroidism can be mistaken for primary psychiatric disease. Carotid bruits suggest advanced atheromatous disease and have special significance if the individual has a history of transient ischemic attacks, reversible neurological deficits due to ischemia, or stroke. Neck stiffness with pain on flexion (meningismus) suggests meningeal irritation. Involuntary torsion of the head and neck to one side (torticollis) may occur as drug-induced dystonia or in association with dystonia musculorum deformans, a rare neurological disorder.

Heart

Congestive heart failure (characterized by a third or fourth heart sound on auscultation) may be associated with hypoxia, anergy, and agitation. Unless the cardiac condition is recognized, "psychiatric signs" may be mistakenly treated with antianxiety, antipsychotic, or antidepressant medications. The midsystolic click of a prolapsed or "floppy" mitral valve is increasingly recognized in association with anxiety attacks. Tachycardia can arise secondary to anxiety or to use of psychoactive medications.

Lungs

Hypoxia from any cause (including asthma, congestive heart failure, pneumonia, pneumothorax, or pulmonary embolism) may produce either quiet or agitated confusional states. Pneumonia is a reversible cause of dementia syndromes in the elderly.

Abdomen

The presence of multiple surgical scars may suggest any of a number of psychiatric illnesses (eg, conversion disorder, somatization disorder, chronic factitious illness, repeated ingestion of foreign bodies by schizophrenic individuals or by patients with borderline personality disorder) or may suggest the numerous abdominal crises seen in acute intermittent porphyria. Hepatomegaly and vascular spiders suggest chronic alcohol abuse.

Skeleton

Bony abnormalities may reflect congenital defects or may have arisen slowly in the context of collagen vascular disease. The cranioskeletal abnormalities of gigantism most frequently arise secondary to pituitary dysfunction.

Extremities

Palmar erythema suggests collagen vascular disease or hepatic disease. Multiple laceration scars over the inner aspects of the forearms or wrists are stigmas of multiple suicidal gestures occasionally seen in severely ill patients with borderline personalities. Clubbing of the digits may reflect cardiac or pulmonary disease. Yellowish staining of the fingertips suggests a smoking habit. The tremor of Parkinson's disease is initially a resting tremor of the hands and may be unilateral. Other forms of tremor may be seen with lithium use, in hyperadrenergic states (eg, anxiety, amphetamine abuse, alcohol withdrawal), or in benign familial (essential) tremor. The central obesity of

Cushing's disease is accompanied by peripheral loss of fatty tissue, with the skin of the hands taking on the quality of parchment.

NEUROLOGICAL EXAMINATION

Cranial Nerves

A. Cranial Nerve I (Olfactory): Is there unilateral or bilateral anosmia secondary to trauma and disruption of the olfactory bulb fibers as they travel through the cribriform plate, or is there unilateral anosmia secondary to a meningioma of the olfactory groove? Does the patient report olfactory hallucinations (schizophrenia versus irritation of the medial temporal lobe)?

B. Cranial Nerve II (Optic): If visual acuity is poor, does it improve if the patient puts on glasses or looks through a pinhole (the pinhole corrects for refractive errors)? Is the patient taking anticholinergic drugs that impair the pupillary constriction required for near vision? Is there a homonymous visual field cut, suggesting a lesion of the optic chiasm or tract, visual radiations, or visual cortex; or is there monocular blindness, suggesting lesions anterior to the chiasm (ie, damage to the optic nerve or retina)? Examination of the fundi may demonstrate blurring of the disk margins (associated with increased intracranial pressure) or arteriolar narrowing that suggests hypertension.

C. Cranial Nerves III (Oculomotor), IV (Trochlear), and VI (Abducens): If nystagmus is present, does it reflect therapeutic or toxic levels of drugs (eg, barbiturates or phenytoin) or alcohol intoxication or withdrawal? Is the nystagmus secondary to phencyclidine ingestion? If gaze paralysis is present, is it caused by thiamine deficiency associated with Wernicke's encephalopathy or by abducens palsy (often a nonspecific sign of increased intracranial pressure), or does it reflect the internuclear ophthalmoplegia seen in multiple sclerosis? Is there limitation of vertical gaze, as seen in progressive supranuclear palsy or with pineal tumors (Parinaud's syndrome)?

D. Cranial Nerve V (Trigeminal): Is facial sensation intact over all three branches of the trigeminal nerve? In cases of conversion (hysterical) anesthesia, sensory loss usually extends to the mandibular angle (innervated by the second cervical nerve).

E. Cranial Nerve VII (Facial): Is there facial asymmetry either at rest or on spontaneous motion? Is the entire hemiface involved (peripheral lesion), or is the forehead spared (central lesion)? Is a cortical lesion suggested by aphasia with right facial paralysis or by aprosody (loss of speech melody) with left facial palsy?

F. Cranial Nerve VIII (Acoustic and Vestibular Components): Is there sensorineural or conductive hearing loss? High-frequency hearing loss (presbycusis) is common in the elderly. Before diagnosing "hysterical" gait disorder, be certain the patient does not have position-induced vertigo secondary to labyrinthine dysfunction.

G. Cranial Nerves IX (Glossopharyngeal) and X (Vagus): Is the gag reflex intact, absent (patient at risk for aspiration), or overly brisk (associated with the "emotional incontinence" of pseudobulbar paralysis)? Swallowing is a complex act and may be grossly impaired despite an intact gag reflex.

H. Cranial Nerve XI (Accessory): Is there asymmetry of sternocleidomastoid muscle strength or diminished bulk of the trapezius muscle on palpation? In cases of conversion (hysterical) weakness, patients often complain of inability to turn the head toward the side of weakness. Patients with hemispheric lesions producing true weakness of limb movement and head turning will demonstrate weakness on turning the head away from the side of weakness.

I. Cranial Nerve XII (Hypoglossal): Does the tongue deviate from the midline? If so, is this a sign of a brainstem lesion, or does it reflect a supranuclear lesion of cranial nerve VII?

Motor System

A. Muscle Mass: Is there asymmetry of face, body, or limb muscle mass (congenital versus disuse atrophy following stroke versus neuropathic or myopathic)?

B. Muscle Tone: Is there parkinsonian cogwheel rigidity, lead pipe rigidity of an upper motor neuron disease, or the flaccidity of a lower motor neuron disease? Are muscles rigid secondary to dystonia? Is there the "waxy flexibility" of cataleptic catatonia or the rigid resistance of negativistic catatonia? Does the examiner encounter the ratchet-like gegenhalten (paratonia) of frontal lobe disease, characterized by increasing resistance in response to the examiner's attempts to passively move the patient's limbs at increasing speeds?

C. Strength: Strength may be graded on a 6-point scale in which 5 = normal strength, 4 = movement against gravity and applied force, 3 = movement against gravity only, 2 = movement with gravity eliminated, 1 = trace movement, and 0 = no movement. Attention is paid to comparisons of left versus right, proximal versus distal, and upper versus lower motor strength.

D. Coordination: Is performance impaired on testing of finger-to-nose, heel-to-shin, and rapidly alternating (rhythmic) movements (all suggesting cerebellar hemispheric disorders), or does ataxia affect chiefly the lower limbs and trunk (suggesting midline cerebellar disorders)? Beware of inferring coordination deficits in the presence of weakness.

E. Reflexes:

1. Deep tendon reflexes–Are tendon reflexes symmetrical or asymmetrical? Is there hyperreflexia consistent with upper motor neuron disease, or does areflexia accompany flaccid paralysis? A brisk jaw jerk suggests bifrontal disease. Diffusely brisk reflexes may be seen in withdrawal from alcohol, benzodiazepine, or barbiturates; catatonic excitement; hyperthyroidism; or magnesium or calcium deficiency. Diffusely sluggish reflexes may be seen in hypothyroidism and barbiturate or benzodiazepine intoxication.

2. Pathological reflexes–

a. Babinski's sign–Does stimulation of the plantar surface of the foot produce plantar flexion (''down-going'' toe) or dorsiflexion (extension) of the great toe? An ''upgoing toe'' suggests pyramidal tract (upper motor neuron) lesions that may be at the level of the spinal cord, brainstem, or brain.

b. Primitive reflexes–Can reflexive sucking, grasping, rooting, or snouting be elicited? Reappearance of these reflexes suggests diffuse frontal lobe disorders. A unilateral grasping reflex may indicate involvement of one frontal hemisphere.

F. Gait and Station: Does the patient walk in a stooped fashion, with slow shuffling steps and diminished arm swing? If so, is this parkinsonian picture drug-induced or idiopathic? Is gait wide-based and ataxic? Gait ataxia may be due to alcoholic intoxication, permanent ataxia secondary to alcoholic cerebellar degeneration, or intoxication with antipsychotic agents such as phenobarbital. Is one leg moved forward in circumduction and the arm on that side held in flexion over the chest? This occurs most commonly following stroke of the contralateral hemisphere.

G. Movements: Is there asymmetry of movement (paralysis, neglect), poverty of movement, or excess of movement? Are there spontaneous dyskinetic movements (Huntington's chorea, tardive dyskinesia, levodopa-induced dyskinesia, Wilson's disease), tremors (resting parkinsonian tremor, benign familial tremor, cerebellar ''intention'' tremor), myoclonic jerks, or fasciculations?

Sensation

Sensory loss is characterized with reference to location and to the modalities involved. Does the patient fail to respond only to pinprick and changes of temperature, or is there also diminished proprioceptive sensation? Is the deficit limited to one extremity, or are upper and lower extremities involved symmetrically (evidence of polyneuropathy)? Is the loss of sensation a crude'' inability to perceive the stimulus, or is it instead a specific inability to localize or recognize the stimulus? Tests of sensory extinction (failure to perceive sensation on one side of the body when bilateral areas are simultaneously stimulated), stereognosis (ability to recognize and name an object after feeling its shape), or graphesthesia (ability to recognize a number or letter ''written'' on the skin) allow the clinician to recognize syndromes of cortical sensory loss associated with parietal lesions.

LABORATORY EXAMINATIONS & OTHER DIAGNOSTIC TESTS

Just as the physical examination provides an opportunity to confirm or refute hypotheses formulated on the basis of the history and review of systems, the request for laboratory and other diagnostic tests should also derive from and be dictated by findings in the history, review of systems, and physical examination. If utilized in this way, the laboratory provides relevant diagnostic and prognostic data that benefit the patient and allow clinicians to sharpen their observational skills. Indiscriminate ordering of laboratory tests, on the other hand, is costly, short-circuits the traditional medical practice of careful examination leading to formulation of hypotheses, and can be detrimental to the patient-physician relationship.

Laboratory tests are essential elements of the modern psychiatrist's diagnostic and therapeutic resources. Even as recently as a decade ago, this was not the case.

Biological tests in psychiatry may be anatomic (CT scan of the head), functional (EEG, dexamethasone suppression test, thyroid function tests, creatinine clearance, positron emission tomography), or diagnostic (Venereal Disease Research Laboratories [VDRL] test for syphilis). Advances in psychopharmacology in the last two decades have demanded refined quantitative measures of medication levels. Over the next decade, research advances in psychiatry and neuroimmunology may require psychiatrists to become conversant with biological probes of the immune system.

This section discusses the role of laboratory and other diagnostic studies in general psychiatric practice. Some of the laboratory tests described are used primarily as research tools and are not in routine use in clinical practice (eg, dexamethasone suppression test, PET scan). It cannot be emphasized too strongly that negative test results do not constitute proof that organic disease is not present. Normal findings on neurological examination, for example, do not rule out a demyelinating process that is in remission any more than negative findings on electroencephalography rule out a seizure disorder. Thus, test results must always be viewed as part of the larger clinical picture.

Diagnostic Workup

A. Delirium: The workup of a delirious patient is similar to that of a demented patient (see below). Special concern, however, is directed toward the toxicology screen. Among the substances for which psychiatrists most often screen are the following: heavy metals (mercury, lead, arsenic); hallucinogens (LSD, phencyclidine, tetrahydrocannabinol); atropinic substances (phenothiazines, antidepressants, sedatives, antiparkinsonism drugs); stimulants (amphetamines, cocaine, methylphenidate); central nervous system depressants (alcohol, phenobarbital, phenytoin); anxiolytics (benzodiazepines, meprobamate); and pain medications (morphine, heroin, hydromorphone, meperidine).

B. Dementia: The following is a list of tests that should be considered before the diagnosis of senile dementia of the Alzheimer type is made.

1. Blood, plasma, or serum values–Hemoglobin, hematocrit, white blood cell count, vitamin B_{12}, folic acid (red blood cell), sodium, calcium, magnesium, creatinine, urea nitrogen, glucose (fasting), bilirubin (direct and indirect), total protein, partial thromboplastin time, aspartate aminotransferase, thyroxine, erythrocyte sedimentation rate, arterial blood gases, and ceruloplasmin (in patients under 50 years of age).

2. Antigen and antibody tests–Fluorescent antinuclear antibody (FANA) test, VDRL test for syphilis, *Treponema pallidum* hemagglutination (TPHA) test, and fluorescent treponemal antibody absorption (FTA-ABS) test.

3. HIV testing–HIV testing is an essential element in the workup, especially for patients in high-risk groups (ie, intravenous drug users, patients with a history of blood transfusions, and homosexuals).

4. Other studies–

a. Chest x-ray.

b. Electrocardiography–A baseline ECG is important before starting treatment with drugs, because many psychotropic medications may produce tachycardia or other arrhythmias.

c. Electroencephalography–The EEG may be helpful in documenting dysrhythmia or epileptic discharge. Provocative maneuvers such as sleep, sleep deprivation, and photic stimulation may be used to lower the seizure threshold. Nasopharyngeal leads may facilitate detection of medial temporal lobe spike activity.

Epilepsy is ultimately a clinical diagnosis, and findings on the EEG may or may not corroborate the diagnosis. Abnormal electroencephalographic tracings may be seen in patients who never have clinical seizures. Likewise, patients with frank clinical seizure disorders may have unremarkable electroencephalographic tracings. Many patients with hysterical seizures (pseudoseizures) also have a history of true seizures. Observation of a clinical seizure with concomitant electroencephalographic tracings that show no epileptic discharge makes possible a diagnosis of pseudoseizure. It does not exclude a coexisting true seizure disorder, however.

The EEG is extremely helpful in assessing toxic, metabolic, and infectious causes of confusion. In the vast majority of organically-induced confusional states the EEG will show slowing. One important exception is barbiturate delirium, in which the EEG is characterized by excessive fast activity.

d. Computerized tomography (CT)–CT scan of the head allows the clinician to examine serial sections of brain. Computerized calculation of tissue density not only identifies abnormal structures but also indicates their nature (eg, cerebrospinal fluid, air, bone, blood). The psychiatric evaluation of any patient over the age of 40 years with no prior psychiatric illness should include a CT scan of the head.

CT scan of the head is an essential tool in the investigation of dementia syndromes. Although generalized atrophy of the brain correlates poorly with the degree of cognitive dysfunction, focal atrophy of the frontal and temporal lobes may suggest a history of Pick's disease or significant closed head injury. Isolated infarction of strategic brain regions (eg, dominant inferior parietal lobe, hippocampus, or dorsomedial thalamus) may produce dementia or amnestic syndromes, whereas numerous infarctions can combine to produce the picture of multi-infarct dementia. Other structural abnormalities to be excluded in the workup of dementia include brain tumors (primary or metastatic), subdural hematomas, and normal-pressure hydrocephalus. Chronic abusers of alcohol, some schizophrenics, and a subpopulation of elderly patients with depression (but without dementia) have abnormal findings on CT scan of the head. Findings such as these, along with possible applications in the treatment of patients with neurobehavioral disorders, indicate that brain imaging will become increasingly important in psychiatric assessment.

e. Magnetic resonance Imaging (MRI)–The advent of MRI presents an attractive alternative to CT scanning, Because this new imaging method does not rely on ionizing radiation, it may be safely performed on the same individual repeatedly. Other advantages of MRI over CT scanning include (1) enhanced resolution of gray-white boundaries; (2) greater sensitivity to edema; and (3) absence of bone-induced artifact in studies of the spinal cord, posterior fossa (brainstem and cerebellum), and orbital frontal regions (which are frequently contused in closed head injury).

f. Lumbar puncture–This procedure is usually performed to detect evidence of hemorrhage, infection, or cancer involving the central nervous system. In the presence of an unrecognized space-occupying lesion of the brain, a sudden drop in cerebrospinal fluid pressure following lumbar puncture may result in herniation of the uncus through the tentorial notch. This in turn compresses the brainstem, leading to stupor, coma, or death. Therefore, lumbar puncture is performed only after a CT scan of the head has been done. A needle is inserted in the L4–5 interspace, and 5–10 mL of fluid is withdrawn. Opening and closing pressures, as well as gross appearance (color and turbidity) of the fluid, are noted. Samples are assayed for cell count, cell type, and protein and glucose levels; submitted for VDRL and FTA-ABS tests for syphilis; and stained and cultured for bacterial and fungal organisms. Special studies such as protein electrophoresis and viral antigen tests may also be performed.

g. Positron emission tomography (PET)–In contrast to the CT scan of the head, which provides static or structural information, the PET scan (currently a research tool) offers a means of monitoring local central nervous system metabolism, ie, examining brain function in vivo. PET scanning offers tremendous promise for finding physiological correlates of psychiatric disorders in which no gross structural deficits exist.

h. Pneumoencephalography–This procedure essentially has been replaced by CT scan of the head.

C. Depression:

1. Levels of 3-methoxy-4-hydroxyphenylglycol (MHPG)–In the mid 1970s, it was suggested that urinary or cerebrospinal fluid levels of MHPG (a metabolic breakdown product of norepinephrine in the central nervous system) could be useful to the clinician in selecting an appropriate tricyclic antidepressant. Original hypotheses suggested that patients with low urinary MHPG levels would be more likely to respond to imipramine than to amitritpyline. Recent work has shown that amitriptyline and imipramine both increase serotonin levels at the synaptic cleft, while their demethylated analogues (nortriptyline and desipramine) primarily potentiate increases in norepinephrine. Thus, it seems reasonable that depressed individuals with low MHPG levels may respond best to tricyclic antidepressants such as nortriptyline and desipramine, which have relative specificity for noradrenergic systems.

2. Dexamethasone suppression test–The development of the dexamethasone suppression test as a biological probe of the hypothalamic-pituitary-adrenal axis (eg, for diagnosis of Cushing's disease) was initially hailed as a landmark for biological psychiatry, Proceeding from the observation that some depressed patients have high serum cortisol levels, researchers soon discovered that these levels failed to be suppressed in response to exogenous corticosteroid administration, a response also found in patients with Cushing's disease.

The dexamethasone suppression test (as modified for psychiatric use) is performed by giving 1 mg of dexamethasone orally at 11:30 PM, obtaining serum samples at 4 and 11 PM the following day, and measuring serum cortisol levels. If either of these two cortisol levels is 5 μg/dL or greater, the patient is described as "failing to suppress" and thus is said to have a positive, or abnormal, response.

Although at first the test was thought to have high specificity (few false-positive results), it is now known that many patients with dementia (without depression) have abnormal dexamethasone suppression test results. Moreover, the test is only 50% sensitive, yielding a significant number of false-negative results.

Because of the increasing number of false-positive results (eg, in patients with dementia and schizophrenia), few indications exist at present for clinical diagnostic use of the dexamethasone suppression test.

Nevertheless, since suppression of cortisol levels correlates with a good response to both electroconvulsive treatment and antidepressant agents, serial tests may be helpful in monitoring drug responses.

a. Causes of false-positive results–These include pregnancy (high doses of estrogens), Cushing's disease or syndrome, major physical illness (as well as trauma, fever, dehydration, nausea), severe weight loss (malnutrition, anorexia nervosa), hepatic enzyme induction (eg, with use of phenytoin, barbiturates, meprobamate), and uncontrolled diabetes mellitus.

b. Causes of false-negative results–These include Addison's disease, corticosteroid therapy, hypopituitarism, and therapy with high doses of benzodiazepines.

3. Thyrotropin-releasing hormone (TRH) stimulation test–TRH, a tripeptide released from the hypothalamus, stimulates secretion of thyroid-stimulating hormone (TSH) from the pituitary. In normal patients, injection of synthetic TRH (protirelin) produces an increase in TSH level of about 5 μU/mL. About 25% of depressed patients have an increase of less than 5 μU/mL, and 60–70% have an increase of less than 7 μU/mL. Recent work suggests that the TRH stimulation test and the dexamethasone suppression test detect different *subpopulations* of depressed patients, since there is only a 30% overlap in results.

The protocol is as follows: The patient should be instructed to take nothing by mouth for 8 hours prior to the test. A baseline TSH level is obtained before administration of protirelin, 0.5 mg intravenously, infused over 1 minute. The TSH level is determined at 30 minutes. An increase of less than 5 μU/mL (blunted response) is abnormal.

A major question about the test is whether it detects trait or state abnormalities, since blunted TSH responses persist following treatment.

Psychiatric conditions that may cause false-positive results (blunted response) include mania, alcohol withdrawal, and anorexia nervosa. Other conditions causing false-positive results include old age, starvation, chronic renal failure, Klinefelter's syndrome, and testing repeated too frequently (pituitary TSH levels may be depleted if the test is done more often than once a week).

4. Thyroid function tests–Thyroid function tests are an integral part of the assessment of both depression and mania as well as dementia syndromes.

Monitoring Therapeutic Drug Levels

A. Lithium: Careful monitoring of serum lithium levels is essential in the management of any patient receiving this medication. Different individuals tolerate or require different levels of lithium. While acutely manic patients may require and tolerate blood levels of 1–1.8 meq/L, a therapeutic blood level for one individual may be a toxic blood level for another.

Elderly individuals, for example, are occasionally maintained effectively at a blood level of 0.4 meq/L and show signs of toxicity when levels rise to 0.6 or 0.7 meq/L. Because lithium is cleared from the central nervous system more slowly than from the peripheral circulation, it may be prudent to discontinue (rather than simply lower the dosage of) lithium if toxicity occurs. 1 here are well-documented reports of toxicity continuing for as long as 1 week after serum lithium levels have fallen well below the therapeutic range.

B. Tricyclic Antidepressants: Methods to evaluate blood levels of tricyclic antidepressants have been available in research settings since the early 1970s. With the exception of nortriptyline, however, they have generally not been used. Nortriptyline is unique in that it appears to possess a "therapeutic window." Specifically, it has been observed that depressed patients do best when they have nortriptyline blood levels of 50–150 ng/mL.

Studies of tricyclic antidepressants have indicated that there may be as much as a 20-fold difference in blood levels among age-matched individuals receiving the same dosage. Thus, failure to respond to an antidepressant medication may reflect not only lack of patient compliance but also individual differences in absorption, metabolism, or excretion of the drug.

C. Anticonvulsants: Methods are available to evaluate blood levels for all of the well-known anticonvulsant medications. Regular monitoring of serum levels is essential in managing individuals with seizure disorders. Levels may fluctuate, depending on other drugs taken by the patient. The physician should determine patient compliance before evaluating whether seizures are refractory to certain medications. Carbamazepine (Tegretol) is a tricyclic anticonvulsant medication that also has psychotropic effects and is emerging as a mainstay in the treatment of complex partial (temporal lobe) seizures. Early reports suggest that a subset of individuals with bipolar affective disorder (manic-depressive illness) also respond to treatment with carbamazepine.

REFERENCES

Bailey H: *Demonstration of Physical Signs in Clinical Surgery,* 15th ed. J. Wright & Sons, 1973.

DeJong RN: *The Neurologic Examination,* 4th ed. Harper & Row, 1979.

Fisher CM: Quantitation of deficits in clinical neurology. Trans Am Neurol Assoc 1969;94:263.

Lee SH, Rao KCVG: *Cranial Computed Tomography.* McGraw-Hill, 1983.

Patten J: *Neurological Differential Diagnosis.* Harold Starke, 1978.

Plum F, Posner JB: *The Diagnosis of Stupor and Coma,* 3rd ed. Davis, 1982.

Rowland LP (editor): *Merritt's Textbook of Neurology,* 7th ed. Lea & Febiger, 1984.

Weiner HL, Levitt LP: *Neurology for the House Officer,* 2nd ed. Williams & Wilkins, 1978.

13

Intelligence Testing & Neuropsychological Assessment

Edward L. Burke, PhD

A diagnostic test may be defined in the broadest sense as an attempt to ascertain the presence or absence—or the excess or deficiency—of some function or condition. Medical research has led to the development of a great number of tests for a wide variety of conditions, and a parallel development can be traced in psychology during the last century.

The attempt to apply scientific methods to human behavior, which gave rise to the modern discipline of psychology, began in the latter part of the 19th century.

INTELLIGENCE TESTING

The early "psychologists" received their first professional training in a variety of other disciplines. Many were educators with special interests in the applications of psychology to the problems of the mentally retarded or of the gifted. They set out to define the criteria for intelligence and to normalize them on large samples of subjects, but controversies arose—still not entirely resolved—concerning the nature of intelligence and how it might be measured. The most basic argument was whether intelligence consisted of a single general factor, designated **g,** which might manifest itself in a variety of ways, or whether what we call intelligence in fact consists of a number of correlated but distinct skills.

However one resolves the controversy theoretically, in practice the most widely used individually administered intelligence tests measure performance in several different areas. The Wechsler intelligence scales serve as an example.

The original Wechsler-Bellevue Intelligence Scale (1939) has gone through several stages of change. The currently used tests are the **Wechsler Adult Intelligence Scale–Revised** (WAIS-R) and the **Wechsler Intelligence Scale for Children–Revised** (WISC-R). The scales for adults and children have the same structural design, but the material used is adapted to different age levels. The WAIS-R and the WISC-R are each divided into two sections, verbal and performance, each with its separately calculated intelli-

gence quotient (IQ). These sections are further divided into subtests: the verbal section into information, comprehension, similarities, arithmetic, digit span, and vocabulary; the performance section into digit symbol, block design, picture completion, object assembly, and picture arrangement. Each of these subtests has also been normalized, with a mean score of 10 and a standard deviation of 3.

Administration of the test to children has the advantage of providing indications for remedial or educational interventions. While such interventions may also be available for adults, they inevitably become less useful with the passage of time.

The Wechsler scales yield a standardized IQ that is normalized separately for each age group. The Stanford-Binet test based the IQ on "mental age" as a percentage of "chronological age." For example, IQ = 100 when mental age and chronological age are the same; IQ = 150 when mental age is 1.5 times chronological age; and IQ = 50 when mental age is 0.5 times chronological age. As a result, IQ declines steadily as chronological age increases once adult mental age has been achieved. On the Wechsler scales, subjects' IQ scores are compared with those of other individuals in the same age group. This makes the WAIS-R useful in measuring the intelligence of older people.

Controversies regarding intelligence tests have not been limited to the question of whether or not what we call intelligence is a single factor or a function of many. Important social issues have been raised regarding the cultural bias of tests (in favor of certain ethnic or socioeconomic groups) and the way in which test scores might be used in making decisions about access to educational opportunity.

The stratification of the sample used to normalize the 1981 edition of the WAIS-R represents an attempt to eliminate such bias. For the most part, data from the 1970 United States census were used. Equal numbers of men and women were included for each age group. Whites and nonwhites were included in approximately the same proportion in which they occur in the population, as reflected in census data collected in 1975 and 1977. The population samples were drawn pro rata according to population density from four major geographic areas. The sample was additionally stratified according to occupational groups and for educational levels. Even after all these efforts, the sample would not be perfect, but the complexity involved shows the problems that confront test designers and the ways in which they try to overcome them. Examples of updating and cultural broadening of material in the information subtest are questions related to Amelia Earhart, Marie Curie, Martin Luther King, Albert Einstein, and Louis Armstrong, replacing questions regarding Longfellow, Homer, and others.

The distribution of IQ scores in the actual sample of the WAIS-R closely parallels that of a theoretical normal curve. With a score of 100 as the mean and a standard deviation of 15, scores from 90 to 109 are characterized as "average." Scores from 80 to 89 and 110 to 119 are considered "low average" and "high average," respectively. Scores from 70 to 79 are "borderline," and scores from 120 to 129—the corresponding scores on the upper side—are "superior." Finally, scores of 69 or below are categorized as "mentally retarded," whereas at the upper end, scores of 130 and above are called "very superior." About 2.5% of the total sample falls in each of the latter two categories.

The most obvious misuse of an intelligence test such as the Wechsler would be to reduce its findings to a single numerical result—the IQ. From what has been said about the standardization of each subtest, it is clear that a person might conceivably have a mean score of 100 but subtest scores almost entirely in the "very superior" and "borderline" ranges.

It should be clear also that factors other than intelligence may influence performance on an IQ test. Consider the apathetic or rebellious adolescent who is required to take the test. Fatigue, illness, or medication may also adversely affect performance, as well as personality traits that cause one subject to "freeze" at the sight of a stopwatch while another becomes energized by the prospect of a timed test.

In practice, the WAIS-R or WISC-R is most frequently administered as one part of a battery of psychological tests. Just how the test results are used will depend upon what the diagnostic question is. As with all other tests, the results are most meaningful in the context of a carefully elicited history.

The information and vocabulary subtests strongly reflect educational experience and family milieu. A bright person might score low on these subtests if illness, isolation, or other factors have impoverished these aspects of life. Arithmetic and digit span can be interfered with by anxiety. Similarities test the capacity for abstraction, while comprehension tests the subject's understanding of what is appropriate or effective in a variety of problem situations. All of these subtests are called **verbal tasks** because the medium of the response is words. In contrast, the **performance tasks**—such as reproducing designs

with blocks, arranging pictures in a meaningful sequence, and assembling parts of a puzzle—are responded to in nonverbal ways.

While almost everyone will do better on one section of the test than the other, scores for the verbal and the performance sections are usually in the same general range. Any notable disparity (eg, 15 points) requires investigation. Given the mainly left-brain and right-brain tasks of the respective parts of the test, one might suspect organic brain damage in such cases, but the possible interpretations are by no means limited to that one explanation. Thought disorders may be detected in bizarre or idiosyncratic answers on the information, comprehension, similarities, or picture arrangement subtests.

Although the Wechsler scales are not expressly designed to detect organic deficits as such, they can be useful as screening devices. As discussed in the next section, Wechsler performance subtests such as digit symbol, block design, and object assembly may confirm or refine findings on simple neuropsychological tests.

NEUROPSYCHOLOGICAL TESTING

Impairment of psychological functions such as perception, concentration, memory, reasoning, or speech may occur at any age, suddenly or gradually, and may be transient or permanent. Impairment may be related to some event such as an injury or accident or may not be attributable to any apparent cause.

In such cases it is important to establish, to the extent possible, the relative contributions of psychological and organic factors. Since these factors may interact in complex ways, most test batteries include tests aimed at identifying both elements. A test battery may be designed to explore the area suspected of being more important, with additional tests aimed at picking up indications of other deficits. If such indications are positive, the lead can then be pursued by further testing.

Screening Tests for Gross Organic Deficits

A number of relatively simple tests frequently included in psychological test batteries are helpful in identifying gross indications of organic mental disorder. One of the most frequently used tests of this type is the **Bender Gestalt Test,** which consists of a series of nine geometric patterns to be copied from models by the subject. Most people can draw the figures without great difficulty. The size and arrangement of the figures may occasionally suggest specific personality characteristics, but one may also encounter rotations of figures or gross distortions suggestive of perceptual or motor difficulties.

A simple test that presents little difficulty for most subjects but may prove extremely difficult or impossible for organically impaired patients to perform is the **Trail-Making Test,** which has two parts. The first part (Trails A) consists of a series of numbers, each enclosed in a circle, spread out on a page. The task is to connect the numbers in proper sequence by drawing a line from one circle to the next until all the circles have been joined. The second part (Trails B) presents a more complicated variant of the same task: The subject is asked to connect the circles in sequence alternating back and forth between numbers and the letters of the alphabet—1, A, 2, B, 3, C, etc.

Several subtests of the WAIS-R (described above) are useful in picking up gross organic deficit. Examples are **block design** (reproducing designs with blocks), **object assembly** (arranging parts of a puzzle), and **digit symbol** (pairing arbitrarily assigned symbols with numbers), the latter being the most sensitive. If scores on these subtests are notably low either absolutely or relative to verbal subtests or to previous scores on these same subtests, organic impairment is strongly suggested.

Halstead-Reitan Battery

The tests and subtests described above are used mainly as screening devices. Other tests explicitly intended to assess neuropsychological impairment in greater detail are available but are costly and time-consuming; they are not ordinarily requested unless there is clear evidence of an organic deficit that requires more detailed examination. The best known set of tests of this type is the Halstead-Reitan battery, an elaborate and complicated series of tests that requires extensive training in its administration and interpretation. It is usually done on referral to a specialist in neuropsychology.

The Halstead-Reitan battery grew out of Halstead's research, begun at the University of Chicago in the 1930s. Halstead employed a battery of 27 behavioral tests in his studies of the effects of brain lesions. About ten have come to be known as the **Halstead Impairment Index.** The impairment index for an individual subject is determined simply by counting the number of tests on which the results fall in the range characteristic of the performance of brain-damaged rather than of normal subjects.

Ralph Reitan set up a program at Indiana University Medical Center aimed at an experimental study of the effects of brain lesions, using several of Halstead's tests. Reitan and his associates administered this elaborate battery individually to almost 2000 patients (usually requiring 1–1½ days for testing each subject). In addition to assessing the presence or absence of brain damage on the basis of test findings, Reitan has gone on to investigate patterns of psychological test results that seem to identify locations and types of brain lesions.

The battery includes the Minnesota Multiphasic Personality Inventory (see Chapter 14), the Wechsler-Bellevue Intelligence Scale (Form I), both parts of the Trail-Making Test (see above), and the following tests:

A. Category Test: This test utilizes a projection apparatus for presenting stimulus material. It is a complex concept-formation test that requires the subject to note similarities and differences in stimulus material; to put forward hypotheses to explain recurring similarities and differences in the stimulus material; to test these hypotheses following positive and negative reinforcement; and to adapt hypotheses as a function of the reinforcement received. The main purpose of the test is to determine the subject's ability to use both negative and positive experiences as a basis for altering performance. Each successful interpretation of the set pattern receives a positive score.

B. Test of Critical Flicker Frequency: The subject is asked to indicate the point at which a variably intermittent light is perceived as a steady light. An additional score is based on the subject's deviation from the first score on five successive trials. This test by itself shows no significant differences between groups with and without brain damage. It remains, however, in the Halstead-Reitan battery.

C. Tactual Performance Test: This test utilizes blocks of various shapes, each of which has a correspondingly shaped space cut into a board. The subject is blindfolded and not permitted to see the board or blocks at any time. The ability to place the variously shaped blocks in their proper spaces depends upon tactile form discrimination, kinesthesia, manual dexterity, and visualization of the spatial configuration of the shapes in terms of their spatial interrelationships on the board.

D. Rhythm Test: This is a subtest of the Seashore Test of Musical Talent. The subject is required to differentiate between pairs of rhythmic beats that are sometimes the same and sometimes different. The subject receives a positive score for each correct discrimination. The test requires alertness, sustained attention to the task, and the ability to perceive and compare rhythmic sequences.

E. Speech-Sounds Perception Test: This test consists of 60 spoken nonsense words that have a syllable containing the sound / ee / . The words are played from a tape recorder. Several variant spellings of each word are listed on a printed sheet (''theeks,'' ''zeeks,'' ''theets,'' ''zeets''). The subject listens to each word and then selects the corresponding spelling from the multiple-choice form.

F. Finger Oscillation Test: This test is a measure of tapping speed, using the index finger, first of the dominant hand and then of the other hand. The subject is allowed five consecutive trials of 10 seconds each for both hands. Performance on this test is dependent almost purely on motor speed. This subject's score is the average of the five trials.

G. Time Sense Test: In this test of visual perception and memory, the subject is required to depress a key that permits a sweep hand to rotate on the face of a clock. The task is to allow the hand to rotate ten times and then to stop it as close to the starting position as possible. The face of the clock is then turned away, and the subject is asked to duplicate the visually controlled performance as closely as possible. The memory component score consists of the number of deviations from the initial perception.

H. Aphasia Examination: This is an adaptation of the Halstead-Wepman Aphasia Screening Test. It samples the subject's ability to name common objects, spell, identify individual numbers and letters, read, write, calculate, enumerate, understand spoken language, identify body parts, and differentiate between right and left. Each of these various abilities is examined in terms of the particular sensory modalities through which the stimuli are perceived. The test also provides an opportunity for judging whether the deficit is receptive or expressive in character. (See Chapters 5 and 11 for more information on aphasia and aphasia testing.)

The interpretation of test battery results is a complex procedure that cannot be described briefly. In a study of 50 patients with brain damage and 50 control subjects with no evidence of brain damage (matched in pairs for race, age, sex, and education), Reitan found that none of the brain-damaged persons had lower impairment indices than their matched controls. Using the best cut-off point in the two raw score distributions, he determined that only 4% of the brain-damaged group had been misclassified. He concluded that the Halstead Impairment Index serves as a valid and reliable basis for inferring the presence or absence of brain damage in individual subjects.

One cannot predict in individual instances which test or tests may be of crucial help. While the impairment index, category test, and localization component of the tactual performance test are generally the most helpful measures, one of the other tests sometimes proves to be particularly important for assessment of individual patients. For the fine points of the clinical application of the individual tests, one may consult Reitan's extensive writings (see references).

Reitan's work has not been limited to an effort to determine the type and location of brain lesions. Additional investigations in his laboratory have been invaluable not only in providing hypotheses for formal investigation but also in furnishing insights into the complexity of brain-behavior relationships in human beings and the limitations and qualifications that must accompany most generalizations.

Batteries Based on Luria's Approach

An alternative approach to the evaluation of local injuries to the brain has been developed by A.R. Luria of the Soviet Union. In Luria's opinion, current psychological tests are too complex and provide no more than gross evaluations of cognitive processes.

He has assumed that complex behavioral processes are in fact not localized but distributed in broad areas of the brain and that the contribution of each cortical zone to the organization of the whole functional system is quite specific. He has accordingly undertaken a careful analysis of specific disturbances in the neuropsychological examination for diagnosis of focal brain injury. Luria's approach has been gaining adherents, but his methods are not yet widely used in the USA.

On the basis of Luria's approach and techniques, Christensen (1979) developed a battery to test ten neuropsychological functions. Many common tests are incorporated into this battery, including elements of the mental status examination such as digit span, certain memory tests, and serial 7s (see Chapter 11). Detailing the variety of tests in Christensen's adaptation of Luria's neuropsychological investigation is beyond the scope of this text. The reader is referred to the writings of Christensen (1979) and Lezak (1983).

Christensen's battery adapts its tests to the needs of each patient (as does Luria's "experimental" approach); thus, the results are difficult to interpret. The battery is not comprehensive, and most patients will require further testing—eg, of intelligence and some memory functions not already covered in the battery.

Golden and his colleagues at the University of Nebraska (1981) developed a standardized battery from the many tests used by Luria and Christensen. The battery, called the **Luria-Nebraska Neuropsychological Battery,** tests the ten functions referred to above. The scales for scoring correspond to the ten functions but with reading and writing placed on separate scales and with motor and tactile functions scored on right-hemisphere, left-hemisphere, and pathognomonic scales. Although standardized, this battery suffers from some of the same limitations as Christensen's battery. The Luria-Nebraska battery distinguishes between normal controls and neurologically impaired patients, but its reliability and usefulness have been questioned (Lezak, 1983).

Luria's contributions to neuropsychological assessment are the flexibility and individualized approach to test subjects. Christensen's battery captures the process; the Luria-Nebraska battery standardizes the tests used.

Other Batteries

In *Neuropsychological Assessment,* Lezak (1983) describes several other batteries and composite tests for brain damage, including one of her own design. In addition, she describes many other neuropsychological tests. Of interest and relevance are the aphasia tests developed by Kaplan and associates (Goodglass and Kaplan, 1972; Kaplan et al, 1978). The reader is referred to these works and to the discussions on aphasia testing in Chapters 5 and 11.

REFERENCES

Bender L: *A Visual Motor Gestalt Test and Its Clinical Use.* Research Monograph No. 3. American Orthopsychiatric Association, 1938.

Christensen AL: *Luria's Neuropsychological Investigation,* 2nd ed. Wiley, 1979.

Golden CJ et al: A standardized version of Luria's neuropsychological tests. In: *Handbook of Clinical Neuropsychology.* Filskov S, Boll TJ (editors). Wiley, 1981.

Goodglass H, Kaplan E: Assessment of Aphasia and Related Disorders. Lea & Febiger, 1972.

Halstead W: *Brain and Intelligence: A Quantitative Study of the Frontal Lobes.* Univ of Chicago Press, 1947.

Kaplan E, Goodglass H, Weintraub S: *The Boston Naming Test.* Lea & Febiger, 1978.

Lezak MD: *Neuropsychological Assessment,* 2nd ed. Oxford Univ Press, 1983.

Matarazzo JD: *Wechsler's Measurement and Appraisal of Adult Intelligence,* 5th ed. Oxford Univ Press, 1972.

Reitan R: The comparative effects of brain damage on the Halstead Impairment Index and the Wechsler-Bellevue Scale. Clin Psychol 1959;15:281.

Reitan R: An investigation of the validity of Halstead's measures of biological intelligence. Arch Neurol Psychiatry 1955; 73:28.

Reitan R: The relation of the Trail Making Test to organic brain damage. J Consult Psychol 1955;19:393.

Reitan R: The validity of the Trail Making Test as an indicator of organic brain damage. Percept Mot Skills 1958;8:271.

Reitan R, Davison L (editors): *Clinical Neuropsychology: Current Status and Applications.* Winston, 1974.

Wechsler D: *The Measure and Appraisal of Adult Intelligence.* Williams & Wilkins, 1961.

Wechsler D: *Wechsler Adult Intelligence Scale-Revised.* Harcourt Brace Jovanovich, 1981. Wechsler D: *Wechsler Intelligence Scale for Children–Revised.* Harcourt Brace Jovanovich, 1981.

Zimmerman I, Woo-Sam J: *Clinical Interpretation of the Wechsler Adult Intelligence Scale.* Grune & Stratton, 1973.

Personality Assessment

14

Daniel S. Weiss, PhD

When Osler suggested that the patient was more important than the disease, he was emphasizing the importance of understanding the life circumstances and personality of the individual patient. When physicians make diagnoses, whether of somatic or psychiatric disorders, they must also consider the nature of the person who has the disorder. Concern with the psychological context in which the symptoms appear helps the clinician understand the meaning and implications of the presenting complaint and the particular symptom pattern. What the current episode of illness means to the patient and what coping resources and personal strengths and weaknesses the patient possesses will influence the clinician's approach to evaluation, setting of treatment objectives, and choice of treatment plans.

Personality is the composite of enduring attributes of an individual's psychological makeup. Today, despite agreement on the importance of a patient's personality in understanding the presentation of symptoms and the choice of treatment for virtually any mental disorder, there are still fundamental questions about what personality is and how it should be defined.

DEFINITIONS OF PERSONALITY

There are probably as many definitions of personality as there are authors who have written about the subject. Allport's (1937) definition is as apt as any: "Personality is the dynamic organization within the individual of those psychophysical systems that determine his unique adjustments to his environment." Two German terms, representing two views of personality, further explain the concept. *Persönlichkeit* denotes the distinctive impression that someone makes on another. This word derives from the Latin *persona* and connotes the sense we get about how individuals choose and perform their social roles. Behind the mask, however, is a complex player donning various roles. The term *personalität* denotes this more fundamental or basic concept of personality used in psychiatric clinical situations. This definition of personality, which goes beyond exhibited behaviors to reach the core of identity, is considered by some to be synonymous with the term *self* and is a key concern in psychodynamics.

DSM-III-R CLINICAL EVALUATION OF PERSONALITY TRAITS & DISORDERS

In *DSM-III-R,* axis II is used to record observations about personality, including personality traits and, when appropriate, personality disorders. *Personality traits* are defined as "enduring patterns of perceiving, relating to, and thinking about the environment and oneself, and are exhibited in a wide range of important social and personal contexts." The diagnosis of *personality disorder* is made "only when personality traits are inflexible and maladaptive and cause either significant impairment in social or occupational functioning or subjective distress." In addition, a person may meet diagnostic criteria for a personality disorder (eg, borderline personality disorder) and also demonstrate histrionic or avoidant personality traits. All of this information is recorded on axis II in a complete clinical evaluation according to *DSM-III-R.*

The major clinical and diagnostic dilemma is determining when (at what point or under what circumstances) a set of personality traits (or the patient's "personality") becomes "maladaptive" or is "overly rigid." Personality assessment is one tool the clinician employs in making decisions about the nature and range of a patient's personality.

The major use of personality assessment, however, is in the context of an overall request for diagnostic psychological testing. In these circumstances, not only are personality measures employed, but some ability testing is also used (see Chapter 13). The most frequent use of this type of assessment procedure is for evaluation of the patient with a myriad of problems and possible causes. Psychological testing is often used to rule in or rule out some potential diagnoses. For example, some personality disorder may occur along with moderate brain dysfunction and a profound learning disability. A second typical occasion for personality assessment is in the forensic arena for custody evaluations, parole decisions, or criminal responsibility evaluations.

PERSONALITY ASSESSMENT PROCEDURES

This chapter will focus on the standardized procedures used by properly trained and experienced clinicians to describe an individual's personality. This description may be in terms of either the more overt impression made by the patient *(Persönlichkeit)* or the more basic temperament of character *(Personalität)*. Most frequently, assessments incorporate aspects of both views of personality. The goals of assessment usually consist of one or more of the following: (1) to assess psychological processes, (2) to assess personality traits, (3) to assess psychological structures, (4) to aid in diagnosis, and (5) to formulate treatment plans.

FEATURES OF PSYCHOLOGICAL TESTS FOR PERSONALITY ASSESSMENT

Standardization

The greatest advantage of using psychological tests for personality assessment is that both the stimuli used to elicit information and the conditions under which the stimuli are administered are standardized. This means that differences in response may be attributed to differences in the respondents. Using standardized procedures eliminates this undesirable source of variability in personality assessment.

Another important feature of standardization is the use of "fixed-choice" responses. This limitation on how responses may be made—for example, answering only "true" or "false" to the questions on the Minnesota Multiphasic Personality Inventory (MMPI)—facilitates comparison of personality assessments by one individual with that of others. Because another source of information that might vary is held constant, other types of information about personality are made clearer.

In personality assessment tools with fixed-response formats, the scoring or keying of responses is also fixed. For example, the patient may respond only "true" or "false" to item 181 on the MMPI: "When I get bored, I like to stir up some excitement." The manner in which the choice affects the score is also standardized: If the patient responds "true," this scores a point on the basic clinical scale measuring hypomania. If the patient answers "false," the score on this and all other scales is not affected. The meaning of this single response in terms of personality assessment is not subject to interpretation by the examiner or by the clinician. With the MMPI, the clinician's contribution lies in interpreting the pattern of scale scores (see below).

Although stimuli (eg, the ten inkblot cards of the Rorschach test) are standardized, each card is not just one more of the same thing; ie, the stimuli are not interchangeable. In the Rorschach inkblots, there is a range of variation in certain dimensions (color, clarity, form). Used as a set, they are standardized, but certain stimuli tap certain personality processes. Similarly, in the MMPI, some items are scored on more than one scale (eg, on scales of depression and schizophrenia), while others are scored only on one scale or only on the other. In personality assessment, this explains the usual clinical practice of using a battery of psychological tests that vary in types of procedures, stimuli, response formats, and scoring methods. The end result is a test battery that evokes a wide range of responses indicating different aspects of personality.

Reliability & Validity

An essential feature for psychological tests of personality function is that they be both reliable and valid. If a measure is **reliable,** its results are stable or consistent across administrations assuming that nothing about the patient's personality has changed. Without reliability, a purported measure of personality is useless.

A measure or set of measures is said to be **valid** if it actually measures what the authors claim it does. For example, a measure of defensiveness should be related to other indices of being defensive, such as being reluctant to acknowledge failings or presenting an exaggerated socially desirable self-description. At the same time, to be valid a measure should not be related to indices that are conceptually independent. The measure of defensiveness, for example, should not be related to intelligence or degree of depression.

Careful research is required to establish the reliability and validity of measures of personality so that their use can assist in diagnostic assessment and treatment planning. Caution is required in the use of any but the most established and well-researched measures.

CLASSIFICATION OF PSYCHOLOGICAL TESTS FOR PERSONALITY ASSESSMENT

Psychological tests are most easily classified as either objective or projective. A clever explanation of the distinction is offered by the psychologist George Kelly (1958): "When the subject is asked to guess what the examiner is thinking, we call it an objective test; when the examiner tries to guess what the subject is thinking, we call it a projective device." There are, of course, psychological tests and assessment devices that do not neatly fit into these categories, but most are predominantly one or the other.

Objective Tests

Objective tests are tests whose scoring (numerical results) can be produced mechanically. This generally implies that the response format is standardized. Examples of such tests in personality assessment are the MMPI, the California Psychological Inventory (CPI), Millon Clinical Multiaxial Inventory. Another objective test familiar to medical students is the Medical College Admission Test. What is not objective in such tests is the meaning of the results or scores. As shown in the clinical example in Chapter 15, the training, experience, and skill of the psychologist come into play in the interpretation and synthesis of the results of the various tests.

Projective Tests

Projective tests are less structured than objective tests in response format and in scoring. The term projective was coined by Frank (1939), based on the following assumption: Because of the unstructured and ambiguous nature of the stimuli and response options available to the respondent, the responses must be *projections* of the patient's "way of seeing life, his meanings, significances, patterns, and especially his feelings." In projective methods, the kinds of responses are not fixed, scoring is usually time-consuming, several scoring systems often exist for each technique, scoring may differ from clinician to clinician, and the interpretation of the results of projective methods frequently requires integrative thinking on the part of the clinician. The best-known example of a projective test is the set of inkblots developed by Rorschach.

MINNESOTA MULTIPHASIC PERSONALITY INVENTORY (MMPI)

The MMPI is the most thoroughly researched objective personality assessment instrument. Item development and testing began in the late 1930s. The test authors, Hathaway and McKinley (a psychologist and a psychiatrist), undertook the mammoth task of test construction, recognizing the acute need for an objective measure of various dimensions of psychopathological disorders to aid clinicians in diagnosis and treatment planning. The MMPI was designed to provide for multiphasic assessment of psychopathological changes in much the same way that medical checkups are multiphasic.

In 1989, MMPI-2 was introduced, an updated version designed to preserve the best of the original measure but to address some of the dated item phrases and mechanics of administration and to add some new items so that assessment would be in accord with current diagnostic conceptions. Many psychologists have applauded the appearance of MMPI-2, but others are cautious about recommending its use until more data are gathered. The scoring and some of the normative data are different enough from the origi-

nal version so that many clinicians who have used MMPI routinely are not ready to switch.

Administration

The MMPI comprises 556 True or False items; the MMPI-2 has 567. In the most popular version of the MMPI, the items were arranged in booklet form so that the first 399 were all that were needed for the basic scales. The patient is instructed to read each item and decide "if it is true as applied to you or false as applied to you." Typically, test subjects use a computer-scannable answer sheet.

Scoring & Scales

The items comprising the various scales were selected by empirically determining which ones distinguished between groups of interest. In this way, the authors of the MMPI and the MMPI-2 did not decide at the outset how paranoid patients would respond to different items. Scoring is based on data that indicate how paranoid patients respond to the items as compared to controls.

The results from either the MMPI or the MMPI-2 are scores on three validity scales and seven clinical scales. These scores are expressed in T-scores and typically plotted on a profile. T-scores have a mean of 50 and a standard deviation of 10. One major difference between the original MMPI and the MMPI-2 is how the T-scores are calculated; this is why many clinicians are still cautious in using the MMPI-2. For an individual patient tested with both the old and the new versions, the same scores may not mean the same thing.

The validity scales of both versions indicate how likely it is that the patient responded truthfully and accurately. Some patients respond in a pattern indicating a wish to appear healthy; others respond as if they want to appear disturbed. Finally, the validity scales can pick up random responding—eg, when a patient loses his or her place on the answer sheet so that the marks are off by one or two items for the last hundred. Finally, problems in reading and comprehension may be spotted by the validity scales.

The clinical scales of MMPI and MMPI-2 index a variety of useful personality dimensions. The hope that they would be truly multiphasic has now been abandoned. Nonetheless, it would be very rare for a personality assessment to be conducted without the MMPI or MMPI-2. The clinical scales are Hypochondriasis, Depression, Hysteria, Psychopathic Deviate, Masculinity-Femininity, Paranoia, Psychasthenia, Schizophrenia, Hypomania, and Social Introversion. The scale names are only broad labels, and detailed information about exactly what they measure is beyond the scope of this chapter.

In addition to the standard scales, there are scales for Alcoholism, posttraumatic stress disorder, and a whole set of Personality Disorder Scales. For these additional scales as well as for the standard scales, it should be emphasized that they are not like a medical diagnostic test. There is no instances where a certain score establishes a specific diagnosis. Rather, the scales assemble a pattern of tendencies that probably characterize that patient and may help a clinician or judge make a decision about management or disposition in an individual case.

Interpretation

It is probable that about 90–95% of MMPI and MMPI-2 tests scored are also interpreted with the aid of some type of computerized formula. These are an outgrowth of the early use of MMPI code-types on the profiles in the 1950s and 1960s. Some of the current programs can be used on a personal computer; others are commercially and centrally operated and generate a four- or five-page single-spaced report. These computerized interpretive reports have the advantage of being done blind to everything about the subject except age, sex, and perhaps educational level and marital status. Thus, the conclusions cannot be influenced by other clinical information. However, they also have the disadvantage of being uninformed about certain trends that could modify conclusions. In any case, almost all reports rightly emphasize that the results are not specific but are based on statistical trends observed in other patients with very similar score profiles. In this respect, such results need to be viewed more as hypotheses to be synthesized with other data rather than "facts" about the patient.

RORSCHACH PSYCHODIAGNOSTICS

The set of ten published Rorschach inkblots is part of a series developed and used by the Swiss psychiatrist Hermann Rorschach in his clinical research. Rorschach was interested in fantasy, and he noticed that specific kinds of blots evoked fairly consistent responses from certain groups of patients. These findings were published in his monograph (1942), but his work was cut short by his death at the age of 38.

The Rorschach technique is probably the best-known personality assessment measure. This is due not only to the extremely widespread use of the technique but also to early claims and hopes that it could and would provide an "x-ray" of the mind. Despite this mystique about the Rorschach technique, it is actually among the most thoroughly researched measures used in all of psychological testing, and today there is good documentation of its range of usefulness as well as its limitations. Much of the credit for this work is due to the psychologist John Exner, whose system of administration and scoring is now the standard in the field (Exner, 1974; Exner, 1990).

Administration

The ten inkblots are ambiguous stimuli that provoke associations. The standard series is reproduced on cards that are 18 × 24 cm (7 × 9½ inches) and numbered from I to X. Card I is shown in Figure 14–1. Five of the blots (I, IV, V, VI, and VII) are in black and white; the others include colors. The examiner gives the patient a statement of directions explaining that a series of inkblots will be shown and that the patient will be asked to tell what they look like. When the first card is offered, the patient is asked, "What might this be?"

During the first phase of the test, the **free association phase,** the examiner records each response as nearly verbatim as possible, notes the orientation of the blot for each response (eg, upside down), and interferes as little as possible.

After all ten blots have been presented, there is usually an **inquiry phase.** Each blot is given back to the patient, and the examiner reads back the patient's response and asks what about the blot prompted that response. During this phase of the procedure, patients may give additional responses. These are noted, and the same inquiry procedure is followed for these additional responses. Even though new responses may be made during the inquiry phase, *only free association responses are scored.*

Scoring

The great bulk of the work is devoted to scoring the responses. There is no one "official" scoring procedure. Major scoring systems were developed in the late 1930s and early 1940s. More recently, Exner (1974;1990) has proposed an integrative scoring system with more detailed normative data, and this system has become the standard for scoring.

All of the major scoring systems follow Rorschach original scheme in noting these four categories: (1) location, (2) determinants, (3) contents, and (4) popularity. Exner uses two other categories: organizational activity and form quality. Exner's scoring system is presented below.

A. Location: Scoring of location is based on the part of the inkblot used as the basis for the response. The common categories of location are (1) the whole blot, (2) a common detail, (3) an unusual detail, and (4) the white space around or in the middle of

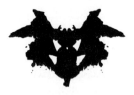

Figure 14–1. Card 1 of the Rorschach Psychodiagnostics, reduced to one-sixth of actual size. (Reproduced with permission of the copyright holder, Hans Huber AG Buchhandlung Verlag.)

the blot. (All of the scoring categories use abbreviated symbols, such as W for whole, but the full set is only of interest to advanced examiners.)

B. Determinant: Scoring of determinants is based on the qualities of the blot that were used in forming the percept, ie, what made it look like the object described by the patient. The major categories of determinants are (1) form, (2) movement, (3) color (chromatic), (4) color (achromatic), (5) texture (shading-derived), (6) dimensionality (shading-derived), (7) shading (general or diffuse), (8) dimensionality (form-derived), and (9) pairs and reflections.

C. Content: There are 27 content categories. Examples with Exner's numbers are (1) whole human, (7) animal detail, (14) blood, (19) fire, (25) sex, and (26) x-ray.

D. Popularity: There are specific responses given frequently to specific cards. Exner has tabulated 13 popular responses; several are listed here, with popularity number shown in parentheses and Rorschach card number shown in brackets: (1) [I] bat or butterfly; (6) [IV] animal skin or human figure dressed in fur; (10) [VII] human heads or faces, usually those of women or children; and (13) [X] crab, lobster, or spider.

E. Organizational Activity: The scoring of organizational activity is indexed by the symbol Z. It is a complex feature to score, and it deals with the patient's process of integrating the various features of the inkblot to form an organized and coherent percept.

F. Form Quality: Most scoring systems evaluate how well the percept "fits" the actual blot. Exner uses a 4-level system for scoring quality of fit: superior (+), ordinary (o), weak (w), and minus (–). The minus response is defined as "the distorted, arbitrary, unrealistic use of form as related to the content offered, where an answer is imposed on the blot area with total, or near total, disregard for the structure of the area."

Interpretation

Despite the heavy and involved emphasis on scoring, conclusions about personality structure and functioning have come less from formal scoring and more from a movement back and forth between what theory suggests about psychopathological disorders and what the responses to the Rorschach inkblots suggest about the patient's style of processing information. Although Exner's scoring system is quite detailed and empirically based, his instructions for interpretation are much less mechanical. They emphasize a 2-stage process of (1) initially generating many hypotheses about defenses, contact with reality, intelligence, fantasy life, and sexuality, based on the formal scoring of the whole record, the specific scoring of each response, the sequence of responses, and the content of the verbalization; and (2) integrating the hypotheses and modifying or ruling out the contradictory ones.

After this process, a coherent personality description is written.

Although some writers have argued that interpretation of the Rorschach record should be blind, without reference to any other information about the patient, this method is not recommended. The Rorschach technique is not a parlor game; it is an aid to understanding personality functioning. As such, all available information about the person's functioning is useful. If several psychological tests have been used, Exner recommends that the Rorschach record be examined first, so that some hypotheses are not prematurely ruled out by non-Rorschach information.

Issues in the Use of the Rorschach Technique

Despite the great strides made by Exner in standardizing scoring, the value of the Rorschach technique in personality assessment continues to depend almost exclusively on the clinician's write-up of the record, which involves some degree of subjectivity. This makes it difficult to evaluate the technique, but some conclusions are possible.

First, by itself, the Rorschach record *cannot* provide a diagnosis. Hypotheses about personality styles or defenses can be entertained, but it is inappropriate to use the Rorschach record to validate these hypotheses. Second, Exner's work amply demonstrates that there are *no universal meanings* for any card. There is no "father card," "mother card," or "sex card," as many writers have argued. Third, the administration process is as ambiguous as the blots are. The record of responses may be influenced by characteristics of the examiner or by the context in which the examination takes place. Fourth, like psychodynamic formulations of conflict and defense, the yield from a Rorschach record must be viewed as a working formulation to be modified on the basis of other information as it becomes available.

THEMATIC APPERCEPTION TEST (TAT)

The TAT was designed to elicit important personality themes from fantasy-based stories told by the patient in response to somewhat ambiguous pictures. Like the Rorschach technique, the TAT is a projective test designed to assess underlying personality processes—in this case, underlying needs. The procedure was developed by Morgan and Murray (1935) as part of a study of normal personality done at the Harvard Psychological Clinic.

Administration

The test materials consist of 31 cards (30 drawings and fuzzy photographs plus one blank card). Murray suggested that each subject be shown only 20 cards, and he designated some to be used only for boys

(B), others for girls (G), and others for male or female adults (M or F). The following are a few examples of pictures (descriptions and numbers are taken from the TAT manual): *Card 2:* Country scene: In the foreground is a young woman with books in her hand; in the background, a man is working in the fields and an older woman is looking on. *Card 3BM:* On the floor against a couch is the huddled form of a boy with his head bowed on his right arm. Beside him on the floor is a revolver. *Card 6GF:* A young woman sitting on the edge of a sofa looks back over her shoulder at an older man with a pipe in his mouth who seems to be addressing her. *Card 12F:* The portrait of a young woman. A weird old woman with a shawl over her head is grimacing in the background. *Card 13MF:* A young man is standing with downcast head buried in his arm. Behind him is the figure of a woman lying in bed.

In clinical practice today, most examiners use fewer than 20 pictures and limit the testing to a single administration. The pictures selected depend upon the examiner's personal preference and intuitive notions about what important dynamic areas of the patient's personality may be illuminated by particular cards. The examiner records verbatim the story given by the patient and should attempt to be as unobtrusive as possible throughout the session. Some writers recommend that patients be prompted to give outcomes for their stories if these are not produced spontaneously; opinions on this procedure vary.

Scoring & Interpretation

Unlike the Rorschach technique, the TAT does not separate scoring from interpretation. Murray's original suggestions involved conceptualizing the story material in terms of (1) the **hero** of each story (presumably the individual with whom the subject identifies); (2) the **needs** (inner states) of the subject for various activities or gratifications (need for aggression, need for achievement); (3) **the press,** ie, the environmental context in which the subject assumes the hero is operating and which influences the hero's needs; and (4) the **thema,** a term indicating the motivational Lends of the hero in responding to the combination of needs and stress.

Other methods of interpreting the TAT are linked to conceptual or theoretic systems, such as psycho-analysis or jungian typologies, or to specific content areas of academic research in psychology, such as motivation to achieve and need for power.

BROAD ISSUES IN PERSONALITY ASSESSMENT BY PSYCHOLOGICAL TESTING

Three themes have run through the discussion of psychological tests in this chapter.

(1) Despite the search for standardization and uniformity in the use of psychological tests for personality assessment, different clinicians have different systems. Thus, the interpretation of a battery of psychological tests depends upon who does the interpreting. In an analogous fashion, the test results depend upon who the patient is; results may be accurate indicators of personality, or they may reflect *individual differences in responses that are not primarily indicative of personality*. This is why tests do not have perfect predictability and why it is difficult to determine with high accuracy a complete picture of a patient's personality.

(2) The research evidence about the utility of testing has been disappointingly mixed. It is not clear how much more information is gained by using the MMPI, the Rorschach technique, and the TAT, for example, rather than just one or two of the tests. In this area, clinicians have been somewhat resistant to take seriously the research evidence, viewing it as simplistic, naive, and not in touch with clinical realities. There are clinical examples in which results of the battery of tests have suggested a personality assessment that is not what any one test would have suggested. The issue here is one of cost- and time-effectiveness. Like laboratory tests in clinical medicine, psychological tests must be evaluated for redundancy, cost, and possibility of yielding incremental information.

(3) The major area requiring more careful scrutiny is the area of agreement among clinicians—not in scoring of psychological tests but in interpreting the results. If trained clinicians cannot reach an acceptable level of agreement about interpretation, then more structured formats for interpretation must be developed to aid in standardizing the kinds of categories used and inferences made from the testing results.

REFERENCES

Allport GW: *Personality: A Psychological Interpretation.* Holt, 1937.

Butcher JN et al: *Minnesota Multiphasic Inventory (MMPI-2). Manual for Administration and Scoring.* Univ Minnesota Press, 1989.

Exner JE: *The Rorschach: A Comprehensive System.* Vol 1. Wiley, 1974.

Exner JE: *A Rorschach Workbook for the Comprehensive System,* 3rd ed. Rorschach Workshops, 1990.

Frank LK: Projective methods for the study of personality. J Psychol 1939;8:839.

Hathaway SR, McKinley JC: *Minnesota Multiphasic Personality Inventory Manual.* Psychological Corporation, 1951.

Kelly GA: Man's construction of his alternatives. In: *The Assessment of Human Motives*. Lindzey G (editor). Rinehart, 1958.

Morgan CD, Murray HA: A method for investigating fantasies: The Thematic Apperception Test. Arch Neurol Psychiatry 1935;34:289.

Murray HA: *Thematic Apperception Test Manual*. Harvard Univ Press, 1943.

Rorschach H: *Psychodiagnostics*. Huber, 1942; Grune & Stratton, 1951.

15

The Clinical Case Summary: The Mayor of Wino Park

Howard H. Goldman, MD, PhD

The following is a case study of the Mayor of Wino Park, briefly introduced as a character sketch in Chapter 9. The standard sequence for presenting clinical psychiatric cases is set forth in Table 15–1. The hypothetical data needed to complete this clinical case summary would have been collected during the Mayor's 3-week hospitalization, when he underwent an extensive evaluation, including all of the elements presented in Chapters 10–14. Although the case is presented here primarily to demonstrate the form and content of a case summary, the details of the case also illustrate the complex interaction of biological, psychological, and social factors in medicine and psychiatry.

CASE SUMMARY

Identifying data: John F. ("Red") Kimball is 54 years old, divorced, unemployed, currently subsisting on Social Security Disability Insurance (SSDI) benefits, and living on the streets or in Wino Park, a protected urban camping ground in San Francisco. The night manager of the Billings Hotel on Pine Street receives and holds the patient's monthly

check. The patient prefers to be addressed as Mayor and referred to as the Mayor.

Informant: The patient is a poor historian. Throughout his hospital stay, his responses to inquiries have been marked by inconsistencies, gaps, and confabulation. His ability to give a useful past history has improved as his attention span increases with treatment, but his history of the present illness continues to be marred by deficits in short-term memory.

To supplement the history, we obtained medical records from previous hospitalizations, outpatient clinic records, and school and military records. No work history documentation could be obtained, nor could any family member be located to verify the history. During an earlier admission, a lifelong acquaintance corroborated much of the patient's early life history as presented in this case study.

Chief complaint: "They closed Wino Park—and I'm yellow, have the shakes, and somebody's trying to poison me. . . ."

History of the present illness: While living in Wino Park off and on for the past 5 years, the Mayor had been in good health except for a few episodes of depression treated with tricyclic antidepressants and supportive psychotherapy. During the past year, he appointed himself mayor of all of the homeless alcoholics and other unemployed and mentally ill people who slept in the park. He felt he was their spokesman, and during the past 3 months, after it was announced that the park was to be closed, he felt under constant pressure to "save" their haven. He began giving impromptu "news conferences" to anyone who would listen at downtown intersections during rush hour—or before groups of tourists waiting for cable cars. He also began to drink more heavily than ever at that time, consuming several quarts of wine daily.

About 10 weeks prior to the present admission, the Mayor was arrested for threatening an officer who attempted to take him into custody when he was found drunk, wandering the streets. He was released the next morning, but the desk sergeant

Table 15–1. Suggested format for a clinical case summary.

Identifying data
Informant (sources of information) and assessment of
  reliability
Chief complaint
History of the present illness
Past medical and psychiatric history
Review of systems
Habits
Family history
Social history
Developmental history
Physical examination
Neurologic examination
Mental status examination
Diagnostic tests
Differential diagnosis
Provisional psychosocial formulation
Hospital course
Multiaxial diagnosis
Psychosocial formulation
Continuing treatment plan and disposition

thought he seemed depressed and perhaps in need of medical evaluation, so he was sent to the hospital in a police ambulance. He admitted he had been in a "black mood" for the past couple of weeks, with no appetite, and had been losing weight, waking up at night, and then unable to get back to sleep. He was obviously agitated and said he could not concentrate and thought a lot about death when he wasn't casting about for some magical solution to the Wino Park "crisis," as he saw it. His preoccupation with death and veiled threats of suicide ("Maybe I'll end it") led to his admission to a psychiatric inpatient unit for observation and protective detention. He signed himself out after 72 hours, proclaiming, "There's nothing wrong with me!" His discharge diagnosis was recurrent unipolar depression. He refused to stay in the hospital for a trial of treatment with antidepressant medication. He could not be committed, because he denied suicidal intentions and had not developed delirium tremens. He also refused referral to an outpatient clinic.

The Mayor continued to be depressed and drank "to kill the pain of going insane" and to stop the "shakes." There was no apparent change in his condition until 2 weeks before the present admission, when he became jaundiced, more agitated, confused, and paranoid. He was afraid that someone had contaminated the wine with some kind of poison or "Yellow Dye Number Nine," and he was organizing people to march to the liquor stores to pull the wine off the shelves. At that point he was sleeping only a few hours a night. He became extremely irritable (euphoric one moment, angry the next), and his scheming, grandiosity, and paranoid ideation increased. His speech was pressured, tangential, and at times almost incomprehensible. The "people's press conferences" at downtown intersections became disruptive, and the police were called on several occasions, but there were no arrests or contacts with the health care system until the day of admission.

On the day of admission, Wino Park was closed, and all of the homeless men and women were being turned out or relocated. The Mayor refused to go. When the police said they would have to arrest him if he did not leave, he became agitated, running around furiously and talking loudly. All of the pathological thought, affect, and behavior of the previous 2 weeks intensified. He threatened loudly that he would kill anyone who touched him and then kill himself. When he seemed close to collapse from exhaustion, the police grabbed him, handcuffed him, called for an ambulance, and drove him to the hospital again.

Past medical and psychiatric history: Medical records indicate that the patient was the 35-week product of a difficult pregnancy and labor compli-

cated by abnormal maternal bleeding secondary to multiple small uterine fibroid tumors. The patient's mother had a hysterectomy following delivery; she was separated from her baby for 4 weeks, unable to nurse him, and then was hospitalized for depression for 4 months postpartum.

During childhood, the patient had measles, mumps, and chicken pox but no other infectious diseases except for an occasional cold. A fractured clavicle at age 8 years was inflicted by his alcoholic father. He had an appendectomy at age 13, shortly after his mother died. (The appendix was normal, according to the pathology report.)

At age 20, the patient received a medical discharge from the navy for a "character disorder" and was noted to be an alcoholic and occasional binge drinker. Between the ages of 20 and 35, he was working, married, and in excellent health. He was divorced at age 35, and his drinking increased. (For details, see Social History.) For the next 5–10 years, his work history was interrupted by several admissions to alcohol treatment centers, outpatient alcohol counseling, and periods of ambulatory psychiatric treatment for depression. Once, while depressed, he was treated with thyroid hormone; he became acutely psychotic and agitated and was thought to have bipolar affective disorder (manic depressive illness).

At age 45, the patient became severely depressed and suicidal. He was committed to a state mental hospital because he had refused treatment in a voluntary general hospital psychiatric unit. On admission, he was heavily sedated with antipsychotic medication because of agitation and auditory hallucinations consisting of voices commanding him to kill himself. Because of the imminent danger of suicide, he underwent a course of 12 electroconvulsive treatments, which dramatically improved his mental status, especially his agitation and suicidal ideation. He remained somewhat depressed and stayed in the hospital for 3 months. A trial of tricyclic antidepressants and supportive psychotherapy was successful in further reducing his symptoms, and he was discharged with a prescription for amitriptyline, 200 mg daily at bedtime. He went to live in a single-room occupancy hotel in the "Tenderloin district" of San Francisco. He was seen as an outpatient for several years in a clinic operated by the county, but his drinking was not controlled, and he stopped his medication. He was readmitted to various hospitals several times. As noted earlier, his sole source of support was SSDI funds. The night manager at the hotel serves as his conservator.

The patient became so mentally disorganized, paranoid, and unmanageable that he could no longer stay at the hotel. He was accepted at a board and care home for alcoholic men but would not agree to the restrictions. He could not be committed to a hospital, because he was not dangerous to himself or others, and so he began his life on the streets and in Wino Park 5 years prior to the current admission.

The Mayor has no documented history of endocrine disorders, including thyroid disease and Cushing's syndrome. He has no history of acute liver disease, gastritis, or other gastrointestinal disorders, although his liver enzyme levels have been elevated in the past. There is no record of jaundice prior to this illness. He has never had delirium tremens or any seizure disorder, and he has no known allergies.

Review of systems: In addition to having the symptoms and signs mentioned in the history of the present illness, the patient admits to seeing double from time to time and losing his footing occasionally. Pertinent negative findings include the absence of focal neurological and endocrinological signs and symptoms (other than those mentioned above, eg, diplopia, tremor) and no abnormalities in stool color.

Habits: The Mayor drinks up to 2 quarts of wine daily. He has been drinking since he was 12 years old; he admits to having been a binge drinker as a teenager and an alcoholic since his 20s. There is no other history of drug abuse. He has smoked one package of cigarettes daily since age 15, plus occasional cigars.

Family history: The patient is the only child of Francis Kimball and Jean-Marie Thibodeau Kimball. Francis Kimball died at age 55, when the patient was 35, of injuries sustained in an accident at the state mental hospital where he had been a patient for nearly 5 years. Mr Kimball had been away without leave from the hospital, had gotten drunk, started a fight with another patient, was pushed over a wall, and fell 10 feet and struck his head. He had been hospitalized for bipolar affective disorder (manic-depressive illness) and alcoholism. He had no other known disorders. Jean-Marie Kimball died at age 32 of breast cancer. She had no other known illnesses other than postpartum depression and uterine fibromyomas. All of the grandparents died before they reached age 50: one by suicide, one from "heart disease," one from influenza in 1918, and one from tuberculosis.

Social history: As a child, John F. Kimball lived with both parents, although their occasional extended absences from home (due to parents' illnesses and father's alcoholism) necessitated informal foster care with neighbors and with "aunts and uncles" for up to 3 months at a stretch. John attended parochial school for 6 years and then completed junior high and attended high school in the

public schools in San Francisco. His performance was uneven; he did well with some subjects and teachers and poorly with others. He was good in dramatics, athletics, and public speaking, had many friends, and was elected class treasurer as a sophomore. He became depressed as a senior, did poorly, and dropped out before graduation. He entered the navy and served for 3 years. He spent time in the "brig" for insubordination, drunkenness, and being AWOL. He was never promoted above the rank of Seaman First-Class and was discharged for medical reasons with a diagnosis of "character disorder and alcoholism."

Building on some skills he learned in the navy and on his persuasive manner, the patient got a union card and a job as a machinist. He worked in a dry dock, repairing ships. He was liked by his work mates; they drank and caroused together, and Kimball became union shop steward. For a time he was involved in union politics and attended local election rallies.

"Red" Kimball married a girl from his old neighborhood shortly after discharge from the navy. They lived in a flat and "got along fine," but he insisted they have no children. She acquiesced reluctantly until she turned 30. At that time, she began to complain about "feeling empty" and wanting a family. He began to spend less time at home, more time with "the boys," and his drinking increased. He became impotent, and they stopped having sexual relations altogether. Their marriage slowly deteriorated as he became more depressed and his alcoholism worsened. They began to fight, and he abused her physically on two occasions. She filed for dissolution of the marriage, and the patient had not seen his wife since the decree became final.

The remainder of the social history is conveyed along with the past history, discussed earlier. As noted, the patient is homeless, unemployed, and supported by SSDI.

Developmental history: The Mayor's life began with a 5-month separation from his mother, who was hospitalized with postpartum complications, including a hysterectomy and postpartum depression. As a newborn, he was raised by a neighbor and supported by his father, whose alcoholism made him an undependable caretaker. Mrs Kimball returned home and took up the child-rearing responsibility with renewed energy, but she never seemed able to get emotionally close to her son. The same was true of Mr Kimball, although when he was sober, he was a great "pal" to his son, teaching him to box and play games.

Little is known of the Mayor's childhood from age 2 to 6 years. In spite of never feeling emotionally close to her son, his mother tended to "spoil him" with small favors and took him with her everywhere. As his father's absences became more frequent and longer in duration, "Red" Kimball became protective of his mother. The Mayor's earliest traumatic memories are of his father's physical assaults on his mother. He was terrified and felt guilty that he couldn't help her. Once he did step in the way of his father's blows and sustained a fractured clavicle. He began to "hate" his "old man" and felt confused when his father confessed to him in tears—drunk and begging forgiveness. The image of the "pal" was incongruent with the hated "old man." As a child, "Red" thought almost everything was his fault because he had been "bad."

Ages 7–12 were marked by minor school difficulties and further troubles at home. "Red" took his first drink at age 12 and became drunk easily at first but soon developed tolerance to large quantities of alcohol. His mother died when he was 13 years old, and he was extremely quiet, withdrawn, and guilty. He had no one to talk to, and his sadness turned to anger and resentment toward his parents, who had neglected him. And the anger turned quickly to guilt for having hateful feelings toward his parents. A few months later, he complained of intense stomach cramps and was operated on for suspected appendicitis, but the surgical specimen was normal.

The patient reached puberty at about age 14, engaged in homosexual horseplay (group masturbation) with some friends at age 15, and had his first heterosexual experience at age 16. He related no history of sexual dysfunction other than episodes of impotence during his marriage (described above) and while drunk. Other details of social and sexual relationships are discussed in the social history.

Physical examination: On admission the patient was a plethoric man who seemed older than his stated age, with a barrel chest, thin limbs, and protruding abdomen. He was in apparent distress, shouting and waving his arms. His scleras were yellow and his skin jaundiced where it was not tanned from prolonged exposure.

Vital signs: Pulse 120 and regular, respiration 24, labored; blood pressure 169/90 left arm, sitting; temperature 100° F. At the time of admission, only a limited examination could be performed because of the patient's lack of cooperation. A cursory examination of the lungs, heart, and abdomen revealed no acute disease. The examination was completed the following morning, when pulse was 88 and regular, respiration 12 and regular, blood pressure 140/90 in both arms with orthostatic drop of 25 mm Hg, and temperature 99° F.

Head, eyes, ears, nose, and throat: Several scars on the face and scalp healed by secondary intention, marked scleral icterus, spider angiomas and injected veins on the nose, nasopharyngeal congestion.

Neck: Supple, no thyromegaly, no lymphadenopathy.

Thorax and lungs: Increased anteroposterior diameter, lungs clear to percussion and auscultation, although breath sounds were distant and the chest was slightly hyperresonant. No gynecomastia.

Heart and great vessels: The point of maximum impulse was felt in the fifth intercostal space 2 fingerbreadths to the left of the midclavicular line; the impulse was hyperdynamic. Heart sounds were all within normal limits, with no murmurs, rubs, or clicks. All peripheral pulses were felt; no bruits.

Abdomen: Icteric skin, appendectomy scar. Abdomen distended with ascites fluid wave (1/4). Tenderness in the right upper quadrant, with an enlarged liver felt 4 cm below the costal margin. No splenomegaly, no masses, no costovertebral angle tenderness. Bowel sounds were normal.

Rectum: Prostatic hypertrophy (2/4) with no discrete mass. Stool test for occult blood was negative.

Genitourinary tract: Normal adult male with slight testicular atrophy. Normal pattern of pubic hair.

Extremities: No bony abnormalities, full range of motion.

Neurological examination:

Mental status: (See below.)

Cranial nerves: I, II, V, VII–XII tested and all within normal limits; III, IV, VI, pupils equal, round, and reacting to light and accommodation, but abduction and conjugate gaze were paralyzed; diplopia was evident.

Motor system:

Muscle mass and tone–Normal.

Strength–Full strength (5/5).

Coordination–Slight asterixis and dysdiadochokinesia, demonstrated in difficulties with finger-to-nose and heel-to-shin tests.

Reflexes–All 3/4 without clonus, except that ankle jerks were absent; Babinski, Hoffmann absent.

Gait and station–Wide-based gait.

Movements–Normal fluidity without tics, chorea, or dyskinesia; mild resting tremor in both hands (1/4).

Sensation: Diminished pain and vibration sense in the extremities, feet worse than hands; no extinction on simultaneous stimulation.

Mental status examination:

Overview: Exaggerated alertness and easy distractibility; disheveled, with poor personal hygiene but a certain flair to his carriage and disarray; uncooperative at times but with perseverance able to complete the exam; hyperactive, unable to sit for more than 3–4 minutes at a time.

Emotion: Labile, expansive, irritable, with rapid shifts from tearful sadness to red-faced anger. Affect was appropriate. (Thoughts were consistent with affect.)

Attention: Failed the 7-digit screening test, only able to recall 3 digits on second try. Unable to perform serial 7s or 3s.

Orientation: To person, place (that it was a hospital only), and time (only to year, not month or day).

Memory: Attention deficit made memory assessment difficult. With effort and repetition, the patient was able to immediately recall three items, but he could not remember any of them at 5 minutes even with prompting and reinforcement. Visual memory was similarly impaired. The patient confabulated to fill in the gaps in recent memory. Long-term memory was adequate for a period prior to 4 or 5 years ago. He knew the United States presidents and current events of the period.

Speech and language: Pressured and incessant, but fluent, with normal comprehension; repetition and naming both intact. Two- and 3-step commands could not be assessed because of memory deficits.

Constructional ability: Unable to perform tests requiring memory. The patient was able to copy test figures when they were in front of him.

Calculations: Able to pass the screening test (5 × 13).

Thought:

Thought process–Thought process markedly disturbed, occasionally incoherent. When coherent, the patient had flight of ideas, was tangential, but did not demonstrate looseness of association.

Thought content–Content marked by mood-congruent auditory hallucinations saying "you are to blame" or laughing derisively. The patient was preoccupied by guilt and images of death alternating with "grandeur." He had paranoid delusions that someone was trying to poison the wine in the liquor stores: "Yellow Dye Number Nine is making me yellow all over!" He denied ideas of reference, thought broadcasting, or other delusions of control. He also denied complex hallucinations of several voices conversing and had no visual, tactile, or gustatory hallucinations, illusions, or other preoccupations.

Cognitive functions–Refused to interpret proverbs or answer screening questions: "Don't bother me with that nonsense. . . . My time is too valuable." Judgment grossly impaired. Did demonstrate some ability to abstract when he tried to take over a nurse's responsibility of explaining to a patient why he should take his medication. He implored the patient, "Take that stuff and your mood might get to be like mine. Besides, it'll help you get out of here quicker if you do like they say!"

Fund of knowledge–Knew the presidents and current events up to 4–5 years ago.

Insight–Aware of the reasons for hospitalization but expended considerable energy denying problems and displacing them onto the politics of the demise of Wino Park.

Diagnostic tests:

Laboratory tests: Serum electrolytes and blood urea nitrogen were normal, Blood ammonia was trivially elevated to 120 μg/dL on admission but fell into the normal range within 3 days. Thyroid studies were normal. Serum aspartate aminotransferase, alkaline phosphatase, and bilirubin were all elevated on admission and returned toward normal by discharge. Bilirubin fell from 4.1 mg/dL to 1.8 mg/dL (mostly direct). Serum albumin was depressed; gamma globulin was elevated. Prothrombin time was in the high normal range. Hematological evaluation showed a mild macrocytic anemia and moderate leukocytosis with a shift to the left. Erythrocyte sedimentation rate was mildly elevated. Serum iron was normal; serum folate was low. Urinalysis and electrocardiography were normal.

X-rays: Chest films showed slight cardiomegaly and evidence of mild emphysema; there was no evidence of congestive heart failure. A CT scan of the head was normal, with no evidence of tumor, infarct, or subdural hematoma.

Neuropsychological tests: Full-scale WAIS had been 110 on a previous evaluation. On this admission, the patient's concentration and memory were so impaired that a complete reexamination was impossible. All tests requiring short-term memory were failed. Results of the screening Bender Gestalt Test, however, were normal. The examiner noted that when the patient was tested near the end of his manic episode, he copied the test figures flamboyantly and large in size.

Personality assessment: No testing was done on this admission. Previous tests included an MMPI; results showed high scores on psychasthenia, masculinity, paranoia, and hysteria. On one administration, he also showed an elevation on the depression scale; at another time, the hypomania scale was elevated.

Differential diagnosis: The differential diagnosis on admission was not complicated, because of the well-established prior diagnoses of affective disorder and alcohol dependence, the recurrence of classical symptoms and signs during this episode of illness, and a strong family history of affective illness. For the sake of completeness, other diagnoses were considered: organic affective syndrome, delirium tremens, and especially the nonaffective psychotic disorders (eg, schizophrenia, acute paranoid disorder). No organic cause could be identified, although it is possible that encephalopathy and transiently elevated blood ammonia levels associated with the patient's alcoholic hepatitis may have exacerbated or precipitated his psychosis. The same may be said of his alcohol intoxication. Upon alcohol withdrawal, there was no worsening of his mental status, no increase in tremor, and no seizures—effectively eliminating delirium tremens from the diagnosis. The pattern of the Mayor's illness without persistent psychosis and with prolonged intervals free of illness precluded a diagnosis of schizophrenia; delusional disorder and the other psychotic illnesses were ruled out only by the presence of the full-blown manic episodes and depressive episodes in the Mayor's history and by current findings on mental status examination. On admission, he demonstrated most of the symptoms and signs of manic episode (Table 22–1); shortly after admission, he developed a major depressive episode (Table 22–1). This pattern replicated at least one earlier cycle of bipolar affective disorder.

A diagnosis of alcohol dependence could also be made unequivocally (Table 18–2). The diagnosis of alcohol amnestic syndrome was straightforward (see Chapter 17 and Table 18–2), having been made in the presence of a gaze palsy characteristic of Wernicke's encephalopathy often associated with Korsakoff's psychosis (amnestic syndrome). The diagnosis of alcoholic hepatitis was based on the acute onset of jaundice in an alcoholic and marked abnormalities in hepatic function. Alcoholic cirrhosis was suggested by the presence of ascites; however, *definitive* diagnosis can only be based on liver biopsy, which was not performed, since it was considered too dangerous and because the Mayor was uncooperative. Hematological evaluation revealed a macrocytic anemia, also probably due to chronic alcoholism.

Provisional psychosocial formulation: Too little information was available on admission to develop a formulation, although the initial psychological themes centered on losses and self-esteem.

Hospital course:
Week 1: The first week was devoted to a thorough evaluation, reported in this case summary, and to initial treatment of the patient's many problems. Treatment of agitation and insomnia began with oxazepam, 30 mg 4 times daily, reduced to 15 mg 3 times daily by the end of the week. When baseline renal and endocrine studies were completed, the patient was started on lithium carbonate, 600 mg orally 3 times daily for 5 days until a therapeutic level of 1.1 meq/L was achieved, and a maintenance dose of 300 mg 3 times daily was established. In evaluative and supportive psychotherapy, the patient revealed many important losses and separations in his life. The psychological themes are discussed in the psychosocial formulation below. The Mayor appeared to become depressed by the end of the first week, as his manic signs and symptoms abated with aggressive treatment. During this period, he was confined to the ward. Attempts to contact family and friends were unsuccessful. Social service personnel set about finding the patient a place to live after discharge.

Oxazepam had been selected initially for the control of agitation for two reasons: It is less toxic to the liver than the antipsychotic medications, and it would help to control alcohol withdrawal symptoms and seizure activity associated with delirium tremens if any of these should occur. The patient was observed closely for delirium tremens, but this did not develop. He was also given thiamine, 50 mg intravenously on admission, followed by 50 mg intramuscularly daily thereafter to reverse the Wernicke-Korsakoff syndrome (gaze paralysis and memory disturbance). The gaze paralysis cleared rapidly, but the patient was left with an impairment in memory. Folic acid was given orally, 1 mg daily, for the anemia.

It was decided not to treat the apparent alcoholic hepatitis and hope that abstinence and improved nutrition would permit the patient's liver to heal and that laboratory values would return toward normal and the jaundice would subside. A definitive diagnosis could not be made; a biopsy was not advisable owing to poor cooperation and the risk of excessive bleeding (prothrombin time in high normal range).

Week 2: The Mayor's affect deteriorated into a depressive episode. He complained of a return of agitation, loss of appetite, thoughts (but no plans) of death and suicide, and difficulty concentrating. Feelings of guilt and failure dominated his individual therapy sessions and his comments in ward group therapy meetings. At the beginning of the week, he was involved in ward activities; by the end of the week, he had lost interest in everything and seldom left his room. He was watched closely to prevent a suicide attempt. In spite of only 1 week of symptoms and signs of depression, he was started on amitriptyline, 150 mg orally at bedtime, since this drug had been effective in treating his depressive episodes in the past. Although a higher dose had been necessary before, a lower dose was advised because of the impaired hepatic function. Oxazepam was discontinued.

Week 3: The third week was characterized by slow improvement in mental status. Concentration and attention improved. There was no psychosis. Affect lightened slightly. The patient's sleep improved, and he was taking two meals daily by the end of the week. He still felt guilty and was negative, but he stopped ruminating about death and suicide. Arrangements were made for him to go to a board and care home for alcoholics, but he could not obtain a bed for 2 weeks. Plans to keep him until his depression had completely resolved had to be dropped because he insisted on discharge, as did the utilization review committee at the hospital. He was not suicidal and could not be committed involuntarily to a state mental hospital for further care. His conservator at the single-room occupancy hotel agreed to look after him and let him stay there again. The Mayor also agreed to take his medication and continue in treatment in the hospital's outpatient department. He was making progress in treatment and was beginning to see that he needed to forgive himself for his imagined wrongdoings and to develop a less intense and extreme style in dealing with other people.

By the time of discharge, the patient still had signs of impaired memory and depressed affect, but he was free of psychosis, and his attention span was normal. His jaundice was clearing, and his liver function was returning toward normal.

Multiaxial discharge diagnosis:

Axis I: Bipolar affective disorder (Table 22–1).
Manic episode on admission.
Depressive episode by discharge.
Alcohol dependence (Table 18–2).
Alcohol amnestic syndrome (Korsakoff's psychosis) (Chapter 17 and Table 18–2).

Axis II: Histrionic and passive-aggressive traits are probably secondary to affective disorder.

Axis III: Alcoholic hepatitis with jaundice.
Wernicke's syndrome (gaze palsy and encephalopathy).
Alcoholic cirrhosis (suspected clinically).
Peripheral neuropathy.
Macrocytic anemia.

Axis IV: Psychosocial stressors rated severe—5/7.
Loss of "home" and status as "Mayor."
Acute physical illness perceived as threat.

Axis V: Global assessment of function.
Current: 20 (in danger of harm).
Past year: 35 (inability to function).

Psychosocial formulation: The Mayor is an angry, guilt-ridden man with bipolar affective disorder complicated by alcoholism and its psychological and physiological concomitants. His life story represents a cyclic struggle to achieve a sense of self-worth and self-forgiveness in the face of hardships, losses, separations, and failures. One can only speculate on the interplay of heredity and environment in the evolution of this man's psychopathology; he has a strong family history of affective disorder and alcoholism. In many ways he has repeated the history of his father—in his illness and in his personal life.

The Mayor's depression may be viewed as a response to his losses and separations, beginning at birth: His mother's hospitalizations and depression, his father's repeated absences and ultimate institutionalization and death, and his mother's death all provoked sadness, anger, and a feeling that perhaps he was unloved, unlovable, or perhaps even so "bad" that he made these terrible events and problems happen. The anger fed his guilt, and when it became too intense, it triggered a morbid retreat into depression and alcohol abuse or an angry flight into mania. Manic euphoria, grandiosity, and the projection of his anger onto others in paranoid fantasies briefly protected him from pain and guilt. (For example, *others* were trying to poison him with Yellow Dye Number Nine, not *he* who was intoxicating himself and his liver with wine.)

The Mayor's sense of guilt and inadequacy appears to stem from the confusion, terror, and helplessness he felt while witnessing his mother's abuse at the hands of his father. He also fell victim to his father's wrath, which hurt him and confused him further. His alliance with his mother may be viewed as overdetermined (ie, having many causes.) His failure to develop a bond with his mother during infancy and her resentment at the loss of her ability to have more children following his birth set up a cycle of reaction formations leading to a studied closeness between them. In other words, they tried unconsciously to overcome their own unconscious resentments toward each other and to compensate for the bond that did not develop in infancy.

The father, too, worked at being a "pal" when he wasn't drunk, depressed or "away." During childhood, the patient felt doubly guilty about his mother (causing her unhappiness and not protecting her from attack)—a pain he says he felt in his "gut." In retrospect, his symptoms of appendicitis shortly following his mother's death may be seen as a manifestation of this pain. In spite of anger toward his father, he emulated him—all the way to the hospital.

The patient's marriage was also in many respects patterned after that of his parents. It was a hostile dependent relationship lasting 15 years. In contrast, the Mayor's marriage ended not with the death of his wife but in divorce following injury and abuse. In this case, the abusiveness stemmed from his wife's wish to have children and the Mayor's adamant opposition. One can speculate that his violent opposition derived from a fear that were he to be a father, he might abuse his "son" (he could only imagine a boy child) and disappoint him ("as my father disappointed me").

The Mayor wants everyone to love him but is unable to get close to anyone. He lacks the capacity for intimacy. His charm, dramatic style, and engaging personality have brought him no closeness and no increase in self-esteem. These he has manufactured in flights into mania—an escape from his severe depression. His disappointments, failures, and anger he projects onto others out to get him, especially authority figures, teachers, superiors in the navy, his bosses at work, the police, alcohol manufacturers, his wife, and his doctors.

Bipolar affective disorder and alcoholism have isolated the Mayor from the things he wanted most but were denied him by fate, circumstance, and heredity. A biological predisposition to affective disorder coupled with environmental circumstances and emotional deprivation and trauma combine to explain the man and his illness.

The patient's sensitivity to loss and stress precipitated this episode of illness with the loss of his "home" in the park and his status as Mayor. He says, "I *was* the Mayor of Wino Park!" The park had been an asylum for a homeless man who needed his expansive fantasies to feel a sense of worth.

The Mayor will soon be 55, the age at which his father died in a mental hospital. Whether the Mayor survives will depend in part on the ability of health care professionals to control his disorder biomedically, understand his illness and his defenses psychologically, help him find a new home and social support, and capitalize on his strengths in his wit, charm, and capacity for leadership.

Continuing Treatment Plan & Disposition:

Biomedical treatment plan:

Lithium carbonate, 300 mg orally 3 times daily.

Amitriptyline, 150 mg orally at bedtime.

Thiamine, 100 mg orally 3 times daily.

Folic acid, 1 mg orally daily.

General internal medicine follow-up in 2 weeks.

Psychotropic medications to be monitored by psychiatrist.

Lithium levels to be determined weekly or until stabilized.

Psychological treatment plan:

Continue in weekly individual supportive treatment focusing on interpersonal skills; sessions limited to 30 minutes, as tolerated.

Referral to Alcoholics Anonymous.

Visit from nurse if patient fails to comply with his appointments.

Social treatment plan:

Transfer to alcoholism board and care home from his discharge residence at the hotel in San Francisco.

Alcoholics Anonymous will help him to build a new social network as well as reinforce his abstinence.

SSDI checks to be transferred from the hotel to the board and care home after a 1-month trial. Conservatorship might also be transferred to the board and care home operator.

Section III. Mental Disorders

Classifying Mental Disorders: *Diagnostic and Statistical Manual of Mental Disorders: (DSM-III-R),* Third Edition (Revised)

16

Howard H. Goldman, MD, PhD, & Jack A. Grebb, MD

Note to Reader on Use of *DSM-III-R* in This Text

By arrangement with the American Psychiatric Association, the authors of *Review of General Psychiatry* have borrowed freely from *DSM-III-R*. Most of what we have taken from *DSM-III-R* is identified as such in the tabular matter, eg, "Table 22–1. *DSM-III-R* diagnostic criteria for mood disorders." Language from the diagnostic criteria of *DSM-III-R* reproduced in this text otherwise than in the tables is in quotes. The quoted passages are reproduced exactly as they appear in *DSM-III-R*. The tables have been normalized to the style of the book in small matters of punctuation and spelling.–HHG.

The *Diagnostic and Statistical Manual of Mental Disorders (DSM-III,)* 3rd edition (American Psychiatric Association, 1980), together with its 1987 revision *(DSM-III-R),* contains a standard classification of mental disorders widely used in North America and gaining international acceptance. It is the product of a thorough review of the current state of psychiatric nosological data and thus serves as a valuable guide to the diagnosis of mental disorders. It contains no information about treatment, individual or family psychodynamics, social issues, or—except in a few specific cases described below—the causes of the syndromes. The word "statistical" in the title refers only to the numbering system used for coding purposes and not to statistical data. The *DSM-III-R* diagnoses and their appropriate code designations are presented at the end of this chapter.

As discussed in Chapter 8, diagnosis is the process of evaluating patterns of signs and symptoms and thus identifying specific disorders. The diagnostic model implies the existence of some problem severe enough to require professional intervention. There-

fore, a compendium of psychiatric diagnoses should not include normal variations in personality styles, mood, or anxiety. For example, normal grief following the death of a close friend or family member is not an entity in *DSM-III*, and an antisocial act (eg, stealing a car) by a person with no psychopathological symptoms does not justify a diagnosis of mental disorder.

Until *DSM-III* was published, the lack of an explicit inventory of mental disorders with specified diagnostic criteria was an impediment to research in the field. Accurate diagnosis is the essential first step toward predicting the course and outcome of mental illness, planning treatment, and devising strategies for prevention. A precise classification system focuses attention on more homogeneous populations of sick people, permitting more refined tests of theories of etiology and pathogenesis of the mental disorders. These characteristics make *DSM-III* a valuable resource for research, clinical care, and psychiatric education. Although *DSM-III* facilitates diagnosis, it does not help with the process of psychosocial formulation. There is a danger that a preoccupation with precise diagnosis, embodied in *DSM-III*, will distract the student and clinician from individual psychosocial assessment. Both processes are essential; only diagnosis has been standardized in *DSM-III*. (See Chapter 8.)

RECENT HISTORY OF OFFICIAL CLASSIFICATIONS

DSM-III is the third classification system to be published by the American Psychiatric Association (APA). DSM-I (1952) emphasized the concepts of "reaction" and "defense mechanisms." The use of "defense mechanisms" reflected the strong influence of psychoanalysis in the development of *DSM-I*. *DSM-II* (1968) dispensed with the term "reaction" and tried (with some success) to avoid implying a specific theoretic framework. Whereas *DSM-I* discouraged multiple diagnoses, *DSM-II* clearly encouraged them.

DSM-III was published in 1980 and represents the most exhaustive attempt to date to reach a consensus about psychiatric diagnosis. Extensive field trials involving 550 clinicians also were conducted. A revision, *DSM-III-R*, was initiated in 1983 to "clarify ambiguities, resolve inconsistencies, and incorporate factual changes" and was published in 1987.

The history of the *International Statistical Classification of Diseases, Injuries, and Causes of Death (ICD)* has somewhat paralleled that of the *DSM*. The *ICD* is published by the World Health Organization and contains the official system for recording all diseases, injuries, impairments, symptoms, and causes of death. Nine editions, *ICD-I* through *ICD-9*, have been published. The latest version of *ICD-9*--clinical modification (*(ICD-9-CM)*—includes some of the new categories from *DSM-III;* however, it retains many of the old categories from *DSM-II* that were not included in *DSM-III*. *ICD-10* is scheduled for publication in 1993, as is *DSM-IV*.

BASIC CONCEPTS

Table 16–1 lists the three basic concepts underlying the philosophy of *DSM-III*. Each of these concepts is further discussed below.

Definition of Mental Disorder

According to *DSM-III*, ". . . each of the mental disorders is conceptualized as a clinically significant behavioral or psychological syndrome or pattern that occurs in an individual and that is typically associated with either a painful symptom (distress) or impairment in one or more important areas of functioning (disability). In addition, there is an inference that there is a behavioral, psychological, or biological dysfunction, and that the disturbance is not only in the relationship between the individual and society. (When the disturbance is limited to a conflict between an individual and society, this may represent social deviance, which may or may not be commendable, but is not by itself a mental disorder.)" The concept of "disorder" represents a level of diagnostic and theoretical conceptualization (see Chapter 8). Table 8–1 lists other levels of conceptualization, along with their definitions and examples from *DSM-III-R*. Although most *DSM-III-R* conditions are in fact syndromes, they are called disorders somewhat in the hope that they represent relatively homogeneous conditions.

Descriptive & Nontheoretical Approach

Only the patient's behavior and subjective reports about his or her internal state provide data for the formulation of *DSM-III* diagnoses. There are no biologically based diagnostic criteria in *DSM-III*. *DSM-III* describes the phenomenology of the disorders; therefore, its approach is often called "descriptive" or "phenomenologic."

DSM-III does not explain how or why a certain disorder exists. The cause of most mental disorders is simply not known, and their descriptions do not properly include theories of origin. In this way, *DSM-III* avoids stating more than is known about mental disorders and makes itself acceptable to mental health professionals with different theoretical backgrounds. Table 16–2 lists the four *DSM-III-R* conditions that

Table 16–1. Basic concepts and major characteristics of *DSM-III*.

Basic concepts
  Definition of mental disorder
  Descriptive and nontheoretic approach
  Reliable and valid categories and criteria
Major characteristics
  Diagnostic criteria (inclusion and exclusion)
  Levels of diagnostic certainty
  Hierarchical organization of diagnostic classes
  Multiaxial diagnosis (and multiple diagnoses)
  Complete and systematic descriptions of diagnostic classes
  Glossary of technical terms

Table 16–2. *DSM-III-R* conditions with specific etiologic considerations.

Condition	Etiologic Factor
Organic Organic mental disorders associated with a specific substance (eg, barbiturate withdrawal)	Specific substance (eg, barbiturate).
Psychologic Conversion disorder	"Psychologic factors are judged to be etiologically related to the symptoms." This criterion clearly describes an intrapsychic dynamic problem as the cause of the condition.
Stressor (rare and extreme) Posttraumatic stress disorder	"The person has experienced an event. . . distressing to almost anyone." This criterion clearly describes an environmental event leading to a mental disorder.
Stressor (common) Adjustment disorders	"A reaction to an identifiable psychosocial stressor." An environmental or social event is considered to be part of the cause of the syndrome.

do in fact include etiological considerations in their descriptions and diagnostic criteria.

Reliable & Valid Categories & Criteria

DSM-III was written with a commitment toward increased reliance on actual data rather than completely subjective impressions. Existing research data were used to ensure the soundness of specific diagnostic categories and criteria. This led to the exclusion of several previously recognized diagnostic categories and the inclusion of several new ones.

The concept of reliability refers to the extent to which different users of a classification system can agree on diagnoses in a series of cases. The concept of diagnostic validity has different levels of meaning. The lowest level is a consensus among professionals that certain characteristics describe a specific subgroup of patients and that these characteristics are somewhat specific to this subgroup. This is the level of validity of most of *DSM- III* and is the result of the many meetings and discussions of the Task Force on Nomenclature and Statistics. The next step in the process of validating the *DSM-III* categories is the focus of much current research addressing the following questions: (1) Does a specified disorder have a single course or outcome? (2) Does it respond consistently to a specific treatment? (3) Does it have a genetic or other biological basis? (4) Does it have a common psychosocial basis? Affirmative answers to these questions indicate higher levels of validity. The advance *DSM-III* makes is that it reliably defines the subgroups of patients about whom these questions can be asked.

MAJOR CHARACTERISTICS OF *DSM-III*

The major characteristics of *DSM-III* are listed in Table 16–1 and described below.

Diagnostic Criteria

For each disorder in *DSM-III-R*, there are specific diagnostic criteria. Most of these are inclusion criteria describing signs or symptoms that must be present before the diagnosis can be made. For example, criterion A of organic hallucinosis is "prominent persistent or recurrent hallucinations." Other criteria are exclusion criteria which, if present, exclude the individual from that particular diagnostic category. For example, criterion C for organic hallucinosis is "not occurring exclusively during the course of delirium."

The criteria are presented as guidelines. Although strict adherence to the criteria is suggested, clinical judgment will of course enter into the diagnostic process. The more research-oriented the situation, the less variation should be permitted in interpretation of the criteria. The criteria themselves are presented

at the lowest level of inference, which means that very little should have to be "read into" them; however, for some diagnostic categories, particularly the personality disorders, more interpretation and subjective judgment are required. For example, criterion 7 of obsessive compulsive personality disorder is "restricted expression of affection." Here the clinician must evaluate what is a normal versus an abnormal expression of affection.

Levels of Diagnostic Certainty

DSM-III-R allows the user to state the diagnosis at the level of certainty appropriate to the amount of information available about a particular patient. Table 16–3 summarizes these levels. The physician should never decide on a diagnosis beyond a level of certainty that is justified by the information (subjective and objective) available. The reader should note that Conditions Not Attributable to a Mental Disorder That Are a Focus of Attention or Treatment (also called the "V" codes) are coded on axis I (see Chapter 25).

Multiaxial Diagnosis

There are five diagnostic axes in *DSM-III-R*, and the inclusion of all appropriate diagnoses (ie, multiple diagnoses) is encouraged on the first three of these. Table 16–4 summarizes the five axes.

Axes I and II contain all of the mental disorders listed in *DSM-III-R*, with axis II containing only the developmental disorders and personality disorders. In addition, personality *traits*, which are not officially coded, are recorded on axis II when a patient does not meet the criteria for a personality *disorder*. All diagnostic classifications for which a patient meets the criteria should be included on these two axes.

Axis III is operationally defined as potentially including all of the diagnoses in *ICD-9-CM* not listed in its section on mental disorders. Given the current

Table 16–3. *DSM-III-R* diagnoses representing levels of diagnostic certainty.

When even the presence or absence of a mental disorder is uncertain:
 Diagnosis deferred on axis I or axis II.
When general class of disorder is known but more specific diagnosis cannot be made:
 Atypical psychosis.
 (Personality) disorder not otherwise specified.
When specific diagnosis is strongly suspected but not confirmed:
 Specific diagnosis (provisional, rule out . . .). *Example:* Schizophrenia, paranoid, unspecified (provisional, rule out amphetamine delusional disorder).
When a specific diagnosis is known:
 Specific diagnosis.
When a mental disorder is definitely not present:
 Codes for conditions not attributable to a mental disorder that are a focus of attention or treatment, eg, malingering.
 No diagnosis on axis I or axis II.

Table 16–4. Summary of 5 *DSM-III-R* axes.

Axis	Content
I	All mental disorders (except 2 classes contained on axis II). Conditions not attributable to mental disorders that are a focus of attention or treatment (V codes). Additonal codes: unspecified mental disorder (non-psychotic): no diagnosis; diagnosis deferred.
II	Developmental disorders. Personality disorders. Personality traits (no numerical diagnostic codes).
III	Any current physical disorder or condition that is potentially relevant to the understanding of the individual.
IV	Severity of psychosocial stressors.
V	Global assessment of functioning (GAF).

Table 16–5. *DSM-III* codes for axis IV.

Axis IV*	
Code	**Term**
1	None
2	Minimal
3	Mild
4	Moderate
5	Severe
6	Extreme
7	Catastrophic
0	Inadequate information or no change in condition

*Severity of psychosocial stressors.

state of knowledge, it is better to be overinclusive on axis III, since most physical conditions are likely to have some effect on mental functioning (via the brain, in particular). Some conditions on axis III might have a direct relationship to axis I, eg, hepatic failure on axis III resulting in delirium on axis I. Other axis III diagnoses (eg, diabetes mellitus or Cushing's disease) might have a less obvious or accepted relationship with the axis I diagnoses (eg, generalized anxiety disorder or major depressive episodes).

Axes IV and V are for use in special clinical or research settings. The code numbers for axis IV are listed in Table 16–5. Axis V is presented in Table 16–6. Specific clinical examples for each code level on these two axes are given in *DSM-III-R*. In the formal *DSM-III* diagnosis, the major psychosocial stressors should actually be listed. Clinicians should distinguish between acute events and enduring circumstances. Axis V, Global Assessment of Functioning, should assess the period of best function lasting at least a few months during the past year as well as the current status. Social relations, occupational functioning, and the use of leisure time should be taken into account in this assessment. This optimum period may in fact be due to optimum treatment at

Table 16–6. Axis V: Global assessment of functioning (GAF).

Consider psychologic, social, and occupational functioning on a hypothetic continuum of mental health–illness. Do not include impairment in functioning due to physical (or environmental) limitations. Use intermediate codes when appropriate, eg, 45, 68, 72.

Code	Level of Functioning
90–81	Absent or minimal symptoms (eg, mild anxiety before an examination, an occasional argument with family member), good functioning in all areas, interested and involved in a wide range of activities, socially effective, generally satisfied with life, no more than everyday problems or concerns.
80–71	If symptoms are present, they are transient and expectable reactions to psychosocial stressors (eg, difficulty concentrating after family argument); no more than slight impairment in social, occupational, or school functioning (eg, temporarily falling behind in schoolwork).
70–61	Some mild symptoms (eg, depressed mood and mild insomnia, occasional truancy, or theft within the household) OR some difficulty in social, occupational, or school functioning, but generally functioning pretty well, has some meaningful interpersonal relationships.
60–51	Moderate symptoms (eg, few friends and conflicts with peers, flat affect and circumstantial speech, occasional panic attacks) OR moderate difficulty in social, occupational, or school functioning.
50–41	Serious symptoms (eg, no friends, unable to keep a job, suicidal ideation, severe obsessional rituals, frequent shoplifting) OR any serious impairment in social, occupational, or school functioning.
40–31	Some impairment in reality testing or communication (eg, speech is at times illogical, obscure, or irrelevant) OR major impairment in several areas, such as work or school, family relations, judgment, thinking, or mood (eg, depressed man avoids friends, neglects family, and is unable to work; child frequently beats up younger children, is defiant at home, and is failing at school).
30–21	Behavior is considerably influenced by delusions or hallucinations OR serious impairment in communication or judgment (eg, sometimes incoherent, acts grossly inappropriately, suicidal preoccupation) OR inability to function in almost all areas (eg, stays in bed all day; no job, home, or friends).
20–11	Some danger of hurting self or others (eg, suicide attempts without clear expectation of death, frequently violent, manic excitement) OR occasionally fails to maintain minimal personal hygiene (eg, smears feces) OR gross impairment in communication (eg, largely incoherent or mute).
10–1	Persistent danger of severely hurting self or others (eg, recurrent violence) OR persistent inability to maintain minimal personal hygiene OR serious suicidal act with clear expectation of death.

that time, eg, when a patient with neuroleptic-responsive schizophrenia is taking his or her medication. Axes IV and V may have important prognostic implications. In general, the more specific the stressor and the higher the recent level of functioning, the better the prognosis.

APPLICATION

DSM-III-R sets forth the following procedural guidelines for arriving at a diagnosis for a particular patient: (1) Record all diagnoses from *DSM-III-R* for which the patient meets the criteria on axes I and II; (2) record all pertinent physical disorders (listed in *ICD-9-CM)* on axis III; (3) if appropriate, assess psychosocial stressors and global assessment of functioning on axes IV and V; and (4) state diagnoses at the appropriate level of certainty. By convention, diagnoses should be listed in descending order of importance within each category or axis. The first axis I diagnosis is considered the major focus of treatment unless the words "principal diagnosis" in parentheses follow an axis II diagnosis. Two examples of complete *DSM-III-R* diagnoses, complete with *DSM-III-R* code numbers, are presented below.

Example 1:

Axis I:	295.14	Schizophrenia, disorganized, chronic, with acute exacerbation.
	305.02	Alcohol abuse, episodic.
	305.33	Hallucinogen abuse, in remission.
Axis II:	V71.09	No diagnosis on axis II.
Axis III:	Right lower lobe pneumonia, unspecified organism.	
Axis IV:	Psychosocial stressors: (1) Lost disability check; (2) evicted from apartment. Severity: 5–Severe. Acute.	
Axis V:	Current GAF: 25. Highest GAF past year: 30.	

Example 2:

Axis I:	300.90	Unspecified mental disorder (nonpsychotic).
	305.62	Cocaine abuse, episodic.
Axis II:	301.81	Narcissistic personality disorder.
Axis III:	None.	
Axis IV:	Psychosocial stressors: No information. Severity: 0–Inadequate information.	
Axis V:	Current GAF: 75. Highest GAF past year: 85.	

Caution Regarding Use

The clinician must remember three major caveats when using *DSM-III*. First, treatment for any specific patient must be individualized regardless of the *DSM-III* diagnosis. For example, not every patient with a diagnosis of major depression is a suitable candidate for treatment with antidepressant drugs. Second, clini-

cians, researchers, and students must avoid grouping people together as "schizophrenics" or "autistics," since this implies homogeneity in all aspects of their lives. A *DSM-III* diagnosis refers to only part of a patient's functioning. It is much more accurate to refer to an individual as "the patient with schizophrenia," for example. Third, researchers and theorists must not assume that each *DSM-III* disorder has a single cause. As already noted, these actually are syndromes that may have multiple causes.

SUMMARY & FUTURE DIRECTIONS

The *Manual* is an evolving document. It continues to be revised. Nothing in *DSM-III* is written in stone. In fact, the major purpose of being clear and specific in *DSM-III* is to facilitate further examination of the disorders and continued testing of the validity and reliability of the diagnostic criteria.

INTRODUCTION TO FOLLOWING CHAPTERS

This text largely conforms to *DSM-III-R* in its classification of disorders, use of diagnostic criteria, and format. Chapters 17–29 generally follow the sequence and content of *DSM-III-R,* including discussions of most of the disorders. There are, however, a few exceptions: Because of their importance in general medicine as well as psychiatry, substance use disorders are discussed separately from the other organic mental disorders in Chapter 18, and alcoholism is discussed in both Chapter 18 (organic aspects of alcohol abuse) and Chapter 19. Psychological factors affecting physical conditions are discussed in Chapter 3 as well as in Chapter 41.

The disorders of infancy, childhood, and adolescence are discussed in Chapter 30. Although *DSM-III-R* nomenclature is also used, the chapter takes its organization from the Group for the Advancement of Psychiatry classification system. The *DSM-III-R* diagnostic criteria of several important or common childhood disorders are presented, but the chapter provides an overview of child psychopathology through a series of illustrative cases. The eating disorders, listed with these disorders in *DSM-III-R,* are discussed separately in Chapter 28—again because of their significance in general medical practice.

This text goes beyond *DSM-III* in its discussion of each of the mental disorders. In addition to a presentation of the clinical features of each disorder (ie, symptoms and signs, including diagnostic criteria and natural history or course), differential diagnosis, and prognosis, there is usually an illustrative case, followed by a discussion of epidemiology, etiology and pathogenesis, and treatment. Occasionally, some of these sections (eg, natural history or prognosis) are deleted or condensed because of lack of information, but this format is the general pattern of Chapters 17–30.

REFERENCES

American Psychiatric Association: *Diagnostic and Statistical Manual of Mental Disorders (DSM-III)*, 3rd ed. American Psychiatric Association, 1980.

American Psychiatric Association: *Diagnostic and Statistical Manual of Mental Disorders (DSM-III-R)*, 3rd ed. (revised). American Psychiatric Association, 1987.

American Psychiatric Association: *Reference to the Diagnostic Criteria from DSM-III-R*. American Psychiatric Association, 1987.

Kendell RE: The choice of diagnostic criteria for biological research. Arch Gen Psychiatry 1982;39:1334.

Spitzer RL, Williams JBW, Skodol AE: *International Perspectives on DSM-III*. American Psychiatric Press, 1983.

Williams JBW, Spitzer RL: Research diagnostic criteria and *DSM-III*. Arch Gen Psychiatry 1982;39:1283. PSYC-17: Updated 3/18

All official DSM-III-R codes are included in ICD-9-CM. Codes followed by an asterisk are used for more than one DSM-III-R diagnosis or subtype in order to maintain compatibility with ICD-9-CM.

A long dash following a diagnostic term indicates the need for a fifth digit subtype or other qualifying term.

The term specify following a diagnostic category indicates qualifying terms that clinicians may wish to add in parentheses after the name of the disorder.

NOS = Not Otherwise Specified

The current severity of a disorder may be specified after the diagnosis as:

mild ——⎤
moderate ⎬ currently meets diagnostic criteria
severe ——⎦

in partial remission
(or residual state)
in complete remission

DISORDERS USUALLY FIRST EVIDENT IN INFANCY, CHILDHOOD, OR ADOLESCENCE

DEVELOPMENTAL DISORDERS
Note: These are coded on Axis II.

Mental Retardation
317.00   Mild mental retardation
318.00   Moderate mental retardation
318.10   Severe mental retardation
318.20   Profound mental retardation
319.00   Unspecified mental retardation

Pervasive Developmental Disorders
299.00   Autistic disorder
         Specify if childhood onset
299.80   Pervasive developmental disorder NOS

Specific Developmental Disorders
         Academic skills disorders
315.10   Developmental arithmetic disorder
315.80   Developmental expressive writing disorder
315.00   Developmental reading disorder

         Language and speech disorders
315.39   Developmental articulation disorder
315.31* Developmental expressive language disorder
315.31* Developmental receptive lan-

---

guage disorder

Motor skills disorder
315.40   Developmental coordination disorder
315.90* Specific developmental disorder NOS

Other Developmental Disorders
315.90* Developmental disorder NOS

Disruptive Behavior Disorders
314.01   Attention-deficit hyperactivity disorder

         Conduct disorder,
312.20   group type
312.00   solitary aggressive type
312.90   undifferentiated type
313.81   Oppositional defiant disorder

Anxiety Disorders of Childhood or Adolescence
309.21   Separation anxiety disorder
313.21   Avoidant disorder of childhood or adolescence
313.00   Overanxious disorder

Eating Disorders
307.10   Anorexia nervosa
307.51   Bulimia nervosa
307.52   Pica
307.53   Rumination disorder of infancy
307.50   Eating disorder NOS

Gender Identity Disorders
302.60   Gender identity disorder of childhood
302.50   Transsexualism
         Specify sexual history: asexual, homosexual, heterosexual, unspecified
302.85* Gender identity disorder of adolescence or adulthood, nontranssexual type
         Specify sexual history: asexual, homosexual, heterosexual, unspecified
302.85* Gender identity disorder NOS

Tic Disorders
307.23   Tourette's disorder
307.22   Chronic motor or vocal tic disorder
307.21   Transient tic disorder
         Specify: single episode or recurrent
307.20   Tic disorder NOS

Elimination Disorders
307.70   Functional encopresis

Specify: primary or secondary type

307.60 Functional enuresis
Specify: primary or secondary type
Specify: nocturnal only, diurnal only, nocturnal and diurnal

Speech Disorders Not Elsewhere Classified
307.00* Cluttering
307.00* Stuttering

Other Disorders of Infancy, Childhood, or Adolescence
313.23 Elective mutism
313.82 Identity disorder
313.89 Reactive attachment disorder of infancy or early childhood
307.30 Stereotype/habit disorder
314.00 Undifferentiated attention-deficit disorder

ORGANIC MENTAL DISORDERS

Dementias Arising in the Senium & Presenium
Primary degenerative dementia of the Alzheimer type, senile onset,
290.30 with delirium
290.20 with delusions
290.21 with depression
290.00* uncomplicated
(Note: Code 331.00 Alzheimer's disease on axis III)

Code in fifth digit:
1 = with delirium, 2 = with delusions, 3 = with depression, 0* = uncomplicated
290.1x Primary degenerative dementia of the Alzheimer type, presenile onset,
_____
(Note: Code 331.00 Alzheimer's disease on axis III)
290.4x Multi-infarctdementia, _____
290.00* Senile dementia NOS
Specify etiology on axis III if known
290.10* Presenile dementia NOS
Specify etiology on axis III if known (eg, Pick's disease, Jacob-Creutzfeldt disease)

Psychoactive Substance-Induced Organic Mental Disorders

Alcohol
303.00 intoxication
291.40 idiosyncratic intoxication (128)
291.80 Uncomplicated alcohol withdrawal
291.00 withdrawal delirium
291.30 hallucinosis
291.10 amnestic disorder
291.20 Dementia associated with alcoholism

Amphetamine or similarly acting sympathomimetic
305.70* intoxication
292.00* withdrawal
292.81* delirium
292.11* delusional disorder

Caffeine
305.90* intoxication

Cannabis
305.20* intoxication
292.11* delusional disorder

Cocaine
305.60* intoxication
292.00* withdrawal
292.81* delirium
292.11* delusional disorder

Hallucinogen
305.30* hallucinosis
292.11* delusional disorder
292.84* mood disorder

Posthallucinogen
292.89* perception disorder

Inhalant
305.90* intoxication

Nicotine
292.00* withdrawal

Opioid
305.50* intoxication
292.00* withdrawal

Phencyclidine (PCP) or similarly acting arylcyclohexylamine
305.90* intoxication
292.81* delirium
292.11* delusional disorder
292.84* mood disorder
292.90* organic mental disorder NOS

Sedative, hypnotic, or anxiolytic
305.40* intoxication
292.00* Uncomplicated sedative, hypnotic, or anxiolytic withdrawal
292.00* withdrawal delirium
292.83* amnestic disorder

Other or unspecified psychoactive substance
305.90* intoxication
292.00* withdrawal
292.81* delirium
292.82* dementia
292.83* amnestic disorder
292.11* delusional disorder
292.12 hallucinosis
292.84* mood disorder
292.89* anxiety disorder
292.89* personality disorder
292.90* organic mental disorder NOS

Organic Mental Disorders Associated With Axis III

Physical Disorders or Conditions, or Whose Etiology Is Unknown

293.00	Delirium
294.10	Dementia
294.00	Amnestic disorder
293.81	Organic delusional disorder
293.82	Organic hallucinosis
293.83	Organic mood disorder
	Specify: manic, depressed, mixed
294.80*	Organic anxiety disorder
310.10	Organic personality disorder
	Specify if explosive type
294.80*	Organic mental disorder NOS

PSYCHOACTIVE SUBSTANCE USE DISORDERS

	Alcohol
303.90	dependence
305.00	abuse
	Amphetamine or similarly acting sympathomimetic
304.40	dependence
305.70*	abuse
	Cannabis
304.30	dependence
305.20*	abuse
	Cocaine
304.20	dependence
305.60*	abuse
	Hallucinogen
304.50*	dependence
305.30*	abuse
	Inhalant
304.60	dependence
305.90*	abuse
	Nicotine
305.10	dependence
	Opioid
304.00	dependence
305.50*	abuse
	Phencyclidine (PCP) or similarly acting arylcyclohexylamine
304.50*	dependence
305.90*	abuse
	Sedative, hypnotic, or anxiolytic
304.10	dependence
305.40*	abuse
304.90*	Polysubstance dependence
304.90*	Psychoactive substance dependence NOS
305.90*	Psychoactive substance abuse NOS

SCHIZOPHRENIA

Code in fifth digit: 1 = subchronic, 2 = chronic, 3 = subchronic with acute exacerbation, 4 = chronic with acute exacerbation, 5 = in remission, 0 = unspecified.

	Schizophrenia,
295.2x	catatonic, _____
295.1x	disorganized, _____
295.3x	paranoid, _____
	Specify if stable type
295.9x	undifferentiated, _____
295.6x	residual, _____
	Specify if late onset

DELUSIONAL (PARANOID) DISORDER

297.10	Delusional (paranoid) disorder
	Specify type: erotomanic
	grandiose
	jealous
	persecutory
	somatic
	unspecified

PSYCHOTIC DISORDERS NOT ELSEWHERE CLASSIFIED

298.80	Brief reactive psychosis
295.40	Schizophreniform disorder
	Specify: without good prognostic features or with good prognostic features
295.70	Schizoaffective disorder
	Specify: bipolar type or depressive type
297.30	Induced psychotic disorder
298.90	Psychotic disorder NOS (atypical psychosis)

MOOD DISORDERS

Code current state of major depression and bipolar disorder in fifth digit:
- 1 = mild
- 2 = moderate
- 3 = severe, without psychotic features
- 4 = with psychotic features (*specify* mood-congruent or mood-incongruent)
- 5 = in partial remission
- 6 = in full remission
- 0 = unspecified

For major depressive episodes, *specify* if chronic and *specify* if melancholic type.

For bipolar disorder, bipolar disorder NOS, recurrent major depression, and depressive disorder NOS, *specify* if seasonal pattern.

Bipolar Disorders

	Bipolar disorder,
296.6x	mixed, _____
296.4x	manic, _____
296.5x	depressed, _____
301.13	Cyclothymia
296.70	Bipolar disorder NOS

Depressive Disorders

	Major Depression,
296.2x	single episode, _____

296.3x	recurrent, _____
300.40	Dysthymia (or depressive neurosis)
	Specify: primary or secondary type
	Specify: early or late onset
311.00	Depressive disorder NOS

ANXIETY DISORDERS
(or Anxiety & Phobic Neuroses)

	Panic disorder
300.21	with agoraphobia
	Specify current severity of agoraphobic avoidance
	Specify current severity of panic attacks
300.01	without agoraphobia
	Specify current severity of panic attacks
300.22	Agoraphobia without history of panic disorder
	Specify with or without limited symptom attacks
300.23	Social phobia
	Specify if generalized type
300.29	Simple phobia
300.30	Obsessive compulsive disorder (or obsessive compulsive neurosis)
309.89	Posttraumatic stress disorder
	Specify if delayed onset
300.02	Generalized anxiety disorder
300.00	Anxiety disorder NOS

SOMATOFORM DISORDERS

300.70*	Body dysmorphic disorder
300.11	Conversion disorder (or Hysterical neurosis, conversion type)
	Specify: single episode or recurrent
300.70*	Hypochondriasis (or Hypochondriacal neurosis)
300.81	Somatization disorder
307.80	Somatoform pain disorder
300.70*	Undifferentiated somatoform disorder
300.70*	Somatoform disorder NOS

DISSOCIATIVE DISORDERS
(or Hysterical Neuroses, Dissociative Type)

300.14	Multiple personality disorder
300.13	Psychogenic fugue
300.12	Psychogenic amnesia
300.60	Depersonalization disorder (or depersonalization neurosis)
300.15	Dissociative disorder NOS

SEXUAL DISORDERS

Paraphilias

302.40	Exhibitionism

302.81	Fetishism
302.89	Frotteurism
302.20	Pedophilia
	Specify: same sex, opposite sex, same and opposite sex
	Specify if limited to incest
	Specify: exclusive type or nonexclusive type
302.83	Sexual masochism
302.84	Sexual sadism
302.30	Transvestic fetishism
302.82	Voyeurism
302.90*	Paraphilia NOS

Sexual Dysfunctions
Specify: psychogenic only, or psychogenic and biogenic (Note: If biogenic only, code on axis III
Specify: lifelong or acquired
Specify: generalized or situational

	Sexual desire disorders
302.71	Hypoactive sexual desire disorde
302.79	Sexual aversion disorder
	Sexual arousal disorders
302.72*	Female sexual arousal disorder
302.72*	Male erectile disorder
	Orgasm disorders
302.73	Inhibited female orgasm
302.74	Inhibited male orgasm
302.75	Premature ejaculation
	Sexual pain disorders
302.76	Dyspareunia
306.51	Vaginismus
302.70	Sexual dysfunction NOS

Other Sexual Disorders

302.90*	Sexual disorder NOS

SLEEP DISORDERS
Dyssomnias

	Insomnia disorder
307.42*	related to another mental disorder (nonorganic)
780.50*	related to known organic factor
307.42*	Primary insomnia
	Hypersomnia disorder
307.44*	related to another mental disorder (nonorganic)
780.50*	related to a known organic factor
780.54*	Primary hypersomnia
307.45	Sleep-wake schedule disorder
	Specify: advanced or delayed phase type, disorganized type, frequently changing type
307.40*	Other dyssomnias

Parasomnias

307.47	Dream anxiety disorder (nightmare disorder)

307.46*	Sleep terror disorder
307.46*	Sleepwalking disorder
307.40*	Parasomnia NOS

FACTITIOUS DISORDERS

	Factitious disorder
301.51	with physical symptoms
300.16	with psychological symptoms
300.19	Factitious disorder NOS

IMPULSE CONTROL DISORDERS NOT ELSEWHERE CLASSIFIED

312.34	Intermittent explosive disorder
312.32	Kleptomania
312.31	Pathological gambling
312.33	Pyromania
312.39*	Trichotillomania
312.39*	Impulse control disorder NOS

ADJUSTMENT DISORDER

	Adjustment disorder
309.24	with anxious mood
309.00	with depressed mood
309.30	with disturbance of conduct
309.40	with mixed disturbance of emotions and conduct
309.28	with mixed emotional features
309.82	with physical complaints
309.83	with withdrawal
309.23	with work (or academic) inhibition
309.90	Adjustment disorder NOS

PSYCHOLOGICAL FACTORS AFFECTING PHYSICAL CONDITION

316.00	Psychological factors affecting physical condition *Specify*: physical condition on axis III

PERSONALITY DISORDERS
Note: These are coded on axis II.
Cluster A

301.00	Paranoid
301.20	Schizoid
301.22	Schizotypal

Cluster B

301.70	Antisocial
301.83	Borderline
301.50	Histrionic
301.81	Narcissistic

Cluster C

301.82	Avoidant
301.60	Dependent
301.40	Obsessive compulsive

301.84	Passive aggressive
301.90	Personality disorder NOS

V CODES FOR CONDITIONS NOT ATTRIBUTABLE TO A MENTAL DISORDER THAT ARE A FOCUS OF ATTENTION OR TREATMENT

V62.30	Academic problem
V71.01	Adult antisocial behavior

V40.00	Borderline intellectual functioning (Note: This is coded on axis II.)

V71.02	Childhood or adolescent antisocial behavior
V65.20	Malingering
V61.10	Marital problem
V15.81	Noncompliance with medical treatment
V62.20	Occupational problem
V61.20	Parent-child problem
V62.81	Other interpersonal problem
V61.80	Other specified family circumstances
V62.89	Phase of life problem or other life circumstance problem
V62.82	Uncomplicated bereavement

ADDITIONAL CODES

300.90	Unspecified mental disorder (nonpsychotic)
V71.09*	No diagnosis or condition on axis I
799.90*	Diagnosis or condition deferred on axis I.

V71.09*	No diagnosis or condition on axis II
799.90*	Diagnosis or condition deferred on axis II

MULTIAXIAL SYSTEM

Axis I	Clinical Syndromes V Codes
Axis II	Developmental Disorders Personality Disorders
Axis III	Physical Disorders and Conditions
Axis IV	Severity of Psychosocial Stressors
Axis V	Global Assessment of Functioning

17

Organic Mental Disorders

Renee L. Binder, MD

The term "organic mental disorder" denotes psychological and behavioral abnormalities resulting from transient or permanent cerebral dysfunction. Organic mental disorders are distinguished from functional disorders such as schizophrenia and affective illness in that they have known biological causes and pathophysiological mechanisms, whereas the functional disorders do not.

The term "organic brain syndrome" denotes a specific array of signs and symptoms. There are a variety of different organic brain syndromes. Eight of them—delirium, dementia, amnestic syndrome, organic delusional syndrome, organic hallucinosis, organic mood syndrome, organic anxiety syndrome, and organic personality syndrome—will be considered in this chapter.

Terminology of Organic Mental Disorders

In previous classification systems *(DSM-I* and *DSM-II)*, certain terms that are no longer considered useful were used in describing organic brain syndromes; their definitions are important because they are still in the older medical literature. The terms "psychotic" and "nonpsychotic" were used to characterize severe and nonsevere brain syndromes, respectively. In current usage, the term "psychotic" denotes inability to distinguish what is real from what is unreal; ie, a psychotic patient is one who lacks "reality testing." The terms "acute" and "chronic" were used to characterize reversible and irreversible brain syndromes, respectively. The prototype of acute brain syndrome was delirium, and the prototype of chronic brain syndrome was dementia. This was confusing, because delirium may progress to irreversible brain damage and dementia may in some cases be reversible. It was also confusing because the terms acute" and "chronic" were being used differently than in medicine generally, where the words refer to mode of onset and duration rather than reversibility.

Symptoms & Signs of Organic Mental Disorders

A. Common Symptoms and Signs: In the evaluation of a patient with a psychological or behavioral disturbance, certain symptoms and signs suggest an organic rather than a functional origin.

1. Fluctuating performance on serial mental status examinations.

2. Memory impairment.

3. Disorientation.

4. Cognitive impairment, eg, dyscalculia, or reduced fund of information.

5. Visual hallucinations or illusions.

6. Formication (sensation of bugs crawling under the skin).

7. Floccillation/carphologia (picking at nightclothes or covers).

8. Prior physical illness or current physical symptoms.

9. Autonomic symptoms (tachycardia, fever, sweating, hypertension).

10. History of recent drug or medication intake.

11. Sudden onset without any previous personal or family psychiatric history—at any age, but especially in a patient over 40.

12. Lack of expected response to traditional treatment.

Although any of these symptoms and signs may be present in a functional disorder, when they are elicited, it is important to at least consider an organic cause of behavioral and psychological disturbances.

B. Syndromes of Same Origin: The same cause can result in different organic brain syndromes in different patients. For example, neurosyphilis can cause delirium, dementia, organic delusional syndrome, organic hallucinosis, organic affective syndrome, or organic personality syndrome. Even in the same patient, a given cause may lead first to one organic brain syndrome and then to another. For example, neurosyphilis may first present as an organic affective syndrome or an organic personality syndrome and then progress to dementia. In addition, HIV infection may cause a variety of organic mental disorders, including delirium, dementia, organic delusional syndromes, and organic hallucinosis.

C. Factors Affecting Symptoms and Signs: Even if a specific organic cause is present, the severity and type of signs and symptoms of organic brain syndromes depend on physical, psychological, and social factors.

1. Physical factors affecting symptoms and signs include the following:

a. The degree of organic insult. For example, brain tumor is manifested differently depending on the size and location of the tumor and whether intracranial pressure is increased. Pernicious anemia is manifested differently depending on the serum level of vitamin B_{12}.

b. The rate at which brain involvement occurs, For example, brain tumor is manifested differently depending on whether it grows slowly or rapidly. In the case of heavy metal poisoning, effects depend on whether intoxication is gradual or acute.

c. The physical condition of the patient.

2. Psychological factors affecting symptoms and signs include the following:

a. The patient's personality and psychological defense mechanisms. For example, in response to the same organic insult, a patient with a paranoid personality may become more paranoid and one with an obsessive personality more obsessive. An obsessive medical student developed a steroid psychosis after she was treated for systemic lupus erythematosus. Her symptoms included pinning notes all around her bed and ruminating obsessively, wondering whether she should put a drinking glass 2 inches or 5 inches from the edge of her nightstand.

b. The patient's intelligence and education.

c. The patient's level of premorbid psychological adjustment. For example, a patient who was relatively well adjusted before developing organic brain syndrome may be able to tolerate a mild deficit better than can a patient with preexisting difficulties.

d. Current psychological stress and conflict. For example, a patient who has recently lost a spouse or been forced to retire may already be depressed and have difficulty tolerating even mild organic deficits.

3. Social factors affecting symptoms and signs include the following:

a. Degree of social isolation versus support. For example, a patient with senile dementia functioned adequately while living with his wife, who took care of him; but when she entered the hospital for treatment of medical problems, his condition deteriorated.

b. Degree of familiarity with the environment. For example, patients with organic brain syndrome often function poorly and become easily confused in an unfamiliar hospital environment, although they may be able to take care of themselves fairly well at home.

c. Either insufficient or excessive sensory input may cause confusion in a patient with organic brain syndrome.

DELIRIUM

Symptoms & Signs

The *DSM-III-R* criteria for the diagnosis of delirium are shown in Table 17–1.

One aspect of delirium is a deficit in the capacity

Table 17–1. *DSM-III-R* diagnostic criteria for delirium.

A. Reduced ability to maintain attention to external stimuli (eg, questions must be repeated because attention wanders) and to appropriately shift attention to new external stimuli (eg, perseverates answer to a previous question).

B. Disorganized thinking, as indicated by rambling, irrelevant, or incoherent speech.

C. At least 2 of the following:
  (1) Reduced level of consciousness, eg, difficulty keeping awake during examination.
  (2) Perceptual disturbances: misinterpretations, illusions, or hallucinations.
  (3) Disturbance of sleep-wake cycle with insomnia or daytime sleepiness.
  (4) Increased or decreased psychomotor activity.
  (5) Disorientation to time, place, or person.
  (6) Memory impairment, eg, inability to learn new material, such as the names of several unrelated objects, after 5 minutes, or to remember past events, such as history of current episode of illness.

D. Clinical features develop over a short period of time (usually hours to days) and tend to fluctuate over the course of a day.

E. Either (1) or (2):
  (1) Evidence from the history, physical examination, or laboratory tests of a specific organic factor (or factors) judged to be etiologically related to the disturbance.
  (2) In the absence of such evidence, an etiologic organic factor can be presumed if the disturbance cannot be accounted for by any nonorganic mental disorder, eg, manic episode accounting for agitation and sleep disturbance.

to maintain and shift attention. Thus, the patient has difficulty answering a question because of difficulty remembering the content or because of perseveration about a previous question. Another method of testing for attention deficit is to ask the patient to recite the months or spell a word backward or count backward from 100 by 3s (100, 97, 94, etc). (See Chapter 11 for formal tests of attention.)

Visual hallucinations are especially common. For example, a patient will report seeing his or her dead mother in the room. Patients sometimes report feeling as if they are dreaming when they know they are awake. A patient may attempt to get out of bed, pick at the bedclothes, or strike out at nonexistent objects. On the other hand, the patient may be sluggish or stuporous. The same patient may alternate from one of these extremes to the other.

In delirium, disorientation to time is worse than disorientation to name or place. For example, a patient may know that his name is John Smith and that he is in a hospital but will have no idea what time it is. As he becomes more delirious, he may still know that his name is John Smith, but he may think that he is in school and still have no idea what time it is. Memory impairment is usually tested by asking the patient to repeat the names of three or four objects and then recall them after 5 minutes. Memory testing may be impossible if the patient is uncooperative or mute or cannot attend to questions.

Natural History

According to *DSM-III-R*, the clinical features "develop over a short period of time (usually hours to days) and tend to fluctuate over the course of a day." In fact, the fluctuating course is one of the most significant clinical aspects of delirium. A patient may be totally disoriented during one mental status examination arid have a fairly coherent lucid period later in the day.

The duration of an episode of delirium is usually brief—about a week, rarely more than a month. The duration and course depend upon identification and correction of the underlying cause. If the underlying disorder persists, delirium may lead to dementia or some other form of organic brain syndrome or may end in death.

Differential Diagnosis

The differential diagnosis of delirium includes functional disorders such as schizophrenia and affective disorder. Both delirium and these functional disorders may include perceptual disturbances, disorganized thinking, disturbances of the sleep-wakefulness cycle, and abnormal psychomotor activity. However, in delirium, delusions and hallucinations tend to be more random and not organized into a delusional system. Also in delirium, there is a fluctuating course with cognitive impairment, and there may be a reduced level of consciousness.

Both delirium and dementia are characterized by cognitive impairment. However, in delirium, there is a fluctuating course, whereas in dementia there is a relatively stable cognitive impairment. It is important to realize that both delirium and dementia may be present in the same patient.

A factitious disorder with psychological symptoms in which the patient tries to simulate delirium must also be ruled out. The patient's ability to simulate delirium will depend on knowing what true delirium looks like. In factitious disorder, the symptoms are worse when the patient is aware of being observed; this is not true of delirium.

In true delirium, there is usually generalized slowing of electroencephalographic background activity; this slowing is absent in delirium tremens.

Prognosis

The prognosis of delirium depends on identification and treatment of the underlying cause. If the underlying disorder is treated successfully, complete recovery is the rule. If it persists without treatment or in spite of treatment, the delirium may lead to dementia or other organic brain syndrome or even death.

Illustrative Case

A 43-year-old woman was brought to the hospital by members of her family, who reported that for the last few days she had become increasingly frightened and suspicious. She felt that the people who lived upstairs were threatening her and that it was unsafe to be at home. She said she had seen babies being lowered from the window of the upstairs apartment. Her family stated that these ideas had no basis in reality.

On initial mental status examination, the patient was observed to be agitated and frightened, with pressure of speech, and preoccupied with ideas of persecution. She was fully oriented to time and place, and memory was intact. The admitting third-year medical student and resident thought the patient was having a paranoid reaction. She was admitted to hospital for evaluation and observation. At that time, an organic cause was not suspected.

On the first day of hospitalization, there was a marked change in the patient's mental status, which seemed to improve and then worsen. She became more agitated and tremulous and developed tachycardia, diaphoresis, and hypertension. This progressed to disorientation (she did not know where she was or what time it was), visual hallucinations (she saw her mother in her room), illusions (shadows on the wall were misinterpreted as a person), and problems in memory (she could not recall three objects).

Urine and serum chemical tests showed high barbiturate levels, though the patient had denied chronic drug use. A diagnosis of delirium secondary to barbiturate withdrawal was then made, and the patient was successfully treated with gradually decreasing doses of barbiturates to prevent seizures.

Epidemiology

Delirium is a common condition. It may occur in any patient entering or recovering from coma or recovering from anesthesia. It may also occur in any patient who is overmedicated with psychoactive drugs. Delirium is especially common in children and in persons over age 60, since the immature or aging brain is more susceptible to delirium. Preexisting brain damage, drug or alcohol addiction, and a history of delirium also appear to increase the chances of developing delirium.

Etiology

A. Common Causes:

1. Metabolic imbalance—Examples are hypoxia, hypercapnia, hypoglycemia, hepatic or renal disease, hyper- or hypothyroidism, porphyria, and electrolyte abnormalities such as excess or deficiency of sodium, potassium, calcium, and magnesium.

2. Substance abuse, drug toxicity, withdrawal syndrome—The classical presentation is delirium tremens from alcohol withdrawal or the delirium of barbiturate withdrawal, as in the illustrative case. A cause of delirium not uncommonly seen in emergency rooms is anticholinergic intoxication. Such patients have been traditionally described as "red as a beet, dry as a bone, mad as a hatter, and blind as a stone''—because of peripheral vasodilatation, dry mucous membranes and lack of sweating, delirium, and impaired visual accommodation. Common agents involved in anticholinergic intoxication are scopolamine, antiparkinsonism drugs (trihexyphenidyl, benztropine), tricyclic antidepressants (amitriptyline, imipramine), and antipsychotic medications (thioridazine, chlorpromazine). There are opportunities for diagnostic confusion when a hallucinating patient is known to be taking antipsychotic medication, so that the clinician does not know if the psychosis is a schizophrenic symptom or a toxic drug reaction. However, in the case of psychosis due to anticholinergic drug toxicity, hallucinations are usually visual (sometimes auditory or tactile), and the patient has the additional somatic symptoms mentioned above.

3. Trauma–Head trauma.

B. Less Common Causes:

1. Infections–Either systemic (pneumonia, typhoid fever, malaria) or intracranial (encephalitis, meningitis, encephalomyelitis, eg, HIV infection).

2. Space-occupying lesions in the brain–Neoplasms, abscesses, tumors, hematomas, aneurysms, parasitic cysts.

3. Thiamine deficiency–Wernicke's encephalopathy.

4. Hypertension–Hypertensive encephalopathy.

5. Seizures–Postictal state.

6. Environmental causes–Either sensory deprivation or overstimulation may cause delirium. Two examples of delirium caused by sensory deprivation are ''black patch delirium'' and ''iron lung delirium.'' When patients underwent bilateral cataract surgery (both eyes done at the same time to decrease the anesthetic risk), they often became delirious when both eyes were patched postoperatively; ophthalmologists now operate on one eye at a time. Patients with poliomyelitis in body respirators had limited visual fields and sometimes became delirious; this was prevented by using mirrors to increase the field of vision. Some patients become delirious in intensive care units, perhaps from a combination of sensory overstimulation (frequent attention by nursing and medical staff, noises of life support equipment, and resuscitation efforts in nearby beds), sleep deprivation, and fear of death.

7. Fever–High fever.

Pathogenesis

The pathogenesis of delirium is not clearly understood, but it appears to involve dysfunction of both the cerebral cortex and the subcortical structures that serve arousal, alertness, attention, information processing, and maintenance of the normal sleep-wakefulness cycle. In delirium, the integrated activity of these anatomic structures is disturbed. Studies of the pathogenesis of delirium sometimes give conflicting results, revealing the heterogeneity of the disorder.

For example, delirium is often associated with a reduced cerebral metabolic rate, but in delirium associated with hyperthermia, the rate is increased. Again, delirium is usually associated with slowing of background electroencephalographic activity, but this does not occur in delirium tremens.

Treatment

A. Specific Measures: The most important aspect of management is to identify and treat causative factors. This involves a complete medical history and physical examination and appropriate laboratory tests, including complete blood count and urinalysis, metabolic screening battery (for renal, adrenal, and hepatic disease and for abnormalities in blood glucose and electrolytes, including calcium and magnesium), thyroid function tests, a serological test for syphilis, toxicology screens, and chest x-ray. An electroencephalogram, CT head scan, lumbar puncture, and other tests such as bromide levels, heavy metal screen, serum vitamin B_{12} levels, and an antinuclear antibody (ANA) test should be considered depending on the clinical situation.

Once the cause is identified, prompt treatment should be given. In the illustrative case (see above), barbiturates in diminishing doses were administered for delirium associated with barbiturate withdrawal.

B. General Measures: Ensure sleep, maintain fluid and nutritional intake, and provide supportive nursing care. This involves monitoring vital signs and watching for hyperthermia or circulatory collapse. The patient should be at rest in a quiet, well-lighted room, with a clock and calendar to help maintain orientation. The nursing staff should periodically reorient the patient to time, location, and reason for hospitalization. The restless, agitated, fearful patient should be mildly sedated with haloperidol, 5 mg every hour, or a similar sedative drug.

DEMENTIA

The *DSM-III-R* criteria for dementia (Table 17–2) include loss of intellectual abilities and impairment of memory. These symptoms will be noted on testing of comprehension, calculation, knowledge, and memory during the mental status examination (see Chapter 11). The patient with dementia is forgetful, has difficulty learning new material, and will often try to minimize or deny deficits. Recent memory is worse than remote memory. The patient may not be able to recall the names of three objects after 5 minutes but may have excellent recall of events that occurred in childhood.

Impairment of abstract thinking can be tested by asking the patient to interpret proverbs or state how a chair and a desk or a dog and a cat are similar or different. Other disturbances of higher cortical function (Table 17–2) can also be identified by means

Table 17–2. *DSM-III-R* diagnostic criteria for dementia.

A. Demonstrates evidence of impairment in short- and long-term memory. Impairment in short-term memory (inability to learn new information) may be indicated by inability to remember 3 objects after 5 minutes. Long-term memory impairment (inability to remember information that was known in the past) may be indicated by inability to remember past personal information (eg, what happened yesterday, birthplace, occupation) or facts of common knowledge (eg, past presidents, well-known dates).

B. At least one of the following:
   (1) Impairment in abstract thinking, as indicated by inability to find similarities and differences between related words, difficulty in defining words and concepts, and other similar tasks.
   (2) Impaired judgment, as indicated by inability to make reasonable plans to deal with interpersonal, family, and job-related problems and issues,
   (3) Other disturbances of higher cortical function, such as aphasia (disorder of language), apraxia (inability to carry out motor activities despite intact comprehension and motor function), agnosia (failure to recognize or identify objects despite intact sensory function), and "constructional difficulty" (eg, inability to copy 3-dimensional figures, assemble blocks, or arrange sticks in specific designs).
   (4) Personality change, ie, alteration or accentuation of premorbid traits.

C. The disturbance in criterion A or criterion B significantly interferes with work or usual social activities or relationships with others.

D. Not occurring exclusively during the course of delirium.

E. Either (1) or (2):
   (1) There is evidence from the history, physical examination, or laboratory tests of a specific organic factor (or factors) judged to be etiologically related to the disturbance.
   (2) In the absence of such evidence, an etiologic organic factor can be presumed if the disturbance cannot be accounted for by any nonorganic mental disorder, eg, major depression accounting for cognitive impairment.

of the mental status and neurological examinations. Two good tests for constructional difficulty are to ask the patient to draw a clock face and set the hands at a certain time or to copy a figure such as those shown below:

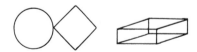

Often, the patient will have an accentuation of premorbid character traits, so that a normally suspicious patient will become more paranoid as dementia develops. With frontal lobe disease, there is loss of inhibition, and the patient may tell obscene jokes or make sexual advances to strangers.

Lability or shallowness of affect may also be noted.

Natural History

Dementia may have a progressive, static, or remitting course. The mode of onset and subsequent course depend on the cause. For example, primary degenerative dementia of the Alzheimer type has a slow onset and progresses to death over a period of several years. Dementia due to head trauma may begin quite suddenly and then remain static for a long time. Dementia due to neurosyphilis or normal pressure hydrocephalus may be completely reversible.

Differential Diagnosis

Normal aging and age-related forgetfulness are part of the differential diagnosis of dementia. In normal aging, memory losses are slight and do not interfere with daily activities. Dementia is not synonymous with aging. In dementia, loss of intellectual abilities is of sufficient severity to interfere with social or occupational functioning.

Delirium is distinguished from dementia by the presence, in delirium, of a widely fluctuating clinical course. In dementia, the cognitive impairment tends to be relatively stable.

Schizophrenia may be confused with dementia, since both conditions are associated with deterioration from previous levels of functioning, impairment of abstract thinking and judgment, and inappropriate affect. In schizophrenia, however, the onset is usually during adolescence and young adulthood, whereas dementia occurs predominantly in the elderly (although dementia may occur at any age, depending on the cause). In schizophrenia, there is no identifiable brain lesion that accounts for the symptoms, and schizophrenia typically presents with no disturbance in sensorium, whereas in dementia there is global cognitive impairment.

Factitious disorders with psychological symptoms may rarely be confused with dementia. In factitious disorders, the symptoms are worse when the patient is aware of being observed, and the symptoms are not consistent with what is observed in dementia. For example, the patient simulating memory impairment will often show equal difficulty with recent and remote memory, whereas in true dementia recent memory is usually worse.

The major differential diagnostic problem in a patient who complains of memory impairment, difficulty in concentrating, and decline in intellectual functioning is between depression and dementia. Much has been written about the syndrome of "pseudodementia," a disorder in which dementia is mimicked or caricatured by functional psychiatric illness, often depression (Table 17–3). Patients who are depressed may perform poorly on mental status examinations and on neuropsychological testing, and patients who are demented may also appear depressed. In depression, there is usually a more sudden onset of cognitive deficit, and its onset can be dated with some precision; in dementia, the onset of cognitive loss is usually more gradual. In depression, there may be a history of previous mental illness; in dementia, this is usually lacking. In depression, there is often a history of

Table 17–3. Differentiation of pseudodementia and dementia.

Pseudodementia	Dementia
Sudden onset.	Gradual onset.
Prior psychiatric illness.	No prior psychiatric illness.
Vegetative signs.	No vegetative signs.
Patients expose cognitive deficits.	Patients conceal cognitive deficits.
Patients respond "I don't know."	Patients give near-miss answers.
Marked variability in cognitive performance.	Consistently poor in cognitive performance.
Recent and remote memory equally poor.	Recent memory worse than remote memory.
Sundowning rare.	Sundowning common.

vegetative signs, such as appetite and sleep disturbances; in dementia, these are usually lacking. In depression, patients expose and exaggerate their defective cognitive performance; in dementia, patients conceal, rationalize, minimize, and compensate for their deficits.

On mental status examination, patients with depression make little effort to perform even simple tasks and will often answer, "I don't know." There will also be marked variability in performance of tasks of similar difficulty. In dementia, patients will struggle to perform tasks and often give near-miss answers, and there will be consistently poor performance on tasks of similar difficulty. In depression, memory loss for recent and remote memory is usually equally severe; in dementia, memory loss for recent events is usually more severe than for remote events. "Sundowning" is rare in depression and common in dementia—ie, the patient becomes more confused and has more cognitive difficultly when the sun goes down at night.

Even with all of these clues to differentiation between pseudodementia of depression and true dementia, it may be difficult to make the distinction. The only definitive way of distinguishing between depression and dementia may be to actively treat the depression and see if the patient continues to show signs of dementia well after the depressive episode ends.

Prognosis

The prognosis of dementia depends on the underlying cause. About 5–15% of all dementias are reversible, and if their cause is identified and is treatable, the prognosis is good. However, Alzheimer's disease (the most common cause of dementia in the elderly) is progressive and usually leads to death in several years. Death is usually preceded by poor nutrition, dehydration, and respiratory infection.

Illustrative Case

The patient was a 65-year-old married and recently retired dentist whose chief complaint was depression. He had experienced a series of professional difficulties

over the years including a prosecution for fraud after billing two insurance companies for the same service. He had never done anything like this in the past, and at a pretrial hearing he claimed he had been confused, and the charges were dropped. The patient later decided to retire and sold his practice impulsively and, as his family thought, improvidently. In retirement, the patient became depressed and suicidal and decided to seek psychiatric help.

The mental status examination showed depressed affect. However, the patient had no vegetative signs and no history of mental illness. He had problems in recent memory and calculation and could not remember where his daughter lived. He had difficulty finding the psychiatrist's office and went to the wrong part of the building several times. A complete medical history revealed that the patient had minor problems with urinary incontinence as well as ataxia. CT scan revealed ventricular dilatation consistent with normal-pressure hydrocephalus. A neurosurgical shunt to divert cerebrospinal fluid from the cerebral ventricular space to the atrium of the heart reversed his dementia as well as his secondary depression.

In the above case, the incident of billing two insurance companies was probably an early sign of deterioration of previously good judgment.

Epidemiology

Dementia is found predominantly in elderly persons, although certain specific etiological factors may cause dementia at any age. The diagnosis may be made at any time after the IQ is fairly stable (usually by age 3 or 4).

In the USA, 5% of people over the age of 65 have severe dementia (unable to care for themselves), and 10% have mild dementia. Therefore, in 1980, with 25 million people over 65, there were 1.2 million individuals with severe dementia and 2.5 million with milder dementia. By 1990, 32 million will be over 65.

Dementia affects 58% of the more than 1 million individuals in nursing homes in the USA. More than half of patients over age 65 in state and county mental hospitals also have a diagnosis of dementia.

Etiology & Pathogenesis

The most common cause of dementia is Alzheimer's disease, which accounts for 65% of dementias in persons over age 65. In Alzheimer's disease, progressive dementia occurs with no identifiable cause (other than aging) and no abnormal laboratory findings. The electroencephalogram is often diffusely slow, and CT scan often shows cerebral cortical atrophy and slight to moderate ventricular dilatation. No correlation has been found between the extent of cerebral cortical atrophy and severity of dementia, and some patients with Alzheimer's disease show no evidence of atrophy. However, most studies have revealed some correlation between the extent of ventricular dilatation and the severity of dementia. Clinically, the diagnosis of Alzheimer's disease is made by excluding other causes of dementia.

The histopathological changes in Alzheimer's disease consist of microscopic senile plaques, neurofibrillary tangles, and granulovacuolar degeneration of neurons. In some texts, a distinction is made between the presenile form of Alzheimer's disease (below age 65) and the senile form (over age 65). However, there is no convincing evidence of morphological or biochemical differences between these two forms of Alzheimer' s disease.

About 10% of cases of dementia in persons over age 65 are so-called multi-infarct dementias, in which cerebral softening occurs following multiple infarctions of brain tissue. There is typically an abrupt onset and a stepwise deteriorating course and patchy distribution of deficits, depending upon which regions of the brain have been destroyed. There are focal neurological signs and symptoms and a history of hypertension and strokes. Another cause of dementia is HIV infection. In fact, 6–14% of HIV-infected patients initially present to a medical clinic with so-called AIDS dementia complex.

Other common causes of dementia are alcoholism and head trauma. *It is important to look for reversible causes of dementia, since 5–15% of all dementias are reversible.*

Examples of causes of reversible dementia include intracranial conditions (meningiomas, subdural hematomas, normal-pressure hydrocephalus), systemic illnesses (pulmonary insufficiency, severe anemia, uremia, hyponatremia, Wilson's disease, porphyria), deficiency states (vitamin B_{12} deficiency, thiamine deficiency, pellagra), endocrinopathies (Addison's disease, myxedema, hyperthyroidism, hypo- or hyperparathyroidism), heavy metal poisoning (mercury, lead, arsenic, thallium), infections (neurosyphilis, chronic tuberculous or cryptococcal meningitis, cerebral abscess), collagen vascular disorders (systemic lupus erythematosus), and drug toxicity (disulfiram, bromides).

In normal-pressure (occult) hydrocephalus, there is usually a triad of dementia, ataxia, and urinary incontinence. The disorder may be idiopathic or due to subarachnoid hemorrhage, meningitis, or head trauma. There is obstruction to the flow of cerebrospinal fluid over the convexities of the cerebral hemispheres, and cerebrospinal fluid absorption through the usual pathways at the superior sagittal sinus is impaired. The ventricles are enlarged, but there is no increase in cerebrospinal fluid pressure. As in the illustrative case (see above), this type of dementia can sometimes be completely reversed with a neurosurgical shunt procedure that relieves the obstruction.

The deficits in dementia result from widespread damage to any part of the brain, but especially the cerebral cortex. There may not be structural changes, but cerebral dysfunction is always present. Neuro-chemical investigations of patients with Alzheimer's disease have shown that central cholinergic neurotransmission is reduced. In consequence, there has been an attempt to treat Alzheimer's disease with acetylcholine precursors such as choline and lecithin, with cholinergic agonists such as arecoline, or with anticholinesterase agents such as physostigmine. All of these methods of treatment have given mixed results and are still experimental.

Treatment

A. Specific Measures: Reversible causes should be sought aggressively in any patient who presents with dementia. This involves a complete history and physical examination, including a history of drug, alcohol, and medication intake. In addition, the following minimal workup should be ordered: complete blood count (look for anemia and evidence of collagen vascular disease); urinalysis; chest x-ray (look for pulmonary disease and congestive heart failure); metabolic screening battery (look for renal, adrenal, and hepatic disease and electrolyte or glucose imbalance); thyroid function tests; serological tests for syphilis, including the Venereal Disease Research Laboratories (VDRL) test and the fluorescent treponemal antibody (FTA-ABS) test (one-third of patients with neurosyphilis have nonreactive serum VDRLs, but FTA-ABS were positive); serum vitamin B_{12} (in pernicious anemia, central nervous system findings may exist without anemia); and CT scan (look for space-occupying lesions, evidence of infarct, and normal-pressure hydrocephalus). Depending on the clinical situation, other tests such as lumbar puncture, toxicology screen, heavy metal screens, serum bromides, HIV, and ANA tests should also be considered.

B. General Measures: Simple advice or psychotherapy will help the patient deal with anxiety and depression. The patient should be given information about the illness as tolerated, help with the process of grieving over losses, and help with the effort to maintain faltering self-esteem. In appropriate circumstances, the patient should be offered advice about a change of situation (job, domicile) and about full utilization of available skills.

Social stimulation and structure must be sustained. The patient should be in a stimulating environment to maximize intellectual capacities. Patients in nursing homes should have free access to television and newspapers and recreational activities, and pets if possible. A structured schedule during the day is important to give a comfortable sense of predictability in life.

Family intervention (such as giving support and advice to the family) is an important part of the treatment of dementia, since family members usually have questions and concerns and may express shame or guilt if given the opportunity.

Prescribe low-dose medication for symptomatic relief. Symptoms that may respond to pharmacological therapy include anxiety, agitation, hyperactivity, depression, irritability, disturbed sleep, and psychotic behavior. (See Chapter 32 for details.)

AMNESTIC SYNDROME

Symptoms & Signs

Table 17–4 sets forth the *DSM-III-R* diagnostic criteria for amnestic syndrome.

Memory loss is both anterograde and retrograde. With anterograde amnesia, the patient cannot recall recent events since the insult to the brain; with retrograde amnesia, the patient cannot recall events before the insult occurred. It is useful to distinguish four kinds of memory: immediate, recent, intermediate, and remote. Memory deficit in amnestic syndrome involves recent and intermediate memory and spares immediate and remote memory. Immediate memory involves the ability to retain new material as long as attention is not distracted—eg, the patient should be able to recite six digits forward. Recent memory involves the ability to retain new material after attention is distracted—eg, by asking the patient to recall the names of three objects after 5 minutes of further interviewing. Impairment of recent memory leads to anterograde amnesia—inability to recall events that have occurred since the insult to the brain, since the patient has not been able to retain new material. Anterograde amnesia covers a variable period of time in different patients, and testing of recent memory is impaired during the period of anterograde amnesia. The somewhat arbitrary term intermediate memory is for events that occurred in the past 3–20 years. This can be tested by asking the patient about events in his or her life or newsworthy events that occurred in the last decade.

Retrograde amnesia is inability to recall events that occurred before the insult to the brain, because of difficulties in intermediate memory. Retrograde amnesia covers variable periods of time in different patients. Remote memory is for events in the more distant past, sometimes arbitrarily defined as what was learned before age 12. This can be tested by asking the patient about events in early life.

In amnestic syndrome, there is no general loss of major intellectual abilities. However, there may be confabulation, where the patient recites imaginary events to fill in gaps in memory. Confabulation is not a constant feature of amnestic syndrome. It tends to occur early in Korsakoff's psychosis but disappears later on. (Korsakoff's psychosis is an amnestic syndrome secondary to thiamine deficiency. Etiology is discussed later.)

Disorientation may be present but is not an invariable feature of amnestic syndrome. Disorientation is usually present in Korsakoff's psychosis but not in amnestic syndrome due to other causes.

Natural History

The mode of onset and the course of amnestic syndrome depend on the underlying cause. Amnestic syndrome secondary to head trauma has a sudden onset with gradual but incomplete recovery. Amnestic syndrome secondary to thiamine deficiency in alcoholics has an acute or subacute onset and may be irreversible, especially if well established.

Differential Diagnosis

The distinction between Wernicke's encephalopathy (a delirium) and Korsakoff's psychosis (an amnestic syndrome) should be clarified, since Korsakoff s psychosis typically appears concomitantly with or following Wernicke's encephalopathy. Wernicke's encephalopathy comes on subacutely in a patient with a history of many years of alcohol abuse. The signs and symptoms include delirium, ataxia, ophthalmoplegia, and nystagmus. The delirium clears in about a month, and in about 85% of survivors the amnestic syndrome becomes manifest if it has not been evident all along. A few patients with thiamine deficiency develop amnestic syndrome without a preceding episode of Wernicke's encephalopathy.

In delirium, there is a fluctuating course; this is absent in amnestic syndrome. In dementia, there are other major intellectual deficits, whereas in amnestic syndrome, only memory deficit is involved. In factitious disorder with psychological symptoms or functional amnesia, there is often a stressful precipitating event, but this may be hard to elicit and, in any case, may also be present in amnestic syndrome. In functional amnesia, the patient may show selective memory impairment (eg, deny being married), although other recent and remote memories are preserved. In another kind of functional amnesia, the patient has global amnesia, ie, professes total amnesia for all events in past life. Failure of a patient without aphasia to state his or her own name is usually functional, and this may help distinguish functional amnesia from amnestic syndrome. Anterograde amnesia is rarely psychogenic and strongly suggests amnestic syndrome.

Prognosis

The prognosis for a patient with amnestic syndrome depends on the underlying cause. Gradual but incomplete recovery may follow amnestic syndrome second-

---

Table 17–4. *DSM-III-R* diagnostic criteria for amnestic syndrome.

A. Both short-term memory impairment (inability to learn new information) and long-term memory impairment (inability to remember information that was known in the past) are the predominant clinical features.

B. No clouding of consciousness, as in delirium; no general loss of major intellectual abilities, as in dementia.

C. Evidence, from the history, physical examination, or laboratory tests, of a specific organic factor that is judged to be etiologically related to the disturbance.

ary to head trauma, subarachnoid hemorrhage, bilateral hippocampal infarction, carbon monoxide poisoning, or other hypoxic states. Permanent memory loss may follow amnestic syndrome secondary to herpes simplex encephalitis and Korsakoff's psychosis. In one study of Korsakoff's psychosis, 21% of patients recovered completely, 53% had incomplete recovery, and 25% showed no appreciable memory improvement. Complete recovery usually occurred within a year. Incomplete recovery may take 5 years to reach its limit.

Illustrative Case

The patient was a 28-year-old married construction worker who was transferred to the psychiatric hospital from a medical ward. Ten days before admission, after learning that his wife was having an affair, he went to the basement and hanged himself with a rope looped over a water pipe. His wife saw him hanging and became confused about what to do. She tried unsuccessfully to burn the rope with a match and then ran to a neighbor for help. By the time the patient was cut down, he had suffered pulmonary and cardiac arrest and had dilated pupils. He had been hanging by the neck for about 10 minutes. He was resuscitated and was having spontaneous respirations within 24 hours of the anoxic episode. Ten days later, he was transferred to the psychiatric unit. Initial mental status examination revealed a patient who was conscious, alert, and feeding himself. He was oriented as to self but disoriented as to place and time. Reading, writing, and spelling were not affected.

The patient was able to repeat six digits forward. However, his recent memory was impaired, and he was unable to recall any of three objects after 5 minutes. Intermediate memory was also impaired, and he did not know he was married and remembered nothing about the suicide attempt. He did not remember past presidents or details of his work history. His remote memory was better, in that he remembered his birthplace and some details of his early life, eg, physical punishment by his stepfather. He was also able to abstract proverbs.

Physical and neurological examinations were within normal limits except for an elevated right hemidiaphragm and right upper extremity weakness from the traction injury of the patient's upper brachial plexus, primarily the C5 root. This weakness improved during the course of his 2-week hospitalization, although the memory impairment remained. The patient was transferred to a long-term rehabilitation hospital. When evaluated 3 months later, he was able to learn new material but had no memory for the period during which he was not storing new information. Intermediate memory had also improved, and he was able to remember more details of his past life.

Since some of this patient's intermediate memory has returned, it appears that his retrograde amnesia was a disorder of retrieval rather than storage.

Epidemiology

Amnestic syndrome is uncommon, and no epidemiological data are available.

Etiology & Pathogenesis

Amnestic syndrome may result from any pathological process that causes bilateral damage to certain diencephalic and medial temporal structures, eg, mammillary bodies, fornix, or hippocampal complex. The most common cause is thiamine deficiency associated with chronic alcoholism. However, thiamine deficiency causing Wernicke's encephalopathy or Korsakoff's psychosis may also result from protracted vomiting, carcinoma of the stomach, and voluntary starvation. The lesions in Korsakoff's psychosis involve the mammillary bodies, the inner portions of the dorsomedial, anteroventral, and pulvinar nuclei of the thalamus, and often the terminal portions of each fornix.

Other causes of amnestic syndrome include head trauma, subarachnoid hemorrhage, surgical trauma, carbon monoxide poisoning, other causes of hypoxia, infarction in the region of the posterior cerebral arteries, bilateral hippocampal infarction, and herpes simplex encephalitis. A syndrome called transient global amnesia has been described (see Chapter 5). Temporal lobe seizures and postconcussive states can also cause an amnestic syndrome of sudden onset and brief duration followed by complete spontaneous recovery.

Treatment

The treatment of amnestic syndrome is supportive, consisting mainly of giving advice and information to the patient and family to help them deal with the deficits. Depending on the severity of the symptoms and the supports available, the patient may or may not be able to lead a supervised existence in the community. Memory therapy, where patients have been taught to use mnemonics, has been successful in some patients.

In a patient with Wernicke's encephalopathy, it is important to prevent or minimize the development of Korsakoff's psychosis. Give thiamine, 100 mg intramuscularly daily for the first 3 days and then 100 mg orally daily until a normal diet is established. Other B complex vitamins should be given for general nutrition.

ORGANIC DELUSIONAL SYNDROME

Symptoms & Signs

Delusions, which are the predominant feature of organic delusional syndrome, may or may not be systematized and may be of different types, eg, delusions of jealousy, grandeur, or persecution. Persecutory delusions are the most common type.

Additional clinical features are outlined in Table 17–5.

Natural History

The mode of onset and the course depend on the underlying cause.

Differential Diagnosis

The differential diagnosis includes delirium, dementia, organic hallucinosis, organic affective syndrome, and the functional psychoses such as schizophrenia or the paranoid disorders. However, in delirium, there is a fluctuating course; in dementia, a significant loss of intellectual abilities; in organic hallucinosis, a predominance of hallucinations; and in organic affective syndrome, a predominance of affective symptoms. The difference between organic delusional syndrome and the functional disorders is that organic delusional syndrome is caused by a specific organic factor. Organic delusional syndrome should be suspected in any patient who presents with a paranoid psychosis with no previous personal or family psychiatric history, especially if the patient is over 40. It should also be suspected if the patient has any physical symptoms, autonomic symptoms, or a history of recent drug or medication intake or an atypical clinical course in terms of mode of onset and responsiveness to treatment.

Prognosis

The prognosis of organic delusional syndrome depends on identification and treatment of the underlying cause. The syndrome often lifts after withdrawal of the toxic agent or recovery from the physical illness; however, delusional psychoses may persist after phencyclidine or amphetamine ingestion and in some other cases, either as a direct effect of the drug or because the drug has unmasked an existing predisposition to a paranoid psychosis such as schizophrenia.

Epidemiology

The prevalence of organic delusional syndrome depends on the underlying cause.

Etiology & Pathogenesis

The causes of organic delusional syndrome include drugs such as amphetamines, phencyclidine, sympa-thomimetic amines, LSD, corticosteroids, and bromides; alcohol (causing alcoholic paranoia); epilepsy (especially temporal lobe epilepsy); brain tumor; encephalitis; neurosyphilis; HIV infection; head trauma; pernicious anemia; systemic lupus erythematosus; endocrine diseases such as hypo- or hyperthyroidism, Cushing's syndrome, Addison's disease, hyperinsulinism, and hypopituitarism; porphyria; and Huntington's chorea.

The pathogenesis of delusional symptoms in these disorders is not well understood.

Treatment

A. Specific Measures: Causative factors must be identified and treated. A patient suspected of having organic delusional syndrome—eg, an older patient with no personal or family psychiatric history who complains of physical or autonomic symptoms and gives a history of recreational drug or medication intake or an atypical clinical course—should have an organic workup including a complete medical history and physical examination, complete blood count, urinalysis, metabolic screening battery, thyroid function tests, serological test for syphilis, serum vitamin B_{12} determination, toxicology screen, and chest x-ray. Lumbar puncture, electroencephalography, ANA test, test for urinary porphyrins, and CT scan should also be considered.

B. General Measures: Give symptomatic relief with medications until the underlying cause can be identified and treated. Chlorpromazine or haloperidol is often used to reduce paranoid symptoms.

ORGANIC HALLUCINOSIS

Symptoms & Signs

Table 17–6 lists the DSM-III-R criteria for organic hallucinosis.

Hallucinations vary from simple and unformed to highly complex and organized. Patients may or may not believe the hallucinations are real. Hallucinations may occur in any modality, but certain causes tend to produce hallucinations in certain spheres; eg, alcohol and otosclerosis tend to induce auditory hallucinations, and hallucinogens and cataracts tend to induce visual hallucinations.

Table 17–5. *DSM-III-R* diagnostic criteria for organic delusional syndrome.

A. Delusions are the predominant clinical feature.

B. Evidence, from the history, physical examination, or laboratory tests, of a specific organic factor that is judged to be etiologically related to the disturbance.

C. Does not occur exclusively during the course of delirium.

Table 17–6. *DSM-III-R* diagnostic criteria for organic hallucinosis.

A. Persistent or recurrent hallucinations are the predominant clinical feature.

B. Evidence, from the history, physical examination, or laboratory tests, of a specific organic factor that is judged to be etiologically related to the disturbance.

C. Does not occur exclusively during the course of delirium.

Natural History

The mode of onset and the course of organic halluci-nosis depend on the underlying cause. For example, organic hallucinosis secondary to alcohol (alcohol hallucinosis) usually comes on acutely while the pa-tient is drinking or after a period of abstinence lasting from a few hours to weeks but-usually within 2 days following the last drink. Alcohol hallucinosis im-proves spontaneously within days to weeks, although hallucinations may last for months or may even be permanent. Patients who are blind as a result of uncor-rected bilateral cataracts may develop chronic visual hallucinations, and patients who are deaf as a result of otosclerosis may develop chronic auditory halluci-nations.

Differential Diagnosis

The differential diagnosis includes delirium, de-mentia, organic delusional syndrome, hypnagogic (upon going to sleep) and hypnopompic (upon waking up) hallucinations, and the functional psychoses such as schizophrenia and affective disorders.

In delirium, there is a fluctuating course; in demen-tia, a significant loss of intellectual abilities; and in organic delusional syndrome, delusions are the pre-dominant feature, though hallucinations may be pres-ent also. Delusions in organic hallucinosis syndrome are restricted to the content of the hallucinations or to the belief that the hallucinations are real. The differ-ence between organic hallucinosis and the functional disorders is that organic hallucinosis is caused by a specific organic factor.

It is sometimes not clear whether a patient with hallucinations and a history of alcohol abuse is experi-encing alcoholic hallucinosis or paranoid schizophre-nia. Patients with alcoholic hallucinosis tend to be older (40s and 50s); have an acute onset of symptoms; have no personal or family history of schizophrenia; have derogatory, persecutory auditory hallucinations or formless hallucinations such as cackling, knocking, whispering, or roaring sounds; have an anxious, de-pressed affect rather than a flat affect; display logical, coherent thought processes; and improve spontane-ously. The distinction from delirium tremens is based on the visual rather than auditory hallucinations and the clouded sensorium in the latter syndrome.

Prognosis

The prognosis of organic hallucinosis depends on the underlying cause. Alcoholic hallucinosis or hallu-cinogen-induced hallucinosis usually resolves sponta-neously but will recur with additional bouts of drink-ing or exposure to hallucinogens. Hallucinosis associ-ated with otosclerosis and cataracts usually is chronic. Patients may harm themselves attempting to flee from terrifying hallucinations.

Epidemiology

The prevalence of organic hallucinosis depends on the underlying cause. Alcoholic hallucinosis is rare and occurs in people who have been drinking for many years.

Etiology & Pathogenesis

The most common causes of this syndrome are prolonged use of alcohol and the use of hallucinogens such as LSD, psilocybin, and mescaline. Other causes include bilateral blindness or bilateral deafness, drug toxicity (levodopa, bromocriptine, amantadine, ephedrine, propranolol, methylphenidate, pentazo-cine), brain tumors and other space-occupying lesions (temporal lobe tumors, meningioma of the olfactory groove, chromophobe adenoma, craniopharyngioma, aneurysm, abscess), temporal arteritis, migraine, hy-pothyroidism, neurosyphilis, HIV infection, Hunting-ton's chorea, cerebrovascular disease, and seizure foci—especially in the temporal and occipital lobes.

The pathogenesis is unclear, but hallucinations are thought to be related to stimulation of specific cerebral sites or to disinhibition of brain areas that store sensory perceptions which are then released and experienced as hallucinations.

Treatment

A. Specific Measures: Identify any underlying causes. If a patient presents with isolated visual, olfac-tory, tactile, or auditory hallucinations, an organic cause should be suspected and ruled out. The workup should include a complete medical history and physi-cal examination, toxicology screen, thyroid function tests, serological tests for syphilis, and perhaps an electroencephalogram and CT scan.

B. General Measures: When indicated, reassure the patient that the hallucinations are temporary and not a sign of impending mental breakdown. for exam-ple, explain that the hallucinations are caused by mi-graine or hallucinogens.

Antipsychotic medications such as haloperidol or sedative-hypnotics such as chlordiazepoxide are often used in patients with alcoholic hallucinosis.

ORGANIC MOOD SYNDROME

Symptoms & Signs

Organic mood syndrome is characterized by a de-pressive or manic mood disorder. Symptoms consis-tent with major depressive disorder include dysphoric mood, appetite disturbance, sleep disturbance, anhe-donia, lack of energy, psychomotor retardation, feel-ings of worthlessness, and suicidal ideation. Those consistent with mania include elated or irritable mood, hyperactivity, pressure of speech, racing thoughts, grandiosity, decreased sleep, distractibility, buying sprees, and reckless decisions.

Table 17–7 lists additional criteria for organic mood syndrome.

Table 17–7. *DSM-III-R* diagnostic criteria for organic mood syndrome.

A. The predominant disturbance is a persistent depressed, elevated, or expansive mood.

B. Evidence, from the history, physical examination, or laboratory tests, of a specific organic factor that is judged to be etiologically related to the disturbance.

C. Does not occur exclusively during the course of delirium.

Natural History

The mode of onset and the course depend on the underlying cause.

Differential Diagnosis

The differential diagnosis includes delirium, dementia, organic hallucinosis, organic delusional syndrome, and the functional affective psychoses.

In delirium, there is clouding of consciousness; in dementia, a significant loss of intellectual abilities (mild cognitive impairment can occur in the organic affective syndrome); in organic hallucinosis, a predominance of hallucinations; and in organic delusional syndrome, a predominance of delusions.

The difference between organic mood syndrome and the functional affective disorders is that the former should be suspected in any patient who presents with an affective psychosis with no personal or family psychiatric history, especially if the patient is over 40. It should also be suspected if the patient has any physical symptoms or a history of recent medication intake or an atypical clinical course in terms of mode of onset and responsiveness to treatment.

Prognosis

The prognosis of organic mood syndrome depends on identification and treatment of the underlying cause.

Epidemiology

The prevalence of organic mood syndrome depends on the underlying cause.

Etiology

A. Drugs: Reserpine, methyldopa, guanethidine, clonidine, propranolol, and oral contraceptives can all cause depression. Amphetamines, cimetidine, isoniazid, levodopa, and bromides can cause mania. Corticosteroids can cause either depression or mania.

B. Endocrine Diseases: Hypothyroidism, hyperparathyroidism, and Addison's disease can cause depression. Cushing's syndrome can cause mania or depression.

C. Infectious Diseases: Infectious mononucleosis and other viral infections can cause depression; influenza and neurosyphilis can cause depression or mania.

D. Neoplastic Diseases: Carcinoma of the pancreas is associated with depression. Brain tumors can cause depression or mania.

E. Miscellaneous Diseases: Pernicious anemia and parkinsonism are associated with depression.

Pathogenesis

Although the pathogenesis of affective symptoms and signs in these disorders is not well understood, many hypotheses exist. Some of these are discussed elsewhere in this text. (See Chapter 22.)

Treatment

A. Specific Measures: Identify and treat causative factors. A patient who presents with late age at onset, physical symptoms, no personal or family psychiatric history, a history of medication intake, or an atypical clinical course should have an organic workup, including a complete medical history and physical examination, complete blood count, urinalysis, metabolic screening battery, thyroid function tests, serological tests for syphilis, serum vitamin B_{12} determination, toxicology screens, and chest x-ray. CT scan should also be considered.

B. General Measures: Symptomatic relief with medications and psychotherapy should be provided until the underlying cause can be identified and treated. Antipsychotic medication such as chlorpromazine, haloperidol, or lithium carbonate can be used to control manic symptoms. Antidepressant medication can sometimes alleviate depressive symptoms.

ORGANIC ANXIETY SYNDROME

The diagnostic criteria for organic anxiety syndrome are listed in Table 17–8. Little is known about this syndrome, which resembles the anxiety disorders but has a variety of specific organic causes, including hyperthyroidism, pheochromocytoma, fasting hypoglycemia, hypercortisolism, intoxication with stimulants (eg, caffeine, amphetamine), withdrawal from central nervous system depressants (eg, alcohol, sedatives), brain tumors of the third ventricle, and epilepsy involving the diencephalon.

Specific treatment requires identification and treatment of the causative factors. Symptomatic treatment with anxiolytic drugs before specific treatment is started may prove helpful.

ORGANIC PERSONALITY SYNDROME

Symptoms & Signs

The *DSM-III-R* criteria for organic personality syndrome are listed in Table 17–9. Patients with emotional lability, impairment of impulse control, and marked indifference often have frontal lobe lesions

Table 17–8. *DSM-III-R* diagnostic criteria for organic anxiety syndrome.

A. Prominent, recurrent, panic attacks or generalized anxiety.
B. Evidence from the history, physical examination, or laboratory tests of a specific organic factor that is judged to be etiologically related to the disturbance.
C. Does not occur exclusively during the course of delirium.

and may be referred for investigation of "frontal lobe signs." Patients with frontal lobe disease are difficult to manage when they are apathetic, euphoric, and irritable. (See Chapter 5.)

Natural History

The mode of onset and the course of organic personality syndrome depend on its underlying cause.

Differential Diagnosis

The differential diagnosis includes delirium, dementia, organic mood syndrome, organic delusional syndrome, organic hallucinosis, and the functional psychoses such as schizophrenia and the affective disorders.

In delirium, there is a fluctuating course; in dementia, significant intellectual deterioration; in organic affective syndrome, signs and symptoms of an affective disorder that dominate the clinical picture; in organic delusional syndrome, predominant delusions; and in organic hallucinosis, predominant hallucinations. The difference between organic personality syndrome and the functional disorders is that in the former there is an organic factor that antedates the personality change and is etiologically related to it. Schizophrenia and affective disorders also cause other symptoms— eg, in schizophrenia, there are delusions, hallucinations, and looseness of associations; in mania or depression, changes in sleep patterns, reduced levels of motor activity and energy, arid loss of self-esteem.

Prognosis

The prognosis depends on the underlying cause. The syndrome may be reversible in the case of chronic intoxication, neurosyphilis, benign brain tumors, or temporal lobe epilepsy; may be static with traumatic injury to the frontal lobes; or may progress to dementia with multiple sclerosis or Huntington's chorea.

Epidemiology

The incidence and prevalence depend on the underlying cause.

Etiology & Pathogenesis

The most common causes of this syndrome are brain neoplasms; head trauma, including postconcussive syndrome; and subarachnoid hemorrhage, especially with anterior communicating artery aneurysm. Other causes include temporal lobe epilepsy, in which the organic personality syndrome is an interictal phenomenon; postencephalitic parkinsonism; Huntington's chorea; multiple sclerosis; endocrine disorders, especially thyroid or adrenocortical disease; chronic poisoning (manganese, mercury); neurosyphilis; arteritis such as in systemic lupus erythematosus; chronic use of drugs such as marihuana, which may cause an a motivational syndrome; and space-occupying lesions of the brain such as abscess or granuloma.

The pathogenesis of personality change in organic disorders is unknown. Some theories about a neuroanatomic basis of these changes are discussed in Chapter 5.

Treatment

In addition to identifying and treating the underlying cause, the clinician should counsel the patient and family with respect to prognosis and other aspects of management. Psychotropic medications such as lithium or phenothiazines may be required to help control violent behavior.

SUMMARY

Important points relevant to the diagnosis and treatment of organic mental disorders can be summarized as follows:

(1) It is often hard to distinguish by clinical presentation whether psychiatric symptoms have an organic or functional basis. Symptoms and signs that suggest organic causes are reviewed at the beginning of this chapter

(2) In all cases that may have an organic basis, it is important to search vigorously for the cause. With appropriate specific treatment, some or all of the psychiatric symptoms can be reversed.

Table 17–9. *DSM-III-R* diagnostic criteria for organic personality syndrome.

A. A persistent personality disturbance, either lifelong or representing a change or accentuation of a previously characteristic trait, involving at least one of the following:
  (1) Affective instability, eg, marked shifts from normal mood to depression, irritability, or anxiety.
  (2) Recurrent outbursts of aggression or rage that are grossly out of proportion to any precipitating psychosocial stressors.
  (3) Markedly impaired social judgment, eg, sexual indiscretions.
  (4) Marked apathy and indifference.
  (5) Suspiciousness or paranoid ideation.
B. Evidence from the history, physical examination, or laboratory tests of a specific organic factor that is judged to be etiologically related to the disturbance.
C. This diagnosis is not given to a child or adolescent if the clinical picture is limited to the features that characterize attention deficit hyperactivity disorder (see Table 41–9).
D. Does not occur exclusively during the course of delirium and does not meet the criteria for dementia.

(3) Two other aspects of treatment are supportive treatment and psychoactive medication to control symptoms.

(4) Organic mental disorders are common. It is important not to miss them in diagnosis, because they are treatable and sometimes curable.

REFERENCES

Beck JC et al: Dementia in the elderly: The silent epidemic. Ann Intern Med 1982;97:231.

Caine ED: Pseudodementia. Arch Gen Psychiatry 1981; 38:1359.

Clarfield AM: The reversible dementias: Do they reverse? Ann Intern Med 1988;109:476.

Coyle JT: Alzheimer's disease: A disorder of conical cholinergic innervation. Science 1983;219: 1184.

Dietch JT, Zetin M: Diagnosis of organic depressive disorders. Psychosomatics 1983;24:971.

Dubin WR, Weiss KJ, Zeccardi JA: Organic brain syndrome: The psychiatric imposter. JAMA 1983;249:60.

Katzman R: Alzheimer's disease. N Engl J Med 1986;314:964.

Kokmen E: Dementia: Alzheimer type. Mayo Clin Proc 1984; 59:35.

Kosik KH, Growdon JH: Aging, memory loss and dementia. Psychosomatics 1982;23:745.

Larson EW: Organic causes of mania. Mayo Clin Proc 1988;63:906.

Lipowski ZJ: Delirium updated. Compr Psychiatry 1980; 21:190.

Lipowski ZJ: A new look at organic brain syndromes. Am J Psychiatry 1980;137:674.

Lipowski ZJ: Transient cognitive disorders (delirium, acute confusional states) in the elderly. Am J Psychiatry 1983; 140:1426.

Mackenzie TB, Popkin MK: Organic anxiety syndrome. Am J Psychiatry 1983;140:342.

Perry SW: Organic mental disorders caused by HIV: Update on early diagnosis and treatment. Am J Psychiatry 1990;146:696.

Peters BH, Levin HS: Effects of physostigmine and lecithin on memory in Alzheimer disease. Ann Neurol 1979;6:219.

Rabins PV: Reversible dementia and the misdiagnoses of dementia: A review. Hosp Community Psychiatry 1983; 34:830.

Reisberg B, Ferris SH, Gershon S: An overview of pharmacologic treatment of cognitive decline in the aged. Am J Psychiatry 1981;138:593.

Schneck MK, Reisberg B, Ferris SH: An overview of current concepts of Alzheimer's disease. Am J Psychiatry 1982; 139:165.

Seltzer B, Sherwin I: Organic brain syndromes: An empirical study and critical review. Am J Psychiatry 1978;135: 13.

Surawicz FG: Alcoholic hallucinosis: A missed diagnosis. Can J Psychiatry 1980;25:57.

Wells CE: Pseudodementia. Am J Psychiatry 1979;136:895.

18 Psychoactive Substance Use Disorders: Drugs & Alcohol*

David E. Smith, MD, & Mim J. Landry

Overview

Substance abuse is one of the major public health problems in the USA. Deaths associated with alcohol abuse and alcoholism now rank third, behind heart disease and cancer. Alcoholism, the most common substance use disorder, affects millions of people each year. Use and cultural acceptance of other psychoactive substances including illegal drugs are increasing significantly. Certain basic principles of diagnosis and treatment apply to all psychoactive substance use disorders. The physician should be familiar with these principles and with the psychopharmacology and toxicology of specific substances. This chapter provides information on the diagnosis and treatment of disorders associated with the use of the following psychoactive substances: alcohol, smokeable stimulants (eg, crack and ice), sedative-hypnotics, hallucinogens, phencyclidine (PCP), opiates, psychotomimetic amphetamines (eg, ecstasy), and marihuana.

Patterns of Psychoactive Drug Use

Use of nonprescription psychoactive drugs can be categorized into five patterns based on the designations utilized by the National Commission on Marijuana and Drug Abuse:

(1) Experimental use is defined as short-term, nonpatterned trials of a drug. The users are motivated chiefly by curiosity and a desire to experience the anticipated effect. Experimental use generally begins socially among friends.

(2) Social-recreational use occurs in social settings among friends or acquaintances who wish to share an experience perceived as acceptable and pleasurable. The primary motivation is social, and use is voluntary.

(3) Circumstantial-situational use is defined as self-limited use of variable pattern, frequency, intensity, and duration. Use is motivated by a perceived need to achieve a known drug effect in order to cope with a specific condition or situation.

(4) Intensified use is characterized by long-term patterned use at least once a day. Such use is motivated by a perceived need or desire to obtain relief from a persistent problem or stressful situation.

(5) Compulsive use is characterized by frequent and intense use of relatively long duration, producing some degree of psychological dependence; ie, the user cannot discontinue use at will without experiencing physiological discomfort or psychological disruption.

Persons at all levels of society (including physicians and other health professionals, who have a disproportionately high rate of alcoholism and prescription narcotic addiction) may fall victim to substance abuse. Addiction to psychoactive substances is not restricted to any particular subgroup or subculture of the population, and proper treatment of addictive disorders requires objective criteria based on clinically sound procedures.

Part of the difficulty in dealing with substance abuse is that recreational drug use is so widespread. Any pattern of drug use involves a complex interaction of physical, psychological, pharmacological, and sociocultural variables. Use of certain psychoactive drugs such as alcohol and tobacco, although culturally accepted, may pose substantial health hazards, while use of other recreational drugs may be illegal and culturally unacceptable but may pose less of a health hazard. The difficulty of defining what constitutes substance abuse causes confusion in diagnosis and treatment.

Definitions

In this chapter, **drug abuse** is defined as use of a psychoactive drug to such an extent that it *seriously interferes* with health or occupational and social functioning. The definition emphasizes "dysfunction" in a way that some definitions of the term "drug abuse" do not. For example, some writers would define as abuse even casual infrequent recreational use of small doses of psychoactive drugs for the pleasurable effects anticipated or for the purpose of enhancing performance. Other definitions are based on cultural norms; eg, Jaffe (1990) defines drug abuse as "the use usually by self-administration of any drug in a manner disapproved by medical or social norms of a given culture." The problem with these definitions is that they offer

---

* For alcohol abuse, see also Chapter 19.

no objective, nonjudgmental criteria that can be used in deciding when intervention and treatment are required.

Although the emphasis in this chapter is on "recreational" drugs, prescribed psychoactive medications can be abused also. Physicians who prescribe such drugs have the responsibility to monitor their effects on the patient to make certain that toxicity and dependence are not developing.

Symptoms of drug abuse (eg, psychological dependence) may evolve into chronic use and physical dependence. Physical dependence, however, is not the chief criterion for defining addictive disease. The key characteristics of addictive disease are compulsion, loss of control, and continued use of the drug despite the adverse physical and social consequences. Compulsive drug abuse is similar in many ways to chronic relapsing physical disease, and emphasis in management should be on the addictive disease as such.

Different individuals may respond in different ways to the same dosage of a particular drug. For example, although diazepam is usually safe in therapeutic doses, individuals with a psychobiological predisposition to addictive disease, as evidenced (for example) by a past or family history of alcoholism, may develop dependence even at ordinary therapeutic dosages. Other predisposed groups may rapidly escalate dosage and develop tolerance, with associated adverse physical, psychological, and behavioral consequences. The psychobiological predisposition of dependency-prone individuals is currently being investigated.

Addiction, as defined by the World Health Organization, is "a behavioral pattern of drug use characterized by overwhelming involvement with the use of a drug, compulsive drug-seeking behavior, and a high tendency to relapse after withdrawal." The World Health Organization stresses that "addiction should be viewed on a continuum relative to the degree where drug use affects the total life quality of the drug user and to the range of circumstances in which it controls his behavior."

Compulsive abuse of certain drugs such as the sedative-hypnotics and narcotic analgesics may produce **physical dependence.** Although stimulants such as amphetamines and cocaine are quite toxic, compulsive abuse does not produce a well-defined pattern of physical dependence; however, it does represent the addictive disease process, since the user becomes compulsive and continues such compulsive use despite adverse effects on health and on occupational and social functioning. Therefore, focusing only on physical dependence is inappropriate because (1) some drugs do not produce the familiar alcohol/heroin dependence and withdrawal phenomena; (2) there may be an absence of physical dependence in spite of compulsive and dysfunctional use of a drug that does cause physical dependence; (3) physical dependence often represents a late stage of addictive disease; and (4) addictive disease is often manifested by binge patterns of use.

The progression and symptoms described for cocaine are almost identical for alcohol and the other drugs. Toxicological and pharmacological differences are pronounced during acute crises and acute medical management.

Addiction and physical dependence have different mechanisms of action, which are only beginning to be understood. Developments in brain chemistry research hold much promise for explaining the addictive process and suggesting treatment strategies. For example, Blum and Trachtenberg (1986) found that the depletion and alteration of neurotransmitter receptor sites in the central nervous system following chronic cocaine and alcohol use may help to explain cocaine and alcohol hunger (treatment involving the use of amino acids was proposed). Some drugs have a higher potential for abuse than others—the potential for abuse of a single drug can vary according to its purity, route of administration, dose, effective duration, and psychopharmacology (including, but not limited to, the user's tolerance and dependence). The mental stability and expectations of the user, other medical and psychological factors, and even social factors affect a drug's potential for abuse.

Principles of Diagnosis

Drug categories associated with substance abuse and dependence are discussed in separate sections below: alcohol; sedative-hypnotics, including barbiturates and benzodiazepines; opiates and opioids; central nervous system stimulants, including amphetamine and cocaine; and hallucinogens, including substances as diverse as LSD, phencyclidine (PCP), and cannabis. Table 18–1 outlines the *DSM-III-R* criteria for abuse of and dependence on these substances, including multiple drug abuse (polysubstance abuse). This section also discusses multiple psychopathological disorders associated with substance abuse.

It is important to note that in polysubstance abuse and addiction, one substance may be the "primary" drug which has more desirable effects (eg, cocaine euphoria). The person often uses a "secondary" drug (eg, alcohol) in order to ease the negative side effects of the primary drug. Thus, the self-described cocaine addict may actually be addicted to both cocaine *and* alcohol. Many people use several drugs simultaneously in order to experience the *combined effect.* Such persons may not describe their intake of cocaine, alcohol, and marihuana as significant, since the intake of each drug may not be very high. The physician should thus focus on **dysfunction** rather than tolerance, physical dependence, or amount when making a diagnosis.

In 1954, the American Medical Association defined alcoholism as a primary disease. The AMA and the American Society of Addiction Medicine, the largest

Table 18–1. *DSM-III-R* diagnostic criteria for psychoactive substance dependence and abuse.

Psychoactive substance dependence:
A. At least 3 of the following:
  (1) Substance often taken in larger amounts or over a longer period than the person intended.
  (2) Persistent desire or one or more unsuccessful efforts to cut down or control substance use.
  (3) A great deal of time spent in activities necessary to get the substance (eg, theft), taking the substance (eg, chain-smoking), or recovering from its effects.
  (4) Frequent intoxication or withdrawal symptoms when expected to fulfill major role obligations at work, school, or home (eg, does not go to work because hung over, goes to school or work "high," intoxicated while taking care of his or her children), or when substance use is physically hazardous (eg, drives when intoxicated).
  (5) Important social, occupational, or recreational activities given up or reduced because of substance use.
  (6) Continued substance use despite knowledge of having a persistent or recurrent social, psychologic, or physical problem that is caused or exacerbated by the use of the substance (eg, keeps using heroin despite family arguments about it, cocaine-induced depression, or having an ulcer made worse by drinking).
  (7) Marked tolerance: need for markedly increased amounts of the substance (ie, at least a 50% increase) in order to achieve intoxication or desired effect, or markedly diminished effect with continued use of the same amount.
      Note: The following items may not apply to cannabis, hallucinogens, or phencyclidine (PCP):
  (8) Characteristic withdrawal symptoms (see specific withdrawal syndromes under psychoactive substance-induced organic mental disorders).
  (9) Substance often taken to relieve or avoid withdrawal symptoms.
B. Some symptoms of the disturbance have persisted for at least 1 month or have occurred repeatedly over a longer period of time.

Psychoactive substance abuse:
A. A maladaptive pattern of psychoactive substance use indicated by at least one of the following:
  (1) Continued use despite knowledge of having a persistent or recurrent social, occupational, psychologic, or physical problem that is caused or exacerbated by use of the psychoactive substance.
  (2) Recurrent use in situations in which use is physically hazardous (eg, driving while intoxicated).
B. Some symptoms of the disturbance have persisted for at least 1 month or have occurred repeatedly over a longer period of time.
C. Never met the criteria for psychoactive substance dependence for this substance.

Polysubstance dependence:
A. A period of at least 6 months during which the person was repeatedly using at least 3 categories of psychoactive substances (not including nicotine and caffeine), but no single psychoactive substance predominated.
B. During this period, the dependence criteria were met for psychoactive substances (as a group) but not for any specific substance.

organization of physicians in the field of addiction treatment, stated in 1987 that all drug dependencies are diseases and should be considered and treated as primary illnesses. In this **disease concept of addic-** **tion,** addiction is a pathological process in its own right, with characteristic signs and symptoms, a reliable diagnosis, prognosis, and treatment and recovery strategies. Traditional psychiatric approaches, however, regard addiction as a symptom of an underlying psychopathological process. In this **psychiatric orientation of addiction,** treatment plans would involve an exploration of underlying illness in the hope that addiction could be overcome indirectly. This controversy regarding the diagnosis and treatment of addiction has a profound effect on treatment as well as on communication and cooperation between health care professionals.

One of the key differences between the two concepts described above centers on their approach to treatment and the importance of complete abstinence from psychoactive drugs. The disease concept of addiction emphasizes sobriety as a tool and as a goal, whereas the psychiatric orientation concept of addiction leaves the door open for learning to use psychoactive drugs responsibly after exhibiting addiction. A problem arises when an individual must be described as having both an addiction and one or more psychiatric disorders **(dual diagnosis).** Some addicts and alcoholics began using psychoactive drugs in an attempt to alleviate psychiatric or social problems, eg, using alcohol to relieve anxiety or cocaine to offset depression. However, once the basic criteria of addiction have been met (compulsion, loss of control, and continued use despite adverse consequences), the addiction should be the primary focus of treatment. Clinical experience has shown that addicts respond best to a treatment approach that emphasizes abstinence.

Guide to Management of Substance Abuse Crises

A. Assessment: This should include the following:

1. Substance used–

a. Type of substance (or availability of sample for identification or testing if the patient does not know the type).

b. Route of administration (inhaled, ingested, injected, etc).

2. Pattern and circumstances of substance use–

a. Self-medication because of physical, mental, or emotional problem.

b. Concomitant use of prescription or over-the-counter medications.

c. Concomitant use of alcohol (type, quantity, duration) and drugs.

d. Alternating or concomitant use of other drugs in the same drug group.

e. Identifiable events, such as loss or celebration, precipitating the substance abuse crisis,

f. If drug is used habitually, pattern of development and method of maintenance of habit.

3. Extent of potential support system—

a. Family or friends available to help the patient follow through on treatment.

b. Community groups or agencies specifically addressing the patient's abuse pattern.

4. History of previous treatment—

a. Type and duration of treatment.

b. Results.

5. Other—

a. Effect of drug use on the patient's life (eg, financial problems, changes in physical appearance).

b. Physical infirmity that could exacerbate the problem.

c. Willingness to change abuse habits.

B. Initial Management of the Crisis: Before treatment is begun, it is important to assure the patient of confidentiality and explain the rationale for treatment and what to expect. The patient's behavior is observed carefully, vital signs are monitored, and the patient is given only symptomatic treatment before the substance is identified. No medication should be given if there is any question about identification of the drug.

The goal of the three approaches listed below is to achieve an alteration in the patient's status or a favorable resolution of the crisis. Judgment must be used in selecting the most appropriate approach in the circumstances.

1. Assistance—The involvement of another individual or authority in the substance abuse crisis often helps patients endure the crisis and work out a personal solution. This gives them an opportunity for growth through mastery of the crisis. Psychiatric emergency clinicians often directly involve others or ask patients to recommend someone with whom they are comfortable to reassure and guide them during the crisis.

2. Complete management—Some cases require complete management of the crisis by the clinician, as in the active treatment of drug overdose. This approach (called ''taking over') is direct and often necessary, but the patient does not participate in resolution of the crisis.

3. Patient education—In some instances, clinicians provide additional information or resources so that patients can resolve their own substance abuse crisis.

C. Follow-Up Strategies: After crisis intervention for the drug overdose, medical management of the complications, and appropriate detoxification procedures (see later sections on specific drugs), the physician should evaluate the patient to determine if there are any associated physical problems, persistent organic mental disorders, or major underlying psychopathological conditions. In most cases, the substance use disorder must be viewed as the primary disease process. Fewer than 10% of patients who have addictive disease have a major underlying psychopathological condition. However, if an underlying problem exists, it is difficult to follow a drug-free abstinence-oriented approach to treatment, since the patient will often require psychotropic medication for management of the psychopathological disorder. Antidepressants may be prescribed for a major depressive episode, or an antipsychotic drug may be given for an underlying thought disorder. For some patients with primary addictive disease, a drug maintenance program (eg, with methadone) may be implemented, but abstinence-based recovery-oriented strategies should be tried first.

Maintenance programs with drugs such as methadone are not considered recovery-oriented strategies, since recovery is defined as living a responsible and comfortable life without the use of psychoactive drugs. However, other drug maintenance strategies that represent exceptions to this definition can facilitate recovery. Clinicians should consider using disulfiram (Antabuse), which blocks the effects of alcohol and produces an adverse reaction when alcohol is used; or naltrexone, which blocks the effects of self-administered opiates. Disulfiram and naltrexone should be used as adjuncts to a full recovery program and should *not* be considered the full extent of treatment.

Most follow-up strategies are psychosocial in nature and include family therapy and individual psychotherapy. Successful strategies include participation in nonmedical self-help groups, such as Alcoholics Anonymous and Narcotics Anonymous; other types of recovery support groups, such as the Cocaine Recovery Support Group and the Impaired Health Professional Support Group, are also available. These programs focus on abstinence and emphasize the principles of recovery, with the group process supporting and maintaining recovery. On occasion, the addict will require residential therapy, typically in a highly structured behavior modification self-help community.

Follow-up care must be tailored to the individual's addictive disease process and must be flexible enough to change as the patient's needs change. The physician should recognize that addiction is a chronic, relapsing disease with potentially fatal consequences but that recovery is possible.

Physicians should be able to diagnose addictive disease both in their patients and in their colleagues, since drug addiction in health professionals is two to three times the national average. Once the diagnosis is established, a treatment plan should be formulated to deal with all aspects of the addictive disease disorder, including crisis intervention, drug detoxification, and follow-up. Consultation with a multidisciplinary health care team is often required to implement such a diverse treatment plan.

ALCOHOL ABUSE
(See also Chapter 19.)

Alcoholism has all of the qualities of substance abuse and dependence. The impairment may involve

Table 18–2. *DSM-III-R* diagnostic criteria for disorders associated with abuse of alcohol.

Alcohol intoxication:
A. Recent ingestion of alcohol (with no evidence suggesting that the amount was insufficient to cause intoxication in most people).
B. Maladaptive behavioral changes, eg, disinhibition of sexual or aggressive impulses, mood lability, impaired judgment, impaired social or occupational functioning.
C. At least one of the following signs: (1) slurred speech; (2) incoordination; (3) unsteady gait; (4) nystagmus; (5) flushed face.
D. Not due to any physical or other mental disorder.

Alcohol idiosyncratic intoxication:
A. Maladaptive behavioral changes, eg, aggressive or assaultive behavior, occurring within minutes of ingesting an amount of alcohol insufficient to induce intoxication in most people.
B. The behavior is atypical of the person when not drinking.
C. Not due to any physical or other mental disorder.

Uncomplicated alcohol withdrawal:
A. Cessation of prolonged (several days or longer) heavy ingestion of alcohol or reduction in the amount of alcohol ingested, followed within several hours by coarse tremor of hands, tongue, or eyelids, and at least one of the following: (1) nausea or vomiting; (2) malaise or weakness; (3) autonomic hyperactivity, eg, tachycardia, sweating, elevated blood pressure; (4) anxiety; (5) depressed mood or irritability; (6) transient hallucinations or illusions; (7) headache; (8) insomnia.
B. Not due to any physical or other mental disorder, such as alcohol withdrawal delirium.

Alchohol withdrawal delirium:
A. Delirium developing after cessation of heavy alcohol ingestion or a reduction in the amount of alcohol ingested (usually within one week).
B. Marked autonomic hyperactivity, eg, tachycardia, sweating.
C. Not due to any physical or other mental disorder.

Alcohol hallucinosis:
A. Organic hallucinosis with vivid and persistent hallucinations (auditory or visual) developing shortly (usually within 48 hours) after cessation of or reduction in heavy ingestion of alcohol in a person who apparently has alcohol dependence.
B. No delirium as in alcohol withdrawal delirium.
C. Not due to any physical or other mental disorder.

Alcohol amnestic disorder:
A. Amnestic syndrome following prolonged heavy ingestion of alcohol.
B. Not due to any physical or other mental disorder.

Dementia associated with alcoholism:
A. Dementia following prolonged heavy ingestion of alcohol and persisting at least 3 weeks after cessation of alcohol ingestion.
B. Exclusion of all causes of dementia other than prolonged heavy use of alcohol by history, physical examination, and laboratory tests.

physiological, psychological, or social dysfunction. As tolerance for alcohol increases, it is common for alcoholics to engage in multiple drug use, typically with barbiturate and other sedative hypnotic drugs. Alcoholism is progressive, so that alcoholics may organize and orient their lives around drinking. Medical authorities and organizations such as the AMA have concluded that alcoholism should be treated as a disease.

Because of its prevalence, alcoholism is discussed

in detail in Chapter 19. In this chapter, basic information and diagnostic criteria will be introduced.

Clinical Features

DSM-III-R diagnostic criteria for the various disorders associated with alcohol use are outlined in Table 18–2. Additional diagnostic considerations are discussed below.

A. Alcohol Abuse and Dependence: A wide range of symptoms and signs of alcoholism may be observed in all parts of the body and may include anxiety, depression, insomnia, impotence, frequent infections, pancreatitis, hypertension, multiple gastrointestinal problems, ulcers that do not heal, behavior disorders and social symptoms indicative of a disrupted life-style, aggressive behavior, and suicide attempts or threats. Laboratory tests may reveal abnormal liver function; decreased levels of serum protein, albumin, magnesium, and potassium; increased levels of blood ammonia; elevated serum uric acid; elevated hemoglobin and red blood cell counts, with or without folic acid or vitamin B_{12} deficiency; drug screen positive for other chemicals; and increased blood alcohol levels.

B. Alcohol Intoxication: The signs of intoxication correlated with progressive blood alcohol levels are summarized in Table 18–3. The relationships between the ingestion of alcohol, the blood ethanol concentration, and the signs of intoxication vary and depend on the history of use, rate of ingestion, and alterations in absorption, metabolism, and excretion.

Table 18–3. Signs of intoxication correlated with blood alcohol levels.*

Blood Alcohol Level (mg/dL)†	Signs of Intoxication
20–99	Muscular incoordination Impaired sensory function Changes in mood, personality, and behavior
100–199	Marked mental impairment Incoordination Prolonged reaction time Ataxia
200–299	Nausea and vomiting Diplopia Marked ataxia
300–399	Hypothermia Severe dysarthria Amnesia Stage I anesthesia
400–700	Coma Respiratory failure Death

*Reproduced, with permission, from Becker CE, Roe RL, Scott RA: *Alcohol as a Drug.* Medcom Press, 1974. Copyright © 1974 by Williams & Wilkins.
†Lethal dose varies. For adults, it is 5–8 g/kg; for children, 3 g/kg. If there is no food intake, lethal dose occurs before above doses are absorbed. Signs of intoxication are more apparent when blood alcohol level is rising than when it is falling.

Alcohol is fully absorbed within 30 minutes to 2 hours, depending on the beverage ingested and on food intake.

C. Alcohol Withdrawal: The most common neurological sign of withdrawal is **tremor.** The tremor of alcohol withdrawal must be differentiated from that of anxiety or thyrotoxicosis and from familial tremor. Tremor from alcohol withdrawal is an exaggeration of a mild tremor that many people have after being frightened, after drinking too much coffee, or after ''a night on the town.'' This tremor is usually benign but slowly worsens as the individual continues to drink over time. Because alcohol ''cures'' the tremor of alcohol withdrawal, it is important that the clinician ask the patient if drinking alcohol eliminates tremor. Some alcoholics claim that the immediate effect of alcohol in stopping their ''shakes'' is the reason they continue to drink. Their tremors can be so severe that they cannot walk or bring a glass to their lips. After several days of withdrawal, the tremor ceases.

The ''rum fit,'' or **seizure,** is generalized and nonfocal. It may be a single seizure but usually is followed by one or more further seizures with interim recovery of consciousness. The postictal period is short, and although multiple seizures and even **status epilepticus** occur in 3% of cases, most of the seizures are over within 6 hours. It is prudent to include a lumbar puncture, electroencephalogram, and skull x-rays in the initial evaluation. Further tests (pneumoencephalography, cerebral angiography, brain scan, etc) are unnecessary if the seizures are clearly the result of withdrawal and the neurological examination is negative for other significant pathological findings.

D. Alcohol Hallucinosis: Clinicians may categorize the hallucinations resulting from withdrawal according to their content (eg, hallucinatory threats) and associated mental state (eg, anxiety in response to these threats). Becker et al (1974) claim that alcoholics have visual or auditory hallucinations or a mixture of both types during withdrawal. Although auditory hallucinations are also typical of functional psychosis, a definitive diagnosis cannot be based on hallucinatory content alone. Final diagnosis can be made only after all signs of alcohol withdrawal have resolved. It is important to rule out a diagnosis of paranoid schizophrenia; this can be done on the basis of the history. The usual age (about 40 years) at the onset of alcohol hallucinosis is later than in schizophrenia, and neither family backgrounds nor premorbid personalities are similar to those of schizophrenic patients.

Hallucinations in an alcohol-dependent patient with a clear sensorium (except for disorientation to time) are indicative of **alcohol hallucinosis.** Hallucinatory behavior is likely to be transient and intermittent, and it usually increases in the evening. The mental status examination shows disorientation only to time, and patients are able to converse rationally and are often aware that they are hallucinating (unlike patients with psychotic disorders).

Patients with **atypical delusional-hallucinatory states** may have relatively secure orientation but may demonstrate marked paranoid ideation and often deny obvious hallucinatory behavior. The type of behavior demonstrated by these patients varies, depending on their premorbid personality, the abruptness of withdrawal, and the meaning of the hallucinations for the patient. Many patients who have hallucinated during prior periods of withdrawal become familiar with the experience and seem able to ignore the hallucinations. Others never seem comfortable with their hallucinations and fear for their sanity.

Transient hallucinosis, like withdrawal seizure activity, is self-limited and tends to occur during the first 24 hours after the patient stops drinking. Many withdrawing alcoholics know that taking a few drinks, diazepam, or other sedative-hypnotic drugs will stop or diminish these hallucinations. However, because most experienced alcoholics also know that alcohol or other sedative drugs will only temporarily alleviate their hallucinations, they will seek medical help once the hallucinations start. Although most patients are usually not a danger to themselves or others during alcoholic hallucinations, some may try to hurt themselves in response to frightening internal voices.

There is a clear difference between the signs of **delirium tremens (DTs)** and the signs of alcohol hallucinosis. Patients with the former have hallucinations and are greatly disoriented and agitated; those with the latter have hallucinations but a clear sensorium. Patients with delirium tremens are disoriented in two or three spheres—time, place, and person. The characteristic hallucinations of delirium tremens are constant, and patients have no awareness that they are hallucinating. There is no means of determining which patients will experience serious delirium tremens and which will have no more than several days of tremulousness with or without transient hallucinations.

E. Alcohol Amnestic Disorder: Psychiatric emergency room staff members occasionally encounter patients who claim that they do not remember how they arrived in this ''strange location.'' These patients may have developed enough tolerance to the effects of alcohol so that they can complete complex tasks and travel many miles but yet have no recollection of having done so. The amnesia results from a thiamine deficiency, and the first stage is called **Wernicke's disease.** Wernicke's disease is a neurological disorder manifested by confusion, ataxia, and abnormalities in eye movement (gaze palsies, nystagmus, and other neurological signs). If Wernicke's disease is not treated with massive doses of thiamine, memory impairment may be permanent (**Korsakoff's psychosis).** Patients who suffer from a confirmed diagnosis of alcohol amnestic disorder usually do not recover but may improve slightly with time. After obtaining a detailed history from these patients (or from their relatives or close friends), particularly regarding drinking habits, the clinician should help the patients reorient themselves. Since amnestic periods caused by drinking are indicators of severe alcohol abuse and since continued drinking jeopardizes brain functioning, it is important that patients with alcohol amnestic disorder seek further treatment for their drinking problem. (See also Chapters 5, 17, and 19.)

F. Drug-Alcohol Interaction: Since approximately 60–70% of the adult population consumes various amounts of alcohol, it is predictable that other drugs, whether prescribed or not, will be taken with alcohol or while alcohol is still present in the body. Clinicians considering the possibility of drug-alcohol reaction should remember that many over-the-counter drugs, including cough remedies, mouthwashes, tonics, and liquid vitamin formulations, contain high concentrations of alcohol. These over-the-counter drugs—as well as sedative-hypnotics, tranquilizers (particularly the phenothiazines), antihistamines, tricyclic antidepressants, and narcotics—have additive depressant effects when taken with alcohol.

Psychiatric emergency room staff may frequently need to assess individuals who have ingested ethanol with methanol (wood alcohol). Methanol is often consumed as a cheap substitute for other alcoholic beverages and is an ingredient in some household and industrial chemical preparations, so that it may be ingested accidentally. Methanol itself is toxic, but its metabolites (formaldehyde and formic acid) are even more toxic, causing metabolic acidosis and damage to the central nervous system and retina. Hyperventilation (precipitated by the acidosis) and visual loss within 12–24 hours of ingesting methanol are the chief signs of methanol poisoning. The patient with methanol poisoning is given ethanol. Alcohol dehydrogenase, the enzyme that metabolizes both ethyl alcohol and methyl alcohol, has a greater affinity for ethanol than for methanol. If an adequate blood concentration of ethanol is maintained, alcohol dehydrogenase will combine preferentially with ethanol. As a result, methanol is not metabolized but safely excreted in the urine.

Treatment

Treatment for the various forms of alcohol abuse is discussed in detail in Chapter 19.

Supportive care, fluid and electrolyte replacement, and monitoring and maintenance of vital signs are basic elements in the management of acute alcohol intoxication. Becker et al (1974) have noted that fructose can be effective in reducing the blood alcohol level in intoxicated individuals who can tolerate this simple sugar, including those with idiosyncratic intoxication. Fructose is converted to D-glyceraldehyde, which is metabolized to nicotinamide adenine dinucleotide, a substance needed to oxidize more ethanol. It is believed that fructose increases the elimination

rate of alcohol from the blood by as much as 80%.

Patients with alcohol hallucinations should *not* be given phenothiazines or other antipsychotic drugs. Phenothiazines lower the seizure threshold, and antipsychotic drugs generally exacerbate the problem.

AMPHETAMINE & STIMULANT ABUSE

General nervous system stimulants are widely used in the USA; the two most prevalent are **nicotine** in tobacco products and **caffeine** in coffee or tea. (Although given diagnostic codes and diagnostic criteria in *DSM-III-R,* tobacco and caffeine abuse are not discussed separately in this text.) Stimulant abuse has become a serious problem, with the major stimulants of abuse being **cocaine** (a derivative of the coca plant) and synthetic stimulants such as **amphetamine** and **amphetamine-like drugs** (eg, methylphenidate) (Table 18–4). Most of the substances have legitimate medicinal value. Cocaine is approved in medicine for topical anesthesia. Amphetamines and amphetamine-like drugs are approved for narcolepsy, hyperkinesia, and short-term diet control.

The management of stimulant abuse is complicated by the availability of cocaine "lookalikes" (eg, ephedrine, lidocaine) that resemble cocaine in appearance, contain no controlled substance, and may themselves be toxic. The potent central nervous system stimulants have a high potential for abuse. In the drug culture, the primary routes of cocaine administration are nasal insufflation, smoking "free base" (crack) cocaine, or ice (a potent form of smokeable methamphetamine), and injection. Administration of amphetamines is by the oral route or injection. Dependence on the stimulant can develop but is primarily of a psychological nature, with no well-defined abstinence symptoms other than depression or lethargy. However, the stimulants can lend themselves to compulsive use and high-dose abuse. Since high-dose abuse of short-acting stimulants such as cocaine lends itself to compulsion, loss of control, and continued use despite adverse consequences, it represents a form of addictive disease.

Because **crack** cocaine is prepared by a simplified basification technique that yields free base cocaine in small, proportionately less expensive dosage units, there are fewer obstacles to involvement with this rapid delivery form of cocaine. Free base cocaine vaporizes at approximately 100 °C and can be easily smoked. The pulmonary route enhances rapid and thorough plasma cocaine concentration. Euphoria is swift and marked, followed by severe depression, which is typically self-medicated with additional cocaine, which in turn leads to a progression and worsening of symptoms.

Amphetamine may be taken orally in low doses

Table 18–4. Characteristics of depressants, hallucinogens, opiates and opioids, and stimulants.

Drug	Usual Route of Administration	Duration of Effects	Potential for Physical Dependence	Potential for Psychologic Dependence	Potential for Tolerance
Depressants					
Barbiturates					
Pentobarbital (Nembutal; "yellow jackets")	Oral (pill or capsule)	4 h	High to moderate	High to moderate	Yes
Secobarbital (Seconal; "reds")					
Barbituratelike substances					
Glutethimide (Doriden)	Oral (pill or capsule)	4 h	High	High	Yes
Methaqualone (Quaalude and others; "ludes," "quaads")*					
Benzodiazepines					
Diazepam (Valium)	Oral (tablet)	8–12 h	Low	Low	Yes
Lorazepam (Ativan)	Oral (tablet)	4–6 h	Low	Low	Yes
Carbamates					
Meprobamate (Equanil, Miltown, others)	Oral (pill or capsule)	4 h	Moderate	Moderate	Yes
Other depressants					
Chloral hydrate (Noctec, Oradrate)	Oral (pill or capsule)	4 h	Moderate	Moderate	Possible
Hallucinogens†					
Indolealkylamines					
DET, DMT ("businessman's special")	Oral (inhalation or smoking)	Up to days	Unknown	Degree unknown	Yes
LSD ("acid," "blotter," "sunshine," "windowpane")	Oral (liquid, pill, capsule, or sugar cube)	12 h	None	Degree unknown	Yes
Psilocin ("magic Mexican mushroom")	Oral (pill, capsule, or sugar cube)	6 h	None	Degree unknown	Possible
Phenylethylamines					
Mescaline ("mescal," "cactus")	Oral	4 h	None	Degree unknown	Yes
Phenylisopropylamines					
DOB, DOM, MDA, MMDA, MDMA, MDE, PCP	Oral (pill or capsule)	4 h–up to days	Unknown	Degree unknown	Yes
Opiates and opioids					
Codeine	Oral (liquid or tablet); injection	3–6 h	Moderate	Moderate	Yes
Heroin	Injection in muscle or vein; inhalation	3–6 h	Very high	Very high	Yes
Methadone	Oral (liquid); injection	12–24 h	High	High	Yes
Morphine	Injection; oral (liquid or tablet)	4 h	High	High	Yes
Opium	Oral (smoking)	4 h	High	High	Yes
Other opioids					
Diphenoxylate with atropine (Lomotil)	Oral (liquid)	4 h	Low	Low	Yes
Hydromorphone (Dilaudid)	Injection	4 h	High	High	Yes
Meperidine (Demerol)	Injection	4 h	High	High	Yes
Propoxyphene hydrochloride (Darvon)	Oral (tablet)	4 h	Moderate	Moderate	Yes
Miscellaneous cough syrups	Oral (liquid)	4 h	Moderate	Moderate	Yes
Stimulants					
Amphetamines	Oral (pill or capsule); injection	4 h	Possible	High	Yes
Cocaine	Inhalation; oral (capsule or smoking)	2 h	Possible	High	Possible
Methylphenidate	Oral (tablet)	4–6 h	Possible	High	Yes
Phenmetrazine	Oral (tablet)	4–6 h	Possible	High	Yes

*Withdrawn in 1983. Not legally available after 1984.
†DET = diethyltryptamine; DMT = dimethyltryptamine; LSD = lysergic acid diethylamide; DOB = 4-bromo-2,5-dimethoxyamphetamine; DOM = 4-methyl-2,5-dimethoxyamphetamine; MDA = methylenedioxyamphetamine; MDMA = N-methyl-3,4-methylenedioxymethamphetamine; MDE = N-ethyl-3,4-methylenedioxyamphetamine; and MMDA = 3-methoxy-4,5-methylenedioxyamphetamine.

to enhance physical or emotional performance; or it may be taken in high doses, either orally or intravenously, to produce euphoria and a "rush" (ie, a burst of energy accompanied by a physical sensation in the head and neck). High-dose oral use can also produce psychotic reactions. Even moderate doses of amphetamine in conjunction with physical exertion at high environmental temperatures may contribute to heat stroke through interference with regulation of body temperature. Several deaths of bicyclists have been attributed to this phenomenon.

Many people are occasional amphetamine users who take low oral doses while studying for an examination or for "treatment" of their obesity. Although obese patients are often under medical care, they are not always carefully supervised, and some actually abuse the drug. Amphetamine is at times used orally or intravenously to counteract effects of other drugs. Once a pattern of amphetamine use is established, the drug is frequently used to counteract the effects of amphetamine abstinence.

Clinical Features

In addition to the effects of euphoria, stimulation, relief of fatigue, and suppression of appetite, other possible effects of stimulant use include excitation, increased pulse rate and blood pressure, and insomnia. Massive overdoses of amphetamine occasionally occur in suicide attempts, in intravenous users who obtain unusually potent preparations, and in children who inadvertently ingest the drug. Patients may be unconscious following seizures, with hypertensive crises or even cerebrovascular accidents.

Differential Diagnosis

There are numerous difficulties in diagnosing acute amphetamine toxicity. Amphetamine use is concealed in some cases, and the clinician encounters an acutely agitated, anxious, paranoid, perhaps belligerent patient whose abnormal behavior is not due to any obvious cause. Differential diagnosis includes the following: (1) paranoid schizophrenia; (2) bipolar affective disorder during the manic phase; (3) anxiety disorders, especially with panic attacks; (4) amphetamine-precipitated psychotic reaction; (5) drug intoxication with psychedelics, phencyclidine (PCP), or other sympathomimetics (eg, ephedrine, cocaine); (6) hyperthyroid crisis, including ingestion of thyroid preparations; and (7) pheochromocytoma.

A history from friends or relatives may provide important clues. A history of recurrent episodes of hyperactivity and paranoia treated for long periods with antipsychotic medication suggests paranoid schizophrenia; however, chronic amphetamine use may account for the recurrent episodes and should be considered. Urine tests may be negative for amphetamine if the urine is alkaline due to markedly reduced urinary excretion. Blood testing for amphetamine is most helpful in confirming the diagnosis;

however, results may not become available for several days.

On physical examination, pupils are usually dilated and heart rate and blood pressure increased. However, psychiatric disorders associated with increased epinephrine or norepinephrine secretion may also dilate pupils or increase heart rate and blood pressure. If the patient's behavior is within tolerable limits for a psychiatric ward and if blood pressure is not dangerously high, a period of observation is frequently helpful in establishing a correct diagnosis. Antipsychotic medications are effective in reducing agitated, hostile behavior but may further obscure the diagnosis, especially if toxicological analysis is not ordered. For this reason, benzodiazepine sedatives are preferred initially for control of behavior. If the individual is suffering from amphetamine toxicity, abnormal behavior will subside over 1–3 days as the blood level of amphetamine falls. An individual who remains actively psychotic after blood and urine amphetamine levels are normal has some other psychiatric disorder rather than—or in addition to—an acute toxic reaction to amphetamine.

Experimental studies confirm the clinical observation that sufficiently large doses of amphetamine will induce paranoid psychosis in all individuals. Methylphenidate (Ritalin) produces a similar reaction. Amphetamine psychosis results from prolonged high-dose amphetamine abuse, often in association with sleep deprivation. The clinical manifestations of full-blown amphetamine psychosis resemble those of a functional paranoid psychosis but are dose-related and have a much shorter course. Unless the individual suffers from a persistent psychotic disorder such as schizophrenia, the psychotic reaction will resolve as the amphetamine or methylphenidate is excreted from the body. When amphetamine is withdrawn, these patients become depressed and anxious and their sleep difficulties intensify. Clinical experience has demonstrated that they do not respond well to phenothiazines, lithium, or antidepressants. Patients arriving at the psychiatric emergency clinic with amphetamine dependence should be referred for outpatient treatment.

Amphetamines can also precipitate latent psychotic reactions that do not necessarily subside on cessation of drug use. It is important to distinguish carefully between acute toxic reactions that are dose-related and amphetamine-precipitated psychotic reactions that continue after blood and urine tests are negative for amphetamine (see above). The prognosis, as well as the long-term treatment, is quite different. A period of observation (24–48 hours) will usually be necessary to differentiate between the two conditions. With a drug-precipitated psychotic reaction, long-term maintenance with antipsychotic medication in conjunction with therapy is the treatment of choice. Therefore, these patients are usually hospitalized.

Treatment

Treatment strategies are largely determined by the initial signs and symptoms (see Guide to Management of Substance Abuse Crises, p 174). Strategies to reduce the amount of drug in the patient's system in cases of acute intoxication (overdose) include emesis in conscious patients, gastric lavage with an acidic solution (ion trapping) in unconscious individuals, and acidification of the urine with ascorbic acid or ammonium chloride to enhance excretion. Hypertensive crises are treated with an alpha-adrenergic blocking agent such as phentolamine. There is an evolving trend toward the use of beta-adrenergic blocking agents such as propranolol in managing acute stimulant reactions. The current antipsychotic drug of choice in treating amphetamine toxicity is haloperidol.

PHENCYCLIDINE (PCP) ABUSE

The phencyclidines are ''dissociative anesthetics'' and have a mechanism of action quite different from that of other hallucinogens. In the drug culture, they are used for ''mind-altering'' experiences. These substances have a high potential for chronic toxicity.

PCP and its analogs, including ketamine, are the ''bogeyman'' drugs of the present day. They can be produced cheaply and easily with readily accessible ingredients. Their use has increased among minority groups and less affluent young people but is rare among ''substance-sophisticated'' populations. About 95% of users experience no crisis, but the 5% who become seriously intoxicated present a difficult management problem. Without warning, the user may alternate between coma and violence.

Clinical Features

The term ''PCP syndrome'' has been used to describe the pattern of PCP toxicity. The PCP syndrome is manifested in the following four stages, which may or may not be successive:

A. Stage 1 (Acute PCP Toxicity): Reactions of acute PCP toxicity are a direct result of PCP intoxication and may include coma, hypertension, seizures, respiratory depression, and psychosis and agitation. Patients with acute toxicity may report to psychiatric emergency units with symptoms of paranoia, thought disorder, negativism, hostility, and grossly altered body image or may be referred for treatment as a result of their assaultive and antisocial behavior.

B. Stage 2 (PCP Toxic Psychosis): Stage 2, development of prolonged toxic psychosis, is apparently not related to toxic blood levels of PCP and does not inevitably follow stage 1.

C. Stage 3 (PCP-Precipitated Psychotic Episodes): In some individuals, PCP may precipitate a psychotic reaction that lasts a month or more and appears to be clinically similar to functional psychosis. Characteristics of PCP-precipitated psychotic epi-sodes are of the schizoaffective type (see Chapter 21), with paranoid features and a waxing and waning thought disorder. Most individuals in stage 3 have odd or eccentric personality disorders, and this is the major prognostic indicator.

D. Stage 4 (PCP-Induced Depression): PCP frequently produces a depressive reaction with severe cognitive impairment. Depression may follow any of the previous stages, but the diagnosis is missed by many clinicians, particularly where depression follows stage 3. The condition lasts from a day to several months but is usually completely reversible with abstinence from PCP.

Treatment

The following protocol is recommended for the various stages of PCP toxicity:

A. Stage 1 (Acute PCP Toxicity):

1. Coma–As in management of any comatose patient, the first step is to stabilize the cardiovascular and respiratory systems and protect the individual from bodily harm, such as may occur during convulsions.

2. Hypertension–Treatment with diazoxide (Hyperstat IV) has been recommended.

3. Seizures–Convulsions may occur and are not necessarily limited to one or two episodes. Therefore, recommended treatment is administration of intravenous diazepam over a period of 2 minutes following the seizure.

4. Respiratory depression–Occurrence of respiratory depression is unusual with pure PCP except in very high dosages. However, respiratory depression may be marked when PCP is taken in combination with alcohol, other sedative-hypnotics, or opiates. If respiration is sufficiently depressed, assisted breathing with a mechanical respirator may be necessary.

5. Psychosis and agitation–Luisada and Brown (1976) have delineated the following five immediate goals of treatment: preventing injury to the patient or others, ensuring continuing treatment, providing a supportive environment with reduced external stimuli, ameliorating the psychosis, and reducing agitation. The reduction of external stimulation through the use of seclusion or a quiet room is of prime importance.

6. Elimination of PCP from the body–Although many clinicians prefer conservative supportive management, Aronow et al (1978) describe the successful use of continuous gastric suction, acidification of the urine with vitamin C and cranberry juice, and a potent diuretic such as furosemide to enhance elimination.

PCP is recycled through the enterohepatic circulation, and introducing a slurry of activated charcoal into the intestine may decrease reabsorption of PCP from the small intestine. This should not be used instead of gastric suction in a comatose patient. However, 100 mg of activated charcoal slurry should be introduced into the stomach just before the nasogastric tube is removed from a comatose patient. The slurry may be given orally to a noncomatose patient.

B. Stage 2 (PCP Toxic Psychosis): After the acute PCP toxicity stage has passed, some individuals develop a prolonged toxic psychosis. Most clinicians recommend the use of haloperidol or other tranquilizer that is not a phenothiazine. Others recommend sedative-hypnotic medication. There is no sound research basis for the use of either of these medications, nor is there any indication that these drugs shorten the course of acute PCP psychosis. It does appear, however, that they make patients more manageable in the ward, which is probably the major reason these medications are used.

C. Stage 3 (PCP-Precipitated Psychotic Episodes): Immediate goals for treatment of psychosis and agitation are the same as those described for acute PCP toxicity, including prevention of injury and reduction of external stimuli.

D. Stage 4 (PCP-Induced Depression): In this form of depression, the individual is at high risk of suicide or may use other types of drugs to alleviate the depression. If antidepressants are prescribed on an outpatient basis, dosage for only two or 3 days should be dispensed at one time. The patient should be cautioned about possible interaction of tricyclic antidepressants with PCP, alcohol, and other drugs and should be advised to discontinue the tricyclic antidepressants if PCP use is resumed. The underlying basis of PCP-induced depression is unknown, and there is disagreement among experienced clinicians about what constitutes the best treatment.

PSYCHOTOMIMETIC AMPHETAMINE ABUSE

Some of the amphetamines include among their properties some that are similar to those of "psychedelic" drugs. MDA (3,4-methylenedioxyamphetamine), MDMA (M-methyl-3,4-methylenedioxymethamphetamine), and MDE (N-ethyl-3,4-methylenedioxymethamphetamine) are some of the more popular psychotomimetic drugs. MDA is known in some areas as the "love drug." MDMA is referred to as "Ecstasy," and MDE is called "Eve." These "designer" drugs have two basic qualities: they enhance insight and empathy and stimulate the central nervous system.

At low doses, MDMA and MDE can produce a state of well-being and self-insight, heightened empathy, and lowered psychological defenses, leading to open communication. These effects have led to their use in therapy by some psychotherapists and psychiatrists. However, at higher doses, the stimulant properties of these drugs emerge.

Research has revealed acute MDMA toxicity syndromes (at low, medium, and high doses), prolonged toxicity syndromes (at high and low doses), and MDMA-induced anxiety syndromes. The acute and prolonged toxicity syndromes are dose-related and can be treated as for stimulant toxicity. However, the MDMA-induced anxiety syndromes, which emerge some time after MDMA ingestion or persist in the absence of MDMA in the bodily fluids, should be treated as anxiety disorders. Unless dysfunctional, patients with these anxiety syndromes should respond to psychotherapy and protocols for nonpsychoactive anxiety. At the upper dosage limits, or in people with underlying cardiac problems, MDMA, MDE, and MDA can result in death caused by hypothermia, cardiac fibrillation, or other complications.

BARBITURATE & OTHER SEDATIVE-HYPNOTIC ABUSE

The category of depressant drugs includes a wide variety of substances which differ markedly in their physical and chemical properties but which share the common characteristic of causing generalized depression of the central nervous system. This drug group includes sedative-hypnotics (eg, barbiturates) and antianxiety agents (eg, benzodiazepines), which are widely prescribed in the USA. Some drugs, such as the barbiturates, are diffuse depressants of the central nervous system, with no specific receptors. Others, such as the benzodiazepines, have a specific receptor in the brain and have more specific action.

Depressant drugs listed in Table 18–4 include the barbiturates, barbiturate-like substances, benzodiazepines, carbamates, and chloral hydrate. In addition to the effects of euphoria and reduction of aggressive or sexual drives, other possible effects of these drugs include drowsiness, respiratory depression, and nausea. Although drugs classified as central nervous system depressants differ in their pharmacological actions and the onset and duration of their effects (Table 18–4), all exhibit some degree of cross-tolerance and cross-dependence. These depressant drugs are also cross-tolerant to alcohol, and their concomitant use with alcohol increases the risk of abuse and overdose.

Barbiturates

The barbiturates are the oldest of the sedative-hypnotics and can be classified as ultrashort-, short-, intermediate-, and long-acting. Ultra-short-acting barbiturates such as thiopental are used for anesthesia because of their rapid onset and brief duration of action. As a consequence, the ultra-short-acting barbiturates are rarely abused. The short- and intermediate-acting barbiturates include secobarbital and pentobarbital and are used primarily for insomnia. Their short duration of action and short to intermediate duration of disinhibition make them the most commonly abused drugs in the barbiturate class. The long-acting barbiturates have an onset of effects of up to 1 hour, and their duration of action is up to 16 hours; thus, they are very useful as anticonvulsant agents. They have a very low abuse potential.

Patients who have taken an overdose of barbiturates or other sedative-hypnotics arrive at emergency its with a variety of signs and symptoms that must interpreted quickly and accurately. A sedative-hypnotic overdose is a life-threatening emergency that cannot be treated definitively by nonmedical personnel. Signs and symptoms of sedative-hypnotic overdose include slurred speech, staggering gait, sustained vertical or horizontal nystagmus, slowed reactions, lethargy, and progressive respiratory depression characterized by shallow and irregular breathing and leading to coma and possibly death.

Most patients treated for an overdose of sedative-hypnotics are acutely intoxicated or in coma following ingestion of a single large dose, but they are not usually physically dependent on the drug. Unless the sedative-hypnotic has been used daily for more than a month in an amount equivalent to 400–600 mg of a short-acting barbiturate, a severe withdrawal syndrome will not develop.

Benzodiazepines

Benzodiazepines have become the most widely used drug group in the USA. The indications for their use are anxiety, muscle spasm, seizures, and treatment of acute alcohol withdrawal symptoms. Benzodiazepines are representative of the broad sedative-hypnotic class. Often inappropriately called "minor tranquilizers" (in contrast to the neuroleptics, or "major tranquilizers'), the benzodiazepines have varying durations of action, including short-acting benzodiazepines such as lorazepam and long-acting ones such as diazepam. All, however, have approximately equal abuse potential.

One of the major reasons for the popularity of benzodiazepines is that they have a much wider therapeutic index than the barbiturates. It is almost impossible to kill oneself with an overdose of benzodiazepines, although the therapeutic index and danger from overdose are greatly altered when benzodiazepines are taken in combination with alcohol. Most cases of benzodiazepine-related overdose seen in emergency rooms are associated with alcohol ingestion.

Dependence

There are substantial variations in individual reactions to the use of benzodiazepines in dosages within the therapeutic range. Most individuals who take benzodiazepines within therapeutic range over long periods experience no significant withdrawal. However, individuals with a psychobiological predisposition to addiction (often with a past history or family history of alcoholism) who take benzodiazepines in dosages within the therapeutic range for over 3 months may manifest severe withdrawal psychosis and seizure upon abrupt cessation of their use.

Some physicians switch from a medium- or longer-acting benzodiazepine such as diazepam to a shorter-acting benzodiazepine such as alprazolam in the mistaken belief that the shorter-acting drug has less potential for abuse. They may lower the equivalent dose as well, prompting the emergence of a sedative-hypnotic abstinence syndrome (anxiety and insomnia) throughout the day and at night. All benzodiazepines have the same potential for abuse; the use of shorter-acting benzodiazepines should be limited to their intended therapeutic purpose (eg, relief of panic). Patients with benzodiazepine dependence should enroll in a formal program of gradual detoxification. Alternatives to psychoactive medications should be sought for patients with both a dependence on benzodiazepines and a diagnosis of anxiety disorder. Therapeutically effective medications that have a lower potential for dependence (eg, imipramine rather than alprazolam in a drug-dependent patient with a history of panic disorder) should also be sought. If these alternatives, as well as stress reduction education, relaxation training and exercise, and biofeedback fail, and if major dysfunction is present, then a benzodiazepine is the drug of choice.

Clinical Features

If a benzodiazepine is taken at several times the therapeutic dosage for approximately 1 month, physical dependence can develop, and abrupt cessation can produce sedative-hypnotic withdrawal symptoms such as withdrawal psychosis and seizures.

Treatment

A. Overdose: Figure 18–1 outlines the ways in which an acute sedative-hypnotic overdose can be managed in an emergency situation. For additional information see Guide to Management of Substance Abuse Crises, p 174.

B. Withdrawal: It should be stressed that both the barbiturate and nonbarbiturate sedative hypnotics can produce physical dependence on the drug for the duration of withdrawal sequelae, determined in part by the differing metabolic properties and duration of action of the primary drug dose. For example, physical dependence on large doses of a short-acting barbiturate may be produced when the drug is abruptly stopped. The peak risk of seizure occurs at about the second day. Conversely, with a longer-acting nonbarbiturate sedative-hypnotic such as diazepam, a large or even standard therapeutic dose over a long period of time produces physical dependence. Abrupt cessation can cause withdrawal seizures as well as withdrawal psychosis, with the peak danger time being the fifth or sixth day. All of these withdrawal syndromes from sedative-hypnotics can be managed by detoxification with phenobarbital, a long-acting barbiturate. In this program of treatment, 30 mg of phenobarbital is initially substituted for each hypnotic dose of a sedative-hypnotic to which the individual is addicted. For example, a 30-mg sedative dose of

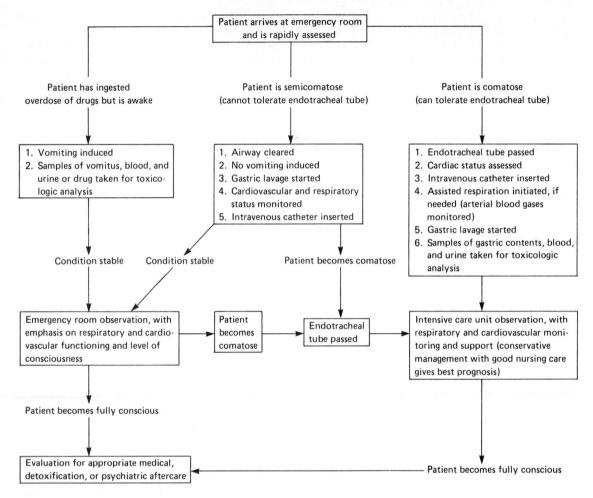

Figure 18–1. Acute treatment for barbiturate or other sedative hypnotic overdose. (Reproduced, with permission, from Smith DE, Wesson DR, Seymour RB: The abuse of barbiturates and other sedative hypnotics. In: *Handbook on Drug Abuse.* DuPont RL, Goldstein A, O'Donnel J [editors]. Basic Books, 1979.)

phenobarbital is substituted for each 100-mg hypnotic dose of the drug to which the individual is addicted. This "phenobarbital stabilization period" should continue for 2 days, followed by graded reduction of phenobarbital dosage over 7–20 days.

If the history of barbiturate abuse is variable or if the patient is using multiple sedative-hypnotics, then a challenge of short-acting pentobarbital (100–200 mg) or of long-acting phenobarbital (100–200 mg) can be used to test the individual's tolerance before starting the detoxification schedule. A person who does not have sedative-hypnotic tolerance will respond to the challenge with signs of sedation, ataxia, and mild intoxication; one who has developed tolerance will show minimal effect.

Addiction to a wide variety of other nonbarbiturate sedative-hypnotic substances—prescribed primarily for insomnia—that have a high abuse potential can occur if the individual takes five to ten times the therapeutic dose for approximately 1 month. This group includes glutethimide, ethchlorvynol, and methaqualone.* Physical dependence on barbiturates and barbiturate-like substances can cause an extremely severe withdrawal syndrome with features of psychosis, seizure, and amnestic disorder. If the individual has been taking these medications for longer than 1 month or has been self-administering them in high doses, they should not be abruptly stopped, and the medication should be either gradually reduced or the phenobarbital substitution and withdrawal technique (detoxification) initiated.

HALLUCINOGEN DRUG ABUSE

Hallucinogen abuse escalated in the 1960s and continues to be a problem. The pharmacological and clinical properties of hallucinogens are presented in

---

* Withdrawn in 1983. Not legally available after 1984

Table 18–4. In addition to effects for which hallucinogens are used (euphoria and altered perception of visual and auditory stimuli), other possible effects include illusions and hallucinations, poor judgment, and impaired perception of time and space.

Clinical Features

A. Acute Toxicity: In acute hallucinogenic drug toxicity, individuals are aware of having taken a drug (eg, LSD) but are in a state of severe anxiety and panic. They feel they cannot control the drug's effects and want to be rescued immediately. The diagnosis depends on a thorough understanding of the phases of the hallucinogenic experience. The course of the hallucinogenic "trip" (based on ingestion of 100–250 μg of LSD) can be described in three overlapping phases. The precise duration of each phase is dependent on dosage, individual idiosyncrasies, and the setting in which the drug is taken.

1. Phase 1 (sensory phase)–This phase, lasting from ingestion to the fifth hour, is characterized by sensory changes—visual, auditory, tactile, olfactory, gustatory, and kinesthetic effects—and awareness of internal bodily functions.

2. Phase 2 (symbolic, recollective, and analytic phase)– From the second to eighth hours, manifestations include visual imagery characterized by vivid colors, "hallucinations" (illusions), and altered visual perceptions; mood and affect changes; and altered communication.

3. Phase 3 (heightened sensibility phase)– From the second to tenth hours, insight, integration, and transformation of perceptions are heightened. Manifestations include concern with philosophy, religion, and cosmology; exaggeration of character traits and psychodynamic conflicts; exaggerated emotion; and feelings of heightened psychological perception and insight.

B. Chronic Toxicity: There are four recognized chronic reactions to hallucinogens or psychedelics:. prolonged psychotic reactions, flashbacks, depression severe enough to be life-threatening, and exacerbation of preexisting psychiatric illness.

Treatment

See Guide to Management of Substance Abuse Crises, p 174 (Seymour, Gorton, and Smith, 1982). External stimuli such as bright lights, loud music, and strangers coming or going may be interpreted as hostile by the patient having a "bad trip." A quiet room in a supportive environment (with "trusted" individuals) is a good place to "talk down" a frightened patient. Sitting on pillows on the floor is recommended for both patient and clinician. A nonthreatening physical setting also allows the clinician to avoid adopting an overly authoritative or threatening style.

Empathy and self-confidence are essential attributes of physicians or others called upon to deal with people undergoing hallucinogenic crises. Anxiety or fear is almost certain to be communicated to the patient, who may perceive the fear in an amplified manner. Physical contact often is reassuring but may be misinterpreted. When approaching patients who have been "tripping," the clinician must be guided by judgment and previous experience.

Psychotic reactions usually occur in patients with preexisting psychological problems. These reactions are similar to functional psychotic states and can be severe and prolonged. Appropriate treatment often requires residential care and then outpatient counseling.

"Flashbacks" are transient, spontaneous recurrences of drug effects long after the hallucinogenic intoxication has dissipated. These episodes cease with time, but in extreme cases the patient should be referred for antipsychotic medication and outpatient therapy.

MARIHUANA ABUSE

Marihuana, hashish, and other cannabis preparations have hallucinogenic and sedative properties. The active constituent is tetrahydrocannabinol (THC). At low to moderate doses, marihuana usually produces a sense of well-being, relaxation, and emotional disinhibition. A range of sensory and perceptual distortions, milder than those associated with LSD, may occur. Increased heart and pulse rates and a small drop in blood pressure are common.

At high doses, marihuana produces LSD-like effects such as hallucinations, disorganized thought, panic, paranoia, agitation, and rare psychotic reactions sometimes accompanied by rage and violence. *DSM-III-R* describes cannabis intoxication and cannabis-induced delusional disorder. Tolerance to cannabis can develop, and a mild withdrawal syndrome of insomnia, anxiety, perspiration, loss of appetite, and upset stomach is also seen. Chronic heavy use compromises pulmonary functioning; it also suppresses testosterone (a particular problem for adolescents). Marihuana also suppresses the immune system. The effects of marihuana and alcohol are additive. Because marihuana is a sedative-hypnotic as well as a hallucinogen, use of marihuana by a person who has developed a tolerance to alcohol will ward off symptoms of alcohol withdrawal. Moreover, a person who has developed tolerance to marihuana or to alcohol may use one drug during abstinence from the other in an attempt at self-medication for symptoms of withdrawal. This practice by persons unsophisticated in the combined use of alcohol and marihuana often leads to alcohol-marihuana overdose.

A small subgroup of chronic marihuana users fulfills the *DSM-III-R* diagnostic criteria for marihuana dependence. These users typically smoke marihuana daily and have family and personal histories of psychoactive substance dependence. Sometimes an individual with a dependence on another drug (eg, alcohol or cocaine) may perceive marihuana as benign and attempt to use it in a controlled fashion while abstaining from the other drug. Invariably, this person will return to the use of the primary drug after using marihuana. It is important to help persons with a dependence upon psychoactive substances to understand that abstinence from all mood-altering drugs is the most critical aspect of recovery.

OPIATE & OPIOID ABUSE

Drugs in the opiate and opioid class include the natural substances derived from the opium poppy, such as opium, morphine, and codeine; semisynthetics, such as diacetylmorphine (heroin); and synthetic narcotic analgesics (opioids), such as meperidine, methadone, and propoxyphene (Table 18–4). Opiates have been used as analgesics since ancient times, and some of them are still the analgesics of choice for severe pain. These drugs are also prescribed for reduction of aggressive or sexual drives. The effects for which these drugs are used illicitly include euphoria and "escape." Adverse effects are drowsiness, respiratory depression, constricted pupils, and nausea.

Clinical Features

The combination of pinpoint pupils and a declining level of consciousness is presumptive evidence of overdose of an opiate (eg, heroin or morphine) or an opioid. While pinpoint pupils are an important diagnostic sign, the pupils may be dilated as a consequence of hypoxia in cases of advanced coma.

Medical complications associated with the direct pharmacological effects of opiates and opioids are relatively rare and include constipation, decrease in sexual desire, and impairment of sexual functioning. However, in the drug culture, opiates such as heroin are usually administered intravenously, producing a broad range of "needle diseases" including abscesses, hepatitis, and endocarditis. Addicts (such as physicians and nurses) who inject meperidine or other pharmaceutical opioids rather than heroin and who use sterile needles have a much lower incidence of "needle disease."

Treatment

A. Overdose: See Guide to Management of Substance Abuse Crises, p 174. Fortunately, overdose with either an opiate or an opioid can be reversed by administration of the narcotic antagonist naloxone (Narcan). This is usually done in the emergency unit. The intravenous route is preferred, with 2–3 mg given initially. If the patient is in shock and has low blood pressure, 1 mg can be injected sublingually initially and the injection repeated sublingually or intravenously to gain a response. The sublingual injection site must be carefully watched for oozing blood, which may be aspirated and cause serious consequences.

In opiate or opioid overdose, pupillary dilation and an elevation in the level of consciousness will occur within 20 seconds to 1 minute following intravenous administration of naloxone. If this response is obtained, a second injection of naloxone, 2 mg intravenously, should follow for prolonged effect. However, for overdose by methadone or propoxyphene napsylate, both long-acting preparations, repeated doses of naloxone will be required every 1–2 hours. (Naloxone is a short-acting narcotic antagonist, and the opiate effect will outlast the antagonist effect of a single dose.)

The availability of a specific reversal agent does not mean that general supportive measures such as clearing the airway, maintaining respiration, keeping the patient warm, and elevating the feet can be neglected.

B. Dependence: Detoxification from opiate dependence usually requires inpatient hospital facilities. In this program of treatment, a long-acting narcotic such as methadone is substituted for the opiate to which the patient is addicted. The methadone dosage during the first 2 days is usually 10–40 mg; this is followed by a gradual dosage reduction over a 3- to 21-day period, until the patient is drug-free. Methadone itself can produce dependence; it is a long-acting narcotic and a drug of abuse in the same drug group.

Nonnarcotic medication may be used on an outpatient basis to relieve symptoms of narcotic withdrawal. This includes the use of a sedative, a hypnotic, and an antispasmodic for relief of anxiety, insomnia, and gastrointestinal upset, respectively. There is a growing trend in outpatient detoxification centers toward the use of effective but less potent narcotic medication, such as propoxyphene. Acupuncture and other nondrug approaches have also been utilized on an outpatient basis for detoxification.

SUBSTANCE ABUSE & AIDS

The substance abuser risks various health complications ranging from drug-related violence and automobile accidents to liver disease. The sharing of needles by addicts carries the risk of direct transmission of hepatitis and acquired immunodeficiency syndrome (AIDS). Unfortunately, psychoactive drug use increases a person's risk-taking behavior, including unsafe sexual practices. For example, the use of intravenous amphetamines is often associated with sexual activity, especially in some homosexual men who use stimulants to sustain erections for many hours. As of the first quarter of 1987, 16.7% of AIDS patients in the USA were intravenous drug abusers, and an additional 7.7% were homosexual intravenous drug abusers. It is critical that such high-risk individuals receive access to both AIDS education and substance abuse education and treatment.

The emergence of AIDS and AIDS-related complex (ARC) adds another dimension to differential diagnosis of chemical dependence and psychiatric disorders. The astute clinician must assess whether psychiatric symptoms (especially anxiety or depression) are (1) symptoms of drug use (or withdrawal); (2) symptoms of an endogenous disorder; (3) a psychological reaction to, or fear of, AIDS; or (4) an indication of the effects (eg, depression and delirium) of the human immunodeficiency virus on the central nervous system. The psychiatrist who has no experience with psychoactive substance use disorders or with AIDS-related psychological disorders should engage in multi-disciplinary cooperation with other health care professionals, including paraprofessional substance abuse and AIDS counselors, when treating psychoactive substance abusers in this high-risk category.

REFERENCES

Aronow R, Miceli JN, Done AK: Clinical observations during phencyclidine intoxication and treatment based on ion-trapping. In: *National Institute on Drug Abuse Research Monograph 21*, 1978.

Becker CE, Roe RL, Scott RA: *Alcohol as a Drug*. Medcom Press, 1974.

Blum K, Trachtenberg MC: Neurochemistry and alcohol craving. California Society for the Treatment of Alcohol and Other Drug Dependencies 1986,13:1.

Done AK, Aronow R, Miceli JN: The pharmacokinetics of phencyclidine in overdosage and its treatment. In: *National Institute on Drug Abuse Research Monograph 21*, 1978.

Dowling GP, McDonough ET, Bost RO: "Eve" and "Ecstasy": A report of five deaths associated with the use of MDEA and MDMA. JAMA 1987;257:1615.

Griffith JS, Cavanaugh J, Oates J: Schizophreniform psychosis induced by large dose administration of amphetamine. J Psychedelic Drugs 1969;2:42

Hayner GN, McKinney HE: MDMA: The dark side of Ecstasy. J Psychoactive Drugs 1986;18:341.

Inaba D et al: *Pharmacological and Toxicological Perspectives on Commonly Abused Drugs*. Medical Monograph Series. Vol 5 National Institute on Drug Abuse, 1982.

Jacobs PE: Emergency room drug abuse treatment. J Psychedelic Drugs 1975;7:43.

Jaffe JH: Drug addiction and drug abuse. Chapter 22 in: *Goodman and Gilman's The Pharmacological Basis of Therapeutics*, 8th ed. Gilman AG et al (editors). Pergamon, 1990.

Katzung BG (editor): *Basic & Clinical Pharmacology*, 4th ed. Lange, 1989.

Luisada PV, Brown BI: Clinical management of the phencyclidine psychosis. Clin Toxicol 1976;9:539.

Manual on Alcoholism. American Medical Association, 1977.

Marks J: The benzodiazepines: An international perspective. J Psychoactive Drugs 1983;15:145.

National Commission on Marijuana and Drug Abuse: *Drug Use in America. Problem and Perspective*. US Government Printing Office, 1973.

Pittel SM, Oppedahl MC: The enigma of PCP. In: *Handbook on Drug Abuse*. DuPont RL, Goldstein A, O'Donnel J (editors). Basic Books, 1979.

Sapira JD, Cherubin CE: *Drug Abuse: A Guide for the Clinician*. Excerpta Medica, 1976.

Schick JFE, Freedman DX: Research in non-narcotic drug abuse. In: *American Handbook of Psychiatry: New Psychiatric Frontiers*, 2nd ed. Vol 6. Arieta S (editor). Basic Books, 1975.

Schick JFE, Smith DE, Meyers FH: Patterns of drug use in the Haight-Ashbury neighborhood. Clin Toxicol 1970;3:19.

Schick JFE, Smith DE, Wesson DR: Analysis of amphetamine toxicity and patterns of use. J Psychedelic Drugs 1972;5:32.

Schuckit MA: *Drug and Alcohol Abuse: A Clinical Guide to Diagnosis and Treatment*. Plenum Press, 1979.

Seymour RB, Gorton JG, Smith DE. The client with a substance abuse problem. In: *Practice and Management of Psychiatric Emergency Care*. Gorton JG, Partridge R (editors). Mosby, 1982.

Showalter CV, Thomton WE: Clinical pharmacology of phencyclidine toxicity. Am J Psychiatry 1977,134:1234.

Siegel RK: Cocaine and sexual dysfunction: The curse of mama coca. J Psychoactive Drugs 1982;14:71.

Smith DE: Benzodiazepine dependence potential: Current studies and trends. J Subst Abuse Treat 1984;1:163.

Smith DE: Cocaine-alcohol abuse: Epidemiological, diagnostic and treatment considerations. J Psychoactive Drugs 1986;18:117.

Smith DE, Gay GR (editors): *It's So Good, Don't Even Try It Once*. Prentice-Hall, 1972.

Smith DE, Milkman HB, Sunderwirth SG: Addictive disease: Concept and controversy. In: *The Addictions: Multidisciplinary Perspectives and Treatments*. Lexington Books, 1985.

Smith DE, Wesson DR: Benzodiazepine dependency syndromes. J Psychoactive Drugs 1983;15:85.

Smith DE, Wesson DR: Low dose benzodiazepine withdrawal: Receptor site mediated. California Society for the Treatment of Alcoholism and Other Drug Dependencies News (San Francisco) 1982;9:1.

Smith DE et al: The diagnosis of the PCP abuse syndrome. In: *National Institute on Drug Abuse Research Monograph 21*, 1978.

Smith DE et al (editors): *A Multicultural View of Drug Abuse*. G.K. Hall & Co. and Schenkman Publishing Co., 1978.

Smith DE et al (editors): *PCP: Problems and Prevention*. Kendall/Hunt, 1980.

Snyder SH: Amphetamine psychosis: A "model" schizophrenia mediated by catecholamines. Am J Psychiatry 1973,130:61.

Wesson DR, Ling W: Naltrexone and its use in treatment of opiate dependent physicians. California Society for the Treatment of Alcoholism and Other Drug Dependencies News (San Francisco) 1980;7:1.

Wesson DR, Smith DE: A clinical approach to the diagnosis and treatment of amphetamine abuse. In: *Amphetamine*

Use, Misuse, and Abuse: Proceedings of the National Amphetamine Conference. Smith DE et al (editors). GK Hall, 1978.

Wesson DR, Smith DE, Linda KL: Drug crisis intervention: Conceptual and pragmatic considerations. J Psychedelic Drugs 1974;6:135.

Whitfield DC, Smith DE, Seymour RB: Psychedelics. In:

The *Patient With Alcoholism and Other Drug Problems: A Clinical Approach for Physicians and Helping Professionals.* Whitfield DC (editor). Year Book, 1980.

Wilford BB (editor): *Drug Abuse: A Guide for the Primary Care Physician.* American Medical Association, 1981.

Williams MH: *Drugs and Athletic Performance.* Thomas, 1973.

Alcoholism* **19**

Nick Kanas, MD

Alcoholism is a major problem in the Unites States. Four percent of American adults suffer from alcohol abuse, and 6% have alcohol dependence. A quarter of hospitalized people have alcohol-related problems, and at least 3% of all deaths can be attributed to causes directly linked to alcohol. In 1983, the cost of alcoholism was estimated at nearly $117 billion, of which 61% was due to reduced work productivity and 13% to medical costs. During 1987, one-half of automobile fatalities were alcohol-related.

There is no single cause of alcoholism. Biomedical, psychological, and social factors (Figure 19–1) all play a role in its development, and stressful events sometimes serve as catalysts of drinking behavior. Increased alcohol use can lead to both psychological and physical dependence, which result in a number of important biomedical, psychological, and social sequelae such as cirrhosis, depression, marital problems, and occupational problems. These sequelae themselves are stressful and lead to more drinking, further dependence, and additional sequelae—and the cycle continues. Treatment should be directed first at the stage of dependence on drinking, then to the important sequelae of drinking, and finally should attempt to explore and modify predisposing causes.

Diagnostic Workup

Some effects of alcoholism are encompassed in the *DSM-III-R* criteria for alcohol dependence and abuse. Table 19–1 lists several biomedical, psychological, and social sequelae.

A. History and Mental Status Examination: Essential to the workup are a complete history and mental status examination in the course of which the possibility of alcoholism is explored in a nonthreatening manner. One should not raise the issue of alcoholism directly at first but instead should look for clues and responses that might indicate a problem with alcohol. For example, the following should alert the physician to the possibility of alcoholism: a history of gulping drinks, blackouts, morning tremor, defensiveness, or dependence on other drugs; a positive family history; or marital or job problems. Indirect questions such as "Do you drink alcohol?" or "When and in what settings do you like to drink?" are much less threatening initially than direct questions such as "Is alcohol a problem for you?" or "Are you an alcoholic?" It is important to start asking questions in general terms and gradually become more specific. If alcoholism is suspected to be a problem, an interview with the spouse or other family members is indicated.

1. Level of alcohol consumption–In 1987, beer accounted for 53% of the per capita alcohol consumed, liquor for 33%, and wine for 14%.† Daily alcohol consumption can be estimated using the following conversion: one 12-oz can of beer (4% ethanol) = one 1-oz shot of hard liquor (43% ethanol) = one 4-oz glass of wine (12% ethanol)—each contains 12–15 mL of ethanol. Alcoholics with tolerance to alcohol may consume the equivalent of a liter or more of hard liquor per day. A high daily consumption rate is but one indication that an alcohol problem exists and should be used in conjunction with other symptoms and signs in making the diagnosis.

2. Denial of drinking problems–Alcoholics usually deny the presence and extent of their problem. In some cases, denial is a characteristic defense mechanism the individual uses in other contexts also. Extreme forms of denial may represent reactions to stress from past traumatic events, sequelae of alcoholism, or even stress associated with the treatment process itself. Denial may vary in intensity, and a patient may deny problems he or she acknowledged previously. If denial is confronted too vigorously, increased anxiety and anger may result, producing more denial or a flight from treatment. Confrontation should be modified in accordance with the therapist's assessment of the patient's ability to face the problem.

3. Blackouts–Blackouts occur in 64–94% of alcoholics. They are a form of anterograde amnesia in which the patient is unable to recall events that occurred during a bout of drinking even though he or she was conscious and active at that time. Blackouts last for minutes to days, and their frequency is an index of the severity and duration of alcoholism. Predisposing factors include gulping drinks on an empty stomach and going without sleep. Blackouts are generally unrelated to organic disturbances as measured by neuropsychological testing. The differential diag-

---

* See also Chapter 18.

† Data from the *Seventh Special Report to the US Congress.*

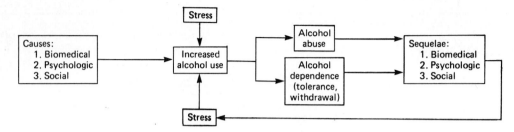

Figure 19–1. A conceptual model of alcoholism.

nosis of alcoholic blackouts includes head trauma, carbon monoxide poisoning, hysteria, and malingering.

B. Physical Examination: A complete physical examination should be performed after the history and mental status examination. In the early stages of alcoholism, pertinent physical findings may be limited to evidence of hepatomegaly, tremor, or mild peripheral neuropathy. In more advanced stages, there may be a number of physical signs consistent with the sequelae listed in Table 19–1.

C. Laboratory and X-Ray Findings: Useful laboratory measurements include the blood alcohol level (see Chapter 18 and Table 18–3); serum levels of aspartate aminotransferase (AST, SGOT), alkaline phosphatase, gamma-glutamyl transpeptidase, and bilirubin (increased levels indicate liver damage); and erythrocyte mean corpuscular volume (macrocytosis indicates liver disease, folate deficiency, or the toxic effect of alcohol on the developing erythroblast). Urinalysis and chest x-ray should be performed in all cases. Fractures, subdural hematomas, pneumonia, tuberculosis, and lung cancer from smoking are often found.

Epidemiology

From 1981 to 1987, total per capita alcohol consumed in the USA has declined from 2.76 gallons to 2.54 gallons. Reasons for this decline include increased public awareness of the dangers of alcohol, the aging population, and the increasingly conservative cultural climate.

Alcoholism rates are considered to be high in the USA, northern France, Poland, northern Russia, Sweden, and Switzerland; they tend to be low in China, southern France, Greece, Italy, Israel, Portugal, and Spain.

In the USA, Kissin (1977) estimated that 20–25% of alcoholics are in the upper and middle social classes; 40–50% are in the lower middle and upper lower social classes; and 25–30% are in the inner city and skid row populations.

Overall drinking rates are lower among blacks than whites, primarily due to the high abstinence rate among black women. However, more black men are at risk for alcohol-related health problems than white men. Hispanic women also have high rates of abstinence, but Hispanic men have high rates of heavy drinking and more alcohol-related problems than either black or white men. Native Americans show great variation in alcohol use, but both men and women have high rates of alcohol-related problems. Asian-Americans have low rates of alcohol use and alcoholism.

Whereas earlier surveys estimated the male:female ratio of alcoholics at 7:1, this ratio has stabilized in recent years at about 3:1. This probably reflects better case reporting of female alcoholics as well as the changing social role of women that allows them to admit having a drinking problem rather than seek help for anxiety or depression.

An interesting survey of 510 adults in the community was reported by Weissman et al (1980). Of the

Table 19–1. Sequelae of alcoholism.

Biomedical	Biomedical (cont'd)
Birth defects	Sexual dysfunction
Blackouts	(impotence,
Bone fractures	amenorrhea)
Cardiomyopathy	Subdural hematoma
Cerebellar degeneration	Tuberculosis
Cirrhosis	Wernicke's syndrome
Delirium tremens	**Psychologic**
Dementia	Angry outbursts
Esophageal varices	Anxiety
Esophagitis	Craving for alcohol
Fatty liver	Denial
Gastritis	Dependency
Hepatitis	Depression
Hypertension	Guilt
Hypothyroidism	Hallucinosis
Increased risk of cancer	Loneliness
(mouth, pharynx, larynx,	Paranoia
esophagus, liver, pancreas)	Suicidal ideation
Intoxication	Use of other drugs
Korsakoff's syndrome	**Social**
Myopathy	Automobile accidents
Nutritional deficiency, espe-	Family problems (marital,
cially vitamin (thiamine,	child abuse)
folate) deficiency	Financial problems
Pancreatitis	Inadequate shelter
Peripheral neuropathy	Legal problems
Pneumonia	Social isolation
Portal hypertension	Vocational problems
Seizures	

6.7% who were alcoholics, 71% had a history of at least one other psychiatric disorder. Over 75% of the subjects had a depressive disorder. The risk for suicide was much higher in alcoholics than in patients with other psychiatric disorders but not alcoholism. About 20% of polydrug abusers have diagnosable alcoholism, and the authors found the prevalence of drug misuse in their survey to be 12% among adult alcoholics.

Alcoholism in Physicians

Alcoholism is a major problem in physicians. Murray (1976) found that 29–39% of British physicians discharged from hospitals in England and Scotland had a problem with alcohol; in addition, first admission rates for alcoholism in his Scottish sample were 2.7 times higher in physicians than in other patients from the same socioeconomic class. In his English sample, 46% of the 41 alcoholic physicians had a family history of psychiatric disorders or alcohol abuse (or both); 29% had attempted suicide; 37% had an additional diagnosed psychiatric disorder; and 56% abused other drugs in addition to alcohol. Thirty-six of these physicians were followed for a mean total of 63 months; 80% continued to have difficulty with alcohol, 67% required further treatment, and 51% were not practicing medicine.

The prognosis for alcoholic physicians is improved if the problem is identified early and they receive intensive treatment for their alcoholism. Bissell and Jones (1976) interviewed 98 United States and Canadian physicians who were members of Alcoholics Anonymous and had been abstinent for at least a year. Many of their characteristics were similar to the physicians studied by Murray, but 75% were able to continue practicing medicine, although one-third of these reported some decline in work status. Kliner et al (1980) studied 67 alcoholic physicians 1 year after they had completed an intensive Alcoholics Anonymous-oriented inpatient program. They found that 76% had been abstinent since treatment; 79% had reported improvement in their professional performance as a result of treatment; and more than 75% reported improvement in all areas surveyed. Experiences such as these have led many states in the USA to establish programs for alcoholic physicians, with emphasis on early identification, adequate treatment, and long-term follow-up.

Etiology, Pathogenesis, & Natural History

Numerous factors have been identified as potential causes of alcoholism. In some patients, one factor may predominate; in others, several factors interact; and in many, no clear-cut cause can be found. In addition, a stressful event may be the final precipitant that initiates the addictive cycle (Figure 19–1).

A. Biomedical Factors: Evidence supporting a role of biomedical factors in alcoholism comes from genetic, physiological, biochemical, and prenatal data.

1. Genetic factors–There have been a number of twin, genetic marker, and adoption studies that support the conclusion that susceptibility to adverse effects of alcohol and predilection for uncontrollable drinking are hereditary. Particularly intriguing are the studies showing that alcoholism is more likely to occur in adopted children whose biological parents were alcoholics than in those whose biological parents were nonalcoholics. Two types of alcoholism emerge from these adoption studies. In type 1, or milieu-limited alcoholism, both genetic predisposition and environmental factors play a role. In type 2, or male-limited alcoholism, genetic factors appear stronger, especially among men. Cloninger (1987) has related type 1 alcoholism to passive-dependent personality traits and type 2 alcoholism to sociopathic personality traits.

2. Physiological factors–Physiological studies have correlated alcoholism with hypofunction of an endocrine gland, eg, the adrenal cortex or the thyroid. In these studies, it is unclear whether endocrine hypofunction leads to alcoholism or vice versa; thus, a clear causal relationship is still unproved. Many Asians have a physiological response to alcohol characterized by facial flushing, headaches, tachycardia, and itching, which may account for the low rate of drinking in this population.

3. Biochemical factors–Because of the association of alcoholism and depression, numerous studies have attempted to relate alcoholism to levels of monoamine oxidase. These studies have generally measured monoamine oxidase levels in platelets and have found that levels are lower in alcoholics than in controls. Since platelet levels of monoamine oxidase are strongly affected by genetic factors, some have speculated that this may be an important biochemical link between hereditary influences and the affective state of alcoholics.

Other brain proteins have been implicated in alcoholism, primarily neurotransmitters (such as GABA, glycine, and glutamate), proteins that control the opening and closing of ion channels, and second-messenger systems. Data are still accumulating in these promising areas of research.

4. Prenatal factors–Infants whose mothers drink heavily during pregnancy often show biological defects such as decreased size and weight. Fetal alcohol syndrome, a neonatal condition characterized by neurophysiological dysfunction and various anatomic malformations, has been described.

B. Psychological Factors: Data supporting psychological causes of alcoholism are from three sources: (1) psychoanalytic case studies, (2) personality assessments using psychological testing, and (3) theories of learning.

1. Emotional conflicts–Psychoanalytic theory holds that early developmental deprivation and trauma may result in painful conflicts that are repressed. Symptoms such as anxiety and depression may occur when these conflicts begin to enter conscious awareness. Reactivation of conflicts may be triggered later in life by stress or by events that are reminiscent of the original conflicts (see Role of Stress, below). Alcohol is seen as releasing inhibitions and allowing for the expression of these repressed conflicts.

2. Personality traits–Psychological testing has been used to explore common personality characteristics found in alcoholics. Several studies using the MMPI have shown that alcoholics demonstrate an abnormal elevation on the D (depression) and Pd (psychopathic deviance) scales. Some of these data on personality traits support the notion that alcoholics exhibit oral-dependent and depressive character traits, which is consistent with the psychoanalytic position mentioned above. Since psychological tests are often administered to adults already identified as being alcoholics, it is possible that years of drinking may encourage the emergence of clinically abnormal character traits later in life. For example, Vaillant (1980) has presented prospective data supporting the notion that oral-dependent traits may result from rather than cause alcoholism.

3. Learned behavior–Learning theory has also been used to develop a causal model of alcoholism. Many alcoholics report that being intoxicated reduces anxiety and replaces it with a feeling of well-being. Since people are drawn toward pleasurable states, drinking behavior is reinforced and gradually becomes a learned behavior (a habit).

C. Social Factors: The importance of social factors as a cause of alcoholism is supported by data from surveys and field studies that show relationships between the particular social variable under study and the rates of alcohol consumption or alcoholism. Some of the most important variables, such as sex, age, and ethnicity, are discussed in the section on epidemiology (above).

Family structure also plays an important role in alcoholism. Using general systems theory, one may conceptualize the alcoholic's family as a maladaptive system whose stability depends on one member fulfilling a sick role. Although the family is dysfunctional, it is in a homeostatic state. Any attempt on the part of the physician, therapist, or others to change the behavior of one family member will disturb the other family members and result in an increase in their anxiety and an attempt by them to resist the disturbing influence. This "systems" view has important implications for treatment, and the entire family should therefore be considered in the treatment plan.

D. Role of Stress: An interaction of biomedical, psychological, and social factors may lead to the gradual development of alcoholism. In some alcoholics, however, an acute traumatic life event (eg, the death of a spouse, physical illness, or even delayed posttraumatic stress syndrome) leads to increased drinking as a coping mechanism in dealing with resultant anxiety and depression. In the diagnostic workup of alcoholic patients, it is useful to make specific inquiry into a history of drinking escalations after stressful events.

Treatment & Prognosis

A. Effect of the Physician's Attitude on Treatment: The physician's attitude affects the treatment of alcoholics. Attitudinal barriers include moralistic views that alcoholics are "bad" people; frustration over the fact that alcoholics are difficult, time-consuming patients who often leave treatment prematurely or offer little financial or ego reward; and pessimism over the "revolving-door syndrome" whereby, despite great expenditure of time and energy on the part of the physician, the patient may later return for treatment in an inebriated state. It is also true that physicians tend to treat those problems that interest them. For example, internists focus on biomedical issues and psychiatrists on psychosocial issues. To properly treat alcoholics, one must give equal attention to biomedical, psychological, and social issues; this is a difficult conceptual stance for many physicians.

Attitudinal barriers begin in the medical school and house staff years. Fisher et al (1975) found a general tendency for pessimism and negative moral views to be expressed as students and physicians ascended the ladder of medical training: House staff members were more negative than second-year medical students, and they, in turn, were more negative than first-year medical students. Chappel et al (1977) found that a course in substance abuse taught to second-year medical students significantly improved their attitudes, so that they took a less moralistic and more therapeutic view of the problem. Since the prognosis for cure of alcoholism is better than for cure of many other conditions, it is important to educate physicians about alcoholism and its treatment so they will know how to deal with this problem.

B. Abstinence Versus Controlled Drinking: A key question in the treatment of alcoholics is whether the goal should be permanent abstinence or moderate, controlled drinking. Alcoholism has been conceptualized as a loss of ability to control consumption, perhaps due to a neurophysiological feedback dysfunction that affects the ability to regulate alcohol intake based on interoceptive cues. It follows that alcoholics must be regarded as inherently unable to control their drinking behavior, so that attempts at controlled drinking are doomed to failure. Furthermore, strict abstinence in the treatment of alcoholics has a long tradition and is a basic philosophic stance of Alcoholics Anonymous, one of the oldest arid most successful treatment programs. Because clinical experience has shown that most alcoholics who attempt controlled drinking ultimately fail, most workers in the field are skeptical about controlled drinking as a basic treatment goal.

C. Disulfiram (Antabuse): Disulfiram produces an unpleasant reaction in the presence of alcohol and is used as a deterrent to drinking. Its primary action is in blocking aldehyde dehydrogenase in the liver. When a patient taking disulfiram drinks ethyl alcohol, acetaldehyde cannot be converted to acetate, and the level of acetaldehyde in the blood may increase five- to tenfold. It is thought that the alcohol-disulfiram reaction is due to this increased level of acetaldehyde.

Nausea and flushing usually occur within 30 minutes, and the full-blown reaction—which may include anxiety, dyspnea, headaches, tachycardia, and hypertension—usually lasts 30–90 minutes. More serious reactions may occur in individuals who are unusually sensitive or have consumed large amounts of alcohol. For this reason, patients undergoing an alcohol-disulfiram reaction should be carefully monitored in an emergency room, and appropriate treatment for possible convulsions, myocardial infarction, or cardiovascular collapse should be available.

Disulfiram has a number of potential side effects. Most of these are rare, with the most common being drowsiness, metallic or garlic taste in the mouth, fatigue, and headaches. Disulfiram has synergistic effects with commonly prescribed medications (eg, benzodiazepines, barbiturates, monoamine oxidase inhibitors), and its use in pregnant women has been associated with fetal abnormalities. It also has been shown to produce psychotic reactions in patients with a history of major depression, mania, borderline personality, or schizophrenia.

The usual dose of disulfiram is 250 mg/d, usually taken in the evening because of the drowsiness it causes. Sensitivity to alcohol develops within 12 hours after taking the firs dose, although antacids and iron decrease its absorption and may prolong this time frame. Disulfiram is eliminated slowly from the body, and patients should be warned that they cannot drink for 1–2 weeks after stopping medication. Disulfiram should seldom be prescribed continuously for more than 3–6 months, because side effects are time-related. Since many of the side effects are also dose-related, the dose should rarely exceed 250 mg/d. Alcoholics taking disulfiram should be carefully cautioned about side effects, the risks of the alcohol-disulfiram reaction, and perhaps unrecognized sources of alcohol such as wine and vinegar sauces and medications that contain alcohol (eg, cough syrup). Occasionally, patients are sensitive to the alcohol in after-shave lotion or aerosol deodorants; therefore, use of talcum powder and alcohol-free deodorants may be advisable.

D. Treatment Settings and Effectiveness: Based on his extensive review, Baekeland (1977) concluded that only 2–15% of untreated alcoholics improve. This is in sharp contrast to the better prognosis for the estimated 15% of alcoholics and problem drinkers who are involved in formal treatment. There are three types of treatment settings for alcoholics: (1) specialized alcoholism treatment programs, (2) Alcoholics Anonymous, and (3) treatment by the individual physician. Each of these settings accounts for treatment of about one-third of the total population in treatment.

1. Specialized alcoholism treatment programs–The number of specialized treatment programs serving the alcoholic population has increased in recent years. Patients are self-referred to these programs or are referred by community agencies, physicians, and other professionals. Many of these programs include detoxification facilities, an inpatient rehabilitation unit, and an outpatient clinic.

a. Detoxification facilities–Detoxification may be done in one of three settings. To prevent late withdrawal reactions, patients should be carefully observed for at least 5 days.

Severely ill patients should be hospitalized and treated in a **general medical ward** or **specialized unit** capable of dealing with potential complications. Indications for admission include impending or frank delirium tremens; medical problems that might be aggravated by the stress of withdrawal; and severe functional problems, such as suicidal or homicidal ideation or a psychotic condition. Patients with a history of medical complications or delirium tremens during previous withdrawals should also be considered for hospitalization.

Since only 5% of alcoholics require hospitalization for detoxification, most can be managed in a **social model detoxification setting.** These centers provide a nonthreatening environment where the patient is kept active and provided with support and attention. Since the centers are usually staffed by nonprofessionals and are not licensed or staffed to handle severe illness or to dispense medications, patients referred to such settings should be ambulatory and physically well.

Finally, some alcoholics may be managed in an **outpatient clinic,** with withdrawal aided by use of benzodiazepines. This type of withdrawal program should be reserved for physically and psychologically stable patients who are well motivated and have friends or relatives who can give them support and monitor their use of benzodiazepines.

b. Inpatient rehabilitation units–Inpatient rehabilitation units have become important settings for dealing with the sequelae of alcoholism. The length of stay may vary from 2 to 4 weeks or even longer. Rehabilitation units offer a variety of services, including general medical workups; disulfiram treatment; individual, group, and family therapy; recreational therapy; educational films and discussions; vocational testing and counseling; Alcoholics Anonymous groups; and careful attention to discharge planning, eg, help with finding a place to live and a temporary source of financial aid. Individuals referred to these units include patients who cannot remain abstinent outside a controlled setting, patients who need a period of hospitalization to stabilize their social situation, and patients who might benefit from an intensive therapeutic experience that may involve up to 10 hours a day of therapeutic work. Alcoholics with severe psychiatric or medical disorders do not do well in these intense, demanding programs.

c. Outpatient alcohol clinics–Many of the treatment services offered by outpatient alcohol clinics parallel those described above. However, since patients often spend years enrolled in outpatient programs, the focus is on long-term management and the uncovering of predisposing causes. Alcoholics in outpatient programs must be able to function outside a controlled environment.

d. Effectiveness of programs–In several reviews of specialized treatment programs, 30–40% of alcoholics were found to be significantly improved after 1–2 years. These results were adjusted statistically to account for program dropouts and patients whose improvement was "spontaneous" (ie, could not be attributed to the treatment program). Success was measured as continuous abstinence or improved biomedical or psychosocial status. Outpatient programs are slightly more successful than inpatient programs, although combined programs give the best results. Treatment programs vary greatly, depending on patient motivation and treatment setting. Poorly motivated alcoholics who are ordered by a judge to participate as a way of retaining a license or staying out of jail improve at a rate of about 10%, whereas improvement rates approaching 70% have been reported in highly motivated patients enrolled in multifaceted programs and receiving support from family and employers.

2. Alcoholics Anonymous–This organization was founded in 1935 by two recovering alcoholics. There are now almost 500,000 members in the USA and Canada alone. Alcoholics Anonymous is a self-help organization of nonprofessionals that emphasizes group support and surrender to a "higher power" to achieve permanent total abstinence. Sponsors and program members are available to help alcoholics 24 hours a day, and sober interactions are encouraged through frequent meetings and club activities.

Although Alcoholics Anonymous surveys usually report a 1-year continuous abstinence rate of nearly 60%, dropout rates are high, approaching 50% in the first 3 months. When these data are considered in the analysis, the 1-year improvement rate approximates that of specialized alcoholism treatment programs. Nevertheless, for those who accept the Alcoholics Anonymous model and remain in treatment, the program offers an important and often lifesaving source of support and abstinence. About half of those who participate for 3 months will be abstinent and continue to participate throughout the next year, and a member who has been abstinent for 1–5 years has a good chance (86%) of completing the following year without drinking. Spin-offs of Alcoholics Anonymous—such as Al-Anon and Alateen for adults and teenagers living with alcoholics—have been helpful in providing support.

3. Treatment by an individual physician–Individual physicians in private, clinic, or hospital-based settings are an important treatment source for alcoholics. Although most physicians concern themselves with aspects of alcoholism treatment that represent their area of expertise, a growing number are taking an eclectic view that integrates biomedical, psychological, and social factors in the treatment plan. It is critical that physicians familiarize themselves with community resources and establish channels for referrals to other professionals who may have more expertise in some aspects of treatment. Treatment approaches should be flexible, supportive, and nonjudgmental. Physicians should remember that alcoholism is a disorder characterized by loss of control over drinking behavior, frequent relapses, a chronic course, and a variety of causes and effects. The physician who takes responsibility for constructing and coordinating all aspects of the patient's care (emotional, physical, etc) will be more likely to have a successful treatment plan.

E. Phases of Treatment for Alcoholism: In planning treatment for the alcoholic, the physician should base priorities on each patient's biomedical, psychological, and social needs. The discussion below approaches treatment in terms of four sequential phases, each with typical problems and possible solutions (Table 19–2). However, not all patients enter treatment in phase 1 or 2, and some patients may skip a phase depending on individual needs.

1. Phase 1 (acute crisis)–In evaluation of an alcoholic, the first consideration is whether or not the patient is experiencing a life-threatening crisis (Table 19–2). The possibility of an acute medical or psychiatric emergency should be considered in every alcoholic. Although the specific details of treatment are beyond the scope of this chapter, measures usually include immediate hospitalization and vigorous medical or psychiatric intervention (eg, administration of intravenous fluids, precautions against suicide attempts, one-on-one nursing care). If family violence has occurred, family therapy and even a home visit by the staff may be useful. Alcoholic patients hospitalized for some other problem must be observed for the appearance of withdrawal symptoms.

2. Phase 2 (withdrawal from alcohol)–After acute crisis is ruled out, safe withdrawal from the effects of alcohol can be started (Table 19–2). Patients admitted to the hospital with delirium tremens should be placed in a well-lighted room and will require frequent observation (and possibly restraints). The principles of care include reassurance, careful monitoring of vital signs, and intravenous fluids with electrolytes and vitamins. Most alcoholics have low thiamine stores, and glucose solutions may cause further depletion of thiamine; therefore, thiamine should be added to intravenous fluids to prevent Wernicke's

Table 19–2. Phases of treatment for alcoholism.

Phase of Treatment	Typical Problems	Possible Solutions
Phase 1 (acute crisis)	Biomedical: Gastrointestinal bleeding; pneumonia; delirium tremens.	Hospitalization; appropriate medical intervention.
	Psychologic: Hallucinosis; paranoia; suicidal ideation.	Hospitalization; appropriate psychiatric intervention.
	Social: Family violence.	Hospitalization; appropriate psychiatric intervention; family therapy; home visit.
Phase 2 (withdrawal from alcohol)	Biomedical: Impending delirium tremens; withdrawal effects; acute medical problems.	Medical or social model detoxification; outpatient detoxification; appropriate medical intervention.
	Psychologic: Denial; worry about health; stressful life events.	Counseling; brief individual or group therapy.
	Social: Inadequate shelter; financial problems.	Counseling; social services referral.
Phase 3 (sequelae of alcoholism)	Biomedical: Chronic medical problems; malnutrition.	Appropriate medical intervention; vitamin supplements, proper diet, and exercise; disulfiram.
	Psychologic: Denial; depression; guilt; stressfull life events; psychologic craving for alcohol.	Counseling; brief individual or group therapy; antidepressants; lithium carbonate; behavior modification techniques.
	Social: Family, housing, vocational, and legal problems; loneliness; unfilled leisure time.	Counseling; social services referral; family therapy; recreational therapy; Alcoholics Anonymous, Al-Anon, or Alateen; alcoholic halfway house.
Phase 4 (focus on predisposing causes)	Biomedical: Genetic factors.	Counseling.
	Psychologic: Neurotic and personality disorders; major affective disorders; schizophrenia.	Long-term individual or group therapy; antidepressants; lithium carbonate; major tranquilizers.
	Social: Sociocultural and familial influences.	Counseling.

syndrome. Intravenous benzodiazepines are generally used, often in high doses, for delirium tremens. The physician must be alert to complications associated with delirium tremens (eg, seizures and marked autonomic hyperactivity) as well as the possibility of associated medical problems (eg, pneumonia or subdural hematoma). With treatment, most alcoholics recover from delirium tremens, although the mortality rate may reach 15%.

In addition to biomedical problems during the withdrawal period, psychosocial issues should also be addressed. Many alcoholics deny or minimize the extent of psychological or social problems. Others are legitimately worried about their health or are recovering from a stressful life event, such as a death in the family or a divorce, that served as the occasion for the latest drinking spree. Supportive counseling or brief individual or group therapy may be instituted as soon as the patient's sensorium clears and the medical status improves. Since compliance with treatment may be affected by problems such as having no money and nowhere else to go, the physician may wish to offer advice about such matters or make referral to appropriate social service agencies.

3. Phase 3 (sequelae of alcoholism)–After acute problems and withdrawal have been dealt with, concern should focus on the sequelae of alcoholism. Some patients in this phase of treatment may be admitted directly to an outpatient clinic. Others with more tenuous biomedical arid psychosocial status should first be admitted to an inpatient rehabilitation unit.

As shown in Table 19–2, chronic medical problems such as peripheral neuropathy, cirrhosis, or organic brain syndrome should be managed appropriately. Vitamins and suitable instructions on the importance of diet and exercise will improve physical status. Disulfiram (Antabuse) should be prescribed for patients who need this added incentive to avoid alcohol.

Psychologically, many alcoholics experience depression, guilt, or the impact of stressful life events during this phase, particularly as the defense of denial begins to crumble. Counseling or brief individual or group therapy may help. Antidepressants or lithium carbonate may be useful for alcoholics with major affective disorders.

Newly abstinent alcoholics are particularly prone to experience a psychological craving for alcohol. The intensity of the craving is correlated with anxiety or environmental factors such as seeing an advertisement for alcohol or experiencing a stressful life event. Behavior modification techniques that utilize aversive conditioning have been used to reduce craving. Mild electric shock or emetics such as apomorphine or emetine are given while the patient drinks in a controlled setting, usually an inpatient or rehabilitation unit. The goal of such treatment is to create an aversion to alcohol that will persist after treatment. Aversive and other behavioral techniques are not effective as the sole form of treatment, but they have been used with success in multifaceted programs that address both drinking behavior and associated psychosocial problems. Covert sensitization (see Chapter 35) and other newer behavioral techniques that use fantasy and imagination to develop conditioned aversion to alcohol have also shown promise, although not all patients can be successfully trained to use these techniques.

Years of alcoholism may lead to family difficulties, inadequate shelter, a poor job history, legal and financial problems, loneliness, and trouble filling leisure time in a nonalcohol context. The physician may wish to counsel the patient on these matters or make referral to appropriate social agencies for food stamps, vocational counseling, etc. Family therapy may be helpful, since patterns of family interaction become more rigid when an alcoholic member is drinking than when he or she is sober. Recreational activities and hobbies may help the alcoholic fill leisure time. Alcoholics Anonymous is useful in giving support as well as encouraging and reinforcing abstinence. Al-Anon and Alateen may be useful for the spouse and children of alcoholics.

In some communities, another referral source is the alcoholic halfway house, which Rubington (1977) defines as "a transitional place of indefinite residence of a community of persons who live together under the rule and discipline of abstinence from alcohol and other drugs." This setting provides the abstinent alcoholic with a sober environment in the company of other recovering alcoholics able to offer support and advice. Food and shelter are provided, and many halfway houses have their own therapeutic programs that may include vocational counseling and informal "rap" groups. Although the stay is usually limited to a few months, many alcoholics are functioning at a higher level by this time and are ready to live independently.

4. Phase 4 (focus on predisposing causes)– After the sequelae of alcoholism have been managed, it is appropriate to focus on predisposing causes of the problem (Table 19–2). The physician should be sensitive to the patient's concerns involving genetic and sociocultural factors. Some alcoholics feel that genetic factors doom them to a life of alcoholism and approach treatment pessimistically for that reason. Others blame their religious or cultural background or are reluctant to seek treatment from physicians of different ethnic backgrounds. Counseling that emphasizes support and reassurance may be effective in alleviating concern, exploring stereotypes, and breaking cultural barriers.

For many alcoholics, psychological issues are important predisposing causes of drinking. Diagnosti-cally, these may include neurotic problems such as dysthymic and generalized anxiety or posttraumatic stress disorder; personality problems such as antisocial, dependent, or borderline disorder; major affective problems such as bipolar or major depressive disorder; and schizophrenia. For alcoholics with neurotic and borderline personality disorders, long-term individual therapy may be useful. Alcoholics with other personality disorders do best in group therapy. Therapy that emphasizes insight and interpersonal learning tends to be stressful for alcoholics, so they need additional group experiences providing support and emphasizing abstinence, such as that offered by Alcoholics Anonymous or a "rap" group. Assertiveness training groups have also been useful for many alcoholics. Finally, for alcoholics with major affective disorders or schizophrenia, treatment with antidepressants, lithium carbonate, or major tranquilizers may be helpful. Minor tranquilizers such as the benzodiazepines have addictive potential and should not be used for long periods.

SUMMARY

Alcoholism is a serious disorder characterized by loss of control over drinking; a chronic, relapsing course; and a number of biomedical, psychological, and social causes and effects. In the diagnostic workup, a complete history, mental status examination, and physical examination are essential, along with appropriate laboratory tests. Since alcoholism affects both sexes and people of all ages, races, and socioeconomic classes, the physician should be alert to its possibility when evaluating any patient. Case finding is made difficult by denial of alcoholism by patients, negative physician attitudes, and the presence of alcoholism among physicians.

Permanent abstinence is a major treatment goal for alcoholics. Therapeutic approaches should be flexible, supportive, and nonjudgmental. Important treatment settings include inpatient and social model detoxification units, inpatient rehabilitation wards, outpatient alcohol clinics, and alcoholic halfway houses. Disulfiram (Antabuse) and Alcoholics Anonymous are important adjuncts to treatment. By addressing issues involving acute crises, withdrawal, and sequelae and causes of alcoholism, the physician may play a key role in coordinating the treatment of alcoholic patients.

REFERENCES

Alexopoulos GS et al: Platelet MAO during the alcohol withdrawal syndrome. Am J Psychiatry 1981;138:1254.

Baekeland F: Evaluation of treatment methods in chronic alcoholism. In: *The Biology of Alcoholism.* Vol 5: *Treatment and Rehabilitation of the Chronic Alcoholic.* Kissin B, Begleiter H (editors). Plenum Press, 1977.

Bissell L, Jones RW: The alcoholic physician: A survey. Am J Psychiatry 1976;133:1142.

Chappel JN et al: Substance abuse attitude changes in medical students. Am J Psychiatry 1977;134:379.

Cloninger CR: Neurogenetic adaptive mechanisms in alcoholism. Science 1987;236:410.

Costello RM: Alcoholism treatment and evaluation: In search of methods II. Int J Addict 1975;10:857.

Eckhardt MJ et al: Health hazards associated with alcohol consumption. JAMA 1981;246:648.

Fisher JC et al: Physicians and alcoholics: The effect of medical training on attitudes toward alcoholics. J Stud Alcohol 1975;36:949.

Kanas N: Alcoholic liver disease: An eclectic approach to the treatment of the chronic alcoholic. In: *Hepatology*. Zakim D, Boyer T (editors). Saunders, 1982.

Kanas N: Alcoholism and group psychotherapy. In: *Encyclopedic Handbook of Alcoholism*. Pattison EM, Kaufman E (editors). Gardner Press, 1982.

Kanas N: Multi-factor group therapy for alcoholics. Curr Psychiatr Ther 1982;21:149.

Kanas N: Stress and alcoholic denial. J Drug Education 1984;14:105.

Kissin B: Theory and practice in the treatment of alcoholism. In: *The Biology of Alcoholism*. Vol 5: *Treatment and Rehabilitation of the Chronic Alcoholic*. Kissin B, Begleiter H (editors). Plenum Press, 1977.

Kliner DJ, Spicer J, Barnett P: Treatment outcome of alcoholic physicians. J Stud Alcohol 1980;41:1217.

Kolakowska T, Swigar ME: Thyroid function in depression and alcohol abuse: A retrospective study. Arch Gen Psychiatry 1977;34:984.

Kwentus J, Major LF: Disulfiram in the treatment of alcoholism: A review. J Stud Alcohol 1979;40:428.

Matthew RJ, Claghom JL, Largen J: Craving for alcohol in sober alcoholics. Am J Psychiatry 1979;136:603.

Murray RM: Alcoholism amongst male doctors in Scotland. Lancet 1976;2:729.

Murray RM: Characteristics and prognosis of alcoholic doctors. Br Med J 1976;2:1537.

Nathan PE, Briddell DW: Behavioral assessment and treatment of alcoholism. In: *The Biology of Alcoholism*. Vol 5: *Treatment and Rehabilitation of the Chronic Alcoholic*. Kissin B, Begleiter H (editors). Plenum Press, 1977.

Rubington E: The role of the halfway house in the rehabilitation of alcoholics. In: *The Biology of Alcoholism*. Vol 5: *Treatment and Rehabilitation of the Chronic Alcoholic*. Kissin B, Begleiter H (editors). Plenum Press, 1977.

Secretary of Health and Human Services: *Seventh Special Report to the US Congress on Alcohol and Health*. US Government Printing Office, 1990.

Shapiro RJ: A family therapy approach to alcoholism. J Marriage Fam Counsel 1971;3:71.

Tarter RE, Schneider DU: Blackouts. Arch Gen Psychiatry 1976;33:1492.

Thompson WL: Management of alcohol withdrawal syndromes. Arch Intern Med 1978;138:278.

Vaillant GE: Natural history of male psychological health. 8. Antecedents of alcoholism and orality. Am J Psychiatry 1980;137:181.

Weissman MM, Myers JK, Harding PS: Prevalence and psychiatric heterogeneity of alcoholism in a United States urban community. J Stud Alcohol 1980;41:672.

20

Schizophrenic Disorders

Bruce Africa, MD, PhD, & Stuart R. Schwartz, MD

The term "schizophrenia" denotes a severe and prolonged mental disturbance manifested as a wide range of disturbed behavior. Though discussed as a disease, schizophrenia is more appropriately considered a group of disorders of uncertain cause with similar clinical pictures—invariably including thought disturbances in a clear sensorium and often with characteristic symptoms such as hallucinations, delusions, bizarre behavior, and deterioration in the general level of functioning. For this reason, the *DSM-III-R* heading—and the title of this chapter—is schizophrenic disorders, though both terms are used in the chapter. In the industrialized world, about one in every 100 persons will develop schizophrenia.

The Concept of Schizophrenia

Descriptions of an illness consistent with the concept of schizophrenic disorders date back to 1400 BC and are found throughout history. Descriptions become frequent only after the social and industrial revolutions of the 18th century, when physicians were given control of the asylums. Emil Kraepelin, a German psychiatrist, attempting to classify all previously described psychoses, introduced the term "dementia praecox" in 1896. Psychotic disorders without known "organic" causes were classified into 3 groups based on clinical presentation and course. Kraepelin used the term **manic-depressive insanity** for the group of disorders characterized chiefly by exacerbations and remissions in disturbances of affect rather than thinking. He linked a second syndrome, **paranoia,** with this group because the psychosis was limited and did not produce severe deterioration of affect or function. **Dementia praecox** was the term used for the third group of disorders, which featured severe disturbances in functioning (eg, **catatonia, hebephrenia**), that began in adolescence and progressively worsened and in which "failure of volition" was a prominent feature. Kraepelin did note that there were variations in course, and he considered **paraphrenia** to be a less complete expression of dementia praecox (Kraepelin, 1909; Barclay, 1919).

In 1911, Eugen Bleuler, a Swiss psychiatrist, was able to reduce the psychiatric psychoses to just two groups by introducing the term **schizophrenia** (meaning "splitting of the mind') to designate a syndrome in which the observable signs and symptoms of both Kraepelin's paranoia and his dementia praecox could

be ascribed to splitting of the normally integrated psychological processes postulated by Freud and Jung. Bleuler believed that four processes were primary to the illness: **autism** (a turning inward, away from the world), **ambivalence,** and primary disturbances in **affect** and **associations.** Like Kraepelin, Bleuler assumed that this syndrome was separate from manic-depressive illness and that underlying biological determinants eventually would be discovered for each (Bleuler, 1911 and 1950). Modern studies of the affective, paranoid, and schizophrenic psychoses began that same year, as serological testing provided a means of identifying patients with tertiary syphilis—which proved to be about one-third of those considered severely mentally ill. Bleuler's psychological criteria were used broadly to designate a group of patients about twice as large as Kraepelin's group. These additional patients were identified by the Norwegian psychiatrist Langfeldt as "schizophreniform," ie, "other than true schizophrenia," and his work in the 1930s established that those who remitted, either spontaneously or after treatment with induced coma or convulsions, were mostly from this group (Langfeldt, 1960) (see Chapter 21).

Adolf Meyer, a Swiss psychiatrist working in the USA early in this century, emphasized the importance of life stress as a modifier of normal development in the genesis of all mental illnesses. He applied his unified psychobiological approach to understanding major psychotic disorders as well as neurotic disorders; his views dominated psychiatry in the USA until the 1940s.

In the 1930s and 1940s, Harry Stack Sullivan, an American, contributed an original explanation of how interpersonal relationships are influenced by—and causally related to—both the development and the treatment of schizophrenia. At the same time, Kurt Schneider, in Germany, attempted to redefine a narrower group within "Bleuler's schizophrenics" by focusing on specific, very severe psychotic symptoms, with less emphasis on either the other functional deficits or the duration of symptom expression. In the 1950s and 1960s, the Bleuler and Schneider criteria dominated thinking in the USA and Germany, and they will continue to be used in *ICD-9* to designate a broader spectrum of schizophrenia than what is found in *DSM-III-R.*

The controversy about the definition and meaning

of the term ''schizophrenia'' has led to different conclusions about the natural course and treatment outcome of the disease. No matter how narrow the initial diagnostic criteria, there is marked variability in both outcomes and in the clinical pictures observed over any individual patient's lifetime. This can lead to contradictory impressions on the part of different observers if each sees the patient at different times. The operational diagnostic criteria of *DSM-III-R* clarified the picture for both clinicians and researchers, as they not only defined a narrower set of symptoms and course but also allowed for reclassification of about half of the disorders in the broader spectrum of schizophrenia into other psychotic diagnoses among the many in *DSM-III-R*. About one-third of those who are reclassified are found to have mood disorders, while the majority remain within the schizophrenia spectrum of schizoaffective, schizophreniform, and atypical psychoses but have better outcomes than the remaining core of *DSM-III-R* schizophrenics. Research using *DSM-III-R* established that the axis II disorders of ''cluster A'' (paranoid, schizoid, and schizotypal personality disorders) but not those of

''cluster B'' (antisocial, borderline, histrionic, and narcissistic personality disorders) are associated with schizophrenia in genetics, course, and response to treatment.

DSM-III-R (Table 20–1) reflects the currently accepted concept of the schizophrenic disorders. Schizophrenia is characterized by disorganization of a previous level of functioning, symptoms involving multiple psychological processes, clear-cut psychotic features during the active phase of the illness, and a tendency toward chronicity.

Onset of Schizophrenia

Schizophrenia after childhood always involves disorganization of a previous level of functioning. First onset of psychosis after age 45 is often related to identifiable organic factors and is not schizophrenia; the remainder of cases are more likely to be mood disorders with psychosis than schizophrenia. Onset of adult schizophrenia is noted when family and friends observe that the person ''has changed'' or is ''no longer the same.'' The individual functions poorly in significant areas of routine daily living,

Table 20–1. *DSM-III-R* diagnostic criteria for schizophrenic disorders.

A. Presence of characteristic psychotic symptoms in the active phase: either (1), (2), or (3) for at least 1 week (unless the symptoms are successfully treated):
　(1) Two of the following: delusions; prominent hallucinations (throughout the day for several days or several times a week for several weeks, each hallucinatory experience not being limited to a few brief moments); incoherence or marked loosening of associations; catatonic behavior; flat or grossly inappropriate affect.
　(2) Bizarre delusions (ie, involving a phenomenon that the person's culture would regard as totally implausible, eg, thought broadcasting, being controlled by a dead person).
　(3) Prominent hallucinations (as defined above) of a voice with content having no apparent relation to depression or elation, or a voice keeping up a running commentary on the person's behavior or thoughts, or 2 or more voices conversing with each other.
B. During the course of the disturbance, functioning in such areas as work, social relations, and self-care is markedly below the highest level achieved before onset of the disturbance (or when the onset is in childhood or adolescence, failure to achieve expected level of social development).
C. Schizoaffective disorder and mood disorder with psychotic features have been ruled out, ie, if a major depressive or manic syndrome has ever been present during an active phase of the disturbance, the total duration of all episodes of a mood syndrome has been brief relative to the total duration of the active and residual phases of the disturbance.
D. Continuous signs of the disturbance for at least 6 months. The 6-month period must include an active phase (of at least 1 week, or less if symptoms successfully treated) during which there were psychotic symptoms characteristic of schizophrenia (symptoms in criterion A), with or without a prodromal or residual phase, as defined below.
　Prodromal phase: A clear deterioration in functioning before the active phase of the disturbance that is not due to a disturbance in mood or to a psychoactive substance use disorder and that involves at least 2 of the symptoms listed below.
　Residual phase: Following the active phase of the disturbance, persistence of at least 2 of the symptoms noted below, these not being due to a disturbance in mood or to a psychoactive substance use disorder.
　Prodromal or Residual Symptoms:
　(1) Marked social isolation or withdrawal.
　(2) Marked impairment in role functioning as wage-earner, student, or homemaker.
　(3) Markedly peculiar behavior (eg, collecting garbage, talking to self in public, hoarding food).
　(4) Marked impairment in personal hygiene and grooming.
　(5) Blunted or inappropriate affect.
　(6) Digressive, vague, overelaborate, or circumstantial speech, or poverty of speech, or poverty of content of speech.
　(7) Odd beliefs or magical thinking, influencing behavior and inconsistent with cultural norms, eg, superstitiousness, belief in clairvoyance, telepathy, "sixth sense," "others can feel my feelings," overvalued ideas, ideas of reference.
　(8) Unusual perceptual experiences, eg, recurrent illusions, sensing the presence of a force or person not actually present.
　(9) Marked lack of initiative, interests, or energy.
　Examples: Six months of prodromal symptoms with 1 week of symptoms from criterion A; no prodromal symptoms with 6 months of symptoms from criterion A; no prodromal symptoms with 1 week of symptoms from criterion A and 6 months of residual symptoms.
E. It cannot be established that an organic factor initiated and maintained the disturbance.
F. If there is a history of autistic disorder, the additional diagnosis of schizophrenia is made only if prominent delusions or hallucinations are also present.

such as work and social relations. There is often a notable lack of concern for self-care in an individual who was previously capable of it. As they lose their grip on reality, patients experience the following feelings:

A. Perplexity: At the onset of illness, patients report a sense of strangeness about the experience as well as confusion about where the symptoms are coming from and why their own everyday experience is so markedly changed.

B. Isolation: The schizophrenic person experiences an overwhelming sense of being different and separate from other people.

C. Anxiety and Terror: A general sense of discomfort and anxiety often pervades the experience. This is sharpened by periods of intense terror, caused by "a world within" that is experienced as dangerous or uncontrollable and often attributed to external sources.

Symptoms & Signs

In schizophrenia, severe disturbances occur in several of the following areas: language and communication, content of thought, perception, affect, sense of self, volition, relationship to the external world, and motor behavior. Any of these symptoms may be seen in other psychological disturbances also, and none by itself is pathognomonic of schizophrenia. Furthermore, individuals who are well adapted and who have no evidence of any underlying psychopathological disorder may, when under stress, exhibit a symptom that is similar to that seen in schizophrenic persons. It is the number of psychological processes involved and the degree of impairment over time that characterize schizophrenia. Disabling symptoms characteristic of schizophrenia do not preclude development of other psychiatric disorders, nor are schizophrenic patients devoid of ordinary human characteristics—feelings, thoughts, and actions.

A. Disturbances in Language and Communication: The schizophrenic individual thinks and reasons according to private and often idiosyncratic rules of logic. The form of thinking is disordered (formal thought disorder). The individual cannot maintain a consistent train of thought, and communication is severely impaired (so-called **derailment** or **looseness of associations**). **Circumstantiality** (irrelevant detours in speech) or **tangentiality** (continuing digression in speech, so that the conversation fails to reach the anticipated goal) may also occur. There may be **poverty of content of speech,** in which little information is communicated, because many words are vague, overly abstract, overly concrete, repetitive, or stereotyped. A more severe symptom is the formation of **neologisms;** the schizophrenic individual's speech is filled with "new words" formed by condensing and combining several known words in a manner unique to the individual, who may often be able to provide a precise definition that may have personal, magical,

or wish-fulfilling properties. Complete incoherence of speech (**word salad**) may occur, with a mixture of words lacking meaning and logical coherence.

The disorder in thought permeates many areas of the patient's life and may be shown not only in language but also in work and personal creative efforts (eg, arts, crafts). Maher (1972) has offered an excellent example of the thought disorder of the schizophrenic patient:

> If things turn by rotation of agriculture or levels in regards and timed to everything: I am referring to a previous document when I made some remarks that were facts also tested and there is another that concerns my daughter she has a lobed bottom right ear, her name being Mary Lou. . . . Much of abstraction has been left unsaid and undone in this product/milk syrup, and others due to economics, differentials, subsidies, bankruptcy, tools, buildings, bonds, national stocks, foundation craps, weather trades, government in levels of breakages, and fuses in electronics to all formerly "stated" not necessarily factuated.

In a case reported by McGhie and Chapman (1961), the patient describes the experience of tangentiality and looseness of association as follows:

> My thoughts get all jumbled up. I start thinking or talking about something but I never get there. Instead, I wander off in the wrong direction and get caught up with all sorts of different things that may be connected with the things I want to say but in a way I can't explain. People listening to me get more lost than I do.

It is important to emphasize that the disturbances in language and communication described above cannot be attributed to lack of education, low intelligence, or a particular cultural background.

B. Disturbances in Content of Thought: Things go on in the mind of a schizophrenic patient that do not go on in the minds of other people. Distortions of reality lead to incorrect conclusions, which are usually defended with high emotion.

A **delusion** is a false belief that may be fixed (ie, maintained over an extended period) or temporary. Certain delusions are particularly characteristic of schizophrenia, such as the notion that one's thoughts are being broadcast into the external world so that others can hear them; or that thoughts are inserted into one's mind by another individual or superior force; or that an individual or machine is dominating and controlling one's life (**delusion of influence**).

Ideas of reference are also common in schizophrenia—ie, events that are in reality not related to the patient are invested with a personal significance (eg, a newspaper article or television program may be perceived as containing a message intended only for the patient). Delusional themes are often persecutory (belief that one is being watched, followed, or plotted against), grandiose (belief that one has a special powers, influence, or wealth), or somatic (belief that something is rotting inside one's body). In normal adolescence, people often experience a feeling of heightened self-consciousness and the feeling that others can read their private feelings. The schizophrenic patient experiences similar feelings with far greater intensity, distress, and conviction. In his autobiography, *Memoirs of My Nervous Illness,* Schreber (1955) has this to say:

> I can put this point briefly: everything that happens is in reference to me. Writing this sentence, I am aware that other people may be tempted to think that I am pathologically conceited: I know very well that this tendency to relate everything to oneself, to bring everything that happens into connection with one's own person is a common phenomenon among mental patients. But in my case, the very reverse obtains. Since God entered into nerve-contact with me exclusively, I become in a way for God the only human being or simply the human being around whom everything turns, to whom everything that happens must be related and who, therefore, from his own point of view, must also relate things to himself.

A psychiatric nurse described her own thought disturbances as follows (McDonald, 1960):

> Not knowing that I was ill, I made no attempt to understand what was happening, but felt that there was some overwhelming significance in all of this, produced either by God or Satan. . . . The walk of a stranger on the street could be a "sign" to me which I must interpret. Every face in the windows of a passing streetcar would be engraved on my mind, all of them concentrating on me and trying to pass me some sort of message.

C. Disturbances in Perception: Hallucinations are false perceptions in the absence of an external stimulus. In schizophrenia, they are usually auditory. Visual, tactile, and olfactory hallucinations can occur in schizophrenia but more often reflect acute or chronic organic brain syndromes. In auditory hallucinations, voices seem to speak directly to the patient or make comments (frequently negative ones) about the patient's behavior. Hallucinations must be distinguished from **illusions,** which are false interpretations of real stimuli.

D. Disturbances in Affect: Affect, or "feeling tone," refers to the outward expression of emotion, as opposed to mood, which is inferred from affect or the patient's own statements. In schizophrenia, affect may be inappropriate, ie, inconsistent with the topic or context of communication. Affect may be extremely labile, showing rapid shifts from tears to joy for no obvious reason; or it may be flattened, with virtually no signs of emotional expression—the voice may be monotonous and the face immobile. Patients may state that they no longer respond to life with normal intensity or that they are "losing their feelings." Physicians must be cautious in evalu-

ating the affect of a patient, because prior use of antipsychotic drugs to treat severe agitation associated with psychosis may have produced a state that is nearly identical to the flattening of affect described above.

E. Disturbances in Sense of Self: Schizophrenic patients have lost touch with who they are. They may have doubts, concerns, and worries about the very nature of their identity. They may feel that the very core of their identity is vulnerable or changing in some mysterious way. The overwhelming sense of perplexity about this feeling is then translated into concerns about the meaning of existence. Two patients' statements, as reported by Mendel (1976), illustrate the point:

> I have experienced this process chiefly as a condition in which the integrating mental picture in my personality was taken away and smashed to bits, leaving me like agitated hamburger, distributed evenly throughout the universe. . . .

> I am like a zombie living behind a glass wall. I can see all that goes on in the world, but I can't touch it. I can't reach it. I can't be in contact with it. I am outside. They are inside, and when I get inside, they aren't there. There is nothing there, absolutely nothing.

F. Disturbances in Volition: In schizophrenia, disturbance in self-initiated, goal-directed activity is invariable and may grossly impair work performance or functioning in other roles. The disruption takes the form of inadequate interest, drive, or ability to complete a course of action successfully. Overwhelming ambivalence, which directs the individual toward two diametrically opposed courses of action, may lead to a stalemate with no goal-directed activity. In contrast, in the early stages of schizophrenia there may sometimes be a sense of mission, with a resulting outpouring of energy to complete a particular task, which often is not only bizarre but also brings the patient into conflict with society.

G. Disturbances in Relationship to the External World: The individual with schizophrenia tends to withdraw from involvement with other people and to direct attention inward toward egocentric and illogical ideas and fantasies. The word "autistic" (from Greek *autos,* "self‘) has been used to describe the overwhelming self-centered concerns of the patient with a schizophrenic disorder.

H. Disturbances in Motor Behavior: Motor disturbances range through both extremes. Decreased reaction to the environment can progress to an almost total reduction of spontaneous movements and activity (catatonic stupor) in which the individual acts "like a zombie" or assumes strange postures. Motion may also become constant, bizarre, or wildly aggressive, continuing until exhaustion, treatment, or death intervene.

Subtypes of Schizophrenia

Schizophrenic disorders in *DSM-III-R* are divided into four active subtypes and one residual subtype on the bases of distinctive symptom clusters (Kendler et al, 1989). These subtypes have been formulated since Kraepelin and Bleuler in an attempt to identify different natural histories and responses to treatment within the schizophrenia spectrum.

A. Disorganized Type: (Formerly called **hebephrenia.**) Features include incoherence, lack of systematized delusions, and blunted, inappropriate, or silly affect. The clinical picture is usually associated with a history of poor functioning and poor adaptation even before illness, an early and insidious onset, and a chronic course without significant remissions. Social impairment is usually extreme.

B. Catatonic Type: Features include either excitement or stupor and mutism, negativism, rigidity, and posturing. The presence of catatonic symptoms alone, without other features of schizophrenic development, suggests a psychotic mood disorder or an organic mental disorder.

C. Paranoid Type: Features include delusions or hallucinations, which need not be restricted to persecutory themes and specifically include somatic themes, as well as absence of the more regressive symptoms. This subtype identifies a patient having a better prognosis—and less family connectedness—than the other subtypes. Onset occurs later in life than in other types, and symptoms persist more stably. Functioning also remains at a more or less constant level without episodes of marked deterioration followed by recovery. Patients in this subgroup may be quite intelligent and well informed. The boundary between the paranoid type of schizophrenia and delusional (paranoid) disorder can be approximated, and this is included in *DSM-III-R*.

D. Undifferentiated Type: Features include grossly disorganized behavior, hallucinations, incoherence, or prominent delusions.

E. Residual Type: Features include current lack of schizophrenic symptoms but definite experience of at least one schizophrenic episode in the past. There may be some delusions and hallucinations, but the person is "burned out" and not caught up in the turmoil of the florid, active phase. These patients often function as long-term outpatients but are usually incapable of maintaining gainful employment.

Type I & Type II Symptoms

Current studies of results of treatment usually follow variables that reflect an important clinical conceptualization of the 1980s, the distinction between type I and type II symptoms of schizophrenia (Crow, 1985), which is incorporated into *DSM-III-R*. **Type I symptoms** are the "positive symptoms" of hallucinations or delusions, bizarre, agitated behavior, and disorganized speech. These symptoms are more frequently seen in the earlier years of psychosis and are usually suppressed by conventional neuroleptics. **Type II symptoms** are those of emotional blunting, social withdrawal, cognitive deficits, and poverty of speech and motor activity; these symptoms imply a poor prognosis even in an acute episode, and they become more common in chronic illness. Type II symptoms are usually associated with a family history of schizophrenia, deficits in premorbid development, and a less favorable response to conventional neuroleptics (Kay et al, 1986). Type II symptoms can be distinguished as "negative" or "deficit": the former are responses of the patient to the psychosis and fluctuate with the illness; the latter are permanent and stable limitations, presumably of the patient's brain (Carpenter and Kirkpatrick, 1988).

Differential Diagnosis

The differential diagnosis must consider organic mental disorders, which often present with bizarre delusions and hallucinations similar to those associated with schizophrenia. Disorientation and memory impairment strongly suggest an organic mental disorder. Toxic psychoses associated with use of amphetamines, LSD, or phencyclidine (PCP) may be characterized by symptoms identical to those of schizophrenia. Any history of drug use provided by such a patient is unreliable, but the diagnosis becomes apparent when a toxic condition clears up dramatically after only a few days of close supervision. Organic disorders associated with alcohol use may mimic schizophrenia, particularly a chronic paranoid type. Metabolic and circulatory diseases such as hyperthyroidism or cerebral arteriosclerosis must be ruled out.

It is important to distinguish schizophrenia from mood disorders, since the course and appropriate treatment of these disorders are different. Until recently, it was not widely appreciated that patients with mood disorders, when acutely psychotic, could present the signs and symptoms of schizophrenia (Pope and Lipinski, 1978). The course of disease in a patient with a mood disorder is generally intermittent, with symptom-free intervals between episodes of illness. The course in schizophrenia, on the other hand, is usually marked by persistent impairment; the schizophrenic patient is always vulnerable to stress, and some thought disorder can usually be found by formal evaluation. A family history of schizophrenia suggests that the diagnosis is other than a psychotic mood disorder; a family history of mood disorder is so common that it should not argue against a diagnosis of schizophrenia.

Other conditions such as schizophreniform or atypical psychosis may resemble schizophrenia at any one point in the clinical picture, but the psychoses are short-lasting (days) and have a different course (by diagnostic definition). Patients with severe personality disorders may have transient psychotic symptoms similar to those of schizophrenia, but, in contrast to schizophrenia, these are very brief (hours), and there are periods of much better functioning. Occasionally, severe neuroses such as obsessive compulsive disorder or phobic disorder may seem to have a delusional component more typical of delusional (paranoid) disorder than of schizophrenia. In mental retardation, the low level of functioning and odd behavior with impoverished affect may suggest long-standing chronic schizophrenia.

Individuals who are members of subcultural or religious groups may have beliefs or experiences that are difficult to distinguish from pathological delusions or hallucinations. When such experiences can be explained because of their known association with such subcultural groups or values, they should not be considered evidence of schizophrenia. The developmental struggles of normal adolescence may resemble the onset of a pattern of abnormal thinking. Even an experienced observer may have difficulty making the correct clinical diagnosis of schizophrenia.

Projective psychological tests such as the Rorschach (inkblots) and TAT (Thematic Apperception Test) may assist in diagnosis (see Chapter 14). Several systems of measuring formal thought disorder can distinguish typical manic and schizophrenic thought processes (Hoffman et al, 1986; Solovay et al, 1987). Although no thought pattern is pathognomonic, the probability of correct diagnosis becomes much more certain when these systems are used (Jampala et al, 1989).

Natural History

The onset of schizophrenia is usually in the second and third decades of life, although paranoid schizophrenia may appear for the first time in childhood or when patients are in their 30s. In some patients, the onset of illness is sudden; in others, prodromal symptoms are present for days, weeks, or months before clear-cut schizophrenic symptoms appear. Depression, anxiety, suspiciousness, hypochondriasis, marked difficulty in concentrating, and restlessness are the usual prodromal symptoms. The patient often presents initially to a family physician and emphasizes hypochondriacal concerns or bizarre somatic delusions. There is commonly some event in the person's life that is identified as the trigger of the development or worsening of schizophrenia. In other patients, it is impossible to define any precipitating event; psychosocial stressors may be understated as the individual retreats from painful reality.

The characteristic presentation of schizophrenia is gradual withdrawal from people, activities, and social contacts, with increasing concern for abstract and sometimes idiosyncratic ideas. The acute stage of psychosis may be florid, with prominent hallucinations, delusions, and severe disorders in thinking. After the active psychotic period, there is often a stage of postpsychotic depression that may last many months, even when treated. Gradually, symptoms may disappear, and the person may recover with no apparent residual deficits; a long remission may follow. Some patients experience only a single recurrence and remain symptom-free for most of their lives. Although the course of illness can fluctuate over several decades following its onset in early adulthood, a characteristic expression of illness is established in 75% of patients within the first 5 years, and few changes in course occur after 15 years.

Each recurrence of illness leads to increasing impairment. Patients who are severely affected are able to function only marginally in the community and usually have periodic relapses requiring rehospitalization. A small proportion of patients whose illnesses are chronic, progressive, and deteriorating require lifetime hospitalization or continuous supervision. Zubin and Spring (1977) have emphasized that the one feature all schizophrenic patients have in common is persistent vulnerability rather than persistent illness. Some patients are highly vulnerable and have repeated or almost continual episodes of illness, whereas others are less vulnerable and have few episodes. When episodes develop in this latter group, they are not lifelong. Eventually the illness may remit, with or without treatment. A majority of schizophrenic patients today spend most of their lives in the community and are superficially indistinguishable from the rest of the population.

After the active phase of illness, impairment may vary widely. During the acute stage, psychotic symptoms are always associated with significant impairment. The individual may require hospitalization to ensure that basic needs are met and that poor judgment does not lead to complications, such as marked failure in social relations, work, and education; gross personal neglect; and suicide or other violent behavior. Although there are many sensationalized accounts of violent acts committed by psychotic individuals, most people with schizophrenia are not dangerous to others. It is not known whether the incidence of violent acts is higher in patients with schizophrenia than in the nonschizophrenic population. The suicide rate is higher than that in the general population, and life expectancy is lower even when only nonsuicidal deaths are considered.

Prognosis

Kraepelin's original cohort proved to have only 4% lasting remissions, and a grim prognosis for schizophrenia was presumed—recovery usually led to a revised diagnosis. Diagnosis of a disease based on its own outcome is logically unsound, and using a period of prolonged illness as a criterion for diagnosis selects for chronicity and poor outcome in schizophrenia. For the first half of this century, outcome was usually measured by discharge from hospital not followed by readmission. Since then, measurements of residual thought disorder, social function, and work function have been included as better descriptors of the patient's quality of life. All four criteria have been found to vary somewhat independently, suggesting that they measure different aspects of the illness.

The clinician attempting to estimate the prognosis for a schizophrenic patient must consider not only the symptoms but also the total picture of that individual—abilities as well as disabilities, assets as well as liabilities. One must evaluate the stresses and demands made on the patient, the world in which the patient lives, and the world the patient creates to live in, often with internal distortion of external reality.

The prognosis is good if the onset of illness is sudden and a precipitating stress is clearly identifiable. The outcome is also more favorable if the patient's social functioning was adequate before illness developed or if the patient performed successfully in a work situation outside the family environment.

The prognosis is poor if the onset of illness is insidious, with slowly emerging symptoms and no clearly identifiable precipitating stress. Likewise, if the individual was not functioning adequately (socially, economically, or intellectually) before the onset of illness, the outlook is unfavorable. Recent data from a 15-year retrospective study of treatment-resistant patients indicate that as the chronic illness progresses, the significance of certain prognostic factors (predictors) changes. For example, previous work and social accomplishments are the major predictors of outcome in the first decade of illness. In the second decade, the presence of affective symptoms (especially depression) is a positive predictor, whereas symptoms of paranoia or assaultiveness and the presence of family overinvolvement are negative predictors. Beyond the second decade, a family history of schizophrenia is the most important negative prognostic factor.

The diagnosis and prognosis become more reliable the longer the follow-up. Studies of the effects of treatment on acute episodes of schizophrenia are usually 2–24 months long (short-term), and 5-year studies (mid-term) are adequate for determining the effects of most interventions. Long-term studies of the complete course of illness require about 15 years, and six comparable studies have appeared in the English literature (Table 20–2). A seventh study primarily describes schizophrenics who survive into their senium.

Though *DSM-III-R* identifies a more chronically symptomatic group of patients, the combined data indicate that both groups have diverse outcomes under all treatment conditions and that the somatic therapies, previously accepted as interrupting the acute exacerbation and improving short-term prognosis, also improve long-term outcome in both the broad and the narrow schizophrenia spectra.

Epidemiology

The major difficulties in epidemiological studies have been the differences in diagnostic criteria, absence of a definitive conceptual framework, and lack of a clearly associated factor that can be quantitated, eg, a biochemical phenotype or genetic marker.

The 1968 United States/United Kingdom study (Cooper et al, 1972) showed that differing diagnostic criteria caused the diagnosis of schizophrenia to be made twice as frequently in New York as in London. The World Health Organization's International Pilot Project for Schizophrenia (IPPS) demonstrated that investigators in nine widely different world cultures could achieve high reliability among themselves (80–90%) when they used agreed-upon diagnostic criteria both within their own cultures and in each of the other cultures studied. Prospective follow-up data are consistent with those summarized in Table 20–2 but show better social outcomes in the less industrialized countries.

The current standard base for psychiatric epidemiology in this country is the NIMH-sponsored Epidemiologic Catchment Area (ECA) Program, which followed over 18,000 persons in four urban centers and one area of towns from 1980 through 1985. Data from all the sites have been published and include

Table 20–2. Studies of long-term outcome in schizophrenia.

| Author | Diagnostic Criteria | At Follow-Up | | Treatment | Outcome[1] | | |
		Years (avg)	N		Good	Fair	Poor
Bleuler	Bleuler	22	176	Social	22	33	47
Huber	Bleuler-Schneider	22	213	Social	15	45	40
		22	287	Social plus ECT	28	41	31
Ogawa	*ICD-9*	24	130	Social plus neuroleptics	31	46	23
Tsuang	*DSM-III*	35	186	Social	20	26	54
McGlashan	*DSM-III*	15	163	Psychosocial	14	23	64
Harding	*DSM-III*	32	82	Psychosocial plus neuroleptics	34	34	32

[1] Outcomes are in terms of overt psychopathology; social functioning outcomes are better in all studies.

sufficient elderly, black, and Hispanic probands to allow extrapolation to the USA population. The ECA "lifetime prevalence rate" of $1.3 \pm 0.2\%$ for *DSM-III-R* schizophrenia is consistent with the 1% figure reported in most other studies. The incidence of both illness onset and first treatment are highest for men between 15 and 24 years of age; for women, the peak appears between 25 and 34 years. Both sexes have an average prodrome of over a year, when psychosocial changes are noted by others but treatment is avoided. Perhaps the most striking feature of schizophrenia documented by the ECA is the history of treatment in only about half of the affected population in spite of the severity of the disorder.

The better outcome of women compared with men with schizophrenia is the single most consistent finding since Kraepelin, and the difference is more pronounced since the neuroleptics and community socialization have become the foundations of treatment. For both sexes, however, the number of those in treatment peaks between the ages of 35 and 44, reflecting the chronicity of the disease. Ninety percent of schizophrenics in treatment are between the ages of 15 and 54 years.

Theories of population biology and cultural complexity had predicted an increase in the treated prevalence of schizophrenia. In fact, since 1970 there has been an actual decrease—beyond that caused by the narrowing of diagnostic criteria. Symptomatic presentations and final outcomes have consistently become less severe since the 1930s, in clear association with the somatic and psychosocial therapies. Though a majority of outcomes still reflect lifelong impairment, the percentage of those severely disabled has decreased, and there is a reciprocal increase in the percentage of less symptomatic patients.

Although patients with schizophrenia represent fewer than 40% of those admitted for psychiatric hospitalization, the morbidity and chronicity experienced by patients with schizophrenia have made it the most serious and disabling mental illness of early and middle adult life. The appearance of schizophrenia during the early adult years and its persistence throughout life heighten the loss to society of productive human beings and underscore the personal tragedy for affected patients and their families.

Etiology & Pathogenesis

The schizophrenic disorders are characterized by thoughts, feelings, and actions that are themselves complex end products of the interaction of the organism and its environment. Despite intensive research, a single causative factor has not been discovered for these schizophrenic syndromes. If schizophrenia does represent a syndrome due to multiple causes and encompassing discrete subtypes, research attempting to arrive at a "unitary hypothesis" of the disorder will continue to be unproductive. Comparing schizophrenic patients with controls in pursuit of a single

causative agent may be as fruitless as comparing "the retarded" with controls or comparing febrile with afebrile patients.

However, many specific findings seem to be different in subgroups of schizophrenic patients compared with normal patients, especially during acute illness. The relationships of these associated findings to the causes and effects of schizophrenia serve as the basis for our current biopsychosocial model of the disease. Studies from the following areas have improved our understanding of schizophrenia and have led to major innovations in treatment: (1) genetics, (2) development of the individual before the illness became apparent, and (3) biopsychosocial states of the patient and the response of these states to treatment throughout the course of the illness. Although information from each of these areas is important, no one or them can by itself explain the development of schizophrenia. Most studies indicate that the disorder is best understood as a heterogeneous "spectrum of schizophrenias." Data are inconsistent with the concept of a single major locus for a "schizophrenic gene."

A. Genetics: Genetic investigations have focused on factors related to consanguinity, adoption, and monozygotic twinning. Consanguinity studies compare the incidence of schizophrenia in the relatives of an index case with the incidence in control families. Closer consanguinity correlates with a higher incidence of schizophrenia (Table 20–3). The two variables of genetics and cultural environment were isolated by studying children who had been adopted shortly after birth and who had subsequently developed schizophrenia. These studies confirmed the existence of a genetic predisposition to schizophrenia. Nine percent of the members of the schizophrenic children's biological families were themselves schizophrenic, whereas only 2% were schizophrenic in the adoptive families of nonschizophrenic children; the incidence of schizophrenia in the adopting families of these two groups of children was the same (ie, 2% and 2%, respectively) (Kety et al, 1971). Whether the schizophrenic parent was the father or the mother made no difference. Independent analyses of these data, using *DSM-III-R* criteria, have confirmed the original findings while suggesting that the genetic expression can manifest itself as schizophrenia or

Table 20–3 Genetic relationship correlated with incidence of schizophrenia.*

Relationship	Incidence
General population	1%
Sibling schizophrenic	8%
One parent schizophrenic	12%
Dizygotic twin schizophrenic	14%
Both parents schizophrenic	39%
Monozygotic twin schizophrenic	47%

*Data from Gottesman and Shields (1976), Kety and coworkers (1976), and Kringlen (1976).

as the "schizophrenia spectrum" of schizoid, schizotypal, and paranoid personality disorders.

A summary of these studies makes it clear that although a genetic factor is involved in the predisposition to schizophrenia, it is not sufficient to mandate development of the disorder, as shown by the discordance in incidence and outcome in monozygotic siblings. Studies of postconception development, adoption, and differing life outcomes among genetically identical siblings have allowed a separation of the effects of the biopsychosocial environment on illness presentation. Only 20% of those who become schizophrenic have a first-degree relative with the overt illness. For others, there seem to be various combinations of "risk factors," including the following: consanguinity with those who have other major psychiatric disorders; identifiable perinatal and developmental stressors; premorbid personality disorders of schizoid, avoidant, or schizotypal disorder; and specific abnormalities in brain anatomy, biochemistry, and physiology. The total effects of the risk factors define the individual's vulnerability. The stressors, occurring before the diagnosis of illness, range from clearly traumatic events such as death of a parent to the normal demands of adult development.

The stress-vulnerability model of schizophrenia assumes that there is a vulnerability to schizophrenia that is present in early childhood, has a pathological effect on development through adolescence, and is expressed as overt illness at about age 20 years. There is controversy about whether specific factors of genetic, uterine, perinatal, or childhood development are linked to specific biopsychosocial findings during illness.

B. Development: (From conception to illness manifestation.)

1. Development of the individual–Attempts have been made to explain the occurrence of schizophrenia in terms of the intrapsychic development of the child, usually using models of psychoanalytic psychology (see Chapters 2 and 4). According to this theory, the normal child goes through a stage of separation from the mother between 1 and 3 years of age and begins to function independently. This process is thought to be essential for the formation of a stable sense of self as separate from the parents and all others. One theory is that the psychological abnormalities noted after the onset of schizophrenia in adolescence result from the young child's failure to develop a mature ego capable of interpreting reality and coping with inner drives and the effects of the resulting deficits on further development. Traditionally, theories of schizophrenia are based on the development of "the self" and focus on the individual patient with symptoms. However, the patient is part of a family system that may also influence the pathogenesis of schizophrenic disorders.

2. Development within the family–Some theories of the pathogenesis of schizophrenia have focused on the immediate environment within the family. Early studies saw the patient as a reflection of disturbed communications among family members, some of whom may themselves have been disturbed. Lidz et al (1965) studied families of schizophrenic patients and identified patterns of dysfunctional interpersonal relationships. Wynne (1978) described families in which the overt content of communication is either unintelligible or distorted by family rules about which thoughts and feelings may be acknowledged or given expression. An example is the "double bind," as described by Bateson et al (1956), in which there is a contradiction between the overt communication of speech and the covert message buried in the emotional tone or nonverbal actions that accompany speech. Rosenbaum (1970) presents the following classical example of the double bind.

> A young man who had fairly well recovered from an acute schizophrenic episode was visited in the hospital by his mother. He was glad to see her and impulsively put his arm around her shoulders, whereupon she stiffened. He withdrew his arm and she asked, "Don't you love me anymore?" He then blushed, and she said, "Dear, you must not be so easily embarrassed and afraid of your feelings."

In all of these patterns of disturbed family relationships, the family also covertly enjoins comment, so that the patient's situation is both unbearable and unchangeable. These logically inconsistent patterns, which are often inconclusive and incomprehensible, have been termed **communication deviance.** The patient cannot win, regardless of the reply or course of action chosen. This theory caused considerable emotional pain for families trying to cope with disturbed family members. Therapists often blamed the family for the patient's illness, further disrupting family relationships. Fortunately, especially for families who remain involved with relatives who have schizophrenia, this theory has been discredited.

A family variable identified in the 1970s was "expressed emotion," defined as "high" when the family consistently directs intrusive, hostile, and overtly critical comments toward the patient. A 15-year prospective study indicates that high levels of communication deviance and expressed emotion are predictors of schizophrenia in persons at high risk, eg, the children of schizophrenic patients.

Although these studies have focused on the family as the most immediate and chronic environmental factor in the development of schizophrenia, other factors from the uterine environment to the larger social environment must also be considered. The importance of some of these factors is shown by studies of monozygotic twins who are discordant for schizophrenia. In one study, the twin with the smaller birth weight became schizophrenic in 10 of 12 cases. Perinatal studies show a higher frequency of difficult births—retrospectively among schizophrenic patients and prospectively for those among their children who develop the illness—compared to nonschizophrenic normal controls.

It is clear that the onset of schizophrenia in young adults coincides with leaving home. This period is for finding a place in society, forming peer relationships, and developing a work role. The onset of schizophrenia is often associated with failure to adapt successfully to the necessary changes required by these new social roles. Once illness begins, a decrease in integration of ego functions and the development of regressive behavioral patterns are almost inevitable.

3. Development within society and the larger environment—The epidemiological studies discussed above not only provide information about the prevalence of schizophrenia within the general population but also identify several factors in addition to those concerned with the patient or the patient's family that clearly have a strong association with schizophrenia. These factors appear to have a major impact on the emergence of schizophrenia in persons genetically susceptible to its development.

a. Population density—Population density has been correlated with prevalence of schizophrenia, though in a manner that seems applicable only to urban settings. There is a strong correlation between the prevalence of schizophrenia and local population density in cities that have a total population greater than 1 million. In cities with populations of 100,000–500,000, the correlation is weaker, and it disappears altogether in smaller towns. These data may reflect differences in the vulnerability of those who live in large cities, in the environmental stresses found in cities, or in the tolerance for deviant behavior that determines case finding.

b. Socioeconomic class—An association of schizophrenia with lower socioeconomic class is consistently confirmed by many studies. It is argued that the stresses of life in hard circumstances may cause schizophrenia to emerge in vulnerable individuals. An alternative theory is that patients who develop schizophrenia tend to drift into the lower strata of society because of the social handicap resulting from schizophrenic symptoms. This "drift hypothesis" is supported by the finding that schizophrenic individuals are more likely to be of a lower social class than their parents.

c. Date of birth—A third factor affecting the incidence of schizophrenia is a birth date in the winter months. In both Europe and the USA, the incidence of schizophrenia is significantly increased in persons born between January and April; and a complementary peak in incidence is found in South Africa during the months corresponding to winter in the southern hemisphere (July, August, September). This finding has led to many intriguing hypotheses, of which the occurrence of prenatal infections in the mother seems best supported by current data.

d. Other factors—Several other factors have been proposed as possible influences on the development of schizophrenia. The data are not as consistent and well established as those for the factors mentioned above. The first of these elements is stress, as subjectively perceived by the patient and reported after the development of illness. The idea is not that stress causes schizophrenia but that the number of identifiable stressful events (particularly loss of a meaningful person or relationship) clearly increases during the time just before the recognized onset of schizophrenia. The causal relationship of these events and the decreased coping skills of the person during the prodrome is unclear. The effects of emigration and the resulting **cultural dislocation** have also been proposed as risk factors likely to increase the incidence of schizophrenia.

Industrialization is another factor that seems to affect the incidence of schizophrenia. In developing countries, the incidence of schizophrenia has risen and the outcome has worsened as they have increased their contact with industrialized nations. As industrial development proceeds, an even more marked difference in the presenting symptoms of schizophrenia occurs: disorganized and catatonic subtypes of schizophrenia become less common, while paranoid schizophrenia becomes more common. This pattern is consistent with the shift that has occurred in the USA over the last 50 years; the number of people presenting with catatonic symptoms has dramatically decreased, while the number of those showing paranoid symptoms has increased.

Many other environmental influences have been explored but have not provided an adequate explanation for the pathogenesis of the schizophrenic disorders.

C. Specific Abnormalities in Patients:

1. Anatomic—Because schizophrenia is not associated with the gross dysfunctions in cognition or sensorium that characterize organic brain syndromes, it was assumed not to be related to abnormalities in gross anatomy of the brain. CT and MRI scans have now shown that a subgroup of schizophrenics has enlarged lateral and third ventricles (which imply changes in the periventricular limbic-striatal area) and smaller frontal and temporal lobes. An MRI study of 15 sets of monozygotic twins discordant for schizophrenia found small anterior hippocampi and enlarged ventricles only in the afflicted twin—on the left in 14 cases and on the right and in the third ventricle in 13 cases—when compared with controls who were monozygotic twins without schizophrenia. The correlations between the structural changes of anatomy and the other variables of genetics, development, biochemistry, physiology, or clinical subtype and outcome are controversial.

2. Biochemical—Biochemical studies have used the selective effects of clinically proved antipsychotic drugs to understand the workings of both the normal human synapse and the altered ones found in the brains of persons with schizophrenia. Most studies have concentrated on the synaptic junction, from presynaptic controls of neurotransmitter release to blockade of the postsynaptic receptors. The relationships between the neuronal surface receptors and the intracellular second-messenger G proteins controlling neuronal metabolism are being studied.

Since 1964, when Carlsson showed that dopamine was a neurotransmitter selectively affected by conventional neuroleptics, most studies of schizophrenia have focused attention on the dopaminergic tracts of the brain. Alterations in the metabolism of dopamine and increases in the number of dopaminergic D_2 receptors in the brains of patients with schizophrenia relative to normal people have frequently been implicated in the pathophysiology of schizophrenia (MacKay et al, 1982). Attention was originally focused on dopamine because it was found that the phenothiazines improved schizophrenia but worsened Parkinson's disease, already recognized as a dopamine deficiency disease. Levodopa, a direct precursor of dopamine, enters the brain, exacerbates schizophrenia, and can be used as a challenge to predict the relapse into psychosis if neuroleptic therapy were to be discontinued. Drugs such as disulfiram that block the conversion of dopamine to norepinephrine also can exacerbate schizophrenia. It has been suggested that the psychosis produced in normal people by amphetamine is related to the blocking of dopamine reuptake. The psychosis associated with ingestion of phencyclidine (PCP) is now recognized to approximate schizophrenia more closely than psychosis associated with amphetamine or LSD. The ingestion of either a stimulant or an hallucinogenic drug is clearly a risk factor—both for the initial episode and for subsequent relapse—in persons vulnerable to the development of schizophrenia, despite the fact that the vast majority of persons having limited experiences using these drugs show no evidence of pathological sequelae. Recent metabolic studies have supported the dopamine hypothesis, because changes in dopamine metabolism often reflect changes in the clinical states of those with schizophrenia (Pickar et al, 1990).

The dopaminergic system consists of only 1% of the neurons in the brain, organized in five discrete tracts. All known neuroleptics affect these dopaminergic tracts sufficiently to explain their antipsychotic effects. Drugs highly selective for the D_2 receptor are among the typical high-potency neuroleptics that have dominated the treatment of schizophrenia for 15 years. Typical neuroleptics are characterized by the production of movement disorders (extrapyramidal symptoms and dystonias), the elevation of serum prolactin, and suppression of the type I symptoms of schizophrenia. "Atypical neuroleptics" characteristically neither produce movement disorders nor result in elevations in serum prolactin.

It must be emphasized that altered levels of dopaminergic function are not considered to be "the cause" of schizophrenia, but they do seem to be implicated in the manifestation of symptoms. In fact, all typical neuroleptics (eg, phenothiazines, butyrophenones, and thioxanthines) are equally effective in reducing acute type I psychotic symptoms, regardless of whether they are manifested as schizophrenia, mania, or organic psychoses. Early evidence indicates that the atypical neuroleptics (eg, clozapine) may provide a better outcome in schizophrenia, both in reduction of type I and type II symptoms and in absence of production of the movement disorders, the most serious adverse side effects of the typical agents.

3. Physiological—Within the last decade, two physiological differences between schizophrenic patients and normal controls have been identified. Abnormalities in saccadic eye movements (seen when the eye tracks a moving object such as a pendulum) are highly associated with schizophrenia. The movements are abnormally jerky in 80% of schizophrenic patients who are not taking medication, in 45% of nonschizophrenic relatives of schizophrenic patients, and in only 7% of controls. The concordance of abnormalities between twins is 71% for monozygotic twins and 54% for dizygotic twins; both rates are higher than the concordance for the actual development of schizophrenia. It has been proposed that this trait is a phenotype for a single major locus on the genome, and that this single major locus both follows mendelian inheritance and is a marker for schizophrenia.

A second source of physiological data relevant to schizophrenia are the neurophysiological correlates of human thought, often called "information processing." Calloway (1982) proposed a model for deficits in information processing as characteristic of schizophrenic thought. Specific deficits have been found in premorbid children at high risk for schizophrenia, in patients with schizophrenia, and in the nonschizophrenic relatives of schizophrenic patients. The increased sensitivities of positron emission tomography and regional blood flow studies have demonstrated decreased metabolism of the medial frontotemporal areas when the schizophrenic patient is challenged with tests that utilize these areas in normals—a result consistent with the anatomical and biochemical data. Weinberger (1989) has summarized the evidence that abnormalities in development of the human brain are associated with "soft neurological signs" and information processing deficits, are present in early childhood, and are deleterious to subsequent development among people who will later become schizophrenic.

Treatment

The consequences of schizophrenia are painful and unacceptable both to the patient and to the community. The magnitude of these consequences has led to a wide range of treatments and protective strategies. Even before the development of a conceptual framework to explain schizophrenia, physical methods were used to protect society and to help families and caretakers minimize the disruption caused by schizophrenia. Treatment during the 19th and early 20th centuries involved sedation, restraint, and confinement. Hospital treatment was a long process, often ending in uninterrrupted institutionalization until death. In over half of cases, however, a combination of psychological, social, and somatic treatments was followed by remission sufficient for discharge.

The probability of eventual discharge from hospitals for patients who have developed schizophrenia for the first time has increased over each decade of this century. The psychosocial therapies and the more accepting attitudes within society have played a major role in this process. The dramatic increase in these release rates since the late 1950s could not have occurred without the introduction of neuroleptics earlier in the decade. Neuroleptic treatment controls acute symptoms, allows the reduction of hospitalization from years to days, prolongs remission, and helps make the outcome of treated schizophrenia much better than that of the untreated disease.

A. Historical Methods of Treatment:

1. Coma–The earliest chemical treatment of schizophrenia induced prolonged coma, either by injection of insulin and subsequent production of hypoglycemia or by infusion of barbiturates. The first method has obvious dangers related to the lowering of blood glucose levels below those associated with coma to those that produce permanent brain damage. Both insulin and barbiturate coma therapies apparently do improve schizophrenic symptoms, but neither is now used to any extent.

2. Electroconvulsive therapy (ECT)–It was originally noted that some institutionalized schizophrenic patients had fewer symptoms after a grand mal seizure. This postictal effect was mistakenly thought to show that epilepsy was incompatible with schizophrenia (and therefore that epileptic convulsions might prevent schizophrenia), and researchers looked for ways to produce seizures in schizophrenics. Seizures were induced initially by a chemical (phenmetrazol [pentylenetetrazol]), but much better control over the induction of seizures was obtained by the use of electric current. Before the use of phenothiazines, electroconvulsive therapy was the treatment of choice for schizophrenia, and many patients improved sufficiently to return to the community. In controlled comparisons, however, electroconvulsive therapy is significantly less effective than the neuroleptics in the treatment of most schizophrenic patients. The current use of ECT is limited to occasional patients who fail to improve after antipsychotic medications have been tried and who require additional symptom control, eg, those who exhibit either catatonic excitement or severe suicidal behavior, each of which has a 20% mortality rate and can be suppressed in a few days by ECT.

3. Psychosurgery–Transection of tracts between the frontal lobe and the midbrain to change thoughts and behavior was developed in the mid 1930s and widely used for about 20 years. The chances of creating a patient who was apathetic and lacked distinctive personality lessened as improved surgical techniques made possible more precise ablations. Recent United States government reports have acknowledged that some conditions may benefit from psychosurgery, but the procedure is rarely used in the treatment of schizophrenia now that the efficacy of neuroleptics has been established.

B. Contemporary Treatment: Treatment of schizophrenia now combines biological, psychological, and sociological methods. The psychiatrist usually works as part of a treatment team, and in many cases the family is actively incorporated into the treatment plan.

1. Psychosocial treatment–The first consideration should always be the physical safety of the patient and the patient's associates. Twenty-four-hour supervision is often necessary during fulminant stages of the illness. With the increasing use of antipsychotic drugs during the past 35 years and the emphasis on treating patients in the least restrictive environment consistent with proper care, most schizophrenic patients have been managed within their own communities after brief periods of hospitalization.

The establishment of a **therapeutic alliance** based on trust between the clinician and patient is of major importance. Schizophrenic individuals are vulnerable and exquisitely sensitive to their environment, even when they appear to be out of touch with reality. Special care must therefore be taken in all interpersonal transactions not to challenge the patient's beliefs too aggressively, to be respectful, and to develop new ideas or suggestions slowly. Working with schizophrenic patients requires a great deal of patience. The clinician must make every effort to understand these patients, even though much of their physical and verbal behavior may be initially repellent. Clinicians must accept these patients as they are and take the position that although patients will not be asked to conform in ways that are not possible for them, they must eventually abandon the maladaptive behaviors associated with their disease and learn to function in ways acceptable to other people. Thus, once the acute phase of illness has passed, patients should begin to attend to their own basic needs and to participate in activities.

Work with schizophrenic patients is supportive in that it not only emphasizes positive reinforcement (appreciation, approval, or justifiable praise) but also "supports" the basic personality structure. Therapy does not try to break down or restructure an already weak and vulnerable ego. The therapist avoids overloading the individual with information about inner motives and frightening impulses or offering interpretations that bring to consciousness early memories that carry a burden of anxiety; this type of insight cannot be usefully assimilated by the overtly psychotic schizophrenic patient. Relief from painful symptoms is essential to successful adaptation, so discussion should focus instead on solving immediate problems and helping patients develop social skills. For example, over time it should be possible to teach the patient to recognize situations that might produce a relapse, to recognize the warning signs of relapse, and to take appropriate action in the event of relapse. The therapist listens carefully but interactively and attempts to understand each patient in a way that fosters development of a more adaptive and mature personality. In effect, the therapist takes the role of a concerned but nonintrusive parent who uses understanding and skill to promote the maximum possible development in a vulnerable individual. Although the diagnosis of schizophrenia carries a guarded prognosis, the situation is never hopeless, and much can be improved. With proper support, many patients can learn to live on their own, and some gain competitive employment or reach other personal goals. The psychiatrist must communicate realistic optimism about what can be achieved both to the patient and to the family.

A 2-year prospective study has shown that the development of a therapeutic alliance between a schizophrenic patient and a therapist favorably influences outcome. Several outcome studies have shown that outpatient psychotherapeutic interventions at a frequency more often than every other week have little additional benefit. This coincides with the interval required to monitor the treatment effects of gradual changes in neuroleptic dosage characteristic of the outpatient treatment of the entire schizophrenia spectrum, a treatment that may involve hundreds of visits spread across many years.

The methods and goals of family therapy in the treatment of schizophrenia have been reconsidered in the last 10 years, following the discovery that high levels of expressed emotion in patients' families contributed significantly to the incidence of relapse. A team approach—often involving a psychiatrist, nurse, and social worker or psychologist—is usually used to educate family and patient about the nature of schizophrenia, the avoidance of stressors, and the recognition of early signs of relapse. Exploration of past emotional conflicts is avoided; instead, the family learns to develop problem-solving techniques. The team approach thus attempts to reduce high levels of expressed emotion within the family while directly coaching the patient in social skills. This approach, in conjunction with neuroleptics, appears to have as significant an impact on delaying relapse as did the introduction of neuroleptics in producing remission 30 years ago. The benefits derived from 9 months of this psychoeducational method were found to extend through a subsequent year when appropriate medications were continued.

2. Drug treatment–(See also Chapter 32.) Initially, phenothiazines emerged as the major drug used in acute hospital treatment of psychosis and the long-term stabilization of schizophrenic patients after their return to the community. Controlled prospective studies from 1965 to 1975 confirmed what had become clinically apparent a decade earlier: that use of phenothiazines achieved remission of symptoms in weeks rather than months or years in 90% of those experiencing an acute schizophrenic episode; that recovery was sufficient to enable patients to return to the community; and that the likelihood of rehospitalization could be reduced by half in those patients who had been treated with phenothiazines in the hospital—regardless of the type of treatment received following discharge (May et al, 1981).

The antipsychotic drugs now used include several other classes of drugs besides the phenothiazines originally used. These are discussed fully in Chapter 32.

a. Choice of neuroleptic–All of the neuroleptic drugs with the exception of clozapine (which is useful in refractory cases) have been found to be equally effective among large groups of patients. Individual patients may respond to one drug better than another, and a history of a favorable response to treatment with a given drug in either the patient or a family member should suggest use of that agent as the drug of first choice. If the initial choice is not effective in 2–4 weeks, one should try another neuroleptic with a different chemical structure. Aside from milligram potencies, the chief differences among the typical neuroleptic agents pertain to side effects, which may improve compliance through advantage to the patient (eg, producing nighttime sedation with chlorpromazine or avoiding appetite stimulation with molindone).

Useful generalizations may be made about the differences between the low- and high-potency neuroleptics. The low-potency drugs have much greater sedative and hypotensive properties, to which the patient often becomes more tolerant within a few weeks; but the greater risk of malignant hyperthermia and obesity associated with this group of drugs continues throughout the period of active drug use. Low-potency drugs also are inherently anticholinergic, so that the use of additional anticholinergic drugs to prevent extrapyramidal symptoms may be unnecessary.

The high-potency drugs, which have been widely used since the 1970s, have little inherent anticholinergic activity and frequently produce extrapyramidal symptoms or dystonia, so that anticholinergic drugs are usually required, at least in the initial weeks of treatment. They may be more likely to produce **neuroleptic malignant syndrome,** a devastating acute illness characterized by fever, delirium, autonomic dysfunction, and muscle rigidity. The incidence of this iatrogenic syndrome may be as high as 1% and may be a grouping of various conditions.

The only long-acting (depot) neuroleptics available in the USA are the esters of fluphenazine and haloperidol, which may be given as infrequently as every 2 weeks to establish adequate drug levels. This type of drug treatment decreases relapse rates for previously stable outpatients but does not produce the same relative benefit in the time immediately following an acute psychotic episode.

Prospective clinical studies with the atypical neuroleptic clozapine have shown that up to one-third of diagnosed schizophrenics proved refractory to conventional neuroleptics will have marked improvement in both type I and type II symptoms when treated with clozapine. Clozapine has been shown to be safe and effective in European studies over the last 15 years, but current use in the USA is restricted by the manufacturer to those who can comply with an expensive system of distribution, involving mandatory weekly monitoring of the white blood cell count. This precaution is an attempt to prevent death from the agranulocytosis that occurs in 1% of clozapine-treated patients, usually in the first 2 months of therapy.

b. Dosage of neuroleptic–The proved efficacy of typical neuroleptics in reducing relapse rates and improving outcome led to some untoward consequences in that patients who had been treated with high doses of antipsychotic drugs to control acute psychotic symptoms continued to receive high doses as maintenance levels in the absence of known contraindications to long-term use and in the belief that this would more effectively prevent relapse. Many patients suffered from unacceptable side effects such as tardive dyskinesia, an often irreversible disfiguring movement disorder, and the psychiatric community recognized that it was essential to determine the minimum effective dose of antipsychotic medications. Fortunately, it was found that except during acute exacerbations of psychosis, lower doses of antipsychotic medications are consistent with excellent long-term control of symptoms in schizophrenia. Studies with both low-potency and high-potency (typical) neuroleptics established that acute psychotic symptoms respond more quickly to moderate doses (600–1200 mg of chlorpromazine or equivalent drug) than to low doses (< 300 mg of chlorpromazine or equivalent).

In the early 1970s, tardive dyskinesia was shown to be a frequent side effect of chronic administration of neuroleptics (see Chapter 32). Tardive dyskinesia is characterized by repetitive involuntary movements, usually of the mouth and tongue but often of the thumb and fingers and occasionally of a limb or the whole trunk. Although movement disorders occasionally occur spontaneously in later life, the major risk factors for the development of tardive dyskinesia are older age and total cumulative exposure to dopamine antagonists, of which typical neuroleptics are the most widely used.

Tardive dysknesia is thought to result from dopamine receptor supersensitivity following chronic receptor blockade by the typical neuroleptics. The question of whether tardive dyskinesia is a later manifestation of changes initially expressed as extrapyramidal symptoms has not been answered. Anticholinergic drugs do not improve tardive dyskinesia and may make it worse. The recommended treatment has been to lower the dosage of typical neuroleptic and hope for gradual remission of the choreoathetoid movements. Increasing the dosage of a typical neuroleptic briefly masks the symptoms of tardive dyskinesia, but symptoms will reappear later as a reflection of the progression of receptor supersensitivity. The atypical neuroleptic clozapine has been found not to produce tardive dyskinesia in over 15 years of use at daily doses of 300–400 mg orally, and the use of clozapine may help resolve tardive dyskinesia related to the prior use of typical neuroleptics.

New dosage strategies have been developed in order to balance the need for adequate levels of neuroleptics in the treatment of psychotic symptoms against the risk from the total lifetime dosage. Three strategies—low dosage, targeted symptoms, and drug holidays—have been used to lower the maintenance doses in the years of illness following acute psychosis and hospitalization. The **low-dose approach** attempts to find the minimum dose effective in preventing relapse. The minimum parenteral dose of fluphenazine decanoate is 5 mg intramuscularly every 2 weeks, and the minimum oral dose of haloperidol is about 5 mg every day; both dosages may have to be doubled at times of symptom exacerbation in order to prevent full relapse. The **targeted symptom strategy** calls for close monitoring of the patient by a treatment team and the use of medications only for specific symptoms. Carpenter et al (1990) have reported that this method can achieve an average daily dose which is lower by 40% than that found with low-dose strategies but that the rate of significant relapse is almost doubled. The use of **drug holidays** (when a long-acting drug is not taken for 1–2 days each week) has fallen into disfavor both because it seems to decrease patient compliance and because it may exacerbate tardive dyskinesia.

c. Duration of drug treatment–The agitated patient with a functional psychosis can usually be calmed in 1–2 days. Low doses of antipsychotics may be used hourly to control initial agitation, but a prospective fixed-dose trial of haloperidol has confirmed the observation of Baldessarini et al (1988) that oral dosages above 20 mg/d of haloperidol may worsen outcome at 6 weeks, probably because of increased side effects (van Putten et al, 1990). The psychosis gradually resolves only after 2–6 weeks of a moderate drug regimen, as outlined above. The dosage used in the hospital should be continued through the time of discharge and the accompanying stress of changing to a new and less structured environment. Major reductions in this dosage should be avoided for at least 6 weeks and are best attempted about 3–6 months after discharge. These decreases should be achieved in stages, and it should be recognized that any new equilibrium in body concentration of the drug will not be reached for at least 2 weeks after the change has been made (since these drugs have half-lives of 1–2 days). The patient should be alerted to note signs of relapse, so that modest increases in dosage may be made, if necessary, to abolish recurrent symptoms. Gradual reduction in dosage should approach a minimum that enables the patient to function at a level in accord with the patient's wishes that is also socially acceptable. The ideal minimum is obviously no medication at all, and for some schizophrenic patients this goal may gradually be achieved. A majority of patients, however, must accept the fact that reduction below a certain minimum dose (usually equivalent to 100–400 mg per day of chlorpromazine) causes return of psychotic symptoms within weeks. For many patients, lifelong maintenance treatment with neuroleptic medications is necessary.

d. Adjunctive drugs–Adjunctive drugs are often used for one of two reasons. The most common reason is to treat a side effect produced by a neuroleptic. Extrapyramidal symptoms are lessened by anticholinergic agents, dystonias are relaxed by diphenhydramine, and akathisia is reduced by propranolol. The other reason is to add another psychoactive drug to treat resistant symptoms: lithium or carbamazepine may stabilize mood, the benzodiazapines may calm anxiety or induce sleep, and nonanticholinergic antidepressants may ease depression in some schizophrenics.

3. Combined treatment–Although neuroleptic medication may effectively normalize a patient's overt behavior, thought processes, and ability to communicate coherently, it does little by itself to enhance the quality of life—eg, the ability to relate to others or to work. The true task of the long-term treatment of schizophrenia is twofold: (1) to establish a psychologically stable baseline free from recurrent psychotic episodes and (2) to help the patient build upon this baseline to lead a life that is qualitatively enriched by personal, social, and vocational achievements.

Hospitalization imposes a regulated social structure to help organize the patient's life. It also provides the constant companionship of trained personnel and supervised medication. Upon return to the community, patients become responsible for complying with medication requirements and organizing their lives. Patients usually remain in contact with a treating physician or an institution over months to years. During this time, patients should assume increasing responsibility for their own well-being as they gain understanding of their illness and life situation.

A major goal in the treatment of patients after discharge is to help them recognize what kinds of stressful situations or internal stimuli signal the beginning of a relapse. When patients become aware of these early signs of psychosis, they can often regain control of their lives merely by increasing the dosage of antipsychotic medication for a few weeks and by increasing their contact with the professionals treating them. This self-help is of major therapeutic benefit to patients, who find that in this way they can exercise some measure of control over their illness and hope for a life that is not interrupted by recurrent hospitalization.

Most schizophrenic patients benefit from prudent use of antipsychotic medication in combination with supportive psychotherapy and work with the patient's family or significant others. Physicians may restrict their involvement to adjusting the dosage of medication, but a therapist may find that increased psychotherapeutic support makes additional medications unnecessary. Unfortunately, although medication is relatively inexpensive, a therapist's time is not. Institutions are rarely able to provide continuing interaction with the same therapist. For many chronically ill schizophrenic patients, one way of overcoming that difficulty is to maintain a relationship with a family physician who understands the patient's vulnerability and needs and can monitor neuroleptic effects. The psychiatrist can be available to consult with the family doctor when required.

Changes observed in improved schizophrenic patients are as follows:

(1) Ability to be alone and yet feel secure.

(2) Development of a more distinct sense of self, independent of other people.

(3) Greatly improved modulation of affect.

(4) Ability to feel genuine pleasure both in aesthetic pursuits and in interpersonal situations.

(5) Improvement in thought disorder, ranging from marked diminution to complete absence of symptoms

(6) Lessened susceptibility to transient psychotic symptoms.

(7) Realistic scaling down of personal ambitions.

(8) Ability to take credit for personal accomplishments.

(9) Improvements in social judgment.

Social Support Services

It is important for clinicians to be aware of the current social context in which patients with schizophrenia are being treated. As management has moved from long periods of institutionalization to brief hospital stays followed by treatment in community settings, there has been a change in the patients' needs. Discharge from institutional settings has meant greater responsibility for patients who not only are impaired but also are typically impoverished and alone. At one time provided with food, clothing, shelter, and medical care in controlled "total institutions," patients with schizophrenia now find themselves exposed to the rigors of life in unsupportive communities. Their basic needs are no longer met, since meeting those needs is often no longer considered the responsibility of the mental health care system. Services are provided in a number of different settings, and resources are scarce. Many patients with schizophrenia are now struggling to survive in the community. They are at increased risk of homelessness, drug abuse, exploitation, suicide, AIDS, and a variety of other illnesses that give them a higher than normal mortality rate. To some observers, the answer is to return these people to the hospital; to others, the answer is improve their access to resources to help them meet their basic needs. This remains an area of controversy.

SUMMARY

Schizophrenic disorders are a complex syndrome characterized by a disturbance in reality testing, marked impairment of social functioning, and severe personality disorganization involving disturbances in thought, affect, and behavior. There is no single cause, though there appear to be genetic and biochemical bases for this illness. Psychosocial factors play an important part in the development of the schizophrenic disorders. Treatment should consist of various biopsychosocial methods in combination and should include the formation of a therapeutic alliance between the therapist and the schizophrenic person as well as contact with friends and family as needed. Although schizophrenia has remained the most serious known psychiatric illness for the last 100 years, a comprehensive approach to the care and treatment of people with schizophrenic disorders can improve the quality of life for the patients and their families and greatly improve the treated outcome as compared to the natural course of schizophrenia.

REFERENCES

Allebeck P, Wistedt B: Mortality in schizophrenia. Arch Gen Psychiatry 1986;43:650.

Andreasen NC et al: Magnetic resonance imaging of the brain in schizophrenia. Arch Gen Psychiatry 1990;47:35.

Andreasen NC et al: Positive and negative symptoms in schizophrenia: A critical reappraisal. Arch Gen Psychiatry 1990;47:615.

Baldessarini RJ, Cohen BM, Teicher MH: Significance of neuroleptic dose and plasma level in the pharmacological treatment of psychoses. Arch Gen Psychiatry 1988;45:79.

Baldessarini RJ, Katz B, Cotton P: Dissimilar dosing with high potency and low potency neuroleptics. Am J Psychiatry 1984;141:748.

Bateson G et al: Towards a theory of schizophrenia. Behav Sci 1956;1:251.

Bleuler E: *Dementia Praecox: Or the Group of Schizophrenias.* (Zinkin J trans.) Internat Univ Press, 1911/1950.

Bleuler M: *The Schizophrenic Disorders: Long-Term Patient and Family Studies.* (Clemens SM, trans.) Yale Univ Press, 1971/1978.

Braff DL: Sensory input deficits and negative symptoms in schizophrenic patients. Am J Psychiatry 1989, 148:1006.

Callaway E, Naghdi S: An information processing model for schizophrenia. Arch Gen Psychiatry 1982;39:339.

Carpenter WT Jr et al: Continuous versus targeted medication in schizophrenic outpatients: Outcome results. Am J Psychiatry 1990;147:1138.

Carpenter WT Jr, Heinrichs DW, Wagman AMIX: Deficit and nondeficit forms of schizophrenia: The concept. Am J Psychiatry 1989;45:578.

Carpenter WT Jr, Kirkpatrick B: The heterogeneity of the long-term course of schizophrenia. Schiz Bull 1988;14:645.

Ciompi L: Catamnestic long-term study on the course of life and aging of schizophrenics. Schiz Bull 1980;6:606.

Cooper JE et al: *Psychiatric Diagnosis in New York and London.* Oxford Univ Press, 1972.

Coryell W, Tsuang MT: Outcome after 40 years in **DSM-III** schizophreniform disorder. Arch Gen Psychiatry 1986;43:324.

Crow TJ: The continuum of psychosis and its implication for the structure of the gene. Br J Psychiatry 1985; 149:419.

Eaton WW: Epidemiology of schizophrenia. Epidemiol Rev 1985;7:105.

Falloon IRH et al: Family management in the prevention of morbidity in schizophrenia. Arch Gen Psychiatry 1985;42:887.

Farde L et al: D_2 dopamine receptors in neuroleptic-naive schizophrenic patients. Arch Gen Psychiatry 1990; 47:213.

Gardos G et al: Clinical forms of severe tardive dyskinesia. Am J Psychiatry 1987;144:895.

Garza-Trevino E et al: Neurobiology of schizophrenic syndromes. Hosp Community Psychiatry 1990;41:9,971.

Gottesman II, McGuffin P, Farmer AE: Clinical genetics as clues to the "real" genetics of schizophrenia. Schiz Bull 1987;13:23.

Harding CM, Zubin J, Strauss JS: Chronicity in schizophrenia: Fact, partial fact, or artifact? Hosp Community Psychiatry 1987;38:477.

Hoffman E, Stopek S, Andreasen NC: A comparative study of manic vs schizophrenic speech disorganization. Arch Gen Psychiatry 1986;43:831.

Hogarty G et al: Dose of fluphenazine, familial expressed emotion, and outcome in schizophrenia: Results of a two-year controlled study. Arch Gen Psychiatry 1988; 45:797.

Holzman PS: Thought disorder in schizophrenia: Editor's introduction. Schiz Bull 1986;12:342.

Jampala VC, Taylor MA, Abrams R: The diagnostic implications of formal thought disorder in mania and schizophrenia: A reassessment. Am J Psychiatry 1989;146:459.

Kales A, Stefanis CN, Talbott JA (editors): *Recent Advances in Schizophrenia.* Springer, 1990.

Kane J et al: Clozapine for the treatment-resistant schizophrenic. Arch Gen Psychiatry 1988;45:789.

Kay R et al: Significance of positive and negative syndromes in chronic schizophrenia. Br J Psychiatry 1986;149:439.

Kendler KS, Gruenberg M: An independent analysis of the Copenhagen sample of the Danish adoption study of schizophrenia. VI: The pattern of psychiatric illness as defined by **DSM-III** in adoptees and relatives. Arch Gen Psychiatry 1984;41:555.

Kendler KS, Spitzer, RL, Williams JBW: Psychotic disorders in *DSM-III-R*. Am J Psychiatry 1989;146:953.

Kety SS et al: Mental illness in the biological and adoptive families of adopted schizophrenics. Am J Psychiatry 1971;128:302.

Kraepelin E: *Dementia Praecox and Paraphrenia*. (Barclay RM trans from the eighth German edition.) RE Krieger, 1971.

Langfeldt G: Diagnosis and prognosis of schizophrenia. Proc Roy Soc Med 1960;53:1047.

Lidz T, Fleck S, Cornelison A: *Schizophrenia and the Family*. Internat Univ Press, 1985.

MacKay AVP et al: Increased brain dopamine and dopamine receptors in schizophrenia. Arch Gen Psychiatry 1982;32:991.

Maher BA: The language of schizophrenia: A review and interpretation. Br J Psychiatry 1972;120:3.

May PRA et al: Schizophrenia: A follow-up study of the results of five forms of treatment. Arch Gen Psychiatry 1981;38:776.

McDonald N: Living with schizophrenia. Can Med Assoc J 1960;82:218.

McGhie A, Chapman J: Disorders of attention and perception in early schizophrenia. Br J Med Psychol 1961;34:218.

McGlashan TH: Predictors of shorter-, medium-, and long-term outcome in schizophrenia. Am J Psychiatry 1986;143:50.

Mendel W: *Schizophrenia: The Experience and Its Treatment*. Jossey-Bass, 1976.

Pickar D et al: Cerebrospinal fluid and plasma monamine metabolites and their relation to psychosis: Implications for regional brain dysfunction in schizophrenia. Arch Gen Psychiatry 1990;47:641.

Pope HG Jr, Lipinski JR Jr: Diagnosis in schizophrenia and manic depressive disease. Arch Gen Psychiatry 1978;35:811.

Regier DA et al: One-month prevalence of mental disorders in the United States. Arch Gen Psychiatry 1988;45:977.

Rosenbaum CP: *The Meaning of Madness*. Science House, 1970.

Salzman C: The use of ECT in the treatment of schizophrenia. Am J Psychiatry 1980;(Suppl 137):1032.

Schreber DP: *Memoirs of My Mental Illness*. Dawson & Sons, 1955.

Schulz SC, Tamminga CA (editors): *Schizophrenia: Scientific Progress*. Oxford Univ Press, 1989.

Solovay MR, Shenton MA, Holzman PS: Comparative studies of thought disorders: I. Mania and schizophrenia. Arch Gen Psychiatry 1987;44:13.

Tsuang MT, Lyons MJ, Faraone SV: Heterogeneity of schizophrenia, conceptual models and analytic strategies. Br J Psychiatry 1990;156:17.

van Putten T, Marder SR, Mintz J: A controlled dose comparison of haloperidol in newly admitted schizophrenic patients. Arch Gen Psychiatry 1990;47:754.

Weinberger DR: Implications of normal brain development for the pathogenesis of schizophrenia. (Letter.) Arch Gen Psychiatry 1987;44:660.

Wyatt RJ et al: Schizophrenia, just the facts: What do we know, how well do we know it? Schizophrenia Res 1989;1:3.

Wynne LL (editor): *The Nature of Schizophrenia*. Wiley, 1978.

Zubin J, Spring B: Vulnerability: A new view of schizophrenia. J Abnorm Psych 1977;86:103.

Delusional & Other Psychotic Disorders

21

Edward L. Merrin, MD

Although most patients with psychosis are suffering from schizophrenia, an organic mental disorder, or a mood disorder, some patients exhibiting psychosis do not precisely fit the diagnostic criteria of the more common disorders. This chapter reviews those other diagnostic entities: schizophreniform disorder, schizoaffective disorder, delusional (paranoid) disorder, brief reactive psychosis, induced psychotic disorder, and atypical psychosis.

The appropriate *DSM-III-R* diagnosis of a patient with psychosis depends upon a detailed history and careful clinical examination. The following issues are particularly important in the differential diagnosis of the psychotic disorders discussed in this chapter: (1) premorbid personality functioning, (2) abrupt versus insidious onset with prodromal symptoms, (3) the presence or absence of specific psychotic and mood symptoms and how they vary over time, (5) the duration and degree of recovery from episodes of illness, and (6) the presence or absence of significant precipitating events.

SCHIZOPHRENIFORM DISORDER

Symptoms & Signs

Schizophreniform disorder is a psychotic illness with symptoms typical of schizophrenia but without the chronic course of that disorder. To satisfy the diagnostic criteria for schizophreniform disorder, patients must display psychotic symptoms sufficient to meet *DSM-III-R* criteria for the active phase of schizophrenia, but they must return to their previous level of functioning within 6 months. See Table 20–1 for the diagnostic criteria for schizophrenia.

Natural History

The long-term course of schizophreniform disorder is variable. In some patients, there is only a single psychotic episode, whereas in others there are repeated episodes separated by varying lengths of time. First episodes usually occur in late adolescence or early adulthood, often in association with a specific precipitating crisis. A better prognosis is associated with adequate social and occupational functioning before the onset of illness, an abrupt rather than insidious onset, and confusion or disorientation during the

most acute phase of the episode. Blunted or flat affect is a poor prognostic sign.

The diagnosis may have to be changed as the patient is followed over a period of months or years. Many patients eventually develop schizophrenia, with recovery being less complete. In others, later episodes may take the form of depression or mania, with or without psychotic symptoms.

Differential Diagnosis

All organic or toxic factors (eg, psychostimulant or hallucinogenic drug intoxication, encephalitis, etc.) should be ruled out by appropriate history, physical and mental status examination, and laboratory tests. Schizophreniform disorder is distinguished from **schizophrenia** by its shorter course (< 6 months for prodromal, active, and residual symptoms combined) and by the absence of deterioration from previous levels of functioning. The diagnosis of **brief reactive psychosis** is suggested rather than schizophreniform disorder when the patient presents with schizophrenia-like features, an abrupt onset, and associated psychological stressors unless the episode persists beyond 1 month. The mood disturbances in schizophreniform disorder, unlike those in **major depression, bipolar disorder,** or **schizoaffective disorder,** are brief in duration relative to the total duration of the episode. Psychotic symptoms in **delusional disorder** are less extensive and do not include prominent hallucinations, loose associations, or bizarre delusions.

Prognosis

When followed longitudinally, about half of all patients with schizophreniform disorder will either improve or recover, whereas only one-third of schizophrenic patients will substantially improve. Those who do less well are often eventually rediagnosed as schizophrenic. Patients whose illness lasts only 1 month are less likely to eventually develop schizophrenia than those with episodes closer to 6 months in duration.

Illustrative Case

A 31-year-old male vocational nurse was hospitalized for his third episode of psychosis. He complained of the recent onset of difficulty focusing his thoughts, intrusive ideas of a bizarre nature ('there's a telepath in my old lady's body'), and auditory hallucinations of the voices of "telepaths" who controlled his body movements. These symptoms had impaired his functioning to the point where he lost his job. Mental status examination revealed pressured speech, loose associations, and occasional idiosyncratic word usage. Various tics and twitches occurred that the patient attributed to the influence of the "telepaths." His symptoms gradually cleared after several weeks of treatment with antipsychotic drugs, and he was able to return to living with his girlfriend and active employment. There were no residual psychotic symptoms.

As a child, the patient had always formed friendships and seemed well adjusted despite frequent family moves. His father was a salesman who was interested in the occult. A younger brother and sister had both suffered from psychotic disorders of an unknown type. The patient's first episode of psychosis occurred at age 25 years after a romantic disappointment. A second episode occurred 3 years later during a period of unemployment and economic distress. In each case, the disturbance remitted completely within a few months.

Epidemiology

Schizophreniform disorder is less common than schizophrenia and occurs with equal frequency in men and women. There appears to be a genetic relationship with schizophrenia, as the risk of developing schizophrenia (2–3%) is similar in first-degree relatives of patients with both schizophrenia and schizophreniform disorder. In contrast, relatives of patients with mood disorder have almost no risk of developing schizophrenia. The same type of analysis indicates that the risk for mood disorder in first-order relatives of patients with schizophrenia and schizophreniform disorder is about 6% versus 13% in relatives of patients with mood disorders.

Etiology & Pathogenesis

The specific causes of schizophreniform disorder are unknown. Neurodevelopmental, traumatic, and genetic models are among those proposed as explanations for these findings but none points to any currently identified specific pathological mechanism.

Treatment

Acute episodes of schizophreniform disorder are best treated in a hospital setting, where a structured supportive environment is provided. Exceptions to this policy may be made if adequate support is present in the home or an alternative facility such as a day hospital is available. Patients who present for treatment in early stages of decompensation may also be treatable on an outpatient basis. Although a few patients improve spontaneously after hospital admis-

sion, most will require medication. The neuroleptic drugs are the usual indicated treatment. Supplementation by benzodiazepines such as lorazepam during the most acute period of treatment may reduce the dose of neuroleptics required and thereby reduce the risk of side effects such as parkinsonism and tardive dyskinesia. Treatment itself proceeds in a fashion identical to that used for schizophrenia, with doses of antipsychotic drugs being gradually increased over a period of days or weeks until maximum benefit is achieved. (See Chapter 32.) Symptoms such as insomnia, agitation, suspiciousness, and disorganized thoughts may recede dramatically during the first few days of treatment, but auditory hallucinations and delusions may clear more gradually. When patients fail to respond in a reasonable period of time, alternative treatments such as lithium carbonate, carbamazepine, and electroconvulsive therapy have been employed. The effectiveness of these agents is controversial; some reports suggest that schizophreniform disorders respond to lithium carbonate, but these were not double-blind trials.

After clinical stabilization, neuroleptic drugs are gradually withdrawn unless symptoms recur. It is useful to instruct patients to recognize early signs of decompensation. Maintenance drugs as well as diagnostic reassessment may be required if relapse occurs.

Suicide is of critical concern in the treatment of patients with schizophreniform disorder, particularly after psychotic symptoms have subsided. Many patients enter into a prolonged depression, which may be part of the natural history of the disorder or represent a psychological reaction to the realization that one has been mentally ill. These postpsychotic depressions respond poorly to antidepressant treatment, and the risk of suicide is high. Patients should be monitored closely after discharge from the hospital and rehospitalized if suicidal ideation becomes apparent.

SCHIZOAFFECTIVE DISORDER

Symptoms & Signs

For decades there has been controversy about whether patients with admixtures of psychotic and mood symptoms were suffering from schizophrenia, an atypical variety of bipolar disorder, or a separate disorder entirely. A number of diagnostic labels have been applied to this group of patients, including (but not limited to) cycloid psychosis, atypical schizophrenia, good-prognosis schizophrenia, and remitting schizophrenia. The term "schizoaffective disorder," first used by Kasanin in 1933, has prevailed, although the boundaries with both schizophreniform disorder and reactive psychosis have often been obscure. In modern diagnostic practice, many of these patients are diagnosed as having psychotic mood disorders. Patients with schizoaffective disorder display persistent delusions, auditory hallucinations, or formal thought disorder consistent with the acute phase of schizophrenia, but these symptoms are frequently accompanied by prominent manic or depressive symptomatology. At other times, schizophrenic symptoms unaccompanied by mood symptoms are present. Schizoaffective disorder is further divided into bipolar (history of manic episodes) and unipolar (depression only) types.

Natural History & Prognosis

Schizoaffective disorder can present at any age, but it is most commonly first seen in young adulthood. Prognosis can be estimated from the relative prominence of schizophrenic and mood symptoms; more prominent and persistent schizophrenic symptoms are associated with poorer outcome, whereas more frequent and persistent mood symptoms predict more positive outcome. The presence of delusions and hallucinations that are mood-congruent (eg, the belief by a depressed woman that she has sinned or a manic individual's belief that he or she is the Messiah) predicts better outcome than mood-incongruent psychotic symptoms.

As with schizophreniform disorder and reactive psychosis, the lack of consistent diagnostic criteria has led to great variability in clinical studies of schizoaffective disorder. Some patients included in older studies would be diagnosed as having mood disorders with psychotic features in *DSM-III-R*. As a result, much of the earlier literature suggested that schizoaffective patients had clinical courses more akin to mood disorders than schizophrenia. More recent evidence suggests that the current definition of schizoaffective disorder characterizes a group of patients who resemble schizophrenics but at the better end of the prognostic spectrum. Premorbid social functioning is better than is commonly seen with schizophrenia.

Differential Diagnosis

A longitudinal rather than cross-sectional approach is necessary to diagnose schizoaffective disorder, since it is the temporal relationship between psychotic and mood symptoms that distinguishes it from schizophrenic and mood disorders. In the absence of such information, a diagnosis of **psychosis NOS** (atypical psychosis) may be necessary. Schizoaffective disorder differs from **major depression** or **bipolar disorder** with psychotic symptoms in that although a full mood syndrome (manic or major depressive episode) is accompanied by psychotic symptoms, delusions or hallucinations have been present alone for at least 2 weeks. It differs from **schizophrenia** or **schizophreniform disorder** in that the total duration of any mood symptoms present is not brief in relation to the total duration of the illness. In more descriptive terms, patients with a predominantly schizophrenic clinical picture who suffer from occasional periods of depression or elation are diagnosed as schizophrenic. For patients whose psychotic symptoms only occur during mood disturbances, the most appropriate diagnosis is major depression or bipolar mood disorder with psychotic features. The remaining patients have schizoaffective disorder.

In **delusional disorder,** mood symptoms are also relatively brief in duration, and psychotic symptoms are limited to nonbizarre delusional systems. **Brief reactive psychosis** is always preceded by psychological stressors and resolves completely within 1 month.

Illustrative Case No. 1

A 65-year-old man of German descent had been hospitalized frequently since his 30s for an illness characterized in part by auditory hallucinations and paranoid delusions. After each hospitalization, he recovered enough to return to his full-time job. Upon retiring, he took up residence in a downtown hotel while receiving injections of depot fluphenazine. Within a few months, he became markedly depressed. A trial of tricyclic antidepressant drugs resulted in a euphoric mood accompanied by pressured speech, insomnia, and poor judgment. The antidepressant medication was discontinued, but the depression returned within a few months, and the patient was hospitalized.

Upon admission to the hospital, the patient was severely slowed in his movements and speech and walked with a stooped gait. He slept poorly and had little appetite. He insisted that therapeutic efforts were best spent on other patients, because he was a worthless person for whom there was no hope. He wanted to be dead but lacked the initiative or "courage" to commit suicide. There were no delusions or hallucinations, and his speech was well organized and logical. He responded dramatically within 10 days after resumption of the antidepressant drug in a lower dosage. A diagnosis of bipolar disorder was made, and prophylactic lithium treatment was begun. The fluphenazine was discontinued.

Several months later, the patient discontinued lithium because of a tremor and began to pace around his hotel, sleeping poorly, and eating only one meal daily. He also stopped bathing and shaving. He presented himself again to the hospital in a filthy, disheveled state; he was lice-ridden and had lost 20 lb. He was not visibly depressed or elated but was negativistic and turned his head and glared frequently as if responding to a voice. After several days of treatment with moderate doses of haloperidol, he began to respond to questioning by his physician. He denied having been depressed and insisted that nothing was wrong with him. He admitted hearing women singing happy German children's songs and often sang along with them. He also discussed his belief that Jews were attempting to harm him and his grandchildren as retaliation for what the Germans had done to them during World War II. He claimed that he had felt this way for years but often avoided discussing it with his doctors. He described a series of seemingly ordinary incidents that had happened through the years that he felt proved his point.

Illustrative Case No. 2

A 44-year-old divorced black male presented with a 20-year history of traveling about the country, virtually annual psychiatric hospitalizations, and alcohol abuse. The usual diagnosis had been paranoid schizophrenia. Two months before his latest request for inpatient care, he had been started on lithium treatment for the first time but discontinued it because of increased urination and dysuria. He also stopped taking the chlorpromazine that had been prescribed. He complained of sleeplessness and weight loss and became loud and belligerent when his need for hospitalization was questioned.

Mental status examination revealed a guarded, somewhat sarcastic, physically thin man who spoke in increasingly loud tones with a considerable degree of pressure and circumstantiality. His behavior on the ward was intrusive and loud, and he slept little. His mood was irritable, and he was frequently pacing, talking, or otherwise active. When questioned about auditory hallucinations, he became extremely defensive and denied hearing voices. He did say, however, that sometimes he picked up information from "the wrong channel" but ignored it. He had gotten "into trouble" in the past when he paid attention to what he had heard.

Treatment was started with lithium. Small doses of haloperidol had to be added temporarily because his pressured, irritable manner caused conflicts with other patients. After 1 week his behavior was considerably subdued, but it became apparent that he was hallucinating. He spent most of the day off the ward in animated conversation with nonexistent persons. Serum lithium levels were within the therapeutic range. Addition of haloperidol in standard doses eliminated the hallucinations, but withdrawal of lithium resulted in a return of manic behavior.

Epidemiology

Estimates of the prevalence of schizoaffective disorder vary widely, but schizoaffective manic patients appear to comprise 3–5% of psychiatric admissions to typical clinical centers. At one point it was widely believed that schizoaffective disorder was associated with increased risk of mood disorders in relatives. This may have been due to the number of patients with psychotic mood disorders who were included in schizoaffective study populations. The current diagnostic criteria apparently define a group of patients more likely to have schizophrenic relatives.

Etiology & Pathogenesis

Although the causes of schizoaffective disorder are unknown, many authorities suspect that this diagnosis represents a heterogeneous group of patients, some with atypical forms of schizophrenia and some with very severe forms of mood disorder. There is little evidence for a distinct variety of psychotic illness. It follows then that the cause is probably identical to that of schizophrenia in some cases or of mood disorders in others.

Treatment

Most schizoaffective patients require neuroleptic medication to control psychotic symptoms, often on a long-term basis. Additional treatment for mood symptoms may be beneficial for some patients. When combined with medications for the signs and symptoms of mood disorder, the dosage of neuroleptic required to achieve clinical stabilization may be reduced.

Adding lithium or carbamazepine to a neuroleptic has been shown to be superior to neuroleptics alone in schizoaffective patients with manic symptoms, though the degree of benefit for an individual patient should be considered carefully, as both of these agents carry additional risks (see Chapter 32). In addition, lithium-neuroleptic combinations may produce severe extrapyramidal reactions or confusion in some patients. Some evidence indicates that manic symptoms in schizoaffective patients may take longer to respond to lithium than would be ordinarily expected. Carbamazepine is generally indicated when lithium is not effective or well tolerated rather than used as a first-line drug. Certain precautions in its use are necessary, since granulocytopenia can occur during the first few weeks of treatment. Valproic acid is also an effective antimanic agent, though clinicians in the United States are less familiar with its use than with that of carbamazepine. Calcium channel blockers such as verapamil may also be effective for manic symptoms. Benzodiazepines such as lorazepam and clonazepam have attained some popularity as adjunctive treatment of acute manic symptoms, but long-term use may result in dependency.

The treatment of the schizoaffective depressed patient has not been as well studied as that of the schizoaffective patient with mania. As in major depression with psychotic features, treatment with antidepressant drugs alone—even at relatively high doses—is not often effective. Administration of a neuroleptic drug is usually required and may have to be continued indefinitely. Patients who are receiving combined treatment of this type should be monitored closely for emergence of delirium secondary to administration of multiple anticholinergic agents and manic symptoms precipitated by the use of an antidepressant. The utility of lithium or carbamazepine in the treatment of schizoaffective depression has not been clearly established. They may be indicated when there is a history of previous positive response, when other drugs have failed, or when there is a history of manic episodes. Both lithium and heter-

Table 21–1. *DSM-III-R* diagnostic criteria for delusional (paranoid) disorder.

A. Nonbizarre delusion(s) (ie, involving situations that occur in real life, such s being followed, poisoned, infected, loved at a distance, having a disease, being deceived by one's spouse) of at least 1 month's duration.
B. Auditory or visual hallucinations, if present, are not prominent (as defined in schizophrenia, criterion A[1][b]).
C. Apart from the delusion(s) or its ramifications, behavior is not obviously odd or bizarre.
D. If a major depressive or manic syndrome has been present during the delusional disturbance, the total duration of all episodes of the mood syndrome has been brief relative to the total duration of the delusional disturbance.
E. Has never met criterion A for schizophrenia, and it cannot be established that an organic factor initiated and maintained the disturbance.

Specify type: The following types are based on the predominant delusional theme. If no single delusional theme predominates, specify as other type.

Erotomanic type: the predominant theme of the delusion(s) is that a person, usually of higher status, is in love with the subject.

Grandiose type: the predominant theme of the delusion(s) is one of inflated worth, power, knowledge, special identity, or special relationship to a deity or famous person.

Jealous type: the predominant theme of the delusion(s) is that one's sexual partner is unfaithful.

Persecutory type: the predominant theme of the delusion(s) is that one (or someone to whom one is close) is being malevolently treated in some way. People with this type of delusional disorder may repeatedly take their complaints of being mistreated to legal authorities.

Somatic type: the predominant theme of the delusion(s) is that the person has some physical defect, disorder, or disease.

Other type: does not fit any of the previous categories, eg, persecutory and grandiose themes without a predominance of either; delusions of reference without malevolent content.

ocyclic antidepressants are effective prophylactic agents in recurrent unipolar depression, but their effectiveness in preventing recurrences of schizoaffective depression is still under study.

DELUSIONAL (PARANOID) DISORDERS

Symptoms & Signs

Delusional disorders are characterized by prominent well-organized delusions and by the relative absence of hallucinations, disorganized thought and behavior, and abnormal affect. Although not as common as other functional psychoses, they are consistently encountered in psychiatric settings. The older name for this disorder, paranoia, was first used by Kahlbaum in 1863 and incorporated as a category of illness in Kraepelin's 1912 textbook. Since it is the delusional beliefs of a persecutory nature that are most commonly described, the term "paranoia" has become associated with suspiciousness or persecutory beliefs. To avoid confusion, the term "delusional disorder" is used in *DSM-III-R*. (See Table 21–1.)

The disorder is usually marked by an insidious onset of delusional ideas that gradually become the focus of the patient's life. The delusional beliefs themselves are internally consistent; in fact, the clinician may have difficulty deciding where legitimate grievances or misfortunes end and psychotic fantasies begin. What may begin as a frustrating experience with a government agency or employer may become a complex conspiracy that involves everyone in the patient's surroundings. These patients may resort to litigation or appeal to public authorities for assistance. As these efforts are frustrated, they perceive those agencies and individuals as having joined the ranks of the enemy. A sense of self-importance and of messianic mission may develop over time as they see themselves standing alone against injustice. Remarkably, these patients behave and communicate in a normal fashion outside of their delusional concerns. Their emotional responses conform to our expectations of a normal person facing the same threat or danger. They may feel strongly motivated to discuss their beliefs and try to engage the clinician as an ally. They rarely have insight into the fact that they are ill, and their attendance in a psychiatric setting is often the result of pressure from family or courts. Depression, perhaps with suicidal ideation, may be present in a patient who has exhausted all personal resources coping with a life that has become a nightmare.

In delusional disorder of the **persecutory** type, patients believe that they are victims of an organized plot. They may feel that they are being pursued, that their telephone is tapped, or that their reputation is being purposely maligned.

Patients with delusional disorder of the **grandiose** type believe that they are special or have very important talents or abilities. Such patients may spend much of their time working on ideas for great inventions. These may be represented as having important potential benefits for humanity but will seem lacking in substance to the listener. They may believe they are persecuted by those who envy their talents; in such cases the boundary between persecutory and grandiose types may become blurred.

Patients with **erotomanic** delusional disorder mistakenly believe that a particular person is deeply in love with them. This person is usually of higher social status (eg, a film star, politician, or college professor). The patient may attempt to communicate with this person by letter, by telephone, or even by forced intrusion into the person's home. The patient may provide idiosyncratic interpretations of the public statements or actions of the target person as evidence his or her attempts to respond.

Patients with delusional disorder of the **jealous** type mistakenly believe that their spouse or lover is unfaithful, often based on mysterious clues that seem to appear everywhere. They may gather evidence based on random events, bits of conversation, or misplaced household items to support their suspicions.

Patients with prominent **somatic** delusions may believe that they have some dread disease or are dying. In one particular manifestation of this type of delusional disorder, patients complain of infestation with insects or parasites; such patients are likely to present for treatment at a dermatologist's office rather than in a psychiatric setting. They frequently offer jars or bottles with "specimens" they have saved for laboratory analysis; often these appear to be pieces of skin or other nonspecific material.

Patients with **unspecified** delusional disorder have more than one type of delusion, without any one clearly predominating. In some cases, grandiose, jealous, and persecutory delusions may share the spotlight. There are also delusions that do not clearly fit other categories (eg, the delusion of doubles [Capgras's syndrome], in which patients believe that a loved one is a double or imposter and is not to be trusted).

Differential Diagnosis

The presence of nonbizarre, superficially plausible delusions for at least 1 month is required for a diagnosis of delusional disorder. The content of the delusions is the basis for classification into erotomanic, grandiose, jealous, persecutory, somatic, and unspecified types. There must also be an absence of prominent hallucinations or bizarre behavior.

Delusional disorder must be distinguished from **organic delusional disorder** (eg, cerebral neoplasm and psychoactive substance-induced delusional disorder), which can also present with prominent delusions. **Schizophrenia, schizophreniform disorder,** and **schizoaffective disorder** differ from delusional disorder in that delusions are accompanied by additional psychotic symptoms such as prominent auditory hallucinations, loosening of associations or poverty of speech, markedly illogical thinking, or delusional content of a bizarre or absurd nature. Although an acute onset of delusional disorder may be associated with a precipitating stressful event, it differs from **brief reactive psychosis** in having a duration of 1 month or longer.

Delusional disorder accompanied by depression differs from major **depression with psychotic features** in that the total duration of the mood symptoms are brief compared to the total duration of the illness. Although depressed patients may experience virtually any type of delusion, persecutory beliefs associated with depression are often thematically related to an exaggerated feeling of guilt—they feel they are being punished for their crimes or otherwise deserve the treatment they are receiving. Both **manic** and delusional disorders can present with exaggerated feelings of self-importance and belligerence, but manic symptoms such as increased motor activity, excessive plans, hypersexuality, racing thoughts, or decreased need for sleep are not prominent or persistent in delusional disorder.

A more subtle distinction is between delusional disorder, persecutory type, and **paranoid personality.** In the case of the latter, the patient may be generally suspicious of the motives of others but does not have frank delusions. In practice, however, it may be difficult to extract delusional ideas from paranoid patients, since they may conceal the extent of their suspiciousness when they do not trust the examiner.

Natural History & Prognosis

Cameron described a typical sequence of events leading to the development of a persecutory delusional system associated with delusional disorder. Initially, the patient experiences feelings of being personally vulnerable and threatened by real or imagined problems. As he tries to discuss his suspicions, he is rebuffed and becomes increasingly isolated. Still unsure of what is going on, he sees evidence of being followed, monitored, or subjected to tests. People indicate by comments or gestures that they are aware of what is going on. Newspapers or television programs may contain concealed messages or references to the patient's situation. The delusional system becomes "crystallized" when the patient develops a hypothesis to account for being singled out and decides who is directing the persecution.

Most cases of delusional disorder are characterized by a gradual onset and chronic course, although more acute forms have been described. The prognosis of chronic forms of delusional disorder is poor. Patients rarely give up their delusional beliefs entirely, and engaging them in treatment is difficult. A satisfactory outcome is achieved if they can function in the community without feeling the need to act upon or discuss their abnormal beliefs.

Illustrative Case No. 1 (Persecutory Type)

A 59-year-old divorced power company engineer became convinced that the design for a new nuclear power plant was faulty and unsafe. Despite 11 years with the company, he was fired, by his account, after repeatedly annoying his superiors with these concerns. Acting as his own attorney, he filed suits against the company, some protesting his firing, some to stop construction of the power plant, and even some to stop utility rate increases. He became well known to company and public officials, who saw him as a ludicrous but somehow tragic figure.

Meanwhile, the patient developed the belief that since he had filed so many suits on his own behalf, he was now an attorney because of a "grandfather" clause in the state law. He also began to believe that his efforts had made him unpopular with certain powerful groups, including the Mafia, the Bank of America, the FBI, and even the Vatican. He squandered his savings on a trip to Europe, where he attempted to pursue his investigations, until he was deported from England. Whenever local authorities would intervene, he would assume that they were involved in the conspiracy, helping to keep track of his whereabouts.

After his personal resources were exhausted and an unsuccessful attempt to convince police that a ''contract'' was out on his life, he requested hospitalization for ''protection.'' At the time of hospital admission, the patient was well groomed and articulate. He rambled on about his delusions and fears unless interrupted firmly. There was no evidence of hyperactivity, hallucinations, or other delusional thinking. During his hospital stay, he was neither overtalkative nor socially intrusive. He slept peacefully, believing that he was safe in the hospital. After treatment with moderate doses of a neuroleptic drug, he felt safe leaving the hospital for a halfway house. Careful questioning revealed his continued beliefs in the conspiracy against him, but he was apparently less compelled to discuss or act upon them.

Illustrative Case No. 2
(Somatic Type)

A 65-year-old Caucasian former prizefighter had been making the rounds of local hospitals for 2 years with the complaint that his nose was shrinking. He feared that if this process progressed too far, he would not be able to breathe and would subsequently die. Although he was at times depressed about this, the depression was transient, whereas his frantic concerns about his nose continued unabated. Attempts by otolaryologists to reassure him were unsuccessful. He had been treated several times on psychiatric units with failed trials of neuroleptics and antidepressants. He had since refused any psychiatric referral. At no time had there been evidence of hallucinations, other delusions, or disorganized thought. His behavior and level of self-care were totally appropriate. Multiple mental status examinations, neurological studies, and laboratory screenings failed to disclose evidence of underlying organic disease.

Epidemiology

Delusional disorder is relatively uncommon, representing 1–4% of all psychiatric hospital admissions. The incidence of the disorder is 1–3:100,000 population annually, while the prevalence is between 0.02% and 0.03%. Onset is typically in middle life or later, with few first hospitalizations before age 35. Women are affected more often than men but not as predominantly so as in mood disorders. Patients are more likely to have been married than schizophrenic patients. Low socioeconomic status and recent immigrant status are common associated factors. Additional populations at risk include older patients with impaired hearing or other physical disabilities that limit social contacts. Genetic studies indicate a lack of familial relationships with either schizophrenia or mood disorder.

Etiology & Pathogenesis

The cause of delusional disorder is unknown, but a number of contributory psychological mechanisms have been proposed, particularly for the persecutory type. Kraepelin and Kretschmer postulated that the disorder resulted from overwhelming stress in a premorbid personality characterized by distrustfulness and hypersensitivity to slights. Later writers have postulated a developmental deficit in the ability to trust others. Cameron (1974) stressed that individuals with delusional disorder have an inability to compare the perspectives of others with their own. They thus seem to be isolated, asocial people who must be vigilant lest something potentially threatening happen. Freud attributed paranoid thinking to **projection,** a psychological mechanism whereby ideas or feelings unacceptable to conscious awareness are disowned and attributed to (projected upon) others. Salzman (1960) and Cameron (1974) both offered alternative models sharing the assumption that delusional symptoms developed from underlying feelings of vulnerability and worthlessness.

These psychological formulations have significant shortcomings. They lack diagnostic specificity; similar psychological themes are identifiable in patients with a variety of psychiatric disorders who happen to have persecutory delusions. Many patients with hypersensitive, asocial personalities develop other disorders (such as schizophrenia). In addition, similar phenomena may occur in otherwise normal individuals, sometimes under conditions of vulnerability such as drug intoxication or fatigue or in social or religious groups whose values isolate them from the larger community. In some circumstances, hypervigilant scanning of the environment for danger or treachery may be adaptive. Nonetheless, social isolation, whether due to maladaptive personality functioning, physical limitations, or cultural dislocation, seems to be an important factor in the pathogenesis of delusional disorders and persecutory symptoms in general. Additional contributory causes obviously are present but are beyond our current understanding.

Treatment

The treatment of delusional disorder usually involves the use of neuroleptic medication. In cases of delusions of infestation, some psychiatrists have claimed that pimozide, a butyrophenone similar to haloperidol, has specific efficacy. There are also anecdotal reports of delusional disorder responding to antidepressants after neuroleptic treatment had failed.

Delusional patients are unlikely to participate willingly in any treatment program unless there is some basis for trust in the physician. Patients with this disorder are wary of any situation they do not control and often suspect that medication may be designed to harm them or lower their resistance to outside influences. The very act of accepting medication may be viewed as an admission that their beliefs are false.

Any side effect, however trivial, may frighten them into refusing further treatment.

Paranoid patients feel that they have been disappointed by people who at first seem to be on their side but later betray them and therefore approach new relationships in guarded fashion. At the same time, they desire human contact and may wish to find someone to trust who can help them. A professional and respectful attitude is necessary to take advantage of this. A paternalistic approach will be perceived as insulting; an informal manner may imply that the physician does not take their concerns seriously. Complete frankness is called for—pretending to give credence to the patient's delusional ideas leads to an appearance of betrayal when the clinician's true feelings emerge. The clinician should make it clear that he or she does not accept as true what the patient asserts *but that disagreement implies no disrespect.* It is pointless and counterproductive to argue or try to talk a patient out of delusions by logical reasoning. As trust develops, evidence for and against the validity of the delusional beliefs can be mutually explored in the hope that the patient will spontaneously begin to question their truth content. In many cases, the best result that can be achieved is to help these patients understand and accept that they have beliefs most others view as illogical and fallacious.

BRIEF REACTIVE PSYCHOSIS

Symptoms & Signs

It has long been recognized that otherwise well-functioning people may develop psychotic symptoms when confronted with overwhelming stress. In certain cultures, symptoms conform to certain patterns that are recognized by the individual's group as legitimate signals of distress. European psychiatrists have recognized the existence of a "nonendogenous" or "psychogenic" form of psychotic illness that is distinct from schizophrenia or manic-depressive illness. American psychiatrists have been less interested in this phenomenon except in cases of "hysterical psychosis" or acute reactions to combat ('3-day schizophrenias'). Previous diagnoses of reactive psychosis may have overlapped somewhat with other "good-prognosis" forms of psychosis such as schizophreniform disorder but are believed to be etiologically distinct.

Brief reactive psychoses are always preceded by a stressful event or series of events such as an automobile accident, divorce or separation, and financial setbacks. The onset of symptoms is abrupt, without the gradually developing prodrome often seen in schizophreniform disorder or schizophrenia. Symptoms are often dramatic and florid and are usually thematically related to the precipitating circumstances and psychologically understandable. There may be emotional turmoil or confusion as well as psychotic symptoms of various types. Delusions, hallucinations (auditory hallucinations are common, but visual hallucinations occur occasionally), loose associations or disorganized speech, and bizarre behavior are all common. Resolution of the precipitating stress results in resolution of the illness.

Natural History & Prognosis

There is no history of premorbid personality functioning suggestive of schizoid or schizotypal personality disorder. The duration of the disorder is brief (no longer than 1 month), and there is no residual deficit. However, many patients will have repeat episodes in response to future stresses, particularly if a basic personality defect is present that serves as a window of vulnerability to psychotic reactions to stress. Upon follow-up, the diagnosis of reactive psychosis is still appropriate for about half of these patients. The rest are rediagnosed at some point as suffering from schizophrenic or mood disorders.

Differential Diagnosis

The diagnostic criteria for brief reactive psychosis distinguish it from various other mental disorders. The presence of **organic** factors, such as withdrawal from alcohol or drugs, should be ruled out by appropriate history taking, physical examination, and laboratory tests. The symptoms of brief reactive psychosis may resemble those of **schizophreniform disorder, mood disorders with psychotic features,** or **delusional disorder,** but these disorders last longer than 1 month and may include prodromal or residual symptoms. However, the diagnosis may be changed, depending on the specific symptoms present, if symptoms persist beyond 1 month. If no precipitating stress can be identified but symptoms clear within 1 month, a diagnosis of **psychosis NOS** (atypical psychosis) may be appropriate. Transient psychotic symptoms may be present in patients with borderline or schizotypal personality disorders, but these are fleeting and not associated with a clear psychosocial stressor (see psychosis NOS, below). The clinician should also be alert to the possibility of **factitious disorder with psychological symptoms;** evasive responses to questions or apparent inconsistencies in the history may suggest this possibility.

Illustrative Case

A 60-year-old widower was admitted to the urology service for evaluation of acute onset of inability to void. While a physician was explaining the nature of a planned diagnostic procedure, bright red blood appeared in the catheter bag in full view of the patient. He became extremely frightened and developed the conviction that he would not survive the procedure. When a psychiatric consultant visited him several hours later, he was sobbing uncontrollably and unable to lie still. He overheard messengers from God telling him he would be dead soon, and he saw visions of his deceased wife, who promised him a reunion.

The patient's psychiatric history dated from World War II, when he had experienced two episodes of psychogenic amnesia and had traveled long distances before finding himself in a strange city. Since then, he had had periods of anxiety, particularly in crowded public situations, and he had finally stopped working at age 50 years. He had never been psychotic.

After 2 days of treatment and frequent reassurance from the medical staff, his symptoms disappeared almost as suddenly as they had begun.

Epidemiology

Although the incidence of brief reactive psychosis is difficult to estimate, family studies suggest that relatives of these patients are themselves prone to develop reactive psychoses but not schizophrenia or mood disorders.

Etiology & Pathogenesis

In contrast to schizophreniform or schizoaffective disorders, brief reactive psychosis is thought to be psychogenic in origin. When confronted with a stressful situation, the natural response is to use familiar problem-solving behavior patterns either to achieve a resolution or to maintain psychological equilibrium until external events change. Psychotic symptoms may emerge when the patient's psychological defenses are completely overwhelmed. For some patients, only chaotic events such as natural disasters or combat experiences are severe enough to upset the equilibrium; other people may be overwhelmed by divorce, physical illness, or financial disaster. Some patients with character defects (ie, personality disorder) may be unable to cope with transitions or disappointments that most would be able to tolerate even though they might find them unsettling.

Treatment

Patients should be assessed carefully for suicidal or homicidal ideation and appropriate steps taken to contain acute symptoms. Psychotropic medications are usually necessary to control agitation and insomnia. Neuroleptic medications should be limited to short-term use only, and symptomatic treatment with benzodiazepines such as lorazepam will often make the use of large amounts of neuroleptics unnecessary. Medication should be tapered off fairly soon after resolution of the acute disturbance. There is ordinarily no indication for maintenance therapy.

Psychological treatment may take several forms. Simply being removed from the crisis and being cared for by the hospital staff may allay the patient's anxiety enough to permit constructive discussion and problem solving. Enlisting the aid of family members may also be important for the same reason. Encouraging the patient to recount the events that led to the breakdown and to discuss their impact and meaning will facilitate recovery. Such discussion offers the patient a model for dealing with crises in the future. Longer-term psychotherapy directed at more fundamental psychological conflicts may be indicated for some patients.

INDUCED PSYCHOTIC DISORDER (Shared Paranoid Disorder)

Symptoms & Signs

Induced psychotic disorder is an uncommon disorder characterized by uncritical acceptance by one person of the delusional beliefs of another. Although two people are most commonly involved (folie à deux), cases have been reported involving three or more and in some instances an entire family. The patients are usually relatives or persons who have lived in intimate contact for a long time.

A characteristic feature of induced psychotic disorder is a pattern of dominance and submission. The dominant partner (primary case) is more seriously ill and suffers from a delusional psychosis—usually paranoid schizophrenia or delusional disorder. This individual is the originator of the delusions, passing them on to the passive partner. The submissive recipient is not otherwise psychotic prior to incorporating the partner's delusional beliefs. The content of the delusions is often persecutory or hypochondriacal and underscores the perceived hostility of the outside world, reinforcing social isolation and interdependence of the parties. This isolation serves as a strong motivation to maintain the close relationship at all costs.

Differential Diagnosis

The primary issue in differential diagnosis of shared delusional disorder is ruling out the presence of schizophrenia or other psychosis in the submissive partner.

Natural History & Prognosis

The prognosis for the submissive "recipient" is quite good if separation from the dominant partner is possible. In approximately 40% of reported cases, the recipient patient has responded to separation from the dominant partner alone. Treatment specific for the underlying illness is necessary for the primary case, with the final outcome depending on the diagnosis.

Illustrative Case

A hotel manager in a small town called the police because a guest family had stopped paying its bills and had been acting strangely. A 48-year-old man, his 25-year-old wife, and their infant son had registered 2 weeks previously and had not left the room except for the wife's trips to the grocery store. These forays had ceased the week before. The rent for the second week had not been paid despite frequent demands. Other guests complained of chanting and yelling during the night.

The husband was an unemployed laborer with a history of psychiatric hospitalizations and arrests for drunkenness and assault. He professed to be receiving messages from God directing him and his family to await the destruction of the world and the beginning of "the new order." His family would be among the few survivors and would play a leading role in the future of mankind. He heard the voice of God and of various angels who gave him instructions.

The wife was an extremely introverted, socially awkward woman who had never dated before meeting her husband. She rarely had contacts with other adults without her husband present; on those occasions, he would invariably speak for her.

The husband had to be forcibly removed from the hotel room and was eventually committed to a state hospital. His wife initially resisted offers of help, fearing that if she left the hotel she would not be saved from the impending Armageddon. She gradually gave up these beliefs in response to simple reassurance. The child was placed in a foster home. The wife and husband were reunited after his release from the hospital and were lost to follow-up.

Epidemiology

There are no data on the incidence or prevalence of induced psychotic disorder, but it is thought to be quite rare. Over 90% of cases involve members of a single family. The most common cases involve two sisters. Mother and child are next in frequency of occurrence, followed by father-child and husband-wife combinations. Pairings between friends are infrequent but have occurred.

Approximately 25% of the submissive (recipient) partners are suffering from a physical disability such as hearing loss or stroke, which may increase their susceptibility to domination by their partners.

Etiology & Pathogenesis

Induced psychotic disorder is believed to arise as a result of interdependency between the partners and serves to preserve their relationship. In order for the mechanism to work, several conditions must be met. The primary case, already mentally ill, must be dominant in the relationship and be able to influence the submissive partner. There must be a distinct advantage for both partners in sharing the delusions. For the inducing partner, maintaining at least one human contact represents a chance to avoid complete isolation. The delusions represent a mode of communication providing a tie with the partner that partially offsets the alienation from outside reality. For the submissive

partner, the delusions become a compromise, allowing a continuation of a dependent relationship.

Treatment

Treatment for the recipient generally consists of separation from the dominant partner. In many cases, the patient then becomes accessible to rational discussion and gives up the delusional system. However, since many patients will return to the same relationship, other steps may be indicated. These might include family or conjoint therapy as well as assistance with developing activities and interests outside the relationship.

PSYCHOSIS NOS
(Atypical Psychosis)

Symptoms & Signs

Psychosis "not otherwise specified" (NOS) is basically a diagnosis for those conditions characterized by psychotic symptoms (delusions, disorganized speech or behavior) that do not meet the criteria for more specific disorders. This diagnosis is appropriate when the data obtained by history taking and clinical examination are incomplete or puzzling or when there are unusual features. When evaluating an acutely psychotic patient, the physician may only be able to manage the patient's agitated or unruly behavior and must forgo more careful diagnostic analysis until later. A diagnosis of psychosis NOS is preferred to "diagnosis deferred" because it communicates more information by implying the presence of psychotic symptoms.

Illustrative Case

A 28-year-old woman presented with ill-defined feelings of depression, insomnia, and fearfulness that came over her daily. There were no apparent signs of psychosis until about 2 weeks after her hospital admission. At that time, she began to believe that all of the other patients and staff knew about her sexual life and were discussing it. She was convinced that the contents of her private discussions with her therapist were being disclosed to the entire ward, and she interpreted the actions and comments of both staff and patients accordingly. She began to feel uncomfortable in the hospital and requested discharge. The request was refused, and after several days of these symptoms, she was given small doses of haloperidol, with improvement occurring almost overnight. A week later, the medication was discontinued, and the symptoms did not recur. No specific stresses could be identified, and a previous history of psychotic disorder was not obtainable.

REFERENCES

Beiser M et al: Refining the diagnosis of schizophreniform disorder. Am J Psychiatry 1988;145:695.

Brotman AW, Jenike MA: Monosymptomatic hypochondriasis treated with tricyclic antidepressants. Am J Psychiatry 1984;141:1608.

Cameron NA: Paranoid conditions and paranoia. In: *American Handbook of Psychiatry,* vol 3. Arieti S, Brody EB (editors). Basic Books, 1974.

Coryell W, Tsuang MT: Outcome after 40 years in DSM-III schizophreniform disorder. Arch Gen Psychiatry 1986;43:324.

Enoch MD, Trethowan WH: Folie à deux (et folie à plusieurs). In: *Uncommon Psychiatric Syndromes,* 2nd ed. John Wright & Sons, 1979.

Goodnick PJ, Meltzer HY: Treatment of schizoaffective disorders. Schizophr Bull 1984;10:30.

Harrow H, Grossman LS: Outcome in schizoaffective disorders: A clinical review and reevaluation of the literature. Schizophr Bull 1984;10:87.

Jauch DA, Carpenter WT: Reactive psychosis I: Does the Pre-*DSM-III* concept define a third psychosis? J Nerv Ment Dis 1988;176:72.

Kasanin JS: The acute schizoaffective psychoses. Am J Psychiatry 1933;90:97.

Kendler KS, Gruenberg AM, Tsuang MT: A *DSM-III* family study of the nonschizophrenic psychotic disorders. Am J Psychiatry 1986;143:1098.

Kendler KS, Spitzer RL, Williams JBW: Psychotic disorders in *DSM-III-R.* Am J Psychiatry 1989;146:953.

Kendler KS: Kraepelin and the diagnostic concept of paranoia. Compr Psychiatry 1988;29:4.

Levinson DF, Levitt MEM: Schizoaffective mania reconsidered: Am J Psychiatry 1987;144:415.

Maj M: Evolution of the American concept of schizoaffective psychosis. Neuropsychobiology 1984;11:7.

McGlashan TH, Carpenter WT: An investigation of the postpsychotic depressive syndrome. Am J Psychiatry 1976;133:14.

Salzman L: Paranoid state: Theory and therapy. Arch Gen Psychiatry 1960;2:679.

Tsuang MT, Levitt JJ: The heterogeneity of schizoaffective disorder: Implications for treatment. Am J Psychiatry 1988;145:926.

Mood Disorders

Victor I. Reus, MD

The British physician Aubrey Lewis once noted that the history of the diagnosis and treatment of melancholia could serve as a history of psychiatry itself. That observation seems particularly relevant today, since advances in the diagnosis and treatment of mood disorders have led to a dramatic increase in their perceived prevalence and to more rigorous criteria for placement in competing nosological categories.

The hallmark of these disorders is a primary pervasive disturbance in mood. In this context, the term "mood" denotes an emotional state that may affect all aspects of the individual's life. The syndromes are characterized by pathologically elevated or depressed mood and should be regarded as existing on a continuum with normal mood. A diagnosis is appropriate when the mood disturbance is "primary" and central to the illness and not secondary to some other physical or psychological state. In the latter instance, the diagnosis would be incomplete without a reference to the precipitating cause. Although historically a precipitating stressful event was thought to be a critical element in the differential diagnosis of mood disorders, current opinion is that data of this sort lack diagnostic specificity and prognostic validity. Even so, when a mood disturbance following a stressful life event is a mild one that does not meet the criteria for any of the disorders discussed in this chapter, a diagnosis of **adjustment disorder with depressed mood** is warranted (see Chapter 25).

In this chapter, the class of mood disorders is divided into disorders in which there is a full major mood syndrome; disorders in which there is only a partial but persistent syndrome; and disorders that cannot be classified in either of these two ways (Table 22–1). Major mood disorders are further classified according to whether the patient has a history of a manic episode. A past or present history of a manic episode justifies a diagnosis of **bipolar disorder,** which may be further subdivided on the basis of the presenting mood state (**manic, depressed,** or **mixed**). Some investigators have suggested that within the spectrum of bipolar illness are distinct subtypes characterized by prominence of either mania or depression. If there is no history of manic episode and if the criteria of severity are met, a diagnosis of **major depressive disorder** is warranted. Major depression is further subclassified according to whether it is a

first episode or a recurrence. Additional clinical features such as the presence of psychotic ideation or vegetative signs should also be specifically recorded. Although not authorized by *DSM-III-R,* the term "unipolar" is sometimes used in describing this group of disorders.

Other specific mood disorders include cyclothymic disorder and dysthymic disorder. In **cyclothymic disorder,** the symptoms resemble those of bipolar disorder but are neither severe enough nor of sufficient duration to meet the criteria for diagnosis of bipolar or major depressive disorder. The term **dysthymic disorder** partially encompasses the group of individuals historically classified as suffering from depressive neurosis. Individuals with this diagnosis have chronic depression that is not of sufficient severity or duration to meet the criteria for major depressive episode.

The terms **bipolar disorder NOS** ("not otherwise specified") and **depressive disorder NOS** are reserved for individuals who do not precisely meet any of the criteria just described. One example would be patients with a history of major depressive episodes and episodes with some manic features not of sufficient severity or duration to meet the criteria for bipolar mood disorder, mixed type.

BIPOLAR DISORDER

Symptoms & Signs

One essential criterion for a diagnosis of bipolar disorder is a past or present history of a manic episode. Manic episodes are characterized by a predominantly elevated, expansive, or irritable mood that presents as a prominent or persistent part of the illness. Manic patients classically have abundant resources of energy and engage in multiple activities and ventures. At baseline and between episodes, the bipolar manic patient may indeed function at a high level of productivity, particularly in areas requiring creative talent. In the initial stages of an episode—and sometimes in attenuated episodes—the ventures may appear genuinely creative and perhaps only mildly eccentric. In time, however, as the investment in these activities becomes excessive, the individual loses the capacity to behave with reasonable caution and judgment and to conform with social expectations and norms. In many manic episodes and particularly in initial stages,

Table 22–1. *DSM-III-R* diagnostic criteria for affective disorders.*†

Manic episode:

Note: A "manic syndrome" is defined as including criteria A, B, and C, below. A "hypomanic syndrome" is defined as including criteria A and B, but not criterion C, ie, no marked impairment.

A. A distinct period of abnormally and persistently elevated, expansive, or irritable mood.

B. During the period of mood disturbance, at least 3 of the following symptoms have persisted (4 if the mood is only irritable) and have been present to a significant degree: (1) inflated self-esteem or grandiosity; (2) decreased need for sleep, eg, feels rested after only 3 hours of sleep; (3) more talkative than usual or pressure to keep talking; (4) flight of ideas or subjective experience that thoughts are racing; (5) distractibility, eg, attention too easily drawn to unimportant or irrelevant external stimuli; (6) increase in goal-directed activity (either socially, at work or school, or sexually) or psychomotor agitation; (7) excessive involvement in pleasurable activities which have a high potential for painful consequences that the person does not recognize, eg, buying sprees, sexual indiscretions, foolish business investments.

C. Mood disturbance sufficiently severe to cause marked impairment in occupational functioning or in usual social activities or relationships with others, or to necessitate hospitalization to prevent harm to self or others.

D. At no time during the disturbance have there been delusions or hallucinations for as long as 2 weeks in the absence of prominent mood symptoms (ie, before the mood symptoms developed or after they have remitted).

E. Not superimposed on schizophrenia, schizophreniform disorder, delusional disorder, or psychotic disorder NOS.

F. It cannot be established that an organic factor initiated and maintained the disturbance.

Note: Manic episodes that are apparently precipitated by somatic antidepressant treatment (eg, drugs, ECT) should be diagnosed as mood disorders.

Major depressive episode:

Note: A "major depressive syndrome" is defined as criterion A below.

A. At least 5 of the following symptoms have been present during the same 2-week period and represent a change from previous functioning; at least 1 of the symptoms is either (1) depressed mood or (2) loss of interest or pleasure. (Do not include symptoms that are clearly due to a physical condition, mood-incongruent delusions or hallucinations, incoherence, or marked loosening of associations.): (1) depressed mood (or can be irritable mood in children and adolescents) most of the day, nearly every day, as indicated either by subjective account or observation by others; (2) markedly diminished interest or pleasure in all, or almost all, activities most of the day, nearly every day (as indicated either by subjective account or observation by others of apathy most of the time); (3) significant weight loss or weight loss or weight gain when not dieting (eg, more than 5% of body weight in a month), or decrease or increase in appetite nearly every day (in children, consider failure to make expected weight gains); (4) insomnia or hypersomnia nearly every day; (5) psychomotor agitation or retardation nearly every day (observable by others, not merely subjective feelings of restlessness or being slowed down); (6) fatigue or loss of energy nearly every day; (7) feelings of worthlessness or excessive or inappropriate guilt (which may be delusional) nearly every day (not merely self-reproach or guilt about being sick); (8) diminished ability to think or concentrate, or indecisiveness, nearly every day (either by subjective account or as observed by others); (9) recurrent thoughts of death (not just fear of dying), recurrent

suicidal ideation without a specific plan, or a suicide attempt or a specific plan for committing suicide.

B. (1) It cannot be established that an organic factor initiated and maintained the disturbance; (2) the disturbance is not a normal reaction to the loss of a loved one (uncomplicated bereavement).

C. At no time during the disturbance have there been delusions or hallucinations for as long as 2 weeks in the absence of prominent mood symptoms (ie, before the mood symptoms developed or after they have remitted).

D. Not superimposed on schizophrenia, schizophreniform disorder, delusional disorder, or psychotic disorder NOS.

Diagnostic criteria for melancholic type:

The presence of at least 5 of the following: (1) loss of interest or pleasure in all, or almost all, activities; (2) lack of reactivity to usually pleasurable stimuli (does not feel much better, even temporarily, when something good happens); (3) depression regularly worse in the morning; (4) early morning awakening (at least 2 hours before usual time of awakening); (5) psychomotor retardation or agitation (not merely subjective complaints); (6) significant anorexia or weight loss (eg, more than 5% of body weight in a month); (7) no significant personality disturbance before first major depressive episode; (8) one or more previous major depressive episodes followed by complete, or nearly complete, recovery; (9) previous good response to specific and adequate somatic antidepressant therapy, eg, tricyclics, ECT, MAOI, lithium.

Bipolar disorder, mixed:

A. Current (or most recent) episode involves the full symptomatic picture of both manic and major depressive episodes (except for the duration requirement of 2 weeks for depressive symptoms) intermixed or rapidly alternating every few days.

B. Prominent depressive symptoms lasting at least 1 full day.

Bipolar disorder, manic:

Currently (or most recently) in a manic episode. (If there has been a previous manic episode, the current episode need not meet the full criteria for a manic episode.)

Bipolar disorder, depressed:

A. Has had one or more manic episodes.

B. Currently (or most recently) in a major depressive episode. (If there has been a previous major depressive episode, the current episode need not meet the full criteria for a major depressive episode.)

Cyclothymia:

A. For at least 2 years (1 year for children and adolescents) presence of numerous hypomanic episodes (criteria A and B but not criterion C of manic episode) and numerous periods with depressed mood or loss of interest or pleasure that did not meet criterion A of major depressive episode.

B. During a 2-year period (1 year in children and adolescents) of the disturbance, never without hypomanic or depressive symptoms for more than 2 months at a time.

C. No clear evidence of a major depressive episode or manic episode during the first 2 years of the disturbance (or 1 year in children and adolescents).

Note: After this minimum period of cyclothymia, there may be superimposed manic or major depressive syndromes, in which case the additional diagnosis of bipolar disorder or bipolar disorder NOS should be given.

D. Not superimposed on a chronic psychotic disorder, such as schizophrenia or delusional disorder.

E. It cannot be established that an organic factor initiated and maintained the disturbance, eg, repeated intoxication from drugs or alcohol.

---

*In order to avoid redundancy, *DSM-III-R* lists criteria for manic and major depressive episodes and their subclassifications and then offers criteria for major affective disorders and other specific affective disorders. This table follows the *DSM-III-R* outline but omits criteria for some subclassifications of episodes.

†Affective disorders are now called mood disorders in *DSM-III-R*.

Table 22–1 (cont'd). *DSM-III-R* diagnostic criteria for affective disorders.*†

Bipolar disorder not otherwise specified:
Disorders with manic or hypomanic features that do not meet the criteria for any specific bipolar disorder. *Examples:* (1) at least one hypomanic episode and at least one major depressive episode, but never either a manic episode or cyclothymia (such cases have been referred to as "bipolar II"); (2) one more hypomanic episodes, but without cyclothymia or a history of either a manic or a major depressive episode; (3) a manic episode superimposed on delusional disorder, residual schizophrenia, or psychotic disorder NOS.
Specify if seasonal pattern.

Major depression, single episode:
  A. A single major depressive episode.
  B. Has never had a manic episode or an unequivocally hypomanic episode.

Major depression, recurrent:
  A. Two or more major depressive episodes, each separated by at least 2 months of return to more or less usual functioning. (If there has been a previous major depressive episode, the current episode of depression need not meet the full criteria for a major depressive episode.)
  B. Has never had a manic episode or an unequivocally hypomanic episode.

Dysthymia (or depressive neurosis):
  A. Depressed mood (or can be irritable mood in children and adolescents) for most of the day, more days than not, as indicated either by subjective account or observation by others, for at least 2 years (1 year for children and adolescents).
  B. Presence, while depressed, of at least 2 of the following: (1) poor appetite or overeating; (2) insomnia or hypersomnia; (3) low energy or fatigue; (4) low self-esteem; (5) poor concentration or difficulty making decisions; (6) feelings of hopelessness.
  C. During a 2-year period (1 year for children and adolescents) of the disturbance, never without the symptoms in criterion A for more than 2 months at a time.
  D. No clear evidence of a major depressive episode during the first 2 years (1 year for children and adolescents) of the disturbance.
Note: There may have been a previous major depressive episode, provided there was a full remission (no significant

signs or symptoms for 6 months) before development of the dysthymia. In addition, after these 2 years (1 year in children or adolescents) of dysthymia, there may be superimposed episodes of major depressive syndrome, in which case both diagnoses are given.
  E. Has never had a manic episode or an unequivocally hypomanic episode.
  F. Not superimposed on a chronic psychotic disorder, such as schizophrenia or delusional disorder.
  G. It cannot be established that an organic factor initiated and maintained the disturbance, eg, prolonged administration of an antihypertensive medication.

Depressive disorder not otherwise specified:
Disorders with depressive features that do not meet the criteria for any specific mood disorder or adjustment disorder with depressed mood. *Examples:* (1) major depressive episode superimposed on residual schizophrenia; (2) recurrent mild depressive disturbance that does not meet the criteria for dysthymia; (3) depressive episodes unrelated to stress that do not meet the criteria for a major depressive episode.

Diagnostic criteria for seasonal pattern:
  A. There has been a regular temporal relationship between the onset of an episode of bipolar disorder (including biopolar disorder NOS) or recurrent major depression (including depressive disorder NOS) and a particular 60-day period of the year (eg, regular appearance of depression between the beginning of October and the end of November). Do not include cases in which there is an obvious effect of seasonally related psychosocial stressors, eg, regularly being unemployed every winter.
  B. Full remissions (or a change from depression to mania or hypomania) also occurred within a particular 60-day period of the year (eg, depression disappears from mid February to mid April).
  C. There have been at least 3 episodes of mood disturbance in 3 separate years that demonstrated the temporal seasonal relationship defined in criteria A and B; at least 2 of the years were consecutive.
  D. Seasonal episodes of mood disturbance, as described above, outnumbered any nonseasonal episodes of such disturbance that may have occurred by more than 3 to 1.

---

the predominant mood is euphoria. The mood is often accompanied by a sense of absolute conviction or certitude, usually involving a self-perceived talent or perception but occasionally centering around more metaphysical and cosmic matters. A newly discovered or dramatically enhanced interest in religious or sexual experiences is a common feature. The euphoria experienced by the manic patient has an infectious quality and may mislead some people—even close associates—into accepting types of behavior that otherwise might not be tolerated. Manic patients can be quite engaging, and their well-known proclivity for buying sprees and improvident business ventures is often accompanied, at least for a time, by a remarkable ability to obtain loans or gifts of money and encouragement from people whose judgment is usually better.

One of the chief early symptoms of a manic episode is decreased need for sleep, so that in many cases the individual may not sleep at all for 3 or 4 days at a time. A "hunger" for social interchange may

be manifested by frequent and inappropriate phone calls to distant acquaintances, particularly during late-night periods when social stimulation is minimal. Hypergraphia (excessive writing) and a fascination with music and playing musical instruments are frequently noted. Manic patients may have a tendency also to wear bright colors and unusual combinations of eccentric attire or may exhibit an attitude of carelessness about clothes or makeup. Public disrobing is also common.

Manic speech is characteristically rapid and discursive. Manic patients are difficult to interrupt and have difficulty not interrupting when others are speaking. The speech itself may involve rhyming, punning, and bizarre associations, but there are no pathognomonic elements. Manic patients are readily distractible and respond to both internal and external stimuli in a self-referential manner. More severe manic episodes and manic episodes observed later in the natural history of the disorder may be characterized by paranoia and irritability rather than euphoria and grandiosity. Anxiety and feelings of suspicion can cause the verbal output of such individuals to be markedly decreased, leading to erroneous diagnostic conclusions. Significant social aggression is rare, although acute mania and hypomania are common diagnoses in individuals with a psychiatric treatment history who commit violent crimes. In some cases, severe depression may occur concomitantly with the manic state or in abrupt alternation with the manic state. True delusions and auditory hallucinations may be present, giving rise to difficult problems of differential diagnosis. The content of the delusions or hallucinations is often consistent with the predominant mood (mood-congruent).

In severe cases, mania can present as a state of catatonia. In such cases, the individual appears "willfully" unresponsive, often assuming a fixed posture and appearing mute except for occasional shouts or guttural sounds. Less severe states may be characterized by primitive delusions, fecal smearing, and extremes of tearfulness and emotional lability.

Natural History

A. Manic Disorder: Now that the use of lithium carbonate in treatment has become widespread, the complete natural history of a manic episode is seldom observed. Speed of onset, severity, and duration of the manic episode vary greatly in different individuals, depending in part, apparently, upon genetic and other factors not clearly understood. Descriptions of past manic episodes are the best source of information about future episodes. Predictions about the future course of a patient experiencing a first manic episode are necessarily vague. In many individuals, the onset will be abrupt, occurring over a period of days or in some cases hours. The onset of the manic episode classically occurs in the early morning hours and is first noted either as early morning awakening or inability to fall asleep. Some patients experience a more protracted onset over a period of weeks. Increases in psychomotor activity, increased energy, and elevated mood are the most common early signs, with manic speech and thought disorder occurring later if at all. Not all individuals pass through the classical sequence of events or progress to the same level of severity. There have been reports of manic individuals who have no complaints of sleep disturbance or obvious euphoria but who appear not to differ either in the natural course of the illness or in response to treatment.

It appears that in many cases manic episodes are self-limiting within days, weeks, or months. The variables that account for the wide reported ranges make assessments based on anything other than the individual's own past history unreliable. Chronic mania has been described and may remain stable at different levels of severity. Although lithium carbonate represents a dramatic advance in the treatment of bipolar disorders, 10–15% of manic patients respond inade-

quately to the medication and continue to present either episodically or chronically with classical signs of the disorder. Even with appropriate treatment, patients who present with rapidly alternating episodes of mania and depression are more likely to remain ill for an extended period of time than are purely manic patients. Bipolar patients experiencing their first episode of depression have approximately a 20% chance of remaining depressed for at least 1 year, a rate comparable to that of individuals with pure depression. In subsequent episodes, the cumulative risk for development of chronic refractory depression rises to 30%.

B. Bipolar Disorder: Although traditional textbooks have associated bipolar illness with a relatively late age at onset, current evidence indicates a peak between 20 and 25 years. Onset after age 60 is rare. Bipolar illness with onset during adolescence is commonly mistaken for an adjustment disorder, a fact that may reflect historical diagnostic bias or diagnostic confusion arising from normal physical and psychological developmental changes during this period.

Differential Diagnosis

Manic symptoms can occur in association with known organic disorders but should in such cases be diagnosed as organic mood disorder (ie, "secondary mania") rather than as bipolar disorder. There appear to be no clinical characteristics that might distinguish the two diagnoses, and it is probable that future research will result in the shifting of many manic diagnoses from a primary to a secondary category. The list of known causal agents is a long one and includes drugs (eg, corticosteroids, levodopa, stimulants), metabolic disturbances (such as those associated with hemodialysis), infections, neoplastic diseases, and epilepsy (particularly partial complex seizures).

In manic patients presenting with prominent delusions and hallucinations, the differential diagnosis is likely to include schizophrenia, paranoid type. Both syndromes can present with identical clinical symptoms, which means that the diagnosis can only be based on the clinical course or on secondary features such as the presence of a family history of mood disorder, the level of premorbid adjustment, a history of manic symptoms, or a prior response to treatment. The diagnosis of schizoaffective disorder is available for cases in which the clinician is unable to choose between manic episode and schizophrenia. Unfortunately, there is at present no agreement on how this category should be defined or on its etiological or prognostic relationship to schizophrenia or mood disorder (see Chapter 21).

Prognosis

Emil Kraepelin, the German psychiatrist who coined the phrase "manic depression," wrote that bipolar illness, in contrast to schizophrenia, usually has a good prognosis. In Kraepelin's original sample of 459 patients, 45% had only one attack, and very few had more than four episodes. The average duration of a pharmacologically untreated manic episode was 7 months, but a wide range was reported. Although most later studies have validated Kraepelin's findings, particularly when the disorder is compared to schizophrenia, it would appear that the prognosis of bipolar illness is less favorable than originally reported. Up to 15% of patients respond inadequately to medication and must endure chronic or recurrent symptoms.

The phases of bipolar illness may differ in their responsiveness to treatment and in their effect on ultimate outcome. Some individuals, for example, experience complete remission of acute manic symptoms and prophylactic benefit from medication but continue to have unmodified or attenuated depressive episodes. Suicide is a significant risk in such individuals. The best predictor of cycle frequency and treatment response is the personal and family psychiatric history. Once the episode has resolved, the duration of the symptom-free interval varies greatly in different individuals. In contrast to Kraepelin's original impression, it is now clear that most patients who satisfy the criteria for bipolar disorder will experience another episode within 2–4 years. The complete cycle—ie, from manic to depressed to manic state—may be as short as 48 hours or so long that the concept of cyclicity becomes meaningless. Patients with bipolar disorder who experience rapid cycles—three or more a year—respond less well to lithium than individuals with longer symptom-free intervals. The few available prospective studies of the course of bipolar illness indicate that for any given individual, the cycles become shorter as time goes on.

The prognosis thus depends on the frequency and duration of individual episodes and the response to medication. Since lithium is effective in moderating the severity of symptoms in most cases, there is always a strong possibility that recurrences represent failure of compliance with the drug regimen. Perhaps because of the quality of the mood experience, manic patients often utilize the psychological defense mechanism of denial, admitting that problems may exist but attributing them to overwork or to job or family stress. Patients with mild bipolar episodes may be able to function adequately during a period in which they demonstrate most of the symptoms of a manic episode. In such cases, factors such as psychological coping mechanisms, social supports, and socioeconomic status influence the outcome as much is response to medication.

Illustrative Case

A 27-year-old male graduate student in molecular biology was brought to the emergency room by his fiancée, who explained that over the preceding 2 weeks he had become increasingly irritable and suspicious and had undergone a "personality change." She noted that he had not slept at all for the past three nights and had become preoccupied by the belief that his research thesis would be regarded as the "new bible of the computer age." Fearing that his ideas might be stolen by government agents, he had constructed an elaborate mathematical code that would allow only him and his appointed "prophets" to understand the documented work. The patient was dressed in a mismatched three-piece suit he claimed was a disguise that would enable him to elude agents assigned to follow him. Although during the initial stages of the interview the patient refused to speak, he suddenly observed that since the interviewing physician was on the faculty of the university, he might be better able to understand the meaning of his research than the resident physician who screened him at the admission desk. He also remarked that the interviewing physician's name contained a syllable similar in sound and spelling to the Latin word for "trust" and suggested that their meeting must have been preordained. Throughout the remainder of the interview, the patient paced around the room, interrupting his responses to questions with associations to the interviewer's style of dress, a paperweight on the desk, and a book whose title he misread.

The history obtained from the fiancée revealed that the patient had never had any symptoms similar to these but that for about 3 months during the past 12 months, the patient had felt too tired to go to class and spent much of the day sleeping. She recalled that the patient had an aunt who was hospitalized twice following the birth of her two children and that an older brother had been married four times and was "quite moody."

After some urging by his fiancée, the patient agreed to enter the hospital and began taking medication, which he called "thought pills." Neuroleptic medication resulted in marked amelioration of symptoms within 5 days. After 2 weeks of treatment with lithium, his suspiciousness and grandiose beliefs diminished significantly. With partial recovery, the patient was mildly depressed and embarrassed about his recent behavior, but he still seemed excessively concerned that his research was important enough so that it might, in the future, require protection from industrial spies.

Epidemiology

Multinational studies indicate that the lifetime risk of bipolar disorder is approximately 1–2%. The concordance rate for bipolar illness in monozygotic twins is approximately 65%; in dizygotic twins the rate is 15%. Bipolar illness occurs in relatives of bipolar patients much more frequently than in relatives of patients with major depression; the rates for depression alone are approximately the same. Adoption studies show that rates of illness clearly depend on the risk associated with biological rather than adopted parents. In general, bipolar probands have more bipolar relatives and more relatives with mood disorder than unipolar probands.

Etiology & Pathogenesis

A. Biochemical Factors: Although many differences in biochemical indices have been described when bipolar patients are compared to normal control subjects, there is no agreement about which alterations have etiological significance and which are secondary effects or epiphenomena. Since the "switch" from depression into mania (and vice versa) can occur in minutes, attempts have been made to identify biochemical changes that might be associated with the switch. Specific changes in brain monoamine neurotransmitter metabolism and receptor function appear to be the most likely mechanisms. Although now regarded as too simplistic, the catecholamine hypothesis suggested that catecholamine (most specifically norepinephrine) deficiency was associated with motor retardation and depression, while catecholamine excess could result in excitement and euphoria. Since all of the major neurotransmitter systems are functionally linked, it is not surprising that changes in other major neurotransmitter systems have also been documented. Increases in dopaminergic function and adrenergic-cholinergic system imbalance have been reported during manic episodes. Trait-dependent alterations in platelet serotonin uptake, in cerebrospinal fluid levels of serotonin metabolites, and in endocrine response to serotonergic agonists have also been found in patients with bipolar illness. Overall, however, there have been few biological studies of *mania,* since the nature of the syndrome interferes with the necessary compliance with research procedures.

Electrolyte disturbances have also been found in bipolar disorders and may represent a defect of cellular membrane function. In general, sodium retention increases during depression, together with increased potassium and water excretion. The reverse is true during manic intervals. A variety of neuroendocrine changes have also been reported for patients with bipolar disorder who are in the depressed phase. About half of both bipolar and unipolar depressed patients show evidence of any or all of the following during a severe depressive episode: increased adrenal glucocorticoid function, decreased thyroid-stimulating hormone response to thyrotropin-releasing hormone, decreased basal prolactin levels, and decreased growth hormone response to insulin challenge.

In light of pharmacological parallels to temporal lobe epilepsy and beneficial responses to several anticonvulsant agents, some investigators have hypothesized that recurrent bipolar mood episodes derive from an endogenous "kindling" of electrical discharges in limbic areas of the brain. Others have emphasized patterns in alteration of circadian rhythmicity. Recently, using DNA markers, one laboratory has shown linkage between bipolar disorder and a locus on the X chromosome.

Another report by an independent group indicated a possible linkage between a marker on chromosome 11 and bipolar disorder in an extended Amish pedigree; initial enthusiasm for this finding was significantly dampened by a subsequent data reanalysis that showed a weaker association. Genetic heterogeneity may account for these disparate findings.

B. Psychosocial Factors: There is no reliable evidence that psychosocial factors cause bipolar disorder, though such influences may precipitate manic or depressed bipolar states and may in fact be necessary for the expression of symptomatology in milder bipolar syndromes. Retrospective analyses are unreliable, since every examined life contains historical matter that could account for behavioral changes. Recent research in biological circadian rhythmicity indicates that subtle changes in the light-dark cycle (eg, seasonal variations) are a better predictor of risk.

Treatment

A. Biomedical Therapies: Treatment of bipolar disorder depends upon the specific form of behavioral disorder at presentation. Lithium carbonate is the treatment of choice for the acute manic state, even though 10–14 days may be required before full effect is achieved. A favorable response to lithium is reported in 80% of bipolar manic patients. Complications are relatively infrequent, but a transient "rebound" depression following resolution of a manic state is not uncommon. Overall response to lithium appears to improve as duration of treatment continues. (For a detailed discussion of the pharmacology of lithium, see Chapter 32.) The degree of psychomotor activation and the fragile structure of the treatment alliance in acute mania require that supplemental treatment with faster-acting neuroleptics be instituted in most cases. Chronic treatment with neuroleptics is to be avoided, as the risk of tardive dyskinesia is increased in mood disorders. For patients who do not respond satisfactorily to lithium, the anticonvulsant drug carbamazepine may be tried; studies show that this drug has both acute antimanic and antidepressant effects on bipolar illness. Valproic acid, clonazepam, and the calcium channel antagonist verapamil have recently emerged as empirical alternatives to lithium, but these should not be considered agents of first choice.

B. Psychosocial Therapies: Some form of psychosocial intervention is almost always indicated in the treatment of bipolar disorder, although its nature and extent will necessarily depend upon the degree of disruption of family and financial situations, the baseline character of the individual, and the response to somatic treatment. The nature of the biological contribution to the disorder (see also Chapter 6) makes it almost impossible to ascertain in advance what the individual's ongoing psychosocial needs might be after acute symptoms subside. Some patients with bipolar disorder have infrequent recurrences, experience long symptom-free intervals, and are able to lead productive lives. Others may have a particularly malignant form of the syndrome or may exhibit pathological degrees of denial and lead turbulent lives calling for active psychosocial involvement by the therapist. Since there is a strong genetic component to bipolar illness, it may be impossible to determine to what extent the patient's problems are referable to the genetic contribution and what aspects reflect environmental and developmental experiences created by a primary disorder in parents and siblings.

CYCLOTHYMIA

Symptoms & Signs

Cyclothymia is characterized by manic and depressive states not of sufficient severity or duration to meet the criteria for either major disorder (Table 22–1). Symptoms must persist for at least 2 years and have no psychotic component. Individuals meeting the criteria for this diagnosis may experience an exacerbation of depression or mania sufficient to warrant a change in diagnosis. Most clinicians presently consider cyclothymia to be an attenuated form of bipolar disorder rather than a personality disorder, as originally thought. Cyclothymia is common in outpatient psychiatric practice and may account for as much as 3–4% of an unselected clinic population.

Cyclothymic patients suffer from short cycles of depression and hypomania that can at times be as *severe* as what are observed in other disorders but which usually fail to meet the criteria for *duration*. It is often difficult to ascertain any regular pattern of mood switching, and patients will commonly describe mood changes that come and go spontaneously over the course of hours or days. Studies of behavioral characteristics of these patients show that they are extroverted sociable individuals who appear self-assured, energetic, and often impulsive. At times this cheerful exuberance turns into irritability and extreme sensitivity to rejection or loss. Cyclothymic patients are frequently described as "stimulus-seeking," a characteristic that leads them to become involved in daring hobbies and results in checkered work and school careers. Promiscuity and drug abuse are also noted, as is a history of repeated romantic disasters. Although many of these characteristics are likely to lead to a socially maladaptive life-style, cyclothymic individuals often achieve substantial success and status in society. This may in part reflect a cultural bias that values "outgoing" personality characteristics, but it is also an outcome of a periodic increase in energies and enthusiasms that leads to accomplishments beyond the reach of more placid individuals.

Natural History

Close examination of the cyclothymic patient's personal history will usually reveal an age at onset of symptoms of early to late adolescence. About a third of patients with this diagnosis will experience an intensification of symptoms during a 2-year follow-up, sufficient to meet the criteria for mania, hypomania, or major depression. The close relationship of cyclothymia to bipolar disorder is supported by the finding that treatment of the depressed phase with tricyclic antidepressants can result in pharmacologically induced hypomania in 40–50% of patients. There seems to be a higher risk for the natural development of formal depressive as opposed to manic episodes.

Differential Diagnosis

As mentioned previously, the main task in differential diagnosis is to determine the severity and duration of the altered mood state. A chaotic life history with poor interpersonal relationships often suggests a diagnosis of borderline personality. Many cyclothymic individuals experience difficulties in ego development and in achieving an integrated sense of self. These issues may come up more frequently in cyclothymia than in formal bipolar disorder, since the milder and more evanescent quality of cyclothymia will make it more difficult for patient and family, friends, and therapist to recognize the constitutional contribution. The deleterious effects on personality development of a constantly changing and autonomous mood state that colors, in random fashion, the critical developmental experiences of childhood and adolescence should be obvious.

Prognosis

Since the syndrome is more broadly defined than either bipolar disorder or major depression, estimates of prognosis depend on assessments of the quality, quantity, and frequency of mood change and the effect of such changes both on the patient and on his or her social and professional world. The lifetime prediction of risk is unknown. Approximately 60% of these patients improve when treated with lithium carbonate.

Illustrative Case

A 34-year-old divorced secretary sought psychotherapy because of her long history of unsatisfactory relationships with men. She was currently employed by an agency that provided temporary secretarial help and admitted that she had quit and been fired from several jobs because of inability to keep regular working hours. She stated that she did not really like secretarial work and hoped to return to fashion modeling, an occupation she had pursued several years previously with modest success. She reported that she encountered difficulties even then from failing to show up for assignments and, on two occasions, from going to an appointment after having had several drinks. Further questioning revealed sporadic recreational use of marihuana, cocaine, and amphetamines. She attributed her difficulty in relationships with men to the fact that most of the men she had been attracted to were too career-oriented and "homebody" types. She acknowledged that several individuals with whom she had been close described her as "moody." She described her life as alternating between times when she felt "buzzed, like on speed" and other times when she felt "blank" and wanted to sleep most of the day. During these latter periods, she stated she felt somewhat better after drinking a bottle of wine but felt especially guilty about the fact that her life was "not going anywhere." The family history revealed a turbulent family environment created principally by an abusive father with a history of binge drinking. Clinical and laboratory evaluation disclosed no organic cause of the mood disorder. The patient was started in psychotherapy and was given a trial of lithium carbonate. Over the succeeding year, she obtained permanent employment and reported an increased sense of emotional stability.

Epidemiology

This disorder seems to be more prevalent than previously acknowledged. It is more common in women, and there is apt to be a family history of mood disorder and "mood spectrum" problems such as alcohol abuse and antisocial personality.

Etiology & Pathogenesis

A. Biochemical Factors: Very little is known about biochemical changes in cyclothymia. Most of the evidence has come from genetic studies linking the disorder to the major mood syndromes and from studies documenting a response to antimanic or antidepressant drug treatment.

B. Psychosocial Factors: Although the primary process responsible for sudden and recurrent mood change in cyclothymia is thought to be biological and genetically transmitted, the psychosocial sequelae of such changes may over time emerge as the most significant aspect of the patient's discontent. This is particularly true for individuals with an early onset of the disorder. Persons who suffer recurrent unpredictable and intense mood upsets, seemingly unrelated to circumstance, develop major themes of loss and low self-esteem. A history of interpersonal conflicts and generalized anger is common, because the character of presentation is often subtle enough to escape the awareness of clinicians and the sympathy of friends.

Treatment

Biomedical treatment of cyclothymia should be empirically derived and should be offered only if the individual's functioning is significantly adversely affected. A trial of lithium carbonate may ameliorate manic symptoms and reduce the frequency of most cycles. Antidepressant medication may relieve de-

pressive symptoms. (See Chapter 32.) Even with successful drug treatment, many patients with this disorder will benefit from psychotherapy that focuses on interpersonal relationships and self-image.

MAJOR DEPRESSION

Depression is one of the most prevalent medical disorders and has been recognized as a distinct pathological entity from early Egyptian times. Common usage of the word "depression" stems principally from the attempts of the 19th century psychiatrist Emil Kraepelin to introduce a term that would have greater diagnostic specificity than "melancholia." Currently, the term melancholia denotes major depressive disorder with changes in endogenous or vegetative function, eg, disturbances of sleep, appetite, and libido.

Throughout most of this century, clinicians have attempted to subclassify the syndrome on the basis of symptoms and causes. Many of the subclassifications proved to be invalid or unreliable. For example, the distinction between depressions that were "reactive" and those that were nonreactive or endogenous—ie, not precipitated by psychosocial stress—has not proved to be of predictive value. Such judgments in any case are highly subjective and depend on how detailed a history is obtained and how much weight is assigned by the patient or clinician to the changes that routinely occur in life, Distinctions on the basis of age have likewise proved suspect, with recent research indicating that depression during the involutional period is qualitatively no different from that experienced during any other stage.

Symptoms & Signs

A variety of studies have distinguished depressed individuals with prominent psychomotor retardation and anhedonia from those who evidence psychomotor activation, guilt, anxiety, and, occasionally, delusional thinking. The number and severity of somatic symptoms generally increase along with the severity of depression. Separating major depressions according to whether they are endogenous or autonomous has not been found to be useful, either in predicting drug response or in improving assessments of general risk. Individuals may in fact show endogenous features in one episode and not in another.

The character of depressive symptoms depends to a large extent on the severity of the disorder. In the most severe cases, patients may present with an extensive paranoid or nihilistic delusional system and the experience of hallucinations, usually self-deprecatory in content and consonant with the underlying mood state. Because such individuals have more psychomotor disturbance and generally respond poorly to antidepressant medication, some investigators have considered psychotic depression as a separate entity and not simply a severe variant of major depression.

Depression occurs at any age and can present with primary symptoms that do not involve obvious mood change. Depression in children may be difficult to diagnose. Because of cognitive and linguistic developmental changes occurring in childhood, emotional states are experienced and projected differently. In old people, the most significant symptom may be a change in cognitive function. The term "pseudodementia" has been applied to a state clinically identical to irreversible senile dementia but which resolves with antidepressant treatment. Recent research questions the utility of this distinction, since an unremitting course and lack of pharmacological response of senile dementia are far from unconfirmed. In "masked depression," a condition in which there is no apparent mood change, the course of illness, prognosis, and response to treatment are the same as those associated with classical major depression. Depression is one of the most common missed diagnoses in the general medical clinic. It may be associated with a primary disorders such as an endocrinopathy, neoplasm, or viral infection, but it more commonly occurs independently in the context of a panoply of multisystem somatic complaints.

Natural History

There is great variation in the clinical presentation and course of major depression. As the individual patient's history accumulates, recurrent episodes tend to develop a cyclic pattern of presentation, so that better judgments about the probable future course can be made.

Depression can occur at any age, but the average age at onset is about 40 years. In general, the earlier the age at onset, the more likely it is that there will be a recurrence. Symptoms develop either gradually over a period of many months or more dramatically over a shorter period, in many cases following a significant loss or episode of stress, although this is not necessary. If untreated, the depressive episode may resolve spontaneously over a period of weeks to months or may become chronic and remain essentially unchanged over a period of years. Although most patients with major depression respond well to somatic treatment, uncontrolled studies have revealed that recovery from major depressive disorder is not as good as once thought. Only about half of patients are completely recovered at 1-year follow-up. The prognosis worsens with increased severity of symptoms at onset, less acute onset, and occurrence of the acute episode superimposed on an underlying state of chronic depression. The risk of relapse after recovery from major depressive disorder is high for a short period—about 25% relapse within 12 weeks. For individuals with recurrent episodes, the question arises how soon another episode can be expected. The presence of a chronic underlying depression or a history of three or more depressive episodes significantly increases the risk of early relapse. In addition, there is evidence that the interval between episodes becomes shorter as the individual ages.

At least 20–30% of patients with major depression and no history of mania will experience a manic or hypomanic episode later in life. Factors positively correlated with eventual bipolar outcome include pharmacological induction of mania, a history of postpartum depression, early onset (< 25 years), and symptoms of hypersomnia and psychomotor retardation.

Differential Diagnosis

Major depression occurs concomitantly with a number of different disease states, such as pancreatic and bronchogenic carcinoma, hypothyroidism, and Cushing's syndrome. As noted, depression and dementia, especially in the elderly, may be confused. However, patients with dementia may develop major depression as well. In some individuals, depression occurs in association with seasonal change, giving rise to the term "seasonal mood disorder." Such individuals have experienced improvement in mood through "phase advance" alteration of their sleep-wake cycle and through the administration of several hours daily of full-spectrum light, usually during morning hours. A regulatory disturbance of pineal gland function and melatonin secretion has been hypothesized in these patients, and the syndrome itself is seen as an evolutionary remnant of the mammalian hibernation cycle. In *DSM-III-R*, a seasonal pattern may be a specific diagnostic feature of *either* bipolar disorder or recurrent major depression.

Schizophrenia commonly presents with significant depressive symptoms, either during the acute phase or shortly following resolution of psychotic symptoms. In such cases the diagnosis of depressive disorder not otherwise specified is added to the primary diagnosis. The differential diagnosis between major depression with psychosis and schizophrenia with depressive signs is exceedingly difficult and can best be made by considering aspects of the patient's premorbid history and a family history of psychiatric disorder. Because a diagnosis of schizophrenia requires a duration of at least 6 months, the date of onset is important.

In dysthymia and cyclothymia, aspects of the depressive syndrome may occur but are not of sufficient intensity or duration to meet the criteria for major depression. It should be remembered, however, that major depression can occur in these or other disorders as an independent, superimposed entity and should be recorded as such.

Patients with bipolar disorder, mixed type, may likewise exhibit features of severe depression but will also present manic symptoms.

Grief syndromes often present with behavioral and physiological changes identical to those observed in major depression. "Major depression" should not be diagnosed until it is determined that the reaction is either too severe or too prolonged to be explained as simple bereavement.

Prognosis

In individual cases, estimates of the degree of recovery and the likelihood of staying well depend mostly upon the patient's age at onset, the number of previous episodes, and the response to somatic and psychosocial treatment. Many individuals have only one depressive episode in a lifetime. The likelihood of recurrence is dramatically increased with the onset of a second episode and continues to rise slightly with each additional episode, eventually reaching a statistical plateau. In cases where suicidal preoccupation is recurrently noted in successive episodes and in those where profound delusional content is noted, the prognosis for recovery is generally poor.

Illustrative Case

The patient was a surgeon referred by an internist for evaluation of complaints of fatigue and hand tremor. During outpatient evaluation, the patient said that 4 months previously he began noticing a significant worsening of manual dexterity during surgery. He attributed his difficulties to a fine tremor that he demonstrated for the examiner. He felt guilty about several patients who had put their faith in him and had suffered for it. He was sure that people in the hospital were making disparaging comments about his condition, though he could offer no specific examples. He had become reluctant to schedule operations but at the same time said that his decreased income was mainly attributable to fewer referrals from colleagues and "the word getting out." Although this was the first occurrence of this kind, he felt that his whole career had been a sham and that his previous accomplishments were undeserved. He could see no medical or psychiatric solution to his difficulties and expressed an intention to retire, though he was only 47 years old and not financially able to do so.

Although the patient had full health and disability insurance coverage, he expressed great concern about the impending hardship to his family from medical expenses and his failure to earn a good income. This concern magnified even trivial expenditures; eg, he felt he could no longer buy a morning paper without jeopardizing his son's college education. He reported poor appetite and a weight loss of 15 lb in less than 2 months. He reluctantly acknowledged that he and his wife had not had sexual relations in 4 months because of his impotence. He was unable to read professional journals or popular reading matter. Direct questioning revealed early morning awakening, but he said this was not a problem. Despite a strong feeling that all of his troubles were due to the hand tremor, he agreed to enter the hospital for a trial of antidepressant medication. On the ward, he received a combination of drug treatment and individual and group therapy. After 10 days of drug treatment (imipramine, 200 mg orally daily), he began sleeping better and eating regularly. He continued to complain of depression but admitted to an increase in energy level, a decrease in tremulousness, and an ability to maintain an erection. A week later, he began to express an interest in returning to work and initiated plans for discharge.

Epidemiology

Although mood disorders are widely acknowledged to be common, their prevalence is difficult to determine because of differences in diagnostic procedures and criteria. Assessments of depressive symptoms—ie, intense, pervasive, and almost daily feelings of sadness or disappointment that affect normal functioning—show prevalence rates of 9–20%. (The relationship of such subjective assessments to the objective diagnosis of major depression is not known.) When more stringent criteria for major depression are used, prevalence of major depression is 3% for men and 4–9% for women. The lifetime risk is 8–12% for men and 20–26% for women. These figures also may be high, since they are largely dependent upon subjective evaluations of individuals who have not sought treatment. There has been a progressive increase in rates of depression in successive birth cohorts throughout this century as well as a progressively earlier age of onset.

About 12–20% of persons experiencing an acute episode develop a chronic depressive syndrome, and up to 15% of patients who have depression for more than 1 month commit suicide.

Etiology & Pathogenesis

A. Biochemical Factors: Genetic studies and studies on the effect of specific antidepressant drugs have led to the conclusion that most cases of recurrent major depression have some biological basis. This does not mean, however, that psychological factors have no role in symptom formation or in precipitation of episodes of depression of lesser severity.

Family and genetic studies indicate that the risk rate among first-degree relatives of individuals suffering from major depression (unipolar) is approximately two to three times the risk in the general population. This, it should be noted, is approximately half the rate reported among first-degree relatives of individuals suffering from *bipolar* illness. The concordance rate is about 11% for dizygotic twins and approaches 40% for monozygotic twins. Biological parents of adopted probands have a much greater prevalence of mood disorder than adopting parents.

The most prominent hypotheses generated to account for the actual mechanism of the mood disorder focus upon regulatory disturbances in the monoamine neurotransmitter systems, particularly those involving norepinephrine and serotonin (5-hydroxytryptamine).

More recently, it has also been hypothesized that depression is associated with alteration in acetylcholine-adrenergic balance and characterized by a relative cholinergic dominance. In addition, there are suggestions that dopamine is functionally decreased in some cases of major depression. Because the central nervous system monoamine neurotransmitter systems are widely distributed and involved in tonic regulation of autonomic functions, arousal, movement, sleep, aggression, and other vegetative functions, they are particularly well suited for their hypothesized role. Original reports suggesting that patients with endogenous depression experienced either decreased nonadrenergic or serotonergic activity now appear to be overly simplistic. All the monoamine neurotransmitter systems are interrelated and subject to compensatory adaptation to perturbation over time. In addition, the discovery that many neuropeptides and hormones may serve as neurotransmitters and neuromodulators in certain contexts has underscored the complexity of the neural regulation of mood (see Chapter 6).

Reports of biological changes in major depression offer potential utility in diagnosis and assessment of treatment response. Foremost among these findings is that a significant number of patients have evidence of either increased or decreased nonadrenergic function, as reflected by urinary levels of 3-methoxy-4-hydroxyphenylglycol (MHPG), the chief metabolite of central nervous system nonadrenergic function. Other major studies have pointed to a decrease in serotonergic activity in certain subgroups, as measured by levels of 5-hydroxyindoleacetic acid (5-HIAA), the principal metabolite of serotonergic activity in the brain. Although these findings derive principally from investigations of the therapeutic effect of antidepressant medication, it has historically been difficult to reconcile the short time course of such changes with the usual 10- to 14-day lag in clinical response. Most current hypotheses of neurotransmitter function in altered mood states have focused on changes in receptor sensitivity and number rather than on changes in the amount of neurotransmitter available. Long-term antidepressant treatment has been found to be associated with reduced postsynaptic beta-adrenergic receptor sensitivity and enhanced postsynaptic serotonergic and alpha-adrenergic receptor activity. Effects on presynaptic receptor sensitivity are more variable. In addition to direct measurement of neurotransmitter and metabolite levels in brain and peripheral fluids, there have been reports that monoamine oxidase (MAO) and catechol-O-methyltransferase (COMT), enzymes important in monoamine metabolism, are lower in depressed patients.

Several specific abnormalities in neuroendocrine regulation may represent evidence of either primary disturbance in hypothalamic-pituitary control or secondary alteration in neurotransmitter function in limbic sites. The most consistent finding is that many patients with severe depressive disorder have an excess secretion of cortisol from the adrenal cortex. This is not simply a stress-related phenomenon, because the actual number of secretory episodes is increased, principally in the early morning hours when the system is normally quiescent. Many cortisol hypersecretors also have levels of norepinephrine, MHPG, and epinephrine in plasma and urine that are several times higher than normal. In addition to alterations in the pituitary-adrenal axis, elevation in serum triiodothyronine and thyroxine have been reported, as has a significant blunting of the response of thyroid-stimulating hormone to an infusion of thyrotropin-releasing hormone. Reports of changes in growth hormone, prolactin, luteinizing hormone, and testosterone regulation in major depressive disorder are contradictory.

From a neurophysiological perspective, the most replicable finding is that sleep in severe depression is characterized by decreased total sleep, decreased REM (rapid eye movement) latency (ie, sleep time from onset of sleep until the first epoch of REM sleep), increased REM density (ie, ratio of REM activity to REM time), and decreased stage 4 delta sleep. Sleep electroencephalography does not differentiate subgroups of depressed patients but may help predict a positive response to antidepressant medication.

Immunological studies have identified a variety of subtle alterations in depression, including change in lymphocyte subsets, response to mitogen, and natural killer cell activity. Thus far, however, there is no clear evidence that such changes have functional significance.

B. Psychosocial Factors: Although psychosocial stress may play a role in precipitation of a major depressive episode and shape the particular constellation of symptoms noted, current research indicates that environmental factors as such do not cause severe depressive episodes. However, depressed individuals are often unable to accept the concept of biological vulnerability and remain convinced that they "themselves" or changes in their environment are principally responsible for their mood state. Self-doubt, guilt, and an overriding sense of worthlessness will often lead to disruption in relationships with friends and family and to a withdrawal from work—actions that have understandable long-term effects on mood. Chronic depression and depressive personality traits may thus emerge as the psychological and social precursors, concomitants, and sequelae of recurrent biological depressive states. Histrionic and hostile character traits are often noted, as is a long history of difficulty in maintaining stable interpersonal relations. The presence of a personality disorder does not affect the symptom profile but does presage a worse outcome.

The observation that many patients with depression have similar distinctive personality traits led Freud and other psychoanalytic writers to see clinical depression as a psychologically reparative mechanism. The loss of a love object and the consequent psychic injury could only be overcome by self-punishment in which the internalized object was devalued. Freud maintained that ego development depended upon successful resolution of object loss. Through a process of narcissistic identification, the ego became the target of revengeful aggressive treatment intended for the original object. Depression thus emerges as the construct of guilt over anger toward an ambivalently perceived (loved, hated) object. Other psychoanalytic writers have elaborated and adapted Freud's views, focusing on depression as an ego response to helplessness rather than internalized anger. Such formulations are undoubtedly useful for conceptualizing the origin of milder depressive episodes in individuals who are still socially functional and for understanding symptom formation in more severe depressive states. However, biological vulnerability is probably an essential prerequisite to the expressions of major depressive disorder.

More recently, investigators have laid stress on the cognitive distortions that dramatically prolong the morbid mood state. The most common cognitive distortions involve negative interpretation of experience, a negative evaluation of the self, and pessimism about the future. Thus, a reverberating loop is established in which a dysphoric affect can give rise to distorted perceptions that in turn exacerbate the dysphoria. This formulation is helpful in understanding the tenacity with which depressed patients seem to cling to the depressive experience even in the face of apparent reward, success, and support.

One cognitive theory based on animal studies is called ''learned helplessness.'' In this formulation, individuals in stressful situations in which they are unable to prevent or alter an aversive stimulus (ie, physical or psychic pain) withdraw and make no further attempts to escape even when opportunities to improve the situation become available. Another theory postulates that a reduction in the rate of positive reinforcement is the principal cause of depression. Low self-esteem is a consequence of the inability of depressed patients to engage in successful goal-seeking behaviors and a resultant low rate of positive reinforcement.

Cognitive and behavioral approaches to the depressive syndrome seem to be more useful for conceptually understanding the psychosocial effects of the depressive state and for planning psychotherapy than for explaining the origin of such episodes. An individual carrying a biological predisposition for recurrent depressive episodes may successfully negotiate critical ''vulnerable'' periods during times of little conflict or stress.

Treatment

A. Biomedical Therapies: A trial of antidepressant medication is indicated for most individuals with major depression, particularly if melancholic features are present (Table 22–1). Most patients with depression are either undertreated or inappropriately treated. Benzodiazepines, which may exacerbate the problem, are prescribed much more often than tricyclic agents. Premature withdrawal of antidepressant medication and symptomatic relapse are also unfortunately common.

The drug of first choice is usually a heterocyclic agent, although new agents of novel structure have recently been developed. Drug selection should be based upon the patient's general medical condition, the drug's side effects, and a personal or family history of therapeutic response to a specific agent. About 70% of patients with major depression respond favorably to antidepressant medication. Most cases of poor response are due either to the patient's failure to take the medication as prescribed or to inadequate dosage. Because the blood level from a given dosage varies as much as 30-fold in different individuals, it is useful in cases of nonresponse to measure plasma drug levels even in patients receiving maximal doses. The value of plasma levels is most clear with nortriptyline and desipramine. Although useful for titrating dosage into a general range, variations in blood levels within that range do not correlate well with clinical response.

Clear therapeutic benefit usually is noticed 10–14 days after starting treatment, although earlier and later responses are not uncommon. In general, objective signs of improvement (increased appetite, weight gain, improved sleep and affect, less agitation, increased purposeful activity) are noted before subjective improvement. A drug of a different class should be considered for patients whose symptoms do not improve after 6 weeks of medication with adequate blood levels. Patients with depression accompanied by delusions require more extended treatment periods (up to 8–9 weeks) and dosage levels higher than those for patients not experiencing delusions. Alternatively, another drug may be added, such as liothyronine, lithium, tryptophan, or MAO inhibitors. A trial of an MAO inhibitor alone might be considered at this point, as might a trial of lithium carbonate.

MAO inhibitors—isocarboxazid, phenelzine, tranylcypromine—can be drugs of first choice for individuals who present with prominent anxiety associated with depression or who complain specifically of fatigue, hypersomnia, and weight gain rather than weight loss. Although lithium does not have as specific an antidepressant effect as more traditional antidepressant agents, it may be the drug that helps in patients with clear periodicity of depressive recurrences and is a better prophylactic agent than traditional tricyclic agents.

It is not always clear how long maintenance treatment should be continued after acute symptoms have subsided.

Patients with very severe depressions and prominent delusional features are relatively refractory to traditional antidepressant treatment. The response often can be enhanced by addition of an antipsychotic agent. Electroconvulsive therapy should be considered in such cases and in cases of nondelusional major depression resistant to drug therapy. Most controlled studies have shown that electroconvulsive therapy is at least as effective as antidepressant medication in the treatment of major depression and often produces a much faster recovery. There are few contraindications to the use of electroconvulsive therapy, and side effects are limited to memory loss for the period just before and after treatment (see Chapter 32).

B. Psychosocial Therapies: Psychotherapy is often indicated for major depression, particularly in improving social functioning following remission of acute symptoms. Controlled studies have indicated that the combination of psychotherapy and antidepressant medication is more effective than either used alone. It should be noted, however, that in most cases of major depression, drug therapy alone is significantly better than psychotherapy alone. Many psychotherapeutic approaches have been utilized, but therapies focused on the depressed patient's interpersonal functioning and cognitive distortions appear to be the most productive. Insight therapy is made difficult by the depressed patient's tendency to interpret therapeutic suggestions as criticism. Cognitive therapy is often didactic in nature and may profitably include "homework assignments" in which the patient is asked to critically examine and test erroneous assumptions deriving from the depressive experience. For example, a patient may say, "I fail at everything I try to do." Asking that patient to keep a log of daily tasks and document the outcome of each effort affords the therapist an effective means of challenging the patient's derogatory self-image. Testimony from others who are able to state that the tasks were performed satisfactorily can be sought if necessary (see Chapter 35).

Family and spouse involvement should not be neglected in treatment planning. This may take several forms, including education about the illness, emotional support, and consideration of interpersonal issues. Although prepubertal children with major depression who receive drug treatment usually show a return to normal functioning in areas such as school performance, ongoing deficits in peer and family relationships frequently continue and require specific intervention.

DYSTHYMIA

Symptoms & Signs

The term "dysthymia" was recently coined to denote in a specific operational way a group of patients formerly described as having "neurotic" or characterological depressions. Clinicians have long observed that such individuals experience chronic feelings of inadequacy and self-denigration and express these feelings in a dramatic manner that defies all attempts at treatment. Such patients describe a loss of interest or pleasure in most activities of daily life but do not have symptoms severe enough to meet the criteria for major depressive episode. Depressed mood may be unremitting or may alternate with short periods of normal mood lasting no longer than a few weeks. Dysthymic patients have a tendency to overreact to the normal stresses of life with depressive mood. They have low self-confidence but can be quite demanding and complaining, blaming others for their failures as much as they blame themselves. Obsessional traits are common. As a result of such attitudes, dysthymic patients tend to lead limited social lives and have unstable relationships with others. Abuse of alcohol and other drugs is common in this group of patients.

Natural History

Dysthymic patients often complain of having felt depressed throughout life. A specific time of onset usually cannot be identified or is described as having occurred very early in childhood or adolescence, with a subsequent history of many therapeutic interventions. In some cases, dysthymia seems to date from a major depressive episode.

Individuals with a characterological predisposition to depressive experience may also be subject to recurrences of major depressive episodes and thus have "double depression" at certain points in their lives. Poor self-esteem, hopelessness, and chronic anhedonia can be viewed as learned phenomena initiated and reinforced at critical junctures by the major depressive event. Since depressive symptoms are usually mild or moderate in severity, morbidity associated with major depression, such as suicide, is less common. Dysthymic patients are voracious consumers of medical and mental health care resources, and a history of participation in self-help organizations can often be obtained.

Differential Diagnosis

Dysthymia is easily distinguished from major depression on the basis of severity and chronicity. Occasionally, individuals with dysthymia experience periods of superimposed major depression, and both diagnoses are warranted during such periods. The personality characteristics of individuals with dysthymia are such that an additional diagnosis of personality disorder may be warranted. Again, both diagnoses should be recorded regardless of the hypothesized causal relationship between the two diagnoses.

The essential feature of this diagnosis is the chronic nature of the depressed mood. Although normal individuals experience mood states similar to what is noted in dysthymia, their depressions are not as persistent or generally as severe as is the case in dysthymic disorder, and there is no ongoing interference with personal or social functioning.

Prognosis

A broad range of impairment is associated with dysthymia. In some cases, social function and job performance are only mildly affected, while others are characterized by recurrent suicidal preoccupation and inability to sustain adequate performance at school or at work. Since the disorder undoubtedly encompasses a heterogeneous group of individuals, the prognosis depends upon the response to psychotherapy, antidepressant medication, or both together.

Illustrative Case

A 34-year-old unmarried computer programmer was referred for evaluation of chronic depression. He stated that he had felt depressed his "whole life" and that previous psychiatric treatment had been of no benefit. The past history revealed that the patient, who had no siblings, had been socially isolated and shy and had avoided participation in athletics and social events during high school. He had a dependent relationship with his mother following the divorce of his parents when he was 4 years old. His college career was uneventful. When asked how he came to choose computer science as a major, the patient replied that it was more "logical" and "real" and did not require participation in small seminar sections, in which he felt he performed poorly.

The patient's chief complaint was that "life is meaningless." He complained of hypersomnia but admitted he often went to sleep a few hours after returning from work because "there is nothing else to do and television is bad." He had no hobbies and stated that he did not like to try things where "I'll look bad." He had been involved in two therapeutic relationships, one lasting 4 months and the other 2 years. He stated that he enjoyed the experience, particularly the longer relationship, but did not feel treatment "really changed anything." He denied ever having experienced any periods of increased energy but did admit that he could "think of being suicidal" if his life did not improve soon.

Epidemiology

Because the term has only recently come into use, the prevalence of dysthymia is not known. Although defined more specifically than the older term "depressive neurosis," the disorder is common in the practice of most clinicians. Dysthymia is somewhat more prevalent in women. Information regarding genetic transmission with familial occurrence of the disorder is lacking, although it is believed that there may be a subgroup of individuals with dysthymia who are experiencing an attenuated form of a biologically based major depressive disorder.

Etiology & Pathogenesis

Biological and psychosocial theories of the causes of dysthymic disorder are similar to those discussed in the section on major depression, the chief distinction being that dysthymia presents as a less severe but more chronic syndrome.

Treatment

Psychotherapy is the principal treatment resource for patients with dysthymia, though a significant number of patients may benefit from a trial of an antidepressant drug or lithium carbonate. The guidelines for assessing the potential utility of drug therapy are a contributory family history and a past history of poor response to other forms of treatment.

Although individual psychotherapy is the most common psychosocial treatment offered, many individuals with dysthymia will benefit from group therapy and from active investigation and restructuring of maladaptive social functioning.

Psychotherapy with chronically depressed individuals is an emotionally draining process for the therapist, and recurrent examination of the therapist's own feelings toward the patient is required. Analysis of one's own anger, boredom, or frustration about some aspect of the patient's behavior can help to isolate the key issue in therapy and lead to symptomatic improvement. The patient's unrealistic and idealistic expectations of himself or herself may, for example, be transmitted to the therapist and give rise to overly optimistic expectations of progress in therapy. If the patient shows no subjective improvement over time, the therapist may inadvertently respond somewhat in the way significant individuals in the patient's life have responded. Interpretation of such personal experiences by the therapist can, in the proper context, be therapeutic.

"Short-term" focused psychotherapy and therapeutic programs that stress changes in interpersonal relationships and cognitive self-awareness are becoming more popular, in part because long-term analytic approaches to personality change are economically unfeasible. Family-centered approaches differ from individual methods in their direct focus on the "role of the sick member" in the family system rather than on the symptoms of the identified patient.

OTHER MOOD DISORDERS

1. BIPOLAR DISORDER NOS

Some individuals with bipolar disorder not otherwise specified experience episodes with manic features not severe enough or protracted enough to meet the criteria for a full manic episode. This syndrome is sometimes referred to as "bipolar II" and signifies a current complaint or history of major depressive episode coupled with a current complaint or history of hypomania. The mild form of mania is often socially acceptable and adaptive for the individual. Hypomanic individuals usually experience benefits from increased energy, decreased need for sleep, increased gregariousness, and greater creativity without the disabling consequences of grossly inappropriate social behavior or delusional preoccupation. Most hypomanic episodes do not call for pharmacological treatment; however, in specific cases a trial of lithium carbonate may be advisable. The subtle nature of many hypomanic episodes results in frequent misdiagnosis. Patients and clinicians alike may see such episodes as "normal" and view only the depressive episodes as pathological. Rarely, bipolar disorder not otherwise specified is used to refer to patients in whom a manic episode is superimposed on schizophrenia or delusional disorder.

2. DEPRESSIVE DISORDER NOS

Depressive disorder not otherwise specified is a diagnosis given to individuals whose depressive symptoms do not meet the criteria for severity or duration noted in the previously described categories. Individuals may experience occasional brief and mild episodes of depression not associated with psychosocial stress or may have dysthymia with periods of normal mood that last longer than several months. Because of the heterogeneous character of the diagnosis and its "by exclusion" feature, no meaningful data are available about prevalence, course, outcome, or treatment response.

Diagnostic problems may arise with depressed individuals whose mood change is either associated with or follows a psychotic process. The rationale for putting patients in this category rather than some other such as schizoaffective disorder (also poorly defined) is unclear (see Chapter 21).

Historically, the diagnosis of depressive disorder not otherwise specified has been most often used to denote individuals with mood disorder with prominent phobic and anxious features. Such individuals may respond to MAO inhibitor medication, though more research is needed.

SUMMARY

It is difficult to conceive of an area in psychiatry in which the clinician's attitude, knowledge, and skills are more severely tested than in the diagnosis and treatment of mood disorders. Knowledge in this area has been accumulating at such a rate that even the most diligent physician would be hard pressed to keep up with all of the new developments in the field. As reviewed in this chapter, there is considerable evidence for a biological basis for most mood disorders. Data supporting this hypothesis have come from genetic, biochemical, psychopharmacological, and neuroendocrinological investigations, and the hope is that psychiatric diagnosis in this area will become a more objective process as these research efforts continue.

Although subgroups of mood disorders seem relatively distinct from one another as described, in clinical practice there is often considerable overlap between symptoms of different disorders as well as ambiguity about which class a given individual belongs in. With the present state of knowledge, predictions about course of illness and response to treatment for patients with mood disorders remain as much an art as a science. Use of the biopsychosocial model in the understanding of mood disorders illustrates the awesome complexity of central nervous system regulation of affect but holds out promise of successful methods of treatment on many different levels.

REFERENCES

Akiskal HS: New insights into the nature and heterogeneity of mood disorders. J Clin Psychiatry 1989;50(Suppl No. 5):6.

Andreasen NC et al: The validation of the concept of endogenous depression. Arch Gen Psychiatry 1986;43:246.

Casper RC et al: Somatic symptoms in primary affective disorder. Arch Gen Psychiatry 1985;42: 1098.

Charney D, Menkes D, Heninger G: Receptor sensitivity and the mechanism of action of antidepressant treatment. Arch Gen Psychiatry 1981;38: 1160.

Consensus Development Panel: Mood disorders: Pharmacologic prevention of recurrences. Am J Psychiatry 1985;142:469.

Coryell W, Endicott J, Keller M: Outcome of patients with chronic affective disorder: A five-year follow-up. Am J Psychiatry 1990;147:12.

Elkin I et al: National Institute of Mental Health treatment of depression collaborative research program. Arch Gen Psychiatry 1989;46:971.

Farmer A, McGuffin P: The classification of the depressions. Br J Psychiatry 1989;155:437.

Frank E et al: Three-year outcomes for maintenance therapies in recurrent depression. Arch Gen Psychiatry 1990;47:1093.

Golinkoff M, Sweeney JA: Cognitive impairments in depression. J Affect Dis 1989;17:105.

Goodwin FK, Jamison KR (editors): *Manic-Depressive Illness*. Oxford Univ Press, 1990

Joyce PR, Paykel ES: Predictors of drug response in depression. Arch Gen Psychiatry 1989;46:89.

Karasu TB: Toward a clinical model of psychotherapy for depression: I. Systematic comparison of three psychotherapies. Am J Psychiatry 1990;147:133.

Katon W, Sullivan MD: Depression and chronic medical illness. J Clin Psychiatry 1990;51(Suppl No. 6):3.

Kupfer DJ, Frank E, Perel JM: The advantage of early treatment intervention in recurrent depression. Arch Gen Psychiatry 1989;46:771.

Meterissian GB, Bradwejn J: Comparative studies on the efficacy of psychotherapy, pharmacotherapy, and their combination in depression: Was adequate pharmacotherapy provided? J Clin Psychopharmacol 1989;9:334.

Nierenberg AA, Amsterdam JD: Treatment-resistant depression: Definition and treatment approaches. J Clin Psychiatry 1990;51(Suppl No. 6):39.

Paykel ES: Treatment of depression. Br J Psychiatry 1989;155:754.

Phillips KA et al: A review of the depressive personality. Am J Psychiatry 1990;147:830.

Post RM et al: Dysphoric mania. Arch Gen Psychiatry 1989;46:353.

Regier DA et al: One-month prevalence of mental disorders in the United States. Arch Gen Psychiatry 1988;45:977.

Rush AJ: Problems associated with the diagnosis of depression. J Clin Psychiatry 1990;51(Suppl No. 6):15.

Sargeant JK et al: Factors associated with 1-year outcome of major depression in the community. Arch Gen Psychiatry 1990;47:519.

Silverstone T, Romans-Clarkson S: Bipolar affective disorder: Causes and prevention of relapse. Br J Psychiatry 1989;154:321.

Tohen M, Waternaux CM, Tsuang MT: Outcome in mania: A 4-year prospective follow-up of 75 patients utilizing survival analysis. Arch Gen Psychiatry 1990;47:1106.

Weissman MM et al: The epidemiology of dysthymia in five communities: Rates, risks, comorbidity, and treatment. Am J Psychiatry 1988;145:815.

Wells KB et al: The functioning and well-being of depressed patients. JAMA 1989;262:914.

Zonderman AB, Costa PT, McCrae RR: Depression as a risk for cancer morbidity and mortality in a nationally representative sample. JAMA 1989;262:1191.

23

Anxiety Disorders

John H. Greist, MD, & James W. Jefferson, MD

Anxiety and fear are ubiquitous emotions. The terms anxiety and fear have specific and scientific meanings, but common usage has made them interchangeable. For example, a phobia is a kind of anxiety that is also defined in *DSM-III-R* as a "persistent or irrational fear." **Fear** is defined as an emotional and physiological response to a recognized external threat (eg, a runaway car or a steep descent in an airplane). **Anxiety** is an unpleasant emotional state, the sources of which are less readily identified. It is frequently accompanied by physiological symptoms that may lead to fatigue or even exhaustion. Because fear of recognized threats causes similar unpleasant mental and physical changes, patients use the terms fear and anxiety interchangeably. Thus, there is little need to strive to differentiate anxiety from fear. However, distinguishing among different anxiety disorders is important, since accurate diagnosis is more likely to result in effective treatment and a better prognosis.

The intensity of anxiety has many gradations ranging from minor qualms to noticeable trembling and even complete panic, the most extreme form of anxiety.

The course of anxiety also varies, with peak severity being reached within a few seconds or more gradually over minutes, hours, or days. Duration also varies from a few seconds to hours or even days or months, although episodes of panic usually abate within 10 minutes and seldom last more than 30 minutes.

The signs and symptoms of anxiety are detailed in the diagnostic criteria for the anxiety disorders (Tables 23–1 to 23–8).

If anxiety arises unexpectedly ('out of the blue'), it is called **spontaneous anxiety** (or if very intense, **spontaneous panic**). When anxiety occurs predictably in specific situations, it is called **phobic** or **situational anxiety** (or when extreme, **phobic** or **situational panic**). **Anticipatory anxiety** (or **anticipatory panic**) is the term used to describe anxiety triggered by the mere thought of particular situations.

The boundary between normal and pathological anxiety cannot be drawn with great precision or confidence. People sometimes seek treatment for anxiety that disappears before they can be seen. Physicians sometimes delay treatment until disruption of functioning is obvious or suffering is severe. These differences are understandable in the context of present knowledge regarding anxiety, attitudinal differences

of both patients and doctors about seeking and giving help, and the effectiveness of various treatments. When anxiety substantially impairs work style or social adjustment, most authorities agree that careful assessment is indicated and that treatment is likely to be worthwhile. Suffering itself is often justification for treatment, even if the person with anxiety can continue to function.

Anxiety commonly occurs as a manifestation of appropriate concern about medical and psychiatric disorders. Medical problems involving any body system can produce anxiety as a symptom. Drugs and dietary factors—particularly caffeine and alcohol—may also provoke anxiety.

Anxiety & Depression

At least three-fourths of patients with primary depression complain of feeling anxious, worried, or fearful. Extreme anxiety may occur in agitated depression in the form of anguished facial expressions; lip biting; picking at fingers, nails, or clothing; handwringing; constant pacing; and inability to sit quietly. Conversely, primary anxiety can be depressing in its own right. If anxiety persists, and particularly if it interferes with functioning, secondary depression is the rule rather than the exception. Some patients have both primary anxiety and primary depressive disorders. While most patients with anxiety or depression fall clearly into the respective *DSM-III-R* categories for anxiety or depression, differential diagnosis can be challenging and require several interviews, further evaluation, and trials of treatment.

Theories of Anxiety

A. Genetic: Isaac Marks (1986) has provided an elegant summary of the genetics of fear and anxiety disorders:

From protozoa to mammals, organisms have been selectively bred for genetic differences in defensive behaviour which are accompanied by differences in brain and other biological functions. Studies of twins indicate some genetic control of normal human fear from infancy onwards, of anxiety as a symptom and as a syndrome, and of phobic and obsessive compulsive phenomena. Anxiety disorders are more common among the relatives of affected probands than of controls, especially among female and first-degree relatives; alcoholism and secondary depression may also be overrepresented. Familial influences have been found for panic disorder, agoraphobia, and obsessive compulsive problems. Panic disorder in depressed probands increases the risk to their relatives of phobia as well as of panic disorder, major depression, and alcoholism. The strongest family history of all anxiety disorders is seen in blood-injury phobia; even though it can be successfully treated by exposure, its roots may lie in a genetically determined specific autonomic susceptibility. Some genetic effects can be modified by environmental means.

B. Psychodynamic: Although Freud at first proposed a physiological basis for anxiety, he later concluded that anxiety serves as a signal to the ego of the emergence of an unconscious conflict or impulse. His theory led to the development of psychoanalysis for the study and treatment of emotional disorders. According to psychoanalytic theory, anxiety is seen as an emotion of the ego (the part of our mental apparatus that balances the impulses and demands of our childlike id, the stern and punitive controls of our parentlike superego, and external reality). Anxiety is also seen as the key indication of hidden psychological conflict.

C. Learned: Behavioral therapists hold that anxiety is a learned response to some noxious stimulus. When a situation or stimulus provokes anxiety in a person who then avoids it, anxiety is diminished and the person learns to reduce anxiety by avoiding situations that provoke it. Generalized anxiety disorder may result from unpredictable positive and negative reinforcement—the person is uncertain which avoidance behaviors will be effective in reducing anxiety.

It is also possible to develop anxiety in response to generally positive or neutral stimuli if these are associated with a noxious or aversive stimulus. This conditioning process is held to be responsible for the avoidance of neutral or benign situations in which distressing anxiety (such as panic) has occurred. Pairing of a recurrent anxiety-inducing thought (such as "contamination") with a compulsive behavior (such as handwashing) that reduces anxiety is thought to explain the development of obsessive compulsive disorder.

D. Biochemical: When compared with normal controls, patients with anxiety disorders have significantly different physiological functioning (eg, higher heart rate, higher blood lactate levels, and greater oxygen debt during moderate exercise). Patients with panic disorders are more sensitive to a number of substances (eg, caffeine, lactate, isoproterenol, epinephrine, yohimbine, and piperoxan). Many of these substances increase activity of the locus ceruleus, the midbrain nucleus which supplies about 70% of the norepinephrine neurons in the central nervous system. Human subjects given these substances report increased anxiety, and monkeys demonstrate fear behaviors similar to those they show when placed in a confrontational setting. Electrical stimulation of the locus ceruleus in monkeys produces a similar fear response, while its ablation reduces fear behaviors. Medications that inhibit locus ceruleus functioning also reduce fear responses in monkeys and anxiety in humans with anxiety disorders as well as in controls. Although α_2 agonists and β-adrenergic receptor blockers have been shown to have some antianxiety properties, the heterocyclic and monoamine oxidase inhibitor antidepressants and benzodiazepine drugs, which down-regulate locus ceruleus (norepinephrine) function, are the most useful clinically.

The benzodiazepines have a second putative mode of action in that they potentiate gamma-aminobutyric acid (GABA), a widely distributed inhibitory neurotransmitter. Discovery of benzodiazepine receptors in the central nervous system led to a search for endogenous benzodiazepines, and these have now been found (see Chapter 5).

The apparent biochemical basis of every behavior, thought, and feeling does not dictate that biochemical abnormalities must be treated with chemicals—brain chemistry can also be changed by behavioral, psychological, and surgical interventions.

Epidemiology

In the recent National Institute of Mental Health epidemiologic catchment area (NIMH-ECA) study (Myers et al, 1984), anxiety disorders were more prevalent over the preceding 6 months than any other mental disorder (8.3% of the populations surveyed in their homes). Of those with anxiety disorders, only 23% were receiving treatment. Other studies have found similar or slightly lower rates of anxiety disorders. The lifetime prevalence of anxiety disorders is uncertain but is probably in the range of 15–25%.

PANIC DISORDER

The emphasis on panic disorder in *DSM-III-R* as an etiological factor in the development of agoraphobia is a reversal of the emphasis in *DSM-III*, which described "agoraphobia with panic attacks" as the most common phobic disorder. There is still substantial debate about the incidence and prevalence of panic episodes or attacks. The NIMH-ECA study found a 6-month prevalence of panic disorder of only 0.7%; the prevalence of agoraphobia was 2.8%. More than one-third of the population may have a panic-like episode during any given year, but fewer individuals develop panic disorder. According to *DSM-III-R*, a diagnosis of panic disorder requires either four panic attacks in a 4-week period or the development of fear, of at least 1 month's duration, of having another panic episode.

Symptoms & Signs

Table 23–1 lists *DSM-III-R* criteria for panic disorder. The distressing constellation of sudden and unpre-

Table 23–1. *DSM-III-R* diagnostic criteria for panic disorder.

Panic disorder:

A. At some time during the disturbance, one or more panic attacks (discrete periods of intense fear or discomfort) have occurred that were (1) unexpected, ie, did not occur immediately before or on exposure to a situation that almost always caused anxiety, and (2) not triggered by situations in which the person was the focus of others' attention.

B. Either 4 attacks, as defined in criterion A, have occurred within a 4-week period, or one or more attacks have been followed by a period of at least 1 month of persistent fear of having another attack.

C. At least 4 of the following symptoms developed during at least one of the attacks:
  (1) Shortness of breath (dyspnea) or smothering sensations.
  (2) Dizziness, unsteady feelings, or faintness.
  (3) Palpitations or accelerated heart rate (tachycardia).
  (4) Trembling or shaking.
  (5) Sweating.
  (6) Choking.
  (7) Nausea or abdominal distress.
  (8) Depersonalization or derealization.
  (9) Numbness or tingling sensations (paresthesias).
  (10) Flushes (hot flashes) or chills.
  (11) Chest pain or discomfort.
  (12) Fear of dying.
  (13) Fear of going crazy or of doing something uncontrolled.

Note: Attacks involving 4 or more symptoms are panic attacks; attacks involving fewer than 4 symptoms are limited symptom attacks (see Table 23–3).

D. During at least some of the attacks, at least 4 of the above symptoms developed suddenly and increased in intensity within 10 minutes of the beginning of the first symptom noticed in the attack.

E. It cannot be established that an organic factor initiated and maintained the disturbance, eg, amphetamine or caffeine intoxication, hyperthyroidism.

Note: Mitral valve prolapse may be an associated condition but does not preclude a diagnosis of panic disorder.

Panic disorder without agoraphobia:

A. Meets the criteria for panic disorder.

B. Absence of agoraphobia, as defined in Table 23–2 below.

Specify severity of panic attacks, as defined above.

---

dicted episodes involving pronounced alteration of physiological functions frequently leads to fears of death, "going crazy," or "doing something uncontrolled." Commonly, patients will experience eight or nine of the 13 symptoms. Panic attacks begin suddenly and usually abate within 10 minutes, rarely lasting 30 minutes or more. Patients may confuse panic with anticipatory anxiety early in the course of the disorder, although most become expert at distinguishing between the two as time passes. Moving about during a panic attack makes many individuals feel somewhat better, but avoidance of situations in which panic has occurred leads to the development of phobias.

Differential Diagnosis

Medical causes of anxiety should not be overlooked, nor should anxiety disorders be overinvestigated or treated as medical disorders. Most medical causes of anxiety symptoms are readily recognized if a careful history, physical examination, and indicated laboratory tests are performed.

Medical problems that may produce anxiety include those affecting the cardiovascular system (angina pectoris, acute myocardial infarction, arrhythmias, congestive heart failure, shock); respiratory problems (asthma, emphysema, pulmonary embolism); neurological disorders (encephalopathy, seizure disorder, benign essential tremor, vertigo); hematological and immunological disorders (anemia, anaphylactic shock); and endocrine dysfunction (diabetes, hypothyroidism, hyperthyroidism, parathyroid disease, Cushing's disease, pheochromocytoma).

Medications may also provoke anxiety symptoms. Antispasmodics, cold medicines, thyroid supplements, digitalis, stimulants, and—paradoxically—antianxiety and antidepressant medicines used to treat panic may all induce anxiety. Discontinuation of certain medications (eg, some blood pressure medicines, sleeping pills, and antianxiety drugs) may lead to withdrawal syndromes in which anxiety may be prominent. Caffeine, alcohol, and marihuana are frequent causes of anxiety symptoms, including panic.

Illustrative Case

A 30-year-old woman had experienced panic episodes since age 20. They usually began spontaneously, "out of the blue," although they often appeared in the context of anger or other emotional extremes of sadness or disappointment. She had awakened from sleep in panic on several occasions. Although she worried initially that the settings or circumstances in which panic occurred might be causing the episodes, she later concluded that no reliable pattern could be detected. She neither smoked nor used alcohol and had discontinued use of caffeine because it made her feel jittery.

Attacks were characterized by rapid heart rate, sweating, nausea, chills, trembling, and a fear of doing something uncontrolled. Early severe episodes had included symptoms associated with hyperventilation, including "smothering," choking, chest discomfort, faintness, and paresthesias, but once she recognized their association with overbreathing, she was able to control them by learning to breathe "slow and shallow."

The patient reported increased frequency but not severity of panic attacks in the premenstruum.

Family history was positive for similar episodes from ages 25 through 45 in her mother and for depression on both sides of her family.

After each of her first few attacks, the patient sought treatment in an emergency room or from her primary care physician, who had carefully examined her and, finding "nothing wrong," attempted to reassure her that her symptoms were a manifestation of anxiety. She had briefly used a benzodiazepine prescribed by her physician but objected to the "drugged" feeling it produced. Panic ceased for one 3-year period and occurred less than once per month for another 3 years. She remained, however, worried that panic could recur at any time. For the 2 years before she sought treatment, panic attacks had occurred at least twice per month. Imipramine in gradually increasing doses (see below) was prescribed, and at levels of 100 mg/d, panic attacks ceased for 6 months. They resumed when the dose was decreased to 75 mg/d.

Epidemiology

The NIMH-ECA study found a 6-month prevalence of panic disorder of only 0.7%, whereas agoraphobia was present in 2.8%. More than one-third of individuals may experience a single episode of panic in any given year. A much smaller proportion will have repeated panic attacks, and less than 1% will develop panic disorder. The peak age at onset of spontaneous panic is between 15 and 25 years, and panic beginning after age 40 would suggest depression or possible medical causes. There is some genetic basis for panic disorder, although many who experience panic attacks come from families with no history of anxiety. Women have been thought to have panic disorder twice as commonly as men, but some of this difference may be due to cultural factors that permit women, more than men, to complain about and seek treatment for symptoms of panic or anxiety.

Etiology & Pathogenesis

The underlying pathophysiology of panic disorder is far from clear. It is commonly held that panic disorder has a biochemical basis, but its precise characteristics have not been elucidated. Many authorities suspect that noradrenergic dysfunction, perhaps mediated through the locus ceruleus (Redmond, 1977), is involved, and drug treatments that alter this system have been shown to be of benefit. Panic appears pathogenetic for phobic complications of anticipatory anxiety and avoidance, which may persist after panic has abated.

There may be an association between early separation anxiety manifested by school avoidance and the later development of agoraphobia.

Treatment

Treatment is largely empirical, since etiological factors have not been clearly established.

A. Psychological Treatment: Many case reports and personal testimonials claim positive benefits from the many varieties of psychotherapy; no one type is clearly any more or less effective than another. In psychotherapy, as well as behavioral therapy and drug therapy, nonspecific factors common to any good patient-clinician relationship (eg, expectation of suc-

cess, belief in treatment, reassurance, encouragement, empathy) probably account for much of the improvement in anxiety disorders achieved with psychotherapeutic approaches.

Cognitive therapy (see Chapter 35) that attempts to modify catastrophic negative thoughts that may accompany panic attacks shows considerable promise and is now the subject of controlled investigations. Thus, an attempt can be made to help a patient whose train of thought runs, "My heart just skipped a beat and my chest feels tight, so I must be having a heart attack and will surely die," to reinterpret these physiological symptoms along a train of thought such as, "My heart just skipped a beat and my chest feels tight. These are familiar symptoms of panic. I can expect several other 'old friends' such as numbness and tingling of my fingers, feeling faint, shortness of breath, and trembling to appear soon. These are all symptoms of panic which I have been through many times before. Panic is unpleasant but not dangerous, and I know this attack will end soon." This reassignment of the physiological components of panic from life-threatening to familiar and manageable may help a larger proportion of patients than other psychotherapies. It also includes elements of exposure therapy (see below).

B. Behavioral Therapy: There is growing evidence that panic attacks can be substantially reduced in frequency and severity by the use of exposure therapy (see Chapter 35). Agoraphobic patients who experience spontaneous panic report marked reduction in the frequency and severity of panic when given exposure therapy without medication. In some studies, panic attacks have stopped altogether in two-thirds of patients. When hyperventilation is a substantial component of panic, teaching patients techniques to control it is often helpful. The voluntary induction of hyperventilation can be coupled with both education linking overbreathing with symptoms and instruction in diaphragmatic breathing. Patients who experience only panic without anticipatory anxiety and avoidance can be exposed, in fantasy or imagination, to the physiological aberrations associated with panic. Thus, they would be asked to imagine that the full constellation of panic symptoms is emerging just as it does during a panic attack and to continue that fantasy until associated anxiety dies down.

When panic attacks are accompanied by anticipatory anxiety and avoidance, exposure is the treatment of choice. Exposure can be simply taught in an office setting in as little as 5 minutes. The patient is instructed to "find and face the things you fear and remain in contact with them until your anxiety subsides." The therapist must reiterate the instruction as treatment progresses and monitor compliance with written records kept by the patient for mutually agreed-upon exposure tasks. Homework assignments constitute the bulk of exposure tasks, and enlistment of a family member or friend who can serve as cotherapist is often helpful. A self-help chapter in a book authored by Greist et al (1986) has been shown to be as effective as sessions with a behavioral therapist in treating individuals with agoraphobia.

C. Drug Therapy: Many consider medications to be the cornerstone of panic disorder treatment (see Chapter 32). Most antidepressants (tricyclics, monoamine oxidase inhibitors, and others) substantially reduce the frequency and severity of panic attacks and often prevent them altogether. They work even if depression is not present. Benzodiazepine anxiolytics are also effective antipanic drugs (alprazolam is the best-studied example but does not appear to be unique) and work more quickly than the antidepressants although they carry a risk of dependence. All antipanic drugs should be started at low dosages and increased gradually until an effective dosage level is achieved. Relapse is the rule rather than the exception when antipanic drugs are discontinued; fortunately, their long-term use appears to be safe in most cases.

While sometimes of ancillary benefit, β-adrenergic blocking agents (eg, propranolol) are not as effective as the above-mentioned drugs. Antipsychotics, barbiturates, meprobamate, and antihistamines are not recommended for treatment of panic attacks.

A combination of medication and behavior therapy is most beneficial for many patients. When the two therapies are combined, relapse rates following medication withdrawal may be substantially lower.

AGORAPHOBIA

Symptoms & Signs

The diagnostic criteria for panic disorder with agoraphobia are listed in Table 23–2. Table 23–3 lists the diagnostic criteria for agoraphobia without a history of panic disorder. Agoraphobia is a fear of being caught in a situation from which a graceful and speedy escape to safety would be difficult or embarrassing

Table 23–2. *DSM-III-R* diagnostic criteria for panic disorder with agoraphobia.

A. Meets the criteria for panic disorder.
B. Agoraphobia: Fear of being in places or situations from which escape might be difficult (or embarrassing) or in which help might not be available in the event of a panic attack. (Include cases in which persistent avoidance behavior originated during an active phase of panic disorder, even if the person does not attribute the avoidance behavior to fear of having a panic attack.) As a result of this fear, the person either restricts travel or needs a companion when away from home or else endures agoraphobic situations despite intense anxiety. Common agoraphobic situations include being outside the home alone, being in a crowd or standing in a line, being on a bridge, and traveling in a bus, train, or car.

Specify current severity of agoraphobic avoidance.

Specify current severity of panic attacks.

Table 23–3. *DSM-III-R* diagnostic criteria for agoraphobia without history of panic disorder.

A. Agoraphobia: Fear of being in places or situations from which escape might be difficult (or embarrassing) or in which help might not be available in the event of suddenly developing a symptom(s) that could be incapacitating or extremely embarrassing. Examples include dizziness or falling, depersonalization or derealization, loss of bladder or bowel control, vomiting, or cardiac distress. As a result of this fear, the person either restricts travel or needs a companion when away from home or else endures agoraphobic situations despite intense anxiety. Common agoraphobic situations include being outside the home alone, being in a crowd or standing in a line, being on a bridge, and traveling in a bus, train, or car.
B. Has never met the criteria for panic disorder.

Specify with or without limited symptom attacks.

if the patient felt discomfort (often in the form of panic). Situations likely to induce fear and avoidance include attendance at auditoriums, eating out (especially at formal sit-down restaurants), shopping in supermarkets, lines, public transportation and driving under conditions where opportunities to pull over, stop, or get off the highway quickly may be restricted. Being accompanied by a trusted family member or friend permits many agoraphobic individuals to increase the number of possibly uncomfortable situations they can endure and to extend the range of their excursions.

For those who panic, fear of fainting during an attack is the most common fear after fear of panic itself. Hyperventilation with its attendant decreases in blood carbon dioxide, ionized calcium, and phosphorus produces paresthesias, light-headedness, visual changes, and feelings of unreality that contribute to the fear of fainting. Actual fainting must be exceedingly rare, since none of the patients seen by the authors has fainted during a panic attack.

By definition, phobias are irrational fears involving avoidance of objects or situations that are extremely unlikely to cause harm and that most people approach without discomfort. Agoraphobic patients lament their inability to face everyday situations and often become discouraged, depressed, and demoralized by the constriction in their lives caused by agoraphobia.

Differential Diagnosis

Avoidance or withdrawal can occur in depression, schizophrenic disorders, and paranoid disorders, some organic mental disorders, other anxiety disorders (eg, social or simple phobia, obsessive compulsive disorder, and posttraumatic stress disorder), and certain personality disorders. This avoidance occurs in the context of other symptoms and signs that usually clarify the underlying diagnosis. A few simple questions (also useful with other anxiety disorders) are likely to point to or away from a diagnosis of agoraphobia:

(1) Are there situations or things you avoid? What are they? (Agoraphobic patients are likely to describe situations in which they would feel caught or trapped.)

(2) What do you feel will happen if you cannot avoid (the situations described in Question 1)? (Expect agoraphobic patients to describe fears of panic, fainting, "going crazy," or dying.)

(3) Do your fears seem exaggerated or out of proportion? (Most agoraphobic patients clearly recognize the unreasonableness of their fears and frequently describe them with words such as dumb, stupid, crazy, goofy, irrational.)

(4) If you must face (avoided situations), how do you bring yourself to do it? (Agoraphobic patients usually describe anticipatory anxiety that leads to excuses to avoid the situation or frank refusal to proceed; frequent requests that others accompany them; or use of alcohol or other sedatives to decrease anxiety.)

(5) Have you ever had the experience of anxiety decreasing if you could not leave the uncomfortable situation for a long time? (Most agoraphobic patients have found themselves in such situations from time to time, and most report a reduction in anxiety with this fortuitous exposure therapy.)

Prognosis

Agoraphobia may remit spontaneously, particularly if panic attacks abate or if life circumstances force or encourage patients to go about their business. Typically, untreated agoraphobia runs a chronic and undulating course with periods of relative exacerbation and remission and with major incapacity associated with anticipatory anxiety and avoidance. Alcohol and other substance abuse becomes a problem for a small proportion of agoraphobic patients who derive initial beneficial antianxiety effects from these substances, rely increasingly upon them, and develop both psychological and physiological dependence.

Agoraphobia can have devastating effects on both sufferers and their families. Roles within the family often change dramatically. For example, spouses work fewer hours after their partners develop the disorder, because of increased family responsibilities. Agoraphobia frequently leads to discouragement and complaints of tension, fatigue, obsessions, and depression.

With treatment, some individuals are cured, and most make substantial gains and resume their previous occupational and social roles with minor residual anxiety. A very small number of agoraphobic patients fail to respond to behavioral and drug treatments.

Illustrative Case

A 23-year-old woman who had experienced panic while driving on an expressway on three separate occasions became worried about driving on the expressway again; worrying about it brought on another panic attack. She stopped driving on the expressway but still experienced extreme anxiety in other situations, such as standing in a supermarket checkout line, sitting in church or under a hair dryer at the beauty parlor, where means of egress were not readily available. She became increasingly worried about panic attacks and avoided more and more settings where they might occur and leave her feeling helpless. She was able to continue working only because a trusted friend conveyed her to and from work.

After reading about agoraphobia in a magazine, she recognized her disorder and sought treatment. Careful history taking revealed that she had last experienced panic 3 months before coming to the clinic but worried about attacks almost constantly (anticipatory anxiety). Treatment was begun with exposure therapy, and she made rapid gains in the range of her activities while experiencing progressively less discomfort. Panic attacks did not recur either in the treatment setting or spontaneously, and at 1-year follow-up she had regained her full range of activities, although she still worried somewhat that panic attacks might recur.

Epidemiology

The NIMH-ECA study reported a 6-month prevalence of agoraphobia of 3.8% for women and 1.8% for men. Some of the higher prevalence in females may be culturally determined. The age at onset peaks in the early 20s, and onset after age 40 is uncommon.

Before agoraphobia begins, people who will develop the disorder and those who will not are similar in terms of social or marital status, marital and sexual adjustment, separation anxiety, dependency, and other personality characteristics. After agoraphobia occurs, many of these attributes change for the worse.

Etiology & Pathogenesis

There is growing evidence that an agoraphobic trait disorder may be inherited. In two studies, specific severe trauma preceded the onset of agoraphobia in only 3% and 8% of people, respectively. However, less severe life stress events were reportedly twice as common in agoraphobic patients as in controls.

Commonly, panic leads to anticipatory anxiety of another panic in the same situation which, in turn, leads to avoidance of that situation. Many patients report this sequence (and would therefore be diagnosed as having panic disorder), but others develop classical agoraphobic avoidance without ever experiencing panic. In some, panic occurs after entering agoraphobic situations (situational or phobic panic). The exact role of panic in the etiology of agoraphobia remains unresolved and is the subject of continuing study.

Treatment

A. Psychological Treatment: The effectiveness of specific psychotherapies for treatment of agoraphobia has not been established. All therapies (including medications and behavioral therapy) should include nonnonspecific but important elements of education and support; this may partly explain the improvement sometimes seen with psychotherapy.

B. Behavioral Therapy: Exposure therapy is the single most effective treatment for agoraphobia with and without panic attacks. Panic, anticipatory anxiety, and avoidance are all reduced by this straightforward approach when it is systematically applied according to simple instructions that many patients can put into practice by themselves or with the help of a family member or friend. Patients are also given suggestions for "coping tactics" to be used when anxiety rises to disturbing levels. Over the past decade, the average number of contact hours spent with an experienced behavioral therapist in the successful treatment of agoraphobia has declined from nearly 20 to less than 4. Patients using exposure therapy develop a new attitude toward the fears they experience and the risks they are willing to take regarding those fears. This change often spreads to other aspects of their functioning, with beneficial results.

C. Drug Treatment: When panic is present, drug treatment is often indicated (see Panic Disorder, above). In the absence of panic, exposure therapy alone is usually sufficient. Some patients have pronounced anticipatory anxiety when they begin exposure therapy; such patients may be given antianxiety medications. The lowest effective dose should be used, since some individuals may fail to learn how to deal effectively with anxiety-causing stimuli when no longer under the influence of anxiolytics. (This phenomenon is known as state-dependent learning, in which what is learned in the drugged state does not generalize to the undrugged state. There is also a risk of dependence on anxiolytics.

SOCIAL PHOBIA

Symptoms & Signs

The *DSM-III-R* diagnostic criteria for social phobia are listed in Table 23–4. Individuals with social phobia have a persistent and recognizably irrational fear of embarrassment or humiliation when performing in social situations. They fear that their performance will be found wanting in some way and lead to embarrassment or humiliation.

Whereas some anxiety can provide people with a performance-enhancing "edge," social phobia is performance anxiety of such great proportions that it interferes with performance. Social phobia can be quite specific (eg, public speaking) or may be generalized to all social aspects of the individual's life.

Individuals asked to face their particular type of social phobia describe anticipatory anxiety and may experience situational panic attacks. Avoidance is a common complication of social phobia.

Table 23–4. *DMS-III-R* diagnostic criteria for social phobia.

A. A persistent fear of one or more situations (the social phobic situations) in which the person is exposed to possible scrutiny by others and fears that he or she may do something or act in a way that will be humiliating or embarrassing. Examples include being unable to continue talking while speaking in public, choking on food when eating in front of others, being unable to urinate in a public lavatory, experiencing hand trembling when writing in the presence of others, and saying foolish things or not being able to answer questions in social situations.

B. If an axis III or another axis I disorder is present, the fear in criterion A, above, is unrelated to it, eg, the fear is not of having a panic attack (panic disorder), stuttering (stuttering), trembling (Parkinson's disease), or exhibiting abnormal eating behavior (anorexia nervosa or bulimia nervosa).

C. During some phase of the disturbance, exposure to the specific phobic stimulus (or stimuli) almost invariably provokes an immediate anxiety response.

D. The phobic situation(s) is avoided or endured with intense anxiety.

E. The avoidant behavior interferes with occupational functioning or with usual social activities or relationships with others, or there is marked distress about having the fear.

F. The person recognizes that his or her fear is excessive or unreasonable.

Specify generalized type if the phobic situation is most social situations, and also consider the additional diagnosis of avoidant personality disorder.

Differential Diagnosis

Marked anxiety and avoidance of social situations may occur in schizophrenia, major depression, obsessive compulsive disorder, and paranoid and avoidant personality disorders. However, the reasons given for such avoidance and anxiety are closely tied to content appropriate for those specific disorders and seldom involve embarrassment or humiliation. For example, a patient who is paranoid may avoid social situations because of delusional fear of being harmed. Substance abuse may occur in a misguided attempt at self-treatment.

Prognosis

Mild social phobias seldom interfere with functioning but may consign sufferers to repeated discomfort when in their phobic situations. More severe social phobia frequently interferes substantially with functioning and causes great suffering. Individuals with social phobia sometimes change professions to avoid situations that give rise to performance anxiety.

Illustrative Case

A medical student ranking in the top 10% of his class sought treatment before making a decision to drop out of medical school during the first clinical rotation in his third year. He had always experienced extreme anxiety whenever called upon to speak in class and had successfully avoided such presentations through high school, college, and the first 2 years of medical school. He had taken pains to select a medical school where he thought formal oral presentations were not required. At the beginning of his junior year, he was informed that he would have to make a "medical advances" presentation 4 months later. Although he quickly developed the topic and was confident of his material, he felt that he could not face the ordeal of making the presentation. Anticipatory anxiety had already begun to mount to a level that interfered with his sleep and performance on the wards.

The student reported that his father had similar anxiety and had given up a career in law for work as an accountant because of his anxiety in mock court during law school.

Treatment was begun with a combination of exposure therapy (videotape feedback) and drug therapy (a beta-blocker). Within 2 weeks (four exposure sessions), the student's anticipatory anxiety abated substantially, and he reported enjoyment of his newfound confidence and improved performance in public speaking. His presentation was a success, and he continued to feel and function well through the rest of medical school.

Epidemiology

Many individuals with social phobia were shy as children; however, most shy children do not develop social phobia. Age at onset is usually around puberty, with peak presentation for treatment in the 20s and few new cases emerging after age 30. Males are almost as likely as females to experience social phobia (the NIMH-ECA study 6-month prevalence is 1.3% for males and 1.7% for females).

Etiology & Pathogenesis

The specific cause of social phobia is unknown. A family history is often discovered, although the relative contributions of heredity and environment have not been determined. As with other phobias, avoidance in a misguided attempt at self-treatment probably increases severity of symptoms and perpetuates dysfunction (Greist et al, 1980).

Treatment

A. Psychotherapy: Many individuals suffering from social and other phobias continue to receive analytic and other dynamic psychotherapies with the ambitious goal of uncovering and working through unconscious psychological causes of the anxiety disorder. There is little research support for the effectiveness of these approaches for phobic disorders. Their continued use in the face of evidence supporting more effective treatments indicates that many clinicians find it difficult to abandon models learned while in training.

B. Behavioral Therapy: Exposure therapy with videotape feedback and in fantasy (for situations that are difficult to produce in real life) is helpful to many individuals with fear of public speaking and other forms of social phobia. At times, paradoxic exaggera-

tion of the feared performance will *decrease* anxiety (eg, asking a patient with fear of writing illegibly to write more illegibly). Although many individuals with social phobias have become convinced that they cannot face their feared situation, a few exposure treatments usually reverse this misapprehension.

C. Drug Treatment: Beta-adrenergic blocking drugs are often helpful in decreasing such peripheral symptoms of anxiety as tremor, tachycardia, and sweating. They may be used in a single dose 1 hour or more before entering situations likely to invoke social phobia. Benzodiazepine antianxiety drugs are sometimes used in combination with beta-blockers. Monoamine oxidase inhibitor antidepressants (usually phenelzine) have been shown to be helpful in treating social phobia, though they must be used regularly and require a diet low in tyramine.

Frequently, a combination of exposure therapy and beta-blocking drugs works well, and patients who have experienced years of disability are helped to substantially higher levels of functioning in a few weeks.

SIMPLE PHOBIA

Symptoms & Signs, Differential Diagnosis, & Prognosis

Simple phobia is something of a misnomer. While less incapacitating than agoraphobia or social phobia, simple phobias can have major effects on sufferers lives. The terms specific phobia and single phobia convey the concept more clearly without diminishing the potential impact of this disorder.

The most common phobic objects or situations that invoke single phobias are snakes, spiders, heights, elevators and other small closed spaces, and flying. Fewer individuals seek treatment for single phobias than for agoraphobia and social phobia, both because many single phobias remit spontaneously and because it is easier to avoid a single phobic situation than the multiple situations often associated with agoraphobia and social phobia.

Flying phobia can cause significant morbidity for those who need to travel because of their work and substantial inconvenience for those who must use surface transportation to cover long distances. Occasionally, insect phobias reach such proportions that individuals remain indoors during the season when the feared insect is active (as with bees). Blood-injury phobia, while less common than some other single phobias, is of particular interest because it commonly causes fainting. While agoraphobic individuals often fear fainting but seldom if ever faint, individuals with blood-injury phobia actually faint owing to vasovagal syncope when exposed to their phobic stimulus. Brought on by sight, experience or discussion of

Table 23–5. *DSM-III-R* diagnostic criteria for simple phobia.

A. A persistent fear of a circumscribed stimulus (object or situation), other than fear of having a panic attack (as in panic disorder), or of humiliation or embarrassment in certain social situations (as in social phobia).
B. During some phase of the disturbance, exposure to the specific phobic stimulus (or stimuli) almost invariably provokes an immediate anxiety response.
C. The object or situation is avoided or endured with intense anxiety.
D. The fear or the avoidant behavior significantly interferes with the person's normal routine or with usual social activities or relationships with others, or there is marked distress about having the fear.
E. The person recognizes that his or her fear is excessive or unreasonable.
F. The phobic stimulus is unrelated to the content of the obsessions of obsessive compulsive disorder or the trauma of posttraumatic stress disorder.

blood, operations, injuries, or even minor pain, blood injury phobia can lead to long-term avoidance of visits to physicians and dentists as well as other situations that have induced fainting. The *DSM-III-R* diagnostic criteria for simple phobia are listed in Table 23–5.

Since individuals with single phobia can usually successfully avoid their feared object or situation ('I know where spiders hang out, so I stay away from those places'), few experience pervasive anxiety. When such individuals know they must face the source of their phobia, they develop anticipatory anxiety, and when they encounter that source, either intentionally or inadvertently, a situational panic indistinguishable from spontaneous panic often occurs.

Differential diagnosis is seldom a problem because of the specific nature of the phobia. Some flying phobia is actually agoraphobia in which the individual fears confinement in the plane's cabin without means of ready egress.

Illustrative Case

A 32-year-old man presented for treatment because he had fainted every time he had had blood drawn since age 12. This experience led to fearful avoidance of doctors and venipuncture in this otherwise healthy and physically fit individual. He sought treatment because he avoided routine health monitoring and might find it difficult to seek care for acute medical problems. He also reported embarrassment about his inability to have blood drawn without fainting unless recumbent. His mother and maternal grandfather also experienced fainting with minor pain.

Epidemiology, Etiology, Pathogenesis, & Treatment

Single phobias are the most common anxiety disorders. Peak onset is in childhood (fears of strangers, large animals, snakes, the dark, and injury are very common), and a rapid and spontaneous resolution

of most of these phobias is the rule, probably because of developmental maturation and natural exposure. In the past, many of these fears had actual survival value for comparatively defenseless small children and would not have been diagnosed as phobias. Their atavistic persistence leads to their definition as phobias. The vast majority of such fears abate without formal treatment. The NIMH-ECA study found that 4.3% of males and 7% of females met *DSM-III* diagnostic criteria for simple phobia. That learning plays a part in some single phobias is most dramatically illustrated by epidemic anxiety (or mass hysteria), such as widespread fainting in schoolgirls after one of their number has fainted.

Treatment of single phobia with exposure therapy is highly successful. Spider phobia, for example, can often be alleviated in a single 2-hour session. One or two "booster" sessions are a prudent follow-up procedure. Patients with flying phobia can be successfully treated in one or two flights in a small plane in which an experienced pilot repeatedly exposes patients to specific phobic stimuli (eg, takeoffs and landings, particular maneuvers, turbulence) until anxiety diminishes to comfortable levels. Blood-injury phobia should first be treated with the patient recumbent; patients seldom faint when recumbent even if bradycardia occurs. Gradual exposure to the evoking stimulus (e.g. a needle) at a rate that does not produce bradycardia is the preferred treatment technique for blood-injury phobia. Most venipuncture phobias can be treated successfully in one or two sessions in a blood-drawing facility.

OBSESSIVE COMPULSIVE DISORDER

Symptoms & Signs

Obsessions are repetitive, intrusive ideas, images, or impulses. Obsessions commonly focus on harming others, acquiring or spreading contamination, doubt about having performed routine tasks properly, and transgressing social norms (eg, making unacceptable sexual overtures).

Compulsive rituals are repetitive acts usually performed reluctantly. The acts may be sensible in the abstract, but the frequency and duration of their repetition make them repugnant and inconvenient, even incapacitating. Attempts are usually made to resist rituals, although children and those who have been performing rituals for years may not resist. If prevented from carrying out a ritual, obsessive compulsive individuals frequently (typically) become anxious. Rituals are usually preceded by obsessions, but obsessions do not always lead to rituals. Rituals of cleaning, repeating, checking, tidying, hoarding, and avoiding may consume almost every waking hour. See Table 23–6 for the *DSM-III-R* diagnostic criteria for obsessive compulsive disorder.

Table 23–6. *DSM-III-R* diagnostic criteria for obsessive compulsive disorder (or obsessive compulsive neurosis).

A. Either obsessions or compulsions:

Obsessions: (1), (2), (3), and (4):

(1) Recurrent and persistent ideas, thoughts, impulses, or images that are experienced, at least initially, as intrusive and senseless, eg, a parent's having repeated impulses to kill a loved child, a religious person's having recurrent blasphemous thoughts.
(2) The person attempts to ignore or suppress such thoughts or impulses or to neutralize them with some other thought or action.
(3) The person recognizes that the obsessions are the product of his or her own mind, not imposed from without (as in thought disorder).
(4) If another axis I disorder is present, the content of the obsession is unrelated to it, ie, the ideas, thoughts, impulses, or images are not about food in the presence of an eating disorder, about drugs in the presence of a psychoactive substance use disorder, or guilty thoughts in the presence of a major depression.

Compulsions: (1), (2), and (3):

(1) Repetitive, purposeful, and intentional behavior performed in response to an obsession, or according to certain rules or in a stereotyped fashion.
(2) The behavior is designed to neutralize or to prevent discomfort or some dreaded event or situation; however, either the activity is not connected in a realistic way with what it is designed to neutralize or prevent, or it is clearly excessive.
(3) The individual recognizes that his or her behavior is excessive or unreasonable (this may not be true for young children; it may no longer be true for people whose obsessions have evolved into overvalued ideas).
B. The obsessions or compulsions cause marked distress, are time-consuming (take more than an hour a day), or significantly interfere with the person's normal routine, occupational functioning, or usual social activities or relationships with others.

Differential Diagnosis

A classical picture of obsessive compulsive disorder can emerge as a secondary complication of major depression. Obsessions alone may appear in the context of either depression or schizophrenia, and the distinction between obsessions and delusions can be difficult. There is a tendency to overdiagnose delusions and underdiagnose obsessions. Other attributes of schizophrenia are usually absent in patients with obsessive compulsive disorder, although some of these patients also suffer from schizotypal personality disorder, which worsens the prognosis.

Obsessive compulsive disorder can usually be differentiated from phobias in the following ways:

(1) Phobics are more fearful about confronting the feared object than are obsessive compulsives, who are usually more concerned about the rituals they will face because of contact with the feared object.
(2) The fears of phobics are usually less complex than those of obsessive compulsives. Phobic fears

are more typically focal (eg, fear of fainting while having blood drawn) than those of obsessive compulsives (there are myriad ways one can become contaminated).

(3) Anxiety of phobics is usually greater than that exhibited by obsessive compulsives when both confront the things they fear.

So-called "compulsive" behaviors such as gambling, drinking, eating, and paraphilic sexual behavior are not true compulsions because they usually provide pleasure.

Prognosis

Dysfunction is defined in terms of the amount of time consumed by obsessions and rituals, interference with functioning, control over obsessions and rituals, and the amount of suffering endured. The disorder usually lasts for decades once it has begun and runs an undulating course, worsening if the individual becomes depressed and temporarily improving if the individual can successfully avoid obsessions that provoke rituals. However, such relief is usually short-lived, as new obsessions and corresponding rituals replace those that have disappeared. At its worst, obsessive compulsive disorder can consume the individual and interfere in a major way with family functioning.

Illustrative Case

Ten years before she sought treatment, a 31-year-old registered nurse noted gradual onset of fears that she would contaminate needles or intravenous apparatus. Nine years before treatment, she changed from inpatient to outpatient nursing because of constant doubt about her skill in safely performing common nursing tasks. For intramuscular injections, she would aspirate two or three times before injecting medication to ensure that the needle was not in a blood vessel. Cleaning instruments was an ordeal because she often repeated the procedure to ensure sterility and still felt anxious about the possibility of contamination. She repeatedly asked for reassurance from physicians regarding the safety of air bubbles in syringes. At this point, her worries were confined to work. As her anxiety and uncertainty in outpatient work increased, she left clinical medicine and became a claims adjuster in an insurance company. Her quest for accuracy led to checking and rechecking of coding, which interfered substantially with the quantity of work performed and produced feelings of guilt about not working to full potential.

As years passed, her concerns spread to the home setting and her person. She worried that she had become soiled by urine and feces, and this led to rituals of repeatedly washing her body and clothing. The latter then became impossible because she felt that she might have put feces, instead of soap, into the washing machine. This "grotesque" thought continued until she was treated with a combination of exposure therapy (she no longer permitted herself to wear gloves or use tissues when touching the telephone, doorknobs, etc) and response prevention, in which she was asked to delay her washing and checking rituals for 3 hours after exposure sessions. With these behavioral treatments, her symptoms diminished rapidly and dramatically, so that she eventually experienced little interference with everyday activities. Common heterocyclic antidepressants had not modified her anxiety or rituals at all, but clomipramine, administered after improvement due to behavior therapy had stabilized, yielded further worthwhile gains.

Epidemiology

In one-third of obsessive compulsive individuals, onset of the disorder occurs by the age of 15. A second peak of incidence occurs during the third decade of life. Once established, obsessive compulsive disorder is likely to persist throughout life with varying degrees of severity. Men are only slightly less likely to suffer this disorder than women. Six-month prevalence of obsessive compulsive disorder in the NIMH-ECA study was approximately 1.5%, and the lifetime prevalence was 2.5%.

Etiology & Pathogenesis

Obsessive compulsive disorder clusters in families and appears to have a partly hereditary basis.

Once an obsessive thought intrudes, the forces maintaining its recurrence are uncertain. Efforts to demonstrate meaningful linkages between obsessions and unconscious conflict have failed to yield useful treatment techniques or to persuade many psychiatrists that such hypotheses have anything to do with the cause or pathogenesis of the disorder. A more credible behavioral explanation is that once the anxiety or discomfort associated with obsessive thought begins, sufferers gain at least temporary partial relief by performing rituals that are tied in a quasilogical way to their obsessions. However, the rituals must be performed to great excess.

The biochemical and anatomic bases of obsessive compulsive disorder have not been fully defined, but exploratory research suggests that they may involve dysfunction of serotonin neurotransmission in the orbital gyri and caudate nuclei.

Treatment

A. Behavioral Therapy: Behavioral therapy employing exposure and prevention of ritualistic responses yields a 60–80% reduction in symptoms for the three-fourths of patients who are able to comply with treatment instructions. Family members are often included as co-therapists. They are instructed to praise the patient when appropriate and to refrain from giving the patient counterproductive reassurance. Many obsessive compulsives become "reassurance junkies" in their quest for certainty; reassurance can be viewed as a ritual avoidance of the anxiety associated with

uncertainty. Behavioral therapy for these patients essentially involves asking them to run the same risks of contamination, uncertainty, and doubt that confront everyone and to stop performing rituals as an excessively costly and ineffective method of gaining transient and illusory certainty of safety.

B. Drug Therapy:

1. Antidepressants–Most antidepressants do not appear to have specific anti-obsessive compulsive properties, but clomipramine does have anti-obsessive compulsive effects independent of its antidepressant properties. Other serotonin uptake-inhibiting agents have also shown promise.

2. Anxiolytics–Antianxiety medications have a limited role in the long-term treatment of obsessive compulsive disorder but are sometimes helpful in the management of acute anxiety.

3. Antipsychotic drugs–Antipsychotic medications are unlikely to be beneficial except for patients with concurrent tics or schizotypal personality disorder.

C. Other Treatment:

1. Electroconvulsive therapy–Electroconvulsive therapy is sometimes helpful in individuals with severe primary depression and secondary obsessions and rituals but it is seldom necessary for patients with mild secondary depression.

2. Psychotherapy– Some obsessive compulsive patients are still treated with dynamic psychotherapy, often for many years, without manifest relief or improvement in functioning. Psychotherapists often point to "intrapsychic" benefits in patients who remain as troubled with obsessions and rituals as when therapy began. While unfortunate, this example of difficulty in changing treatment methods in the face of strong evidence supporting an effective alternative approach has long been recognized (Kuhn, 1962).

3. Psychosurgery–Stereotactic limbic leucotomy (Kelly, 1980) has been shown to be of some benefit in more than 80% of obsessive compulsive patients who have failed to benefit from other treatments.

POSTTRAUMATIC STRESS DISORDER

Symptoms & Signs

The *DSM-III-R* diagnostic criteria for posttraumatic stress disorder are presented in Table 23–7. Many people experience a psychologically traumatic stressor "outside the range of usual human experience," but few develop posttraumatic stress disorder. Many of those subjected to psychologically traumatic stressors reexperience them in dreams or memory with associated unpleasant feelings; changes in affect and reexperiencing of trauma usually diminish in frequency and intensity (just as recall of pleasant events does)

Table 23–7. *DSM-III-R* diagnostic criteria for posttraumatic stress disorder.

A. The person has experienced an event that is outside the range of usual human experience and that would be markedly distressing to almost anyone, eg, serious threat to one's life or physical integrity; serious threat or harm to one's children, spouse, or other close relatives or friends; sudden destruction of one's home or community; or seeing another person who has recently been, or is being, seriously injured or killed as the result of an accident or physical violence.

B. The traumatic event is persistently reexperienced in at least one of the following ways:
   (1) Recurrent and intrusive distressing recollections of the event (in young children, repetitive play in which themes or aspects of the trauma are expressed).
   (2) Recurrent distressing dreams of the event.
   (3) Sudden acting or feeling as if the traumatic event were recurring (includes a sense of reliving the experience, illusions, hallucinations, and dissociative [flashback] episodes, even those that occur upon awakening or when intoxicated).
   (4) Intense psychologic distress at exposure to events that symbolize or resemble an aspect of the traumatic event, including anniversaries of the trauma.

C. Persistent avoidance of stimuli associated with the trauma or numbing of general responsiveness (not present before the trauma), as indicated by at least 3 of the following:
   (1) Efforts to avoid thoughts or feelings associated with the trauma.
   (2) Efforts to avoid activities or situations that arouse recollections of the trauma.
   (3) Inability to recall an important aspect of the trauma (psychogenic amnesia).
   (4) Markedly diminished interest in significant activities (in young children, loss of recently acquired developmental skills such as toilet training or language skills).
   (5) Feeling of detachment or estrangement from others.
   (6) Restricted range of affect, eg, unable to have loving feelings.
   (7) Sense of a foreshortened future, eg, child does not expect to have a career, marriage, children, or a long life.

D. Persistent symptoms of increased arousal (not present before the trauma), as indicated by at least 2 of the following:
   (1) Difficulty falling or staying asleep.
   (2) Irritability or outbursts of anger.
   (3) Difficulty concentrating.
   (4) Hypervigilance.
   (5) Exaggerated startle response.
   (6) Physiologic reactivity upon exposure to events that symbolize or resemble an aspect of the traumatic event (eg, a woman who was raped in an elevator breaks out in a sweat when entering an elevator).

E. Duration of the disturbance (symptoms in criteria B, C, and D) of at least 1 month.

Specify delayed onset if the onset of symptoms was at least 6 months after the trauma.

and are not in themselves signs of posttraumatic stress disorder.

A diagnosis of posttraumatic stress disorder requires the presence of substantial disruption in functioning or suffering associated with reexperiencing the trauma; persistent symptoms of arousal; and signs of numbing or avoidance.

A diagnosis of posttraumatic stress disorder cannot be made unless symptoms persist for at least 1 month; delayed onset should be specified if symptoms became apparent more than 6 months after the trauma.

Differential Diagnosis

Most of the time, the human capacity for recall and associated affect does not provoke substantial dysfunction or suffering and should not be diagnosed as posttraumatic stress disorder.

Adjustment disorders involve "a maladaptive reaction to an identifiable psychosocial stressor" but involve a broader range of less extreme human experiences (eg, the nonviolent death of a relative) and may result in a few of the symptoms found in posttraumatic stress disorder (eg, symptoms of arousal, numbing, or avoidance). Intense reexperiencing is less common with adjustment disorders.

Prognosis

Acute posttraumatic stress disorder usually responds well to simple measures if they are promptly applied. Full recovery is the rule rather than the exception. Chronic posttraumatic stress disorder, however, is more difficult to treat and may last for decades while causing varying degrees of disability.

Illustrative Case

Four years before seeking treatment, a highly successful truck driver with a 21-year history of accident-free driving had been involved in a two-truck accident in which the other driver was trapped and burned to death despite the patient's effort to free him. In addition to burns received in the rescue attempt, he also suffered a concussion, bruises, and a scalp laceration. While still in the hospital immediately after the accident, the man had nightmares involving repetition of the incident. He became wary about falling asleep, was reluctant to discuss the accident with his family or authorities, and claimed he could not remember much of what happened. The patient seemed markedly distant to close family members and expressed the worry that there was not much one could count on in life. Irritability was noted by all, and he appeared to have difficulty concentrating.

Because of the circumstances of the accident, he was not permitted to resume work as a truck driver for more than 9 months until administrative hearings concluded that he had not been at fault. During that interval, his condition remained largely as described, although his nightmares became less frequent and the quality of his relationship with his family improved. When he was allowed to resume work, he felt extreme apprehension and could not bring himself to drive again because of fear that another accident would result. He was also fearful about driving or riding in a car, and he specifically stated that he had "seen what trucks can do." Tricyclic antidepressant medication decreased the frequency of nightmares and improved sleep but had little effect on his anxiety and avoidance. Previous psychotherapy had not been helpful, and exposure therapy did little to ease his distress.

Epidemiology

Since a psychologically traumatic experience is a prerequisite for posttraumatic stress disorder, incidence and prevalence figures would ideally be related to several different types of trauma. However, no uniform classification of trauma has been agreed upon. The prevalence of posttraumatic stress disorder-like phenomena is demonstrated by an 80% incidence of acute posttraumatic syndrome in survivors of the Buffalo Creek flood disaster and a 57% prevalence after 1 year in survivors of the Cocoanut Grove fire; it should be remembered that diagnostic criteria have changed and that some diagnoses were based on unstructured interviews.

A survey of 2500 St. Louis citizens conducted as part of the NIMH-ECA study found a lifetime prevalence of 1% in both sexes. Fifteen percent of subjects in the study had at least one symptom of posttraumatic stress disorder. Of those exposed to psychological trauma "outside the range of usual human experience," 4% satisfied *DSM-III* criteria for the disorder and 20% experienced some symptoms of the disorder. In a group of 15 Vietnam combat veterans who were wounded, 20% fully satisfied *DSM-III* criteria and 60% had one or more combat-related symptoms (Helzer, 1987).

Etiology & Pathogenesis

Since different individuals experiencing the same trauma respond differently, the cause and pathogenesis of posttraumatic stress disorder involve many factors. The relative contributions of genetic endowment, physical development, psychological maturity, social support, cultural expectations, past experience with trauma, and the nature of the trauma itself are unclear. Psychologically, failure to integrate a traumatic experience into a person's life experiences may lead to a pattern of alternating reexperiencing of the traumatic event and defensive numbing when the reexperiencing itself proves traumatic (Horowitz, 1976).

Treatment

A. Acute Posttraumatic Stress Disorder: Excellent evidence gathered in military conflicts from World War II onward indicates that individuals suffering from incapacitating acute posttraumatic stress disorder are highly likely to recover fully if they are treated as follows: As symptoms and signs of posttraumatic stress disorder emerge in combat and are recognized by fellow soldiers, the affected individuals are removed from the front line and sent to the nearest aid station. There, they are kept in uniform, given food, encouraged to talk about their experiences, and told that their reaction is normal for the trauma they

have experienced. They are expected to perform such duties as they are capable of, are not permitted to assume the role of a patient, and are returned to the front line within 24–72 hours. Sedation is unnecessary and may be counterproductive because of the suggestion of a "sick role" and possible induction of state-dependent learning. The Israeli experience in the 1973 Yom Kippur War found these techniques effective in restoring soldiers to combat fitness and preventing development of chronic posttraumatic disorder. This approach appears to include important elements of graduated exposure.

The implications of war experience for acute posttraumatic stress syndromes in civilians are obvious and confirm the old aphorism: "You must climb right back on the horse that throws you."

B. Chronic or Delayed Posttraumatic Stress Disorder: There are no effective treatments for chronic posttraumatic stress disorder. However, some of its manifestations may be treated symptomatically. Exposure in fantasy or, when it may be done with safety, in real life (eg, asking a woman who has been raped to revisit the site of the rape) has been shown to be helpful to some, but not all, patients. For others, exposure seems a form of reexperiencing which they (and some therapists) view as too distressing and possibly sensitizing. Other behavioral therapists experienced in working with patients suffering from posttraumatic stress disorder maintain that exposure is effective for most patients unless they are markedly depressed. Exposure is most helpful for the phobic avoidance and anxiety symptoms associated with this disorder.

Medications are often helpful in relieving dysphoric and depressive symptoms associated with chronic posttraumatic stress disorder. In particular, sleep disturbance and nightmares are often alleviated with heterocyclic or monoamine oxidase inhibitor antidepressant medications. Antianxiety medications may be of benefit as well, although the risk of dependence must be kept in mind. Beta-blocking agents may be helpful if tremor is a major problem.

Psychotherapy aimed at integration of the traumatic experience into the patient's sense of self may be helpful. Such therapy should first employ techniques of catharsis and abreaction, which may properly be viewed as a form of exposure in fantasy. If these brief psychotherapeutic approaches prove ineffective, more extensive exploration of the meanings of the trauma may be undertaken, although evidence for the effectiveness of long-term psychotherapy is scant.

GENERALIZED ANXIETY DISORDER

Symptoms & Signs

The *DSM-III-R* diagnostic criteria for generalized anxiety disorder are listed in Table 23–8. This diagno-

Table 23–8. *DSM-III-R* diagnostic criteria for generalized anxiety disorder.

A. Unrealistic or excessive anxiety and worry (apprehensive expectation) about 2 or more life circumstances, eg, worry about possible misfortune to one's child (who is in no danger), and worry about finances (for no good reason) for a period of 6 months or longer during which the person has been bothered more days than not by these concerns. In children and adolescents, this may take the form of anxiety and worry about academic, athletic, and social performance.

B. If another axis I disorder is present, the focus of the anxiety and worry in criterion A is unrelated to it, eg, the anxiety or worry is not about having a panic attack (as in panic disorder), being embarrassed in public (as in social phobia), being contaminated (as in obsessive compulsive disorder), or gaining weight (as in anorexia nervosa).

C. The disturbance does not occur only during the course of a mood disorder or a psychotic disorder.

D. At least 6 of the following 18 symptoms are often present when anxious (do not include symptoms present only during panic attacks):

Motor tension

(1) Trembling, twitching, or feeling shaky.
(2) Muscle tension, aches, or soreness.
(3) Restlessness.
(4) Easy fatigability.

Autonomic hyperactivity

(5) Shortness of breath or smothering sensations.
(6) Palpitations or accelerated heart rate (tachycardia).
(7) Sweating or cold, clammy hands.
(8) Dry mouth.
(9) Dizziness or light-headedness.
(10) Nausea, diarrhea, or other abdominal distress.
(11) Flushes (hot flashes) or chills.
(12) Frequent urination.
(13) Trouble swallowing or "lump in throat."

Vigilance and scanning

(14) Feeling keyed up or on edge.
(15) Exaggerated startle response.
(16) Difficulty concentrating or "mind going blank" because of anxiety.
(17) Trouble falling or staying asleep.
(18) Irritability.

E. It cannot be established that an organic factor initiated and maintained the disturbance, eg, hyperthyroidism, caffeine intoxication.

sis has been made less frequently in the USA since panic disorder was included in *DSM-III*. In Great Britain and Europe, where panic is usually viewed as extreme anxiety and not as a categorically discrete disorder, a diagnosis of generalized anxiety disorder is more common.

Differential Diagnosis

Several of the symptoms of generalized anxiety disorder are commonly present in mild depression (sometimes called dysphoria or dysthymia). Generalized anxiety disorder usually causes less dysfunction than other anxiety disorders (except simple phobia). Caffeine intoxication and withdrawal from central nervous system depressant substances can mimic generalized anxiety disorder. Because of the substantial overlap in motor tension and autonomic hyperactivity symptoms with those of panic disorder, careful attention to the possibility of panic is essential in distinguishing between generalized anxiety disorder and panic disorder.

Epidemiology

The NIMH-ECA study did not diagnose generalized anxiety disorder, but it is thought to be quite common, affecting approximately 5% of the population and with a female-to-male ratio of approximately 2:1.

Etiology & Pathogenesis

As with all of the anxiety disorders, many factors are probably involved in the etiology and pathogenesis of generalized anxiety disorder.

A. Biochemical Theories: The up and down regulation of noradrenergic function mediated largely through the locus ceruleus (Redmond, 1977), and demonstration of brain benzodiazepine receptors (Squires and Braestrup, 1977) and their interaction with GABA (Paul et al, 1980), have stimulated research on the role played by the GABA-benzodiazepine and noradrenergic-locus ceruleus systems. The GABA-benzodiazepine system may be more active in generalized anxiety disorder, while the noradrenergic-locus ceruleus system is more often implicated in the etiology of panic.

B. Behavioral Theories: Successful avoidance of noxious stimuli (unconditioned stimulus) that reduces discomfort or trauma (unconditioned response) is usually reinforced in both humans and other species (Kandel, 1983). When avoidance in humans produces unpredictable results, avoidance becomes unreliable and generalized anxiety is thought to develop (see Chapter 1).

C. Psychological Theories: A state of general anxiety is thought by many dynamic psychotherapists to reflect an unconscious conflict about dangerous emotions, behaviors, or states (eg, anger, depression, injury or death, sexual arousal, hunger, and anxiety itself). Another theory holds that some individuals with generalized anxiety disorder may seek anxiety-provoking stimuli and maintain themselves in situations likely to evoke high anxiety in order to achieve mastery over anxiety, gain relief through the eventual cessation of such anxiety states, or avoid an even less enjoyable affective state such as anger or boredom.

Prognosis

Generalized anxiety disorder persists for at least 6 months and, commonly, for many years. Untreated, it usually waxes and wanes in response to common stressors and unspecified factors. With treatment (eg, antianxiety medication), symptoms are reduced but usually reemerge when treatment is stopped.

Illustrative Case

For as long as he could remember, a 53-year-old male had "worried" about things that never came to pass; their possible occurrence had little foundation in reality, and if they did occur, they were unlikely to be of serious consequence. He described himself as always feeling tense and restless, sometimes trembling or being on edge, and feeling irritable and easily fatigued. He had trouble falling and staying asleep because of "worries." At times of peak worry, he described symptoms of autonomic distress, including dry mouth, sweating, tachycardia, urinary frequency, and diarrhea. These symptoms were present most days to a greater or lesser degree and never worsened suddenly.

He had engaged in two courses of psychotherapy, each lasting more than 1 year, as well as "relaxation training" and biofeedback. None of these treatments had led to meaningful reduction in symptoms. When benzodiazepines became available, his family physician began treatment with diazepam, which proved remarkably effective over the following 20 years at a dose of 15 mg/d. The patient never increased the dosage, and on repeated occasions, when he or his doctor had attempted to withdraw the medication, symptoms returned.

Treatment

A. Drug Treatment: Benzodiazepine antianxiety drugs are effective in reducing or alleviating symptoms of generalized anxiety in many patients. Return of symptoms is common when benzodiazepines are discontinued. Sedation is the major side effect, and physiological dependence will occur in most patients taking benzodiazepines steadily over several months. Despite this potential, the incidence of benzodiazepine abuse is quite low except in those who abuse other substances, and many patients find these agents effec-tive for generalized anxiety disorder and do not take more than the prescribed dosage.

Buspirone is a nonbenzodiazepine also useful for treating generalized anxiety disorder. It does not have sedative effects, does not interact with alcohol, and does not lead to dependence.

Beta-adrenergic blocking agents and antihistamines have limited roles in the treatment of symptoms associated with generalized anxiety. Barbiturates and meprobamate have been superseded by benzodiazepines, buspirone, and, to a lesser degree, beta-blockers and antihistamines.

B. Behavioral Therapy: Behavioral therapy has not been of particular benefit in the treatment of generalized anxiety disorder because it is difficult to specify situations or stimuli to which the individual should be exposed. Relaxation and biofeedback are commonly advocated, but their efficacy has not been validated in controlled studies of clinically significant generalized anxiety disorder.

C. Psychotherapy: For decades, dynamic psychotherapy was the treatment of choice for generalized anxiety. Unfortunately, evidence from controlled studies supporting the efficacy of this approach is limited at best. Cognitive therapy is being evaluated and has shown some promise (Woodward et al, 1980).

SUMMARY

Anxiety is a common emotion with adaptive value for most individuals most of the time. For some, anxiety is so intense or lasts so long that it becomes maladaptive and is properly diagnosed as a disorder. Treatment of anxiety disorders has improved substantially over the last two decades, with behavioral therapy and drug therapies forming the foundations of effective treatment. Classification is becoming more refined, and understanding of the epidemiological, genetic, developmental, psychological, behavioral, biochemical, and environmental aspects of anxiety is growing steadily (Marks, 1987).

REFERENCES

Baxter LR et al: Local cerebral glucose metabolic rates in obsessive-compulsive disorder. Arch Gen Psychiatry 1987;44:211.

Charney DS et al: Drug treatment of panic disorder: The comparative efficacy of imipramine, alprazolam, and trazodone. J Clin Psychiatry 1986;47:580.

Greist JH, Jefferson JW, Marks IM: *Anxiety and Its Treatment: Help Is Available.* American Psychiatric Press, 1986. [Also available as a Warner paperback, 1986.]

Greist JH et al: Avoidance versus confrontation of fear. Behav Res Ther 1980;11:1.

Helzer JE, Robins LN, McEvoy LT: Post-traumatic stress disorder in the general population: Findings of the Epidemiologic Catchment Area Survey. New England J Med 1987;317:1630.

Horowitz MJ: *Stress Response Syndromes.* Jason Aronson, 1976.

Jenike MA, Baer L, Minichiello WE (editor): *Obsessive-*

Compulsive Disorders: Theory and Management. PSG Publishing Co., 2nd Ed, 1990.

Kandel ER: From metapsychology to molecular biology: Explorations into the nature of anxiety. Am J Psychiatry 1983;140:1277.

Kelly D: *Anxiety and Emotions: Physiological Basis and Treatment*. Thomas, 1980.

Kuhn TS: *The Structure of Scientific Revolutions*. Univ Chicago Press, 1962.

Marks IM: *Fears, Phobias and Rituals: The Nature of Anxiety and Panic Disorder*. Oxford Univ Press, 1987.

Marks IM: Genetics of fear and anxiety disorders. Br J Psychiatry 1986;149:406.

Myers JK et al: Six-month prevalence of psychiatric disorders in three communities, 198- to 1982. Arch Gen Psychiatry. 1984;41:959.

Paul SM, Skolnich P, Gallager DW: Receptors for the age of anxiety: Pharmacology of the benzodiazepines. Science 1980;207:274.

Redmond EE: Alterations in the function of the nucleus locus coeruleus: A possible model for studies of anxiety. Pages 293–306 in: *Animal Models in Psychiatry and Neurology*. Hanin I, Usie E (editors). Pergamon, 1977.

Squires RF, Braestrup C: Benzodiazepine receptors in rat brain. Nature 1977;266:732.

Woodward RP, Jones RB: Cognitive restructuring treatment: A controlled trial with anxious patients. Behav Res Ther 1980;18:401.

24

Somatoform & Dissociative Disorders

Stephen D. Purcell, MD

Although the phenomena that define the two diagnostic categories that are the subject of this chapter are quite different, psychological factors are believed to have primary and essential etiological significance in most of these disorders.

SOMATOFORM DISORDERS

As the name implies, the essential feature of the category of psychiatric disturbances termed the somatoform disorders is the presence of symptoms that suggest physical disorder. In order to establish a diagnosis of any one of the somatoform disorders, however, there must be no demonstrable physical findings or known physiological mechanisms that might account for the symptoms and there must be positive evidence—or a strong presumption—that the symptoms have a psychological origin.

There are four subtypes of somatoform disorders: somatization disorder, conversion disorder, somatoform pain disorder, and hypochondriasis. In each type, though the symptoms are physical, the specific pathophysiological processes involved are not demonstrable or explicable on the basis of laboratory or other physical diagnostic procedures.

It is now well documented that a large proportion of patients in general medical outpatient clinics and private medical offices do not have organic disease requiring medical treatment. It is likely that many of these patients have somatoform disorders, but they do not perceive themselves as having a psychiatric problem and thus do not seek treatment from psychiatrists. It is especially important, then, that nonpsychiatrist physicians be familiar with these disorders so they can be recognized and treated appropriately.

SOMATIZATION DISORDER

Historically, somatization disorder has been known as both hysteria and Briquet's syndrome.

Symptoms & Signs

According to *DSM-III-R,* somatization disorder is characterized by multiple physical symptoms that recur over a period of several years and are either unrelated to an identifiable physical disorder or grossly in excess of physical findings. A diagnosis of somatization disorder cannot be made unless symptoms occur in contexts other than panic attacks and unless symptoms have been severe enough to drive the patient to attempt self-medication with drugs other than aspirin, to seek medical attention, or to make lifestyle changes. The symptoms are often part of a complicated medical history and may be vaguely defined or presented in a dramatic or exaggerated manner. People with this disorder have usually seen many physicians, sometimes simultaneously. Anxiety and depressed mood are common associated symptoms. When mental health care is sought by people with these disorders, it is usually because of these symptoms and not because the physical symptoms are believed to have a psychological basis. Histrionic personality disorder and, less frequently, antisocial personality disorder are sometimes present in addition to somatization disorder; and concurrent occupational, interpersonal, and marital difficulties are common. The hallucination of hearing one's name called (without impairment of reality testing) has been reported in association with this syndrome. Otherwise, however, "psychotic-like" symptomatology does not occur. The most common complaints are of being "sickly," with pain, psychosexual symptoms, and symptoms associated with the neurological, gastrointestinal, cardiopulmonary, and female reproductive systems (Table 24–1).

Natural History

The pattern of multiple, recurrent physical symptoms begins most often during the teen years but (by definition) always before age 30. In women, menstrual problems may signal the onset of this disorder, but a wide variety of symptoms may be observed in both sexes. Somatization disorder is a chronic disorder, and spontaneous remission occurs rarely; fluctuations in the number and severity of symptoms do occur, but it is unusual for a year to pass without medical attention being sought.

Table 24–1. *DSM-III-R* diagnostic criteria for somatization disorder.

A. A history of many physical complaints or a belief that one is sickly, beginning before the age of 30 and persisting for several years.

B. At least 13 symptoms from the list below. To count a symptom as significant, the following criteria must be met:
   (1) No organic pathology or pathophysiologic mechanism (eg, a physical disorder or the effects of an injury, medication, drugs, or alcohol) to account for the symptom or, when there is related organic pathology, the complaint or resulting social or occupational impairment is grossly in excess of what would be expected from the physical findings.
   (2) Has not occurred only during a panic attack.
   (3) Has caused the person to take medicine (other than over-the-counter pain medication), see a doctor, or alter life-style.

Gastrointestinal symptoms: (1) vomiting (other than during pregnancy); (2) abdominal pain (other than when menstruating); (3) nausea (other than motion sickness); (4) bloating (gassy); (5) diarrhea; (6) intolerance of (gets sick on) several different foods.

Pain symptoms: (7) pain in extremities; (8) back pain; (9) joint pain; (10) pain during urination; (11) other pain (excluding headaches).

Cardiopulmonary symptoms: (12) shortness of breath when not exerting oneself; (13) palpitations; (14) chest pain; (15) dizziness.

Conversion or pseudoneurologic symptoms: (16) amnesia; (17) difficulty swallowing; (18) loss of voice; (19) deafness; (20) double vision; (21) blurred vision; (22) blindness; (23) fainting or loss of consciousness; (24) seizure or convulsion; (25) trouble walking; (26) paralysis or muscle weakness; (27) urinary retention or difficulty urinating.

Sexual symptoms for the major part of the person's life after opportunities for sexual activity: (28) burning sensation in sexual organs or rectum (other than during intercourse); (29) sexual indifference; (30) pain during intercourse; (31) impotence.

Female reproductive symptoms judged by the person to occur more frequently or severely than in most women: (32) painful menstruation; (33) irregular menstrual periods; (34) excessive menstrual bleeding; (35) vomiting throughout pregnancy.

Note: Symptoms 1, 7, 12, 16, 17, 28, and 32 may be used to screen for the disorder. The presence of 2 or more of these items suggests a high likelihood of the disorder.

The impact on the lives of people who have this disorder should not be underestimated. Symptoms may be quite severe and persistent to the point of being incapacitating or disruptive to occupational and interpersonal relationships. Because of the continuing search for medical care from different physicians, there is a risk of iatrogenic complications. Physicians who fail to perceive the psychological basis of the patient's physical complaints may perform unnecessary surgical procedures or prescribe medications aimed at treating physiological abnormalities—each procedure or treatment with its own set of adverse reactions or complications. There is also a risk of substance use disorder from prescribed analgesics or antianxiety agents. Because of associated depressive thoughts or moods, suicidal threats and attempts occur; when suicide results, it is usually in association with substance abuse.

Differential Diagnosis

The differential diagnosis of somatization disorder obviously includes physical disorders that present with vague or multiple somatic symptoms. These include multiple sclerosis, systemic lupus erythematosus, hyperparathyroidism, and porphyria. In addition, a recent study has shown an association between Briquet's syndrome and polycystic ovary disease (Orenstein et al, 1986). It is important to remember that somatization disorder begins before age 30 and, conversely, that the onset of multiple physical symptoms later in life usually represents physical disease. Schizophrenia with multiple somatic delusions and major depression with somatic symptoms may occasionally require differentiation from somatization disorder. In panic disorder, physical symptoms may occur, but only in association with panic attacks. Conversion disorder involves certain physical symptoms that occur in the absence of the full clinical picture of somatization disorder. Factitious disorder with physical symptoms is distinguished by the presence of voluntary control of the symptoms. Somatization disorder, which does not involve any demonstrable physiological abnormality, should not be confused with psychological factors affecting physical condition, in which psychological factors contribute to the onset or exacerbation of a physical disorder. These last-mentioned disorders have been called ''psychosomatic'' or ''psychophysiological'' in the past and include such disorders as peptic ulcer disease, rheumatoid arthritis, regional enteritis, and ulcerative colitis.

Prognosis

Without treatment, the prognosis is poor. Spontaneous remission is rare, and a lifelong pattern of seeking medical attention develops with its attendant interference with other aspects of the patient's life and with iatrogenic complications.

Illustrative Case

A 36-year-old divorced woman who worked as a salesclerk entered the hospital emergency room at 2:00 AM complaining loudly that something was wrong with her stomach. She was tearful and agitated, with arms held tightly across her abdomen. She stated that shortly after her evening meal she began to feel nauseated and ''bloated'' and that she vomited some undigested food. Within minutes of vomiting she began to feel a dull pain in her periumbilical area that gradually became sharper and spread throughout her entire abdomen; when the pain became ''unbearable,'' she decided to come to the emergency room.

As the patient calmed down and became more comfortable, she stated that she had had many similar episodes of abdominal discomfort over the past 15 years but that no doctor had been able to determine the cause. At the age of 18 she had had severe salpingitis requiring removal of the left oviduct, and 2 years later, because of persistent abdominal pain, the right ovary was removed. When she was 22, she underwent cholecystectomy, and over the next 10 years she had 3 abdominal surgical procedures to correct "adhesions" causing abdominal pain. At various times, she said, physicians had told her that she had "an ulcer" or "colitis," but despite a variety of medical treatments her symptoms had persisted. On further questioning, she also admitted to sporadic episodes of dizziness, chest pain that awakened her from sleep, chronic dysuria, occasional urinary retention requiring catheterization, and chronic low back pain. As she finished relating her history, she commented that "only someone with a poor constitution could be sick for this long. She admitted taking diazepam (10 mg) 4 times a day for "nerves," phenobarbital (30 mg) 4 times a day for her gastric symptoms, and "some pain pills whenever I need them'—each medication prescribed by a different physician.

Except for voluntary guarding on palpation of the abdomen and the old abdominal surgical scars, physical examination was normal.

Epidemiology

Somatization disorder is estimated to occur in 1–3% of women but seems to be truly rare in men (Cloninger et al, 1986). There is a strong familial tendency. Antisocial personality disorder and alcohol abuse are more common in such families.

Etiology & Pathogenesis

The specific cause of this disorder is unknown, but it is presumed to be psychological in origin. Although the increased incidence among family members suggests a genetic basis, there is no conclusive evidence of that, and no biochemical theories have been adduced to explain the disorder. A history of childhood sexual molestation has been implicated in the pathogenesis of somatization disorder in women (Morrison, 1989).

Most psychiatrists believe that psychological factors play a major role in the genesis of somatization disorder, but there is no consensus about their exact nature. Pathological identification with a parent, immature efforts to deal with dependency needs, and maladaptive resolution of intrapsychic conflict have all been proposed as mechanisms by which symptoms similar to those seen in somatization disorder are produced. Kellner (1990) has reviewed the various theories and the research relating to somatization.

Treatment

In a review of the treatment of somatization disorder, Ochitill (1982) concludes that because of diagnostic confusion and therapeutic controversy, there is no standard effective treatment. Neither biological nor behavioral treatments have had practical success,

and psychotherapy remains the usual therapeutic approach. However, patients usually do not see any relationship between their symptoms and psychological factors, and the psychologically based treatments—individual or group psychotherapies—are usually not helpful. Most patients refuse psychotherapy, and the literature suggests that psychotherapy is not successful when it is used. Thus, the nonpsychiatrist physician often has the only opportunity to engage the patient in a beneficial relationship. The physician must be sensitive to the psychological and social needs and problems of the patient and able to tolerate the patient's "incurable" chronic complaints. A useful management objective in such cases would be to prevent multiple medical consultations and unnecessary somatic treatments with associated costs and iatrogenic complications. In selected cases, when the physician can detect some psychological thinking (insight) or motivation to change, psychiatric consultation may be indicated.

CONVERSION DISORDER

Historically, conversion disorder also has been known as hysterical neurosis, conversion type.

Symptoms & Signs

Conversion disorder is characterized chiefly by loss or alteration of physical functioning that suggests physical disorder but which instead is apparently an expression of psychological conflict or need. The symptom is not under voluntary control and cannot be explained by any physical disorder or known pathophysiological mechanism.

Conversion symptoms suggesting neurological disease of the sensory or motor systems are most common: paresis, paralysis, aphonia, seizures, blindness, anesthesia. Occasionally, the autonomic nervous system or the endocrine system may be involved, as with vomiting or pseudocyesis.

By definition, the diagnosis of conversion disorder is not made when the physical alteration is limited to pain or to a disturbance in sexual functioning—in which case the diagnoses of somatoform pain disorder or sexual dysfunction, respectively, are made. This diagnosis is also precluded when the conversion symptom occurs as one component of somatization disorder (Table 24–2).

Natural History

Conversion disorder may begin at any age but is most likely to make its first appearance in adolescence or early adulthood. There may be only one episode, or episodes may recur over a lifetime. The natural history of the disorder cannot be described with certainty at present, but the onset seems to be most often abrupt and in the context of psychosocial stress; though variable, the duration is probably most often

Table 24–2. *DSM-III-R* diagnostic criteria for conversion disorder (or hysterical neurosis, conversion type.)

A. A loss of, or alteration in, physical functioning suggesting a physical disorder.
B. Psychologic factors are judged to be etiologically related to the symptom because of a temporal relationship between a psychosocial stressor that is apparently related to a psychologic conflict or need, and initiation or exacerbation of the symptom.
C. The person is not conscious of intentionally producing the symptom.
D. The symptom is not a culturally sanctioned response pattern and cannot, after appropriate investigation, be explained by a known physical disorder.
E. The symptom is not limited to pain or to a disturbance in sexual functioning.

Specify: single episode or recurrent.

short, and resolution is rapid. In some instances, the "conversion symptom" is later found to be the first manifestation of a neurological disorder, in which case either the initial diagnosis of conversion disorder was incorrect or the neurological disorder "predisposed" to the development of the conversion symptom. Occasionally, a patient with a chronic neurological disorder (eg, multiple sclerosis) may develop symptoms (eg, paraplegia) without physical evidence of active disease. It is as if the patient "learned" the conversion symptom from previous experience with neurological illness.

As with the physical symptoms occurring in somatization disorder, the symptoms of conversion disorder can be extremely disruptive and can place the individual at risk for the costs and complications of unnecessary medical or surgical treatment. Actual physical problems may result from the conversion symptoms, eg, contractures or disuse atrophy associated with conversion paralysis. A number of factors have been noted to predispose to the development of conversion disorder, including an antecedent physical disorder, exposure to others with physical symptoms, severe psychosocial stress, and histrionic and dependent personality disorders.

Differential Diagnosis

The differential diagnosis includes physical disease and is especially difficult when the underlying disease is one that characteristically presents with vague neurological symptoms, such as multiple sclerosis. A diagnosis of conversion disorder is suggested when the physical symptom does not conform to an actual known physical disorder or does not correspond to the anatomy of the nervous system. An example of this situation would be normal pupillary and electroencephalographic responses to light in someone with "blindness"; another example is "stocking-glove anesthesia," in which numbness in a foot or hand is complete and sharply delimited at the wrist or ankle

rather than conforming to the distribution of sensory nerves. Even when a physical disorder cannot be identified, the diagnosis of conversion disorder should not be made unless there is also evidence that the symptom serves a psychological function. Conversion symptoms may occur as one component of somatization disorder or schizophrenia, and when this occurs, the diagnosis of conversion disorder is not made. Hypochondriasis involves physical symptoms but without any loss or distortion of bodily function. In both factitious disorder and malingering, physical symptoms are under voluntary control, whereas in conversion disorder they are not.

Prognosis

There are no good data on the natural history of conversion disorder, nor have there been large-scale systematic studies characterizing response to treatment. It is believed that many conversion symptoms may resolve over a period of days to months without treatment and, conversely, that some conversion symptoms may persist for years in spite of intense efforts at treatment. The prognosis seems to be highly variable, probably has little to do with the specific symptom involved, and is seemingly dependent on the interplay of the individual's psychological makeup, the social environment, and the response to the symptom by people who are important to the patient.

Illustrative Case

A 21-year-old college student telephoned her physician and, later the same day, appeared (with her mother) at his office with the complaint that she had awakened from sleep 2 days earlier with total numbness and paralysis in both legs. She said she had no idea what was the matter but that she was incapable of caring for herself and had summoned her mother from another state to come and take care of her.

The patient had a history of good physical and mental health except for an episode of bilateral hip pain at age 14 that had resolved spontaneously. For the past 2 years she had shared an apartment with her boyfriend, but after a prolonged series of arguments he had moved out on the day preceding the onset of her symptoms.

On examination, the patient appeared slightly tense but in no acute distress. She stated that she knew she should seek medical help for the paralysis, but her main worry was how she was going to "support" herself without her boyfriend's contributions to the household expenses. She was completely unable to move either leg, and there was total anesthesia and lack of response to painful stimuli (pinprick) in both legs up to the inguinal ligament bilaterally, where sensation abruptly resumed. All deep tendon reflexes and both plantar reflexes were normal, as was the rest of the physical examination.

Epidemiology

There are no firm data on the prevalence or sex distribution of conversion disorder. In the 19th century, the disorder was apparently much more common than it is now and was seen predominantly in women. Cases seen today usually appear in nonpsychiatric settings such as in neurology clinics and among military personnel. Some believe that one particular conversion symptom, **globus hystericus** (impaired swallowing caused by a sensation of a lump in the throat), is more common in women.

Etiology & Pathogenesis

Conversion disorder is unusual in the *DSM-III-R* classification, because a presumed cause (relationship to psychological conflicts or needs) is incorporated into the definition, and it is unique because specific psychological mechanisms to account for the disorder are proposed in the concepts of primary and secondary gain. An unacceptable sexual or aggressive drive is denied expression and repressed and thus becomes unconscious. The mental energy associated with the drive, which would normally push the drive into conscious experience, is converted into a somatic symptom. This allows the individual to remain unaware of the drive and at the same time permits symbolic expression of it. Protection from experiencing the drive is a **primary gain.** The symptom itself elicits from others responses that gratify needs which were not involved in the original symptom production— eg, sympathy and attention, which may gratify dependency needs. This gratification is referred to as a **secondary gain.** The source of the symptom, in other words, is primary gain; once established, both primary gain and secondary gain serve to maintain the symptom.

Historical Note

The story of the discovery of the psychological mechanisms responsible for conversion symptoms is worthy of a brief digression here.

What are now called conversion symptoms were recognized in women by the ancient Greeks and Romans and were explained by them as resulting from a wandering of the uterus from its normal anatomic position into various other parts of the body, which were adversely affected. The term "hysteria," which in the past was used synonymously with conversion disorder, is derived from the Greek word for uterus. In the Middle Ages, conversion phenomena were given various supernatural and religious interpretations. By the late 19th century, conversion symptoms (called hysteria then) had become a legitimate focus of medical and scientific investigation, and there were 2 prominent and opposing European schools of thought regarding their origin. One theory, whose major proponent was Jean-Martin Charcot, was that conversion symptoms were a manifestation of degenerative neurological disease. The other theory held that conversion symptoms derived from psychological factors, some of which were unconscious, and Hyppolyte Bernheim most strongly represented this point of view.

Although he studied with Charcot and was committed to understanding hysteria as a neurological disease, Pierre Janet also made significant contributions to understanding the psychology of conversion symptoms. Specifically, Janet proposed the psychological mechanism of **dissociation,** by which selected mental contents could be removed from consciousness (dissociated from experience) but continue to produce motor and sensory effects. This mechanism was thought to be illustrated by posthypnotic suggestion, in which a directive given to a subject in a hypnotic trance would be carried out after return to the normal waking state of consciousness without any memory by the subject of having received the directive.

Sigmund Freud, at that time a neurologist interested in hysteria, worked with both Charcot and Bernheim. He observed the use of hypnosis in treating conversion symptoms and returned to his own practice of neurology to use the new technique in treating his own patients. Freud was especially interested in the psychological theories of hysteria, and his psychological theorizing was given an important boost by an accidental discovery made by a colleague, Josef Breuer. Breuer was treating a woman with hysteria ("Anna O"), who in a hypnotic trance produced memories of previously unconscious traumatic events that appeared to be directly and causally related to the hysterical symptoms. Furthermore, the expression of these memories and the associated emotions caused the symptoms to disappear. Drawing on the concept of the psychological mechanism of dissociation and these new observations, Freud proposed that emotions associated with the traumatic event were morally unacceptable to the woman and, because of this, the emotions were forced (repressed) into her unconscious. The mental energy associated with these emotions and denied expression was then "converted" into a somatic symptom that symbolically represented the traumatic event. In these early formulations, it was emotions associated with the sexual drive that were subjected to dissociation and "conversion." Subsequent observations have shown that the aggressive drive also is subject to these same processes; therefore, both sexually and aggressively based conflicts may underlie conversion symptoms.

Treatment

During World War II, the use of pentobarbital was common in the treatment of soldiers who developed conversion symptoms as a result of traumatic combat experiences. Sometimes called narcosynthesis, the intravenous use of a barbiturate to place the patient in a trancelike state of complete relaxation was combined with direct encouragement of the patient to remember traumatic events and emotions associated with the onset of the conversion symptom. An emotionally intense reliving of the traumatic experience often occurred which, when accepted and remembered by the patient, caused the symptom to disappear. This method of treatment is uncommonly used today.

Given our present understanding of the origin of conversion disorder, only psychotherapy would be expected to provide lasting benefit. Some patients are effectively treated with psychoanalytically oriented individual psychotherapy, but the appropriateness of this type of treatment has less to do with the conversion symptom per se than with the suitability of the patient. Only a minority of patients with conversion disorder are well suited for psychotherapy aimed at achieving insight. For most patients, individual or group supportive psychotherapy aimed at changing the patient's psychosocial environment is indicated. Environmental manipulation should include adjustments to alleviate the stress that initially precipitated the conversion symptom as well as interventions with important people in the patient's life who may be maintaining the symptom by providing secondary gain.

Successes have been reported with behavior therapy. The role of hypnosis is controversial. It is used most often when rapid relief of symptoms is indicated.

There is no evidence for the effectiveness of any somatic therapy in the treatment of conversion disorder.

SOMATOFORM PAIN DISORDER

Symptoms & Signs

Somatoform pain disorder is essentially the same as conversion disorder except that the symptom involved is limited to physical pain. Because of the relative frequency of this symptom and the special clinical problems associated with the management of pain, separate diagnostic categories are indicated.

Somatoform pain disorder is diagnosed when the major complaint is preoccupation with pain of at least 6 months' duration in the absence of, or grossly in excess of, explanatory physical findings (Table 24–3). In contrast to conversion disorder, there is no evidence of a psychological factor that might be causing the pain. This change from DSM-III reflects a move away from inferred psychological factors and theory.

Natural History

Patients with somatoform pain disorder typically make repeated visits to doctors for diagnosis or pain relief. Many physicians may be consulted successively or simultaneously, and there is an obvious risk of substance use disorder involving prescribed analgesics. Complaints of anxiety or depression are common but are not the predominant symptom, and there is an increased incidence of conversion symp-

Table 24–3. *DSM-III-R* diagnostic criteria for somatoform pain disorder.

A. Preoccupation with pain for at least 6 months.
B. Either (1) or (2):
  (1) Appropriate evaluation uncovers no organic "pathology" or pathophysiologic mechanism (eg, a physical disorder or the effects of injury) to account for the pain.
  (2) When there is related organic pathology, the complaint of pain or resulting social or occupational impairment is grossly in excess of what would be expected from the physical findings.

toms. Histrionic personality disorder is an uncommon associated disorder.

This disorder may begin at any age but usually starts in adolescence and young adulthood. It seems to begin suddenly and increases in severity over days to weeks. It may resolve spontaneously or with treatment or may become chronic despite treatment. Severe symptoms may seriously disrupt overall function and expose the individual to iatrogenic complications of medical or surgical treatment.

Differential Diagnosis

Differential diagnosis includes painful physical disorders, such as atherosclerotic coronary artery disease and lumbar disk disease. The dramatic presentation of physical pain out of proportion to physical findings is not sufficient for the diagnosis, since the manner of expressing pain may reflect individual personality traits or cultural factors. Furthermore, pain that shows temporary improvement with placebo medications or suggestion should not be judged to be of psychological origin, since these phenomena also occur with pain due to physical disease. Complaints of pain in somatization disorder, major depression, and schizophrenia rarely dominate the clinical picture, and the diagnosis of somatoform pain disorder is not made if the pain is judged to be due to any other mental disorder. In malingering, pain is under voluntary control, and that is not the case in somatoform pain disorder.

Prognosis

There are no good data on the prognosis of somatoform pain disorder. Clinical experience suggests a variable course with chronicity as a frequent characteristic.

Illustrative Case

A 32-year-old unemployed college graduate arrived at the emergency room frightened and breathless, complaining of severe substernal chest pain that he characterized as an unbearable "tightness." Except for slight tachycardia, his vital signs and electrocardiogram were normal. Despite reassurance from the physician, he continued to complain of severe pain and demanded "a shot of Demerol." After a time the physician ordered 75 mg of meperidine intramuscularly, after which the patient felt "a little better."

A telephone call to the family physician elicited the following information: There was a strong family history of heart disease, and the patient's father had died suddenly of acute myocardial infarction in his son's presence 4 years earlier. The patient's first episode of chest pain occurred 1 year later, when he was awakened from sleep the night before he was due to appear in court to testify in a legal proceeding contesting his father's will. Since that time he had had bouts of chest pain, usually requiring narcotic analgesia for relief, about twice a month and occasionally as often as 3–4 times a week. Thorough physical evaluation, including coronary angiography, revealed no organic disease.

Epidemiology

The prevalence of somatoform pain disorder is not known, but the disorder seems to be common in general medical practice. It is more common in women than in men. Familial distribution has not been reported. However, there is an increased familial incidence of painful injuries and illnesses, suggesting that some symptomatology may be learned or may result from identification with an ill family member.

Etiology & Pathogenesis

The pain is thought to be of psychological origin. The specific psychological mechanisms involved in pain production are unknown and are probably multiple and variable. It has been proposed that the pain of somatoform pain disorder is a conversion symptom produced by the same mechanisms responsible for the symptoms of conversion disorder. A psychological cause is indicated by the following: (1) a temporal relationship exists between a presumed environmental stimulus (stressor) and pain; (2) the pain enables the person to avoid a noxious activity; or (3) the pain enables the person to obtain added support from the environment. It has also been observed that in certain cases the psychological mechanism appears to be identification, where the individual takes on the attributes (symptoms) of an emotionally significant other person, such as a parent. Pinsky (1978) has proposed that people with somatoform pain disorder have less capacity to directly experience and verbalize emotions; the implication is that emotions are more or less directly translated into physical pain (by unknown mechanisms) rather than being expressed in other ways.

Treatment

In recent years, there has been considerable interest and progress in the treatment of chronic pain. Studies have shown that a multidisciplinary approach (neurologists, internists, and anesthesiologists in addition to psychiatrists) to management in an inpatient setting, which includes treatment with tricyclic antidepressants, can be effective in achieving pain relief and improving depressive symptoms. It is difficult to explain the benefit derived from treatment with antidepressants or the relationship between chronic pain and depression. Because the studies were done on patients with a variety of chronic pain syndromes and not necessarily somatoform pain disorder, it is impossible to generalize about the implications for treatment of the narrowly defined group of patients under consideration here.

There are increasing numbers of multidisciplinary treatment centers for patients with chronic pain, and referral to one of these centers may be appropriate when that is possible. Specialized treatment methods often include group, milieu, and behavioral approaches to the problem and are aimed at "replacing pain-related behavior with normal activity" (Brena and Chapman, 1983) rather than pain alleviation. When specialized treatment resources are not available, the physician should attempt to establish a supportive relationship with the patient that helps to prevent unnecessary medical and surgical procedures and treatments. When drugs are used in treatment, sedative and antianxiety agents should be avoided, and the use of opiates has no place in the treatment of patients with this disorder. Most patients should be given a trial of tricyclic antidepressant medication in the dosages used to treat a major depressive episode. Probably only a few patients will benefit from individual psychotherapy, but with a very small subset of patients who seem to possess characteristics predicting good responses to psychotherapy, direct or indirect psychiatric consultation is indicated for the purpose of deciding whether a trial of individual psychotherapy should be offered.

HYPOCHONDRIASIS

Hypochondriasis was formerly called hypochondriacal neurosis. A "hypochondriac" is a person who complains about minor physical problems, worrying unrealistically about serious illness, and persistently seeks professional care and consumes multiple over-the-counter remedies. This use of the term includes elements of somatization disorder and hypochondriasis.

Symptoms & Signs

The chief manifestation of hypochondriasis is the fear of having (or the belief that one has) a serious physical disease. This fear is based upon actual benign symptoms or signs or normal physiological sensations, and it exists despite the absence of evidence of physical disorder to account for the belief—although there may in fact be a coexistent physical disorder. The misinterpretation of symptoms is quite natural. In hypochondriasis, however, the fear of having a serious disease persists despite medical reassurance, and it interferes with social or occupational functioning.

Table 24–4. *DSM-III-R* diagnostic criteria for hypochondriasis (or hypochondriacal neurosis).

A. Preoccupation with the fear of having, or the belief that one has, a serious disease, based on the person's interpretation of physical signs or sensations as evidence of physical illness.
B. Appropriate physical evaluation does not support the diagnosis of any physical disorder that can account for the physical signs or sensations or the person's unwarranted interpretation of them, and the symptoms in criterion A are not just symptoms of panic attacks.
C. The fear of having, or belief that one has, a disease persists despite medical reassurance.
D. Duration of the disturbance is at least 6 months.
E. The belief in criterion A is not of delusional intensity, as in delusional disorder somatic subtype (ie, the person can acknowledge the possibility that his or her fear of having, or belief that he or she has, a serious disease, is unfounded).

A person with hypochondriasis may interpret normal functions (heartbeat, peristalsis) or minor abnormalities (tension headache, viral respiratory infection) as evidence of serious disease. The fear of serious disease usually involves multiple organ systems simultaneously or in succession, though in some individuals the fear will center on a single organ system, such as in "cardiac neurosis," in which the unrealistic fear is of heart disease (Table 24–4).

Natural History

Anxiety, depression, and compulsive personality traits are commonly associated with hypochondriasis. When asked about their state of health, hypochondriacal patients usually respond at great length, often expressing frustration with physicians and the inadequate medical care they have received.

This disorder usually begins in adolescence but may not begin until the fourth decade in men and the fifth decade in women. It is usually chronic but marked by fluctuation in the intensity with which the belief is held and in the degree of disruption of social and occupational functioning. As with the other somatoform disorders, disruption of the patient's life may be marked (eg, the patient may take to bed and adopt an invalid life-style). The tendency to seek treatment from different physicians involves an increased risk of unnecessary medical or surgical treatments and their associated costs and complications.

Differential Diagnosis

The differential diagnosis of course includes actual serious physical disease. Occasionally, hypochondriasis will require differentiation from schizophrenia or major depression with somatic delusions. In these cases, although the final diagnosis will be based on specific diagnostic criteria, the belief that physical disease exists does not have the rigidly fixed quality of a true delusion, in that the person with hypochondriasis will usually entertain the possibility that the feared disease does not exist. Differentiation from

somatization disorder is usually on multiple physical symptoms rather than on the fear of having a specific disease.

Prognosis

Hypochondriasis is considered by most psychiatrists to be a chronic disorder with a very poor prognosis.

Illustrative Case

A 28-year-old salesman sought a medical appointment for "a complete physical examination." He stated that several months ago he had consulted another physician but now was looking for a doctor who could "get to the bottom" of his problems. He expressed some anger because the other physician had refused to perform tests the patient thought were indicated, and he hoped the new doctor would be more helpful.

When asked what was troubling him, the patient said he was sure he had cancer—probably cancer of the stomach. He reported that 4 or 5 years ago he began to have occasional burning sensations in his upper abdomen after meals. He saw several doctors then, all of whom performed multiple diagnostic procedures and pronounced him healthy except for mild indigestion. He began to scrupulously monitor his diet, keeping records of the frequency and intensity of his gastric symptoms. Gradually he began to "suspect the worst" (cancer) and again saw several different physicians, hoping that his cancer could be diagnosed and treated. He began to feel tired at the end of the workday and occasionally thought he felt "swollen glands" in his neck, which suggested that his cancer might be spreading. He cut back on the amount of work he was doing ('to rest more') and broke off a relationship with a woman.

Recently the patient became angry when his last physician refused to repeat diagnostic procedures already done and instead requested records from other physicians. He then made the startling admission that unless the cancer could be diagnosed this time, "I guess I'll have to give up the idea that I have it. But I feel like I do."

Epidemiology

Hypochondriasis is common in general medical practice and seems to occur with equal frequency in men and women. It is not known if there is an increased incidence among family members.

Etiology & Pathogenesis

Hypochondriasis is believed to have its origin in maladaptive attempts to cope with unmet psychological needs or unconscious psychological conflicts, but there is no agreement about the specific psychological mechanisms involved. Some feel the hypochondriacal patient merely shows an excessive self-concern; others suggest that hypochondriasis represents a physical expression of low self-esteem (sick, weak, defective); and still others have proposed that this way of viewing oneself protects the individual from awareness of destructive impulses toward others (seeing oneself as being damaged rather than as wishing to damage others). Some writers have recently proposed that these symptoms result from serious deficits in the ability of a patient to maintain a "sense of the self" (as well integrated or "put together') and that hypochondriacal symptoms must be viewed as one manifestation of this underlying problem.

Treatment

Psychotherapy appears to be useful for only a few hypochondriacal patients. Most are resistant to the idea of psychiatric treatment, and it should probably be offered only to highly motivated, insightful patients who will readily accept the recommendation. There is no evidence that somatic treatments are effective.

Since people with hypochondriasis usually present to nonpsychiatrist physicians and are opposed to psychiatric treatment, the general medical practitioner has the best opportunity to be of help. In order to benefit a hypochondriacal patient, the physician must give up the idea of cure in the usual sense of relieving symptoms. The physician must be able to accept the patient's fears and complaints as manifestations of a chronic psychiatric disorder that serve an important (if poorly understood) psychological function and which will continue indefinitely. With this approach, the physician may be able to avoid becoming frustrated, angry, or hopeless and will maintain a sensitivity to the patient's social and psychological needs and problems. The possibility exists that as a consequence of this supportive doctor-patient relationship, there will be a reduction in the patient's anxiety, which may result in a lessening of the fears of disease and improved social and occupational functioning. The physician should have fixed, regular appointments of unvarying duration with the hypochondriacal patient and should continue to respond in appropriate ways to physical complaints or true disease while avoiding unnecessary diagnostic or therapeutic procedures. This approach at least prevents "doctor-shopping" by the patient and reduces the risk of iatrogenic complications.

SUMMARY

The somatoform disorders are a group of psychiatric syndromes characterized by physical symptoms suggesting the presence of a physical disorder. There must be no physical findings or demonstrable pathophysiology to account for the symptoms, and there must be direct or strong presumptive evidence of psychological origin. People with these disorders usually do not perceive themselves as psychiatrically disturbed and therefore frequently present to nonpsy-

chiatrist medical practitioners for treatment. It is important that physicians be knowledgeable about these syndromes in order to avoid unnecessary and potentially harmful diagnostic and therapeutic interventions and to minimize secondary gain in the context of the medical treatment or in the patient's other relationships. At present, there are no specific treatments for most of these disorders, although a variety of psychotherapeutic treatments have been effective in some cases.

DISSOCIATIVE DISORDERS

The dissociative disorders are a group of psychiatric syndromes characterized by a sudden, temporary disruption of some aspect of consciousness, identity, or motor behavior. There are four main types: **psychogenic amnesia,** an alteration of the memory function of consciousness; **multiple personality disorder,** a disturbance in personal identity; **psychogenic fugue,** characterized by disturbances in both identity and motor behavior; and **depersonalization disorder,** a more limited disruption of identity in which perception of one's own reality is disturbed.

The functions of memory, personal identity, and motor behavior are crucial for the integrated operation of the complex set of mental and behavioral activities we call personality. Thus, although these syndromes are statistically uncommon, when they do occur they may present very dramatic clinical pictures of severe disturbance of normal personality functioning. These disorders are presumed to share the mental mechanism of dissociation in their pathogenesis.

PSYCHOGENIC AMNESIA

Symptoms & Signs

Psychogenic amnesia (Table 24–5) is characterized by a sudden onset of a single episode of inability to recall important personal data. The memory disturbance is not due to organic mental disorder (see Chapters 5, 17, and 18) and is too severe to be ordinary forgetfulness. There is no associated major disturbance of motor behavior. An individual with psychogenic amnesia is usually aware of the memory deficit but may show indifference to it, and during an amnestic episode, the person may demonstrate disorientation, perplexity, and purposeless wandering.

Four different types of memory disturbance are identified, and any one may occur in this disorder. The most common type is "localized" amnesia, inability to recall *everything* occurring within a brief period (hours to days) surrounding a given event.

Table 24–5. *DSM-III-R* diagnostic criteria for psychogenic amnesia.

A. The predominant disturbance is an episode of sudden inability to recall important personal information that is too extensive to be explained by ordinary forgetfulnes.
B. The disturbance is not due to multiple personality disorder or to an organic mental disorder (eg, blackouts during alcohol intoxication).

"Generalized" amnesia is inability to recall anything that has happened during the individual's lifetime. Both localized and generalized amnesia may be "selective"—ie, the memory loss (whether circumscribed in time or extending over the entire lifetime) may be for some events but not all. "Continuous" amnesia is an unusual memory disturbance in which all events subsequent to a specific time (up to and including the present) are forgotten, so that the individual is unable to form new memories even though apparently alert and aware.

Natural History

An episode of psychogenic amnesia typically begins following a life event that causes severe psychological stress in the affected individual. The precipitating event is often an extraordinary one and severely stressful, eg, something that threatens the patient's life or in which injury or death of others is witnessed. At other times the precipitating event may be only moderately stressful but experienced as extremely threatening because of idiosyncratic personality traits, eg, participation in an extramarital affair in spite of strong moral disapproval of such behavior. The onset and termination of the episodes are usually sudden, followed by complete recovery. Recurrences are unusual.

Differential Diagnosis

The differential diagnosis includes organic mental disorder, in which memory loss is sometimes one feature. In organic mental disorder, the disturbance in memory is usually more severe for recent events than for remote ones, and there is no temporal association with psychological stress. Memory return in organic mental disorder is gradual and usually incomplete if it occurs at all. A circumscribed memory loss is common in substance-induced intoxication (eg, "alcoholic blackouts"), but the ingested substance and absence of full return of memory are distinguishing features. A deficit limited to short-term memory (not immediate recall) is characteristic of alcohol amnestic disorder, also called Korsakoff's disease, and does not occur in psychogenic amnesia. Alcohol amnestic disorder occurs in the context of heavy and prolonged alcohol abuse, often follows an episode of Wernicke's encephalopathy, and is not associated with psychological stress. Postconcussion amnesia follows head injury and if necessary can be distinguished from psychogenic amnesia through the use of hypnosis or amobarbital interview techniques. Under the influence of hypnosis or amobarbital, return of memory is strongly suggestive of amnesia of emotional origin. Psychogenic fugue may include amnesia but is distinguished from psychogenic amnesia by the additional features of travel to a new locale and assumption of a new identity. Malingering involving feigned amnesia may be difficult to distinguish from psychogenic amnesia, but the motivation (secondary gain) is usually obvious. Hypnosis or amobarbital interview will usually make the diagnosis of malingering also.

Illustrative Case

A 25-year-old woman was admitted to the orthopedic service of a general hospital for treatment of a fractured femur, sustained when the car she was driving left the road and struck a utility pole. Her only child, a 2-year-old daughter, was killed in the crash, and the ambulance attendant reported that when he arrived at the scene, the patient was sitting quietly in the car holding her daughter's body and appearing slightly dazed.

There was no evidence of head injury, and the neurological examination was normal. It was apparent to the hospital staff that the patient was suffering from amnesia. She spoke freely of some portions of her past life but did not remember the accident. During a psychiatric interview the next day, she seemed only vaguely disturbed by recent events and made no mention of her daughter's death. Close questioning by the psychiatrist demonstrated that she had no memory of her daughter or of most events subsequent to a vacation trip with her husband about 2½ years ago. In a later discussion with the husband about this trip, the psychiatrist learned that it was then the patient first suspected she was pregnant.

Epidemiology

Psychogenic amnesia is rare, though it occurs more frequently in conditions of war or as a sequela of natural disaster. Adolescent and young adult women appear to be most commonly affected. There is no known familial tendency.

Etiology & Pathogenesis

Although efforts have been made to explain dissociative amnesia (and other dissociative phenomena) on the basis of neurophysiological dysfunction, most psychiatrists believe that psychological theories of psychogenic amnesia have the most credibility and usefulness.

In the discussion of the somatoform disorders, it was proposed that a morally unacceptable or frightening sexual or aggressive drive could be actively repressed and relegated to the unconscious. Although explained by somewhat different theoretical constructs, a similar mental mechanism is the basis for our current understanding of psychogenic amnesia. In the case of amnesia, it is proposed that the memory of a painful event (along with the associated emotions) is segregated from ongoing conscious experience as a protective mechanism. In some cases, escape can be achieved by selective disruption of memory; in others, a much more far-reaching disturbance is required.

The concepts of primary and secondary gain, discussed on p 262, also contribute to our understanding of psychogenic amnesia. The primary gain is protection from painful emotional experience. Responses of others may provide gratification of other psychological needs (secondary gain) and thus serve to maintain the amnesia after it is established. Examples of secondary gain are a soldier who develops amnesia on the battlefield and is sent home or to a hospital in a rear area, and a dependent wife who develops amnesia upon her husband's sudden death so that she is cared for by sympathetic friends and relatives.

The great majority of people experiencing severe psychosocial stress do not develop dissociative disorder. Most are able to cope psychologically with emotional responses in ways that permit adaptive functioning. People who do develop dissociative disorders often have chronic underlying psychiatric problems. A severe personality disorder or an organic mental disorder may prevent a normal adaptive response.

Treatment & Prognosis

Many cases of psychogenic amnesia resolve spontaneously when the individual is removed from the stressful situation.

Intravenous administration of intermediate- and short-acting barbiturates has been used in the treatment of psychogenic amnesia. The amobarbital interview can be useful in differentiating psychogenic amnesia from other types of amnesia, and in some cases therapeutic benefit (symptom relief) also occurs. A patient who under the influence of a barbiturate can recall "forgotten" events and come to terms emotionally with the painful memories (ie, abreact) may be able to retain the memories later in a drug-free state. Most clinicians recommend psychotherapy also to reinforce adjustment to the psychological impact of retrieved memories and the emotions associated with them.

Psychotherapy has also been used as primary treatment for patients with psychogenic amnesia. When relief of symptoms is the main goal of treatment, techniques of persuasion (directly encouraging remembering) and directed association (urging the patient to ruminate freely about events surrounding the amnestic period), gently applied in a supportive manner, have been helpful. Hypnosis, to facilitate recall and abreaction, has been effective in treating some cases and may be used in combination with psychotherapy. (The reader is referred to Nemiah's [1989]

discussion of the case of ''Barbara M'' for an excellent example of the combined use of psychotherapy and hypnosis in the treatment of psychogenic amnesia.)

If the patient is found to have some underlying psychiatric disorder when the episode of amnesia resolves, treatment of the amnesia should be followed by further psychiatric assessment and appropriate treatment. In the case of an underlying personality disorder, psychoanalysis or long-term insight-oriented psychotherapy might be indicated.

MULTIPLE PERSONALITY DISORDER

Symptoms & Signs

Multiple personality disorder is characterized by the existence of two or more personalities within a single individual (Table 24–6). Clinically, only one of the personalities is "present" at any given moment, and one of them is dominant most of the time over the course of the disorder. Each personality is well integrated and is a complex aggregate of unique memories, behavior patterns, and social relationships that control each individual's functioning during its dominant intervals. The transition from one personality to another is sudden, often dramatic, and usually precipitated by stress. Because patients with this disorder may actively conceal evidence of its existence, attention to more subtle signs of dissociation—not included in the formal diagnostic criteria—may facilitate its detection (Franklin, 1990; Putnam, 1989).

The various personalities are almost always quite discrepant and often seem to be opposites—eg, a shy, socially withdrawn, faithful husband may become a gregarious womanizer and heavy drinker. The original personality usually has no knowledge of the other personality or personalities, but when there are two or more subpersonalities, they are usually aware of each other's existence to some degree. When a given personality is dominant and interacting with the environment, the other personalities may not perceive all that is happening.

Natural History

One of the existing personalities may function reasonably well and alternate with another that does not. Studies of individuals with this disorder have shown that various subpersonalities may have measurably different psychological and physiological attri-

Table 24–6 *DSM-III-R* diagnostic criteria for multiple personality disorder.

A. The existence within the person of 2 or more distinct personalities or personality states (each with its own relatively enduring pattern of perceiving, relating to, and thinking about the environment and self).
B. At least 2 of these personalities or personality states recurrently take full control of the person's behavior.

butes such as pulse and blood pressure. A subpersonality may even have a specific, separate mental disorder: Somatoform disorders and psychological factors affecting physical condition are apparently common diagnoses in people with multiple personality. Most often, the various subpersonalities have different names, but they may be unnamed and may be of a different sex, race, and age.

Multiple personality disorder may begin at any age but is usually not recognized before adolescence. It seems to be related to sexual or physical abuse and other types of severe emotional trauma in childhood. The degree of functional impairment is variable, but it is usually at least moderate and may be severe. In contrast to other dissociative disorders, it tends to be more chronic, with only incomplete recovery.

Differential Diagnosis

The differential diagnosis of multiple personality disorders include distinguishing it from schizophrenic disorders, for example, when an individual with schizophrenia reports delusions of multiple personality or when a person with multiple personality disorders reports auditory hallucinations when another personality speaks. The distinction is based on the presence of distinguishing features of the schizophrenic disorders and the absence of subpersonalities that are complex and well-integrated units of unique behavior patterns and social relationships. Malingering may also present a diagnostic problem, but as in the differential diagnosis of the other dissociative disorders, the malingerer's symptoms will serve a recognizable goal and the true nature of the symptoms will be disclosed under hypnosis or during an amobarbital interview. Psychogenic amnesia and psychogenic fugue have similar characteristics but are distinguished, in part, by the repeated shifts of identity and the "interloper's" awareness of the existence of the original identity in multiple personality disorder.

Illustrative Case

A 21-year-old single woman who lived with her parents and attended a local college had been reared in a family that strictly adhered to the teachings of a fundamentalist religious denomination that prohibited drinking and dancing and forbade intercourse for any reason other than procreation. She was a good student but had no close friends and few social acquaintances. She lived a quiet life.

Acting on the advice of their minister, the patient's parents brought her to a psychiatrist after she told them she was pregnant but did not know how it had happened. (The fact of pregnancy was verified by the family physician.) In interviews with the psychiatrist, she seemed to be a painfully shy, soft-spoken, moralistic young woman who evidenced great remorse and apparently genuine perplexity about how her pregnancy had occurred. The psychiatrist asked for the patient's cooperation using hypnosis. The patient agreed and was easily hypnotized; in the hypnotic state, she demonstrated an entirely new personality. She insisted on being called "Dominique" and interacted with the psychiatrist in a provocative and flirtatious manner. She spoke loudly and used clichés and profanity in describing to the psychiatrist her recent escapades as Dominique. She told about slipping out of the house at night, consuming large quantities of alcohol, and having intercourse with men she picked up. When brought out of her hypnotized state, she was her usual self and had no memory of "Dominique." Later, in the course of her treatment, it was revealed by a third personality named "Baby" that an uncle had repeatedly forced her to engage in various sexual activities between the ages of 4 and 8 years.

Epidemiology

Although the relevant data regarding the exact incidence and distribution of multiple personality disorder are not yet available, most authorities no longer consider it a rare condition. It is most common in late adolescent and young adult women. There is no known familial occurrence.

Etiology & Pathogenesis

A complete understanding of the causes and development of multiple personality disorder is not yet possible, but there is now considerable empirical evidence establishing a strong association between reports of childhood physical and sexual abuse and the presence of the disorder in adults (Ross et al, 1990). Many authors see the phenomena of the disorder as reflecting the use of dissociative mental capacities to adapt to the abusive conditions and their psychological sequelae. In some cases, the different personalities seem to represent expressions of or protection against various emotions, attitudes, memories, etc, which in a normal person would be integrated in a single personality.

Treatment & Prognosis

There are now many reports of successful treatment of this disorder with long-term individual psychotherapy. These treatments, which often have stormy courses, are usually difficult for both the patient and the therapist and not infrequently require brief hospitalizations for management of crises and control of self-destructive behavior. Adjunctive pharmacotherapy for the management of anxiety or the concurrent treatment of other complicating psychiatric disorders is often of value in the treatment of these patients.

PSYCHOGENIC FUGUE

Symptoms & Signs

Psychogenic fugue (Table 24–7) is characterized by sudden, unexpected "flights" from home or workplace and assumption of a new identity. It is as if

Table 24–7. *DSM-III-R* diagnostic criteria for psychogenic fugue.

A. Sudden unexpected travel away from one's home or customary place of work, with inability to recall one's past.
B. Assumption of a new identity (partial or complete).
C. The disturbance is not due to multiple personality disorder or to an organic mental disorder (eg, partial complex seizures in temporal lobe epilepsy).

the patient is running away from something but is unaware of fleeing. There is inability to recall one's past, and when the episode resolves, there is inability to recall events of the fugue state. Although apparent disorientation and perplexity may occur, this disorder cannot be diagnosed in the presence of organic mental disorder.

The moving about that is part of psychogenic fugue is purposeful, in contrast to the confused wanderings that may be seen in psychogenic amnesia. In a typical case, the fugue consists of brief, purposeful journeying during which contacts with other people are minimal and in which the new identity is simple and incompletely developed. In rare cases, the assumed identity is quite elaborate, and the individual may take a new name and residence and engage in complex interpersonal relations or occupational activities so that the presence of a mental disorder is not suspected. When a new, complex identity is established, it is often characterized by more gregarious and uninhibited social behavior than was the patient's style before.

Natural History

There is evidence that heavy alcohol abuse may predispose to development of psychogenic fugue, but other predisposing factors have not been identified. The course of this disorder is similar to that described for psychogenic amnesia: An episode most often begins in the context of severe psychosocial stress and typically is of a brief duration (hours to days). Occasionally, an episode may last for months and involve complex social activity. Recovery is usually spontaneous, rapid, and complete, and recurrences are rare.

Although in most cases functional impairment is not severe or long-lasting, the degree of disruption or distress is variable. Violent behavior may occur, but this is not typical.

Differential Diagnosis

The differential diagnosis includes organic mental disorders, although the distinction is not usually difficult. Unexpected wandering from home is unusual in organic mental disorder, and when it does occur it usually has an aimless quality. The memory disturbance of psychogenic fugue may be similar to what occurs in psychogenic amnesia, but the latter does not involve purposeful travel or the assumption of a new personal identity. Complex partial seizures may be associated with a brief journey, but there is no assumption of a new identity and usually no psychoso-

cial precipitating episode. Malingering, which involves an apparent inability to remember one's identity, is difficult to distinguish from psychogenic fugue, but as is the case with all instances of malingering, a practical motive can usually be discerned. Hypnosis or amobarbital interview techniques might be a useful adjunct in distinguishing malingering from psychogenic fugue.

Illustrative Case

A 32-year-old married schoolteacher and minor town official, after learning of his wife's sexual involvement with another man, left home for work and just disappeared. Two months later, an acquaintance stopped for a meal in a small restaurant in the next state and saw him washing dishes behind the counter. The patient claimed not to know the friend and did not respond to his own name. The friend informed the local police, who found that the patient was unable to remember anything about his life prior to the preceding 2 months. He claimed he had found himself in the town 2 months ago not knowing who he was or how he had gotten there and that he invented a name for himself, moved into a rooming house, and took a job as a dishwasher, hoping he would remember who he was. His employer described him as a quiet and secretive man who nonetheless had been a reliable worker.

Epidemiology

Accurate prevalence rates are not available, but psychogenic fugue is rare and occurs most often under conditions of war, natural disaster, or intense personal crisis. No information is available regarding sex distribution or familial patterns of occurrence.

Etiology & Pathogenesis

Psychogenic fugue is thought to be related to some disorder of personality development. Because of severe anxiety or other unpleasant emotional experience (resulting from a traumatic life experience or internal conflict), certain aspects of the personality are psychologically put aside, "dissociated" from the usual complex organization of ideas, memories, emotions, and behavior patterns comprising the personality. The dissociated aspects of the personality are then not a part of the ongoing conscious experience of the individual. The underlying motivation is escape from painful emotional experience. A new identity is substituted. Leaving home might be "necessary" to make the new identity believable to oneself and others.

People who develop psychogenic fugue may have underlying emotional or mental abnormalities, including organic mental disorders, which make them especially vulnerable to psychological stress. These abnormalities also require that they resort to the extreme psychological maneuver of change in personal identity to deal with the stress rather than reacting in normally adaptive ways. The reasons for these underlying problems are thought to lie in early personality development.

Treatment & Prognosis

Recovery is usually rapid, spontaneous, and complete, and no specific treatment is required other than supportive care. Depending on the circumstances, environmental manipulation or supportive psychotherapy might play a role in ameliorating factors related to stress or in helping the patient adapt to stress in the future. If the episode is prolonged, psychotherapeutic techniques such as gentle encouragement or directed association may be helpful, either alone or in combination with other techniques, such as hypnosis or amobarbital interviews, which are also aimed at facilitating recall of the previous identity.

DEPERSONALIZATION DISORDER

Symptoms & Signs

Historically, the symptoms of depersonalization and derealization have been recognized as part of the clinical picture of a wide variety of mental disorders. Common to both of these symptoms is a temporary disturbance in the subjective experience of reality, so that the usual quality of familiarity associated with perception is replaced by a sense of estrangement or unreality. In the case of **depersonalization,** the disturbance is in the perception of oneself; in **derealization,** the alteration is in the perception of the external environment. In depersonalization disorder, the major symptom is that of depersonalization, but as presently defined, the disorder may include the symptom of derealization as well.

Depersonalization disorder is defined in *DSM-III-R* as the occurrence of one or more episodes of depersonalization, not due to any other mental disorder, that causes marked distress (Table 24–8). The major feature is sudden temporary loss of the sense of one's

Table 24–8. *DSM-III-R* diagnostic criteria for depersonalization disorder (or depersonalization neurosis).

A. Persistent or recurrent experiences of depersonalization as indicated by either (1) or (2):
   (1) An experience of feeling detached from and as if one is an outside observer of one's mental processes or body.
   (2) An experience of feeling like an automaton or as if in a dream.
B. During the depersonalization experience, reality testing remains intact.
C. The depersonalization is sufficiently severe and persistent to cause marked distress.
D. The depersonalization experience is the predominant disturbance, not a symptom of another disorder, such as schizophrenia, panic disorder, or agoraphobia without history of panic disorder, but with limited symptom attacks of depersonalization or temporal lobe epilepsy.

own reality, manifested as an experience of being detached from one's body or mental processes or feeling as though one were an outside observer of one's body or mental processes. Patients may also describe feeling as though they were mechanical or as though they were in a dream. Reality testing remains intact, but various feelings of self-estrangement or beliefs that the body's physical characteristics have changed may accompany the episode. Various types of automatism or sensory anesthesias may also occur.

Derealization typically involves the perception that objects in the external world have changed in size or shape, or the subjective feeling that other people are automated, mechanical, somehow inhuman, or dead.

All of these distorted perceptions are experienced as being unpleasant and undesired and may be accompanied by anxiety, dizziness, a fear of becoming insane, feelings of depression, obsessive thoughts, or disturbances in the subjective experience of time.

Natural History

The onset of an episode of depersonalization is usually sudden, and resolution is gradual. The duration of the episode is usually brief, lasting a period of minutes, but complete disappearance of the symptom may take hours.

Differential Diagnosis

When episodes of depersonalization occur as part of another mental disorder, the frequency or intensity of episodes usually parallels the severity of other symptoms occurring as part of the primary disorder. The course of depersonalization disorder as defined here is usually chronic, with exacerbations and remissions.

Mild episodes of depersonalization may occur in people without any mental disorder; the diagnosis of depersonalization disorder is not made, even if episodes are recurrent, unless the symptom causes social or occupational dysfunction. Episodes of depersonalization may also occur in the presence of a variety of mental disorders; examples include schizophrenia, affective disorders, organic mental disorders, anxiety disorders, personality disorders, and epilepsy. In such cases, the diagnosis of depersonalization disorder is not made.

Illustrative Case

A 35-year-old lawyer telephoned a psychiatrist and asked for an appointment, saying, "I don't know what's the matter with me, but I'm afraid I'm going crazy." At the first appointment, he explained that for several years he had been having strange "attacks" about once a month. The "attacks" generally occurred during the course of his work, and on two recent occasions he had had to leave the courtroom in the midst of a legal proceeding "to get control" of himself. He explained that an "attack" usually was heralded by a sudden feeling of nervousness and awareness that his heart was pounding. This was followed by the experience that all objects in his visual field had diminished to about half their normal size and by the perception that people's actions (his own and others) had lost their usual fluid quality and took on a mechanical, jerky character, "as in silent movies." These symptoms occasionally would be accompanied by the experience that he had become someone else ('I don't know who, but not myself'). On the day he telephoned the psychiatrist, an "attack" had begun while he was driving his car, and the usual symptoms were accompanied by the perception that his arms had become detached from his body and continued to steer the car "on their own."

Epidemiology

There is no information on the prevalence, sex ratio, or possible patterns of familial distribution of depersonalization disorder.

Etiology & Pathogenesis

Empirical observations have led some investigators to propose that the phenomenon of depersonalization (as distinct from depersonalization disorder) has a neurophysiological basis. Patients with brain tumors and epilepsy have reported depersonalization episodes in association with their neurological disorder. Electrical stimulation of the temporal lobe cortex has been reported to produce depersonalization phenomena, and some psychotomimetic drugs (eg, LSD) produce various distortions of reality (including the sense of reality in the perception of the self) in some individuals.

Explanations emphasizing psychic conflict and disturbances of ego structure have been offered within the framework of psychoanalytic theory, but they have been incomplete and unsatisfactory. Experiencing the self as "not real" would offer protection or escape from (ie, function as a defense against) anxiety or some unpleasant emotional state resulting from internal psychological conflict. For example, individuals with strong internal prohibitions against aggressive feelings might, when threatened with aggressive impulses, perceive themselves as not "real" and thus in a sense negate the knowledge that they "really" have aggressive impulses.

Attempts to explain depersonalization in terms of constructs regarding the structure of the ego are beyond the scope of this discussion.

Treatment & Prognosis

Little is known about the treatment of depersonalization disorder. Pharmacotherapy with dextroamphetamine or amobarbital has been used, with inconclusive results. Both supportive and insight-oriented psychotherapeutic techniques have been attempted, again with variable success. Evaluation of treatment is complicated by the fact that much of the work has been with patients who experienced depersonalization phenomena in association with a variety of other psychiatric disorders and not with depersonalization disorder as defined here.

SUMMARY

The dissociative disorders are a group of distinct psychiatric syndromes characterized by severe disturbances in one or more of the personality functions of consciousness, personal identity, or motor behavior. The primary disturbance in psychogenic amnesia is of memory; in multiple personality and depersonalization disorders, it is of identity; and in psychogenic fugue, both identity and motor behavior are affected. As a group, the dissociative disorders are relatively uncommon, but psychogenic amnesia occurs frequently enough so that most physicians will encounter it at some time during their careers. Although depersonalization disorder is apparently unusual, depersonalization phenomena are common among normal people as well as among people with other psychiatric disorders. Except for the role of sexual and physical abuse in the etiology of multiple personality disorder, the causes of the various dissociative disorders are not clearly or specifically defined, but psychological theories of causation are widely accepted. The treatment of dissociative disorders is poorly understood and not always effective, and except when resolution of symptoms is spontaneous, referral of patients to a psychiatrist is indicated.

REFERENCES

Braun BB (editor): *Treatment of Multiple Personality Disorder*. American Psychiatric Press, 1986.

Brena SF, Chapman SL: *Management of Patients With Chronic Pain*. Spectrum, 1983.

Breuer J, Freud S: Studies on hysteria (1895). In: *Standard Edition of the Complete Psychological Works of Sigmund Freud*. Vol 2. Hogarth Press, 1955.

Cloninger C et al: A prospective follow-up and family study of somatization in men and women. Am J Psychiatry 1986;143:873.

Combs G Jr, Ludwig AM: Dissociative disorders. Chapter 9 in: *Treatment of Mental Disorders*. Greist JH, Jefferson JW, Spitzer RC (editors). Oxford Univ Press, 1982.

Dysken MW: Clinical usefulness of sodium amobarbital interviewing. Arch Gen Psychiatry 1979;36:789.

Dysken MW: Clinical usefulness of sodium amobarbital interviewing. Am J Psychiatry 1979;36:789.

Greist JH, Jefferson JW, Spitzer RC (editors): *Treatment of Mental Disorders*. Oxford Univ Press, 1982.

Kaplan, HI, Freedman AM, Sadock BJ (editors). *Compre-*

hensive Textbook of Psychiatry/IV, 4th ed. Williams & Wilkins, 1985.

Kellner R: Somatization: Theories and research. J Nerv Ment Dis 1990;178:150.

Kluft RP (editor): *Childhood Antecedents of Multiple Personality*. American Psychiatric Press, 1985.

Morrison J: Childhood sexual histories of women with somatization disorder. Am J Psychiatry 1989;146:239.

Nemiah JC: Dissociative disorders (hysterical neurosis, dissociative type). Chapter 20 in: Kaplan HI, Sadock BJ (editors). *Comprehensive Textbook of Psychiatry/V*, 5th ed. Williams & Wilkins, 1989.

Ochitill H: Somatoform disorders. Chapter 8 in: *Treatment of Mental Disorders*. Greist JH, Jefferson JW, Spitzer RC (editors). Oxford Univ Press, 1982.

Orenstein H et al: Polysymptomatic complaints and Briquet's syndrome in polycystic ovary disease. Am J Psychiatry 1986;143:768.

Pinsky JJ: Chronic intractable benign pain: A syndrome and its treatment with intensive short-term group psychotherapy. J Human Stress 1978;4: 17.

Putnam FW: *Diagnosis and Treatment of Multiple Personality Disorder*. Guilford Press, 1989.

Ross CA et al: Structured interview data on 102 cases of multiple personality disorder from four centers. Am J Psychiatry 1990;147:596. PSYC-25: Updated 3/19

25

Adjustment Disorder

Kathryn N. DeWitt, PhD

Other chapters in this text describe psychiatric disorders that are characterized by identifiable symptom patterns. Although these disorders are important subjects of psychiatric research and teaching, they do not include the emotional problems of a great many individuals who seek help. The patients whose problems comprise the subject matter of this chapter lack some or all of the specific symptoms that would qualify them for the disorders discussed in other chapters. Adjustment disorders are generally associated with difficult life experiences, but the suffering or dysfunction that results is out of proportion to the degree of stress.

The adjustment disorder diagnosis serves three important functions: (1) It draws attention to people who need professional help; (2) it provides a way of collecting data to devise new subcategories of illness; and (3) it describes specific procedures for distinguishing these patients from those with other mental disorders or those with normal responses to the problems of life. Patients with "problems in living" but no mental disorder are classified by use of "V" codes (see below).

Establishing a Diagnosis of Adjustment Disorder

DSM-III-R characterizes adjustment disorder as "a reaction to an identifiable psychosocial stressor or multiple stressors that occurs within three months of the onset of the stressors." The reaction may take the form of "impairment in occupational (including school) functioning or in usual social activities or relationships with others" or "symptoms that are in excess of a normal and expectable reaction to the stressors." The disturbance may not have persisted for longer than 6 months. The diagnosis of adjustment disorder is not used when symptoms conform to the specific criteria for another mental disorder (excluding personality disorder or developmental disorder); nor is it used when current distress represents but one instance of a general pattern of overreaction to stressors. For this reason, adjustment disorder is a diagnosis of exclusion.

Four major decisions are involved in the diagnosis of adjustment disorder: (1) establishing a relationship to a psychosocial stressor, (2) evaluating the level and duration of disturbance, (3) ruling out other mental disorders, and (4) evaluating the context of the patient's total personality.

A. Establishing a Relationship to a Psychosocial Stressor:

Illustrative case. A 64-year-old retired teacher came to an internist, seeking help for a feeling of constant exhaustion. She said that her troubles began months earlier with the death of her husband from kidney disease. She had thought then that her problems were due to sadness at her loss, but now that they had lasted unchanged for nearly 6 months, she wondered whether she had "high blood pressure or low blood sugar or some such." She reported that her sleeping patterns had not changed and she had continued her regular pattern of daily walks. The patient and her husband were both accomplished bridge players, and she was an excellent cook; yet neither playing cards nor cooking was pleasurable any more. She still had a good appetite and attended her bridge club regularly, but her lack of enthusiasm was commented on by club members. The patient admitted that she felt she would be better off if she had died too, though she would not do anything to hurt herself. She was able to get around and take care of herself, but life did not seem to have any meaning.

Physical examination and laboratory tests failed to show evidence of any physical disorder. The physician concluded that the symptoms were of psychological origin.

Before a diagnosis of adjustment disorder can be made, the clinician must determine whether the patient's current problem is causally related to a psychosocial stressor. In many cases, a patient or someone who knows the patient may make a causal connection between the stressor and the disturbance. If the current disturbance represents a change in functioning that coincided with the occurrence of the stressor, there is a good cause for suspecting a connection. Symptoms may have appeared within minutes after the onset of stress or may have been long delayed. The *DSM-III-R* diagnostic criteria require that the dysfunction be evident within 3 months after occurrence of the stressor and persist for no longer than 6 months.

Sometimes there is a logical connection between

the kind of stressor and the content of the patient's disturbance, or the patient may report being consciously preoccupied with the stressor, as was the widow (see above). In other cases, patients may be unaware of a connection or even deny it if asked. In more ambiguous circumstances, discerning a connection may depend on the creativity and clinical experience of the clinician. A diagnosis of adjustment disorder is applicable only to patients whose current disturbance is clearly linked to a specific event, as would appear to be the case with the widow, since her exhaustion, suicidal thoughts, and lack of interest in life activities began soon after her husband's death and were not characteristic of her functioning before the event.

B. Evaluating the Level and Duration of Disturbance: The second decision-making process in the diagnosis of adjustment disorder is evaluation of the patient's specific signs and symptoms. A diagnosis of adjustment disorder is warranted only if the following circumstances apply: (1) The patient's symptoms are more severe than would be expected in the absence of some mental disorder; (2) the disturbance does not meet the criteria established for other mental disorders; and (3) the duration of symptoms does not exceed 6 months. A diagnosis of adjustment disorder is used for patients whose response to a stressor is more severe than normally expected but somehow nonspecific or incomplete.

\ *DSM-III-R* indicates that the clinician should compare the patient's response with that of an "average person in similar circumstances and with similar sociocultural values." However, "the severity of the reaction is not completely predictable from the severity of the stressor. Individuals who are particularly vulnerable may have a more severe form of the disorder following only a mild or moderate stressor, whereas others may have only a mild form of the disorder in response to a marked and continuing stressor." The seriousness of a stressor is evaluated in terms of how much change it has caused, how central it has been to the person's life, how expected it was, whether it was a negative or a positive event, and whether it was shared or not.

The diagnosis of adjustment disorder is considered when a person's stress response is stronger or lasts longer than most other people's. Patients whose reactions exceed expectable limits often are an object of concern to those around them, so that they may come to the physician's office accompanied by a friend or relative, or they may come alone but make a point of having done so at another's urging.

The reactions of others may help the clinician determine whether or not the patient's response to stress should be diagnosed as adjustment disorder. Responses not indicative of mental disorder may be assigned a V code (see below) to identify the condition that was the focus of medical attention. Responses indicative of some mental disorder by virtue of inappropriate severity or duration are examined more closely so that a specific diagnosis may be assigned. In the illustrative case discussed above, the unchanged nature of the widow's disturbance exceeds the expectable reaction following death of a spouse. Her symptoms are interfering with her social functioning and have been commented on by those around her.

C. Ruling Out Other Mental Disorders (Excluding Personality and Developmental Disorders): Patients are not given a diagnosis of adjustment disorder if their stress response meets the criteria for some other mental disorder. Patients for whom a diagnosis of adjustment disorder is inappropriate include those whose disturbances are organically caused, psychotic in nature, or limited to psychosexual problems, amnesia, loss of integration of consciousness, or loss of identity. Also eliminated are those whose current disturbances are a single instance of a continuing psychosexual, substance abuse, or impulse control problem; similarly excluded are manic episodes, panic attacks, or phobic avoidance. Many excluded diagnostic categories are defined in part as an untoward reaction to a psychosocial stressor; examples include brief reactive psychosis, somatoform pain disorder, conversion disorders, psychogenic amnesia, psychogenic fugue, depersonalization disorder, and separation anxiety. Each of these diagnoses has additional specific distinguishing features that differentiate it from the nonspecific category of adjustment disorder.

Patients with adjustment disorder show disturbances of mood (either anxiety or depression) and impaired social and occupational functioning (withdrawal, misconduct, inhibition). They usually satisfy some but not all of the criteria for generalized anxiety disorder, posttraumatic stress disorder, major depressive disorder, dysthymia, cyclothymia, conduct disorder, or avoidant disorder.

In the case of the widow, the symptoms of fatigue, loss of pleasure in formerly satisfying activities, and passive death wishes place her within the spectrum of depressive disorders as set forth in Table 25–1, the depressive disorders include uncomplicated bereavement, adjustment disorder, major depressive disorder, dysthymia, and posttraumatic stress disorder. The patient's symptoms exceed the normal reaction to the death of a spouse. They began soon after her husband's death and continued unchanged for 6 months; they caused concern to her and those around her. Therefore, "uncomplicated bereavement" would be eliminated as a diagnostic consideration, and, by extension, the presence of a mental disorder would be confirmed. The duration of symptoms is insufficient for a diagnosis of dysthymia, which requires that symptoms be continually present for at least 2 years. The death of the patient's husband from kidney disease does not meet the criteria for posttraumatic stress disorder, since the principal stress is not beyond the range of common human experience. A diagnosis

Table 25–1. Differential diagnosis of depressed mood in bereavement.

	Type of Death	Duration of Symptoms	Type of Symptoms
Uncomplicated bereavement	Any type.	2–3 months; longer by social custom or relationship to deceased.	Limited to those normally expected.
Adjustment disorder	Any type.	Begin within 3 months; may be longer than normally expected; may not persist beyond 6 months.	Either impaired social or occupational functioning or symptoms in excess of those normally expected.
Major depressive disorder	Any type.	Every day for at least 2 weeks.	Dysphoric mood plus 4 out of 8 major symptoms (see Table 22–1).
Dysthymia	Any type.	Continually present for 2 years, with remissions of 2 months or less.	Depressive mood, but symptoms not severe enough for major depression; 3 out of 13 key symptoms present (see Table 22–1).
Posttraumatic stress disorder	Outside the range of usual experience.	Immediate or delayed; duration not specified.	Reexperiencing of trauma; numbing of responsiveness plus 2 out of 6 additional symptoms (see Table 23–7).

of major depressive disorder is inappropriate because the patient demonstrates only three of the eight major symptoms. The diagnosis of adjustment disorder is thus reached by a process of exclusion.

D. Evaluating the Context of the Patient's Total Personality:

Illustrative case. A 56-year-old steelworker was brought by his daughter to a family practitioner. The daughter explained that her father had always been considered "difficult" but that lately he had become "nearly impossible," and she was concerned about his health. She reported that her father was known for sayings as, "I wouldn't trust him as far as I could throw him." He usually kept to himself and was touchy about being taken advantage of. For the past 4 months, his suspicions had become frantic— he spent every waking moment worrying about some possible harm that might be done to him until he collapsed exhausted.

The patient did seem haggard and exhausted, though hyperalert during the interview. He nervously scanned the room as he talked and nearly jumped off the examining table when the nurse entered the room. When asked to explain his troubles, he replied that he had come "to get my daughter off my back." He said that although he was very tired, he could not let up, because he knew that "guys from work have it in for me." He had been out of work for 4 months since the local plant had closed. Previously he could "keep those bums in their place" because of his seniority, but now he was less able to defend himself and had to be constantly on the alert.

The patient was in touch with reality. His fears about his coworkers had the flavor of self-fulfilling prophecy and were not out of the realm of possibility, given his customary behavior in social situations. He showed no signs of abnormal thought patterns and was oriented as to time and place. He refused physical examinations and tests. In the absence of additional clinical information, the physician concluded that the patient's symptoms were probably due to psychological causes.

The clinician must assess the patient's personality style to determine whether the current maladaptive response stands out as a unique and striking episode or is simply one aspect of a consistently maladaptive pattern of relating to the environment and oneself, as occurs in personality disorder. In general, a diagnosis of adjustment disorder is made if no diagnosis of personality disorder or developmental disorder alone can account for all of the symptoms and signs or if symptoms of the current stress response are atypical for a preexisting personality disorder.

The functioning of the widow did not meet the criteria for any of the personality disorders. She was capable of warm personal relationships and had a well-developed sense of self. In contrast, the steelworker's usual manner of relating was compatible with a diagnosis of paranoid personality disorder. His current symptoms of exhaustion, suspiciousness, and hypervigilance were judged to be a stress-related exacerbation of a long-standing and stable dysfunctional personality style. Since the patient did not have symptoms that would lead to a diagnosis of organic delusional syndrome, paranoia, or paranoid schizophrenia, diagnoses of adjustment disorder and paranoid personality disorder were made.

Types of Adjustment Disorder

DSM-III-R describes nine main symptom patterns in adjustment disorder and assigns a code to each. The codes and their corresponding symptoms are set forth in Table 25–2.

The diagnosis of the widow would be classified as adjustment disorder with depressed mood, since all of her symptoms (exhaustion, loss of pleasure, death wishes) lie within the spectrum of depression. The steelworker's predominant symptoms of excessive vigilance against possible attack justify a diagnosis of adjustment disorder with anxious mood.

Table 25–2. Types of adjustment disorder.

Code	Predominant Symptom Pattern
309.00	Depressed mood
309.24	Anxious mood
309.28	Mixed emotional features
309.30	Disturbance of conduct
309.40	Mixed disturbance of emotions and conduct
309.23	Work (or academic) inhibition
309.82	Physical complaints
309.83	Withdrawal
309.90	Adjustment disorder not otherwise specified

V Codes for Conditions Not Attributable to Mental Disorder

DSM-III-R includes 13 V codes for "conditions that are a focus of attention or treatment but are not attributable to any of the mental disorders noted previously." These codes were adapted from a longer listing of similar conditions in *ICD-9-CM* (World Health Organization's *International Classification of Diseases, Injuries, and Causes of Death*, 9th ed, with clinical modification codes [CM]) and include such categories as malingering, adult antisocial behavior, noncompliance with medical treatment, and marital problems. The reactions of some patients in whom a diagnosis of adjustment disorder is being considered may fall within the limits of a normal and expectable response to a stressful life event; these patients would be assigned an appropriate V code to show the reason for their contact with a health facility. A V code may also be used when information is insufficient to determine whether a mental disorder is present or when the focus of treatment is not related to a coexisting mental disorder, eg, treatment of an uncomplicated marital problem in a person with simple phobia.

Natural History

A. Course and Outcome: The course and outcome of adjustment disorder are less severe and disabling than those of other major psychiatric disorders. A large study by Looney and Gunderson (1978) showed that the problems of persons with this diagnosis tended to be less severe with regard to chronicity, length of treatment, and disposition than those of other major psychiatric disorders.

B. Differential Course and Outcome in Adolescents and Adults: Studies by Andreasen et al (1980, 1982) found important differences in the expression of adjustment disorder in adolescents and in adults. Adolescents with adjustment disorders showed more serious disturbance than did adults with regard to symptoms, required length of treatment, and duration of symptoms before diagnosis. Adolescents also differed from adults with regard to their main presenting symptoms, with disturbance of conduct being more likely to be reported, whereas adults

were more likely to report depressive symptoms. The patient's age was found to be one of the most significant predictors of the outcome of adjustment disorder. About twice as many adolescents as adults experienced an episode of some other psychiatric disorder during a 5-year follow-up period.

In summary, available empirical evidence does indicate that adjustment disorder is less severe than other disorders with regard to both course and outcome. However, for some patients—especially adolescents—an episode of adjustment disorder may be characterized by distress that is not self-limited and may be recurrent.

Epidemiology

A. General Prevalence: The limited data available on the prevalence of adjustment disorder support the view that the diagnosis is common in the psychiatric population, especially among adolescents. The diagnosis was used in roughly 20% of cases classified in *DSM-III* field trials. About 10% of adults and 30% of adolescents in this sample were assigned a diagnosis of adjustment disorder.

B. Differential Prevalence in Adolescents and Adults: The diagnosis of adjustment disorder is frequently made in adolescents. It is not clear whether the disorder is actually more common during adolescence or whether there are other reasons that the diagnosis is more commonly used for patients in that age group.

In spite of arguments and evidence to the contrary, many clinicians believe that significant distress is a common response to physiological and cultural events that normally occur during adolescence. They may therefore automatically classify cases of adolescent psychological disturbance as examples of adjustment disorder.

Frequent use of the diagnosis of adjustment disorder for adolescents may reflect its function as a provisional diagnosis. A crucial requirement of many alternative diagnoses is that the observed disturbance be long-standing and persistent; however, many psychiatric problems first appear during adolescence and persist from then on. The ambiguous picture may force the use of adjustment disorder as a nonspecific diagnosis until the long-range picture is clear.

Finally, researchers have found that some clinicians overuse the category because they are concerned about the adverse effects of applying psychiatric labels such as alcoholism or antisocial personality disorder to young people. The diagnosis of adjustment disorder is seen as less harmful than lifelong stigmatization by other diagnoses.

Careful epidemiological studies should eliminate such diagnostic inaccuracies, so that a more valid estimate of the prevalence of adjustment disorder can be made. Meanwhile, the diagnosis should be used with discretion. In an adolescent, there should be strong evidence that current problems are related to some specific event or to some identifiable aspect of the adolescent experience. When the diagnosis is unclear after careful assessment, a diagnosis of atypical psychosis or unspecified mental disorder (nonpsychotic) should be used instead.

Etiology & Pathogenesis

A. Presumed Causal Mechanism: Stress-related disorders are a disruption of the normal process of adaptation to stressful life events. Models of normal adaptation have been developed by Lindemann (1944), Pollock (1977), and Horowitz (1976), among others. In the Horowitz model, the person experiencing stress passes through regular stages of response, including **outcry,** in which the person protests that what has happened cannot be true; **intrusion** and **denial,** during which the person is either painfully aware of or oblivious to the new reality; **working through,** when the person becomes better able to integrate the event; and **completion,** which is marked by function at or above the prestress level.

In adjustment disorder, this process of adaptation does not proceed to completion. The presumed cause is **psychic overload,** ie, a level of intrapsychic strain that exceeds the individual's ability to cope.

The pattern of disruption may take many forms. Some persons become caught in a seemingly endless stage of denial; they act as if the stressful event had never occurred, avoid all reminders of the stress, and remain emotionally numb or isolated. In others, intrusive symptoms predominate; individuals become so painfully aware of the stressor that they are unable to sleep or control the flood of incoming emotions and images associated with the event. Still others oscillate between symptoms of intrusion and denial, with no overall change in psychological assimilation of the stressor. Any of these patterns may be accompanied by difficulties in interpersonal relationships.

B. Contributing Factors: Several models have been developed to explain why some people can handle stress and even grow as a result, whereas others develop distress of psychopathological proportions. Most models take into account the interaction of the stressor, the situation, and the person.

1. Stressors– Stressors are of two general types: **Shock-type stressors** are time-limited events; **continuous stressors** are ongoing situations. Most descriptions of adaptation to stress concentrate on shock-type stressors. However, research shows that continuous stressors were more commonly cited as precipitating causes of psychiatric disorders. Adults usually developed adjustment disorder in response to ongoing problems in marriage, finances, work, or school. In adolescents, common stressors were problems with school, parental rejection, or parents' marital problems. Shock-type stressors were less commonly cited precipitating factors.

Research shows that the degree of undesirable change a stressor causes is the most significant aspect

of its ability to cause strain. Other characteristics that influence the amount of strain produced by a stressor include whether the event was sudden or anticipated, central or peripheral to the life of the individual, and culturally shared or experienced in social isolation.

2. Situational context– The presence of material and social supports or handicaps can mitigate or exacerbate the strains of adaptation to stress. Pertinent factors in the material environment include economic conditions, occupational and recreational opportunities, and weather conditions. Factors in the social environment include family, friends, neighbors, and cultural or religious support groups. These elements create a supportive or nonsupportive climate for adaptation.

3. Intrapersonal factors– Intrapersonal factors are considered the most crucial in determining whether the response to stress will be normal or dysfunctional. Not all persons with roughly similar stressors and environmental circumstances have similar responses to stress. Some are vulnerable to even minor stressful events, whereas others show an amazing resilience in the face of the most traumatic experiences.

Intrapersonal vulnerability to stressful life experiences may be general or specific. General factors include limitations in social skills or in intelligence, flexibility, and range of coping strategies. The presence of chronic disorders such as organic mental disorder, mental retardation, psychotic disorder, or personality disorder limits the general adaptive capacity of an individual.

Vulnerability to specific types of stressful events or circumstances may arise from relevant life traumas, unresolved conflicts, or developmental issues. Women who lost their mothers in infancy are more likely to develop serious depressive episodes following adult losses. People who have conflicts about aggression may respond to assault by alternately avoiding and provoking fights with others. Individuals who have difficulty making choices respond to the absence of structure in retirement by feeling helplessly directionless. Each of these intrapersonal factors combines with extrapersonal factors and characteristics of the stressor to produce the individual's stress response.

Treatment

A. Controversy About Treatment: The *DSM-III-R* definition of adjustment disorder has engendered controversy about treatment. On the one hand, the disorder is expected to eventually remit after the stressor ceases or, if the stressor persists, when a new level of adaptation is achieved. This expectation has led some to argue that treatment is unnecessary and wasteful. Some suggest that treatment may actually interfere with normal coping and result in worsening symptoms and delayed resolution.

On the other hand, adjustment disorder is also defined as being associated with exaggerated symptoms and social or occupational impairment. Clinicians who favor treatment suggest that symptoms must be brought within manageable limits before the patient can begin to cope with the stress. They also point out that in adjustment disorder, duration of symptoms may have exceeded the point of spontaneous remission. Such disturbances become self-sustaining and require some means of interrupting the downward spiral if serious effects on work and social relationships are to be avoided. Proponents of crisis intervention theory, such as Caplan (1964) and Langsley and Kaplan (1968), maintain that a crisis offers an ideal opportunity for treatment that will act as a catalyst for positive change in coping strategies.

B. General Recommendations: The general recommendation for treatment of adjustment disorder is for brief treatment with periodic reassessments. The primary goals of treatment are to relieve symptoms and assist patients in achieving a level of adaptation that at least equals their functioning before the stressful event. A secondary goal is to foster positive change whenever possible—especially in areas still vulnerable to recurrent stress-related disorders.

C. Psychosocial Treatment Methods: Mental health professionals most commonly recommend some form of psychosocial treatment for patients with adjustment disorder. Since adjustment disorder is generally thought to arise from vulnerabilities in the patient's psychosocial functioning, treatment measures are designed to have an impact on whatever habits, conflicts, developmental inadequacies, or disturbing social symptoms are thought to be the source of the patient's problem. Such treatments hold the greatest promise for preventing recurrent disorders.

1. Individual psychotherapy is the most common psychosocial treatment for adjustment disorder. The brief psychodynamic psychotherapy developed by Horowitz and Kaltreider (1980) is a good example. In this approach, the patient's problems are thought to result from the meanings assigned by the individual to the stressful event in relation to unresolved conflicts, previously latent negative self-images, earlier traumatic experiences, and developmental inadequacies. Common psychodynamic techniques of supportive and expressive psychotherapy are used to discover and resolve these meanings.

Individual behavior therapy differs significantly in theory and technique from individual psychodynamic psychotherapy. In behavior therapy, the patient's problems are seen as the result of habitually dysfunctional patterns of responding to situations. The goal of treatment is to replace ineffective adaptive response patterns with successful ones. Modeling, coaching, didactic presentations, and carefully designed reinforcement schedules are common techniques. Behavior therapy has usually been considered most appropriate for problems of impulse control, which

may occur in adjustment disorder with disturbance of conduct.

2. Family therapy is the second most common treatment for adjustment disorder. In this approach, the focus of diagnosis and treatment is shifted from the individual to the system of relationships in which the individual is involved. Treatment is designed to alter the functioning of the social network, and when possible, all relevant family members are included in treatment sessions. Family therapy should be seriously considered in adjustment disorder associated with developmental milestones such as birth of a child, mid-life transition, or retirement. It is also helpful in situations such as family bereavements and marital problems.

3. Self-help groups, in which people who have experienced similar stressful life events come together without a professional facilitator, are increasing in popularity. Group members often gain reassurance from discovering that many of their frightening emotional experiences are common and therefore not "crazy," as they had feared. Members also benefit from having an arena in which they can talk about painful topics without feeling like a burden to family and friends. Group members exchange advice, share coping strategies, and provide support and encouragement. They may also develop new social networks to replace those lost through events such as death or divorce. Community service agencies can be a good source of information on self-help groups.

D. Biomedical Treatment Methods: Medication may be the most commonly used treatment for adjustment disorder, since self-medication with alcohol, caffeine, over-the-counter medications, and street drugs is undoubtedly widespread. Treatment of symptoms of depression and anxiety with prescribed medications is common also. Prescription drugs have the potential advantage of being carefully chosen and continually monitored.

Mental health professionals usually do not treat adjustment disorder with medication. Reasons for not using medication include concerns that their effect is temporary; that alleviating symptoms only masks the real problem or interferes with the motivation to find a real, lasting solution; and that patients may develop either psychological or physiological dependence.

Although depressive symptoms are common in adjustment disorder, concerns about side effects of antidepressant medications and the length of time required to achieve effective results persuade most clinicians that their use should be limited to major depressive disorder.

When used, medications are generally considered adjuncts to treatment or as backup treatment when psychological treatments are unavailable or unacceptable to the patient. Medications may be used to bring distress within tolerable limits, so that the patient's coping strategies may be effectively mobilized. When they are used, clinicians should prescribe the lowest effective dosage for the shortest possible duration, together with frequent monitoring of efficacy and side effects.

SUMMARY

Adjustment disorder is one of the more common psychological disorders for which patients seek professional help, especially from general practitioners. For this reason, all clinicians should have a good working knowledge of the four decision-making procedures used to diagnose adjustment disorder:(1) establishing a relationship to a psychosocial stressor; (2) evaluating the level and duration of disturbance; (3) ruling out other mental disorders (excluding personality or developmental disorder); and (4) evaluating the patient's total personality. Patients with adjustment disorder demonstrate inadequate or incomplete adaptation to life stresses. The treatment of choice is brief psychosocial intervention designed to enhance the patient's ability to cope with the stressful event. When patients feel out of control, appropriate medications may be used to alleviate symptoms to the point that the patient can begin to cope with the stressful situation.

REFERENCES

Andreasen NC, Hoenk PR: The predictive value of adjustment disorders: A follow-up study. Am J Psychiatry 1982;139:584.

Andreasen NC, Wasek P: Adjustment disorders in adolescents and adults. Arch Gen Psychiatry 1980;37:1166.

Caplan G: *Principles of Preventive Psychiatry*. Basic Books, 1964.

Horowitz MJ: *Stress Response Syndromes*. Jason Aronson, 1976.

Horowitz MJ, Kaltreider N: Psychotherapy of stress response syndromes. In: *Specialized Techniques in Individual Psychotherapy*. Karasu T, Bellak L (editors). Brunner/Mazel, 1980.

Langsley D, Kaplan D: *The Treatment of Families in Crisis*. Grune & Stratton, 1968.

Lindemann E. Symptomatology and management of acute grief. Am J Psychiatry 1944;101:141.

Looney JG, Gunderson EK: Transient situational disturbances: Course and outcome. Am J Psychiatry 1978; 135:660.

Pollock GH: The ghost that will not go away: Specificity theory today. J Am Acad Psychoanal 1977;5:421.

Pollock GH: The psychosomatic specificity concept: Its evaluation and reevaluation. Ann Psychoanal 1977;5:141.
PSYC-26: Updated 3/20

Personality Disorders

26

Charles R. Marmar, MD

Patients with personality disorder are common both in medical and in psychiatric practice. Such people frequently make pressing demands for treatment of their numerous complaints while at the same time resisting appropriate treatment recommendations. Their lack of cooperation may cause resentment and possibly even alienation and burnout in the health care professionals who treat them. The frequently overriding needs of such individuals for self-aggrandizement, their diminished capacity for understanding and respecting the needs of others, and their mistrust and emotional instability lead to maladaptive behavior, including manipulation and exploitation of others. Such individuals are limited in their capacity to participate in mutual give-and-take with another person.

In this chapter, each major personality disorder is discussed from two perspectives, that of formal psychiatric nosology and that of management of the medically or surgically ill patient with an impaired personality.

Medical illness may have a recurrent, predictable psychological meaning for patients with specific personality disorders. Hidden motives (covert agendas) in the patient's relationship with the physician may lead to problems of overutilization or underutilization of the health care system, substance abuse, and potential negative reactions in the physician. This chapter presents coping strategies for the physician that may increase the chances of patient compliance with medical or surgical treatment and minimize medical complications and interpersonal problems in the care of such patients.

Characteristics of Personality Disorders

DSM-III defines **personality traits** as "enduring patterns of perceiving, relating to, and thinking about the environment and oneself . . . exhibited in a wide range of important social and personal contexts." It is only when these patterns are "inflexible and maladaptive and cause either significant impairment in social or occupational functioning or subjective distress" that they constitute **personality disorders.** Such personality disturbances can be recognized by adolescence or earlier and commonly continue through adulthood; the pathological characteristics have their precursors in early developmental distur-

bances and remain as enduring qualities of a person. A diagnosis of personality disorder is not appropriate if the disturbance in functioning is episodic, since the symptoms of personality disorder should represent the person's *stable* characteristics and social functioning.

Because elements of character disorders appear early in life, childhood and adolescent disorders correlate strongly with adult personality disorders. For example, a child with conduct disorder frequently presents as an adult with antisocial personality disorder. Similarly, schizoid disorder of childhood or adolescence is linked to schizoid personality disorder of adulthood; avoidant disorder of childhood or adolescence may become avoidant personality disorder of adulthood; oppositional disorder of childhood may become passive-aggressive personality disorder of adulthood; and identity disorder of childhood may become borderline personality disorder in adulthood.

Because individuals with personality disorders exhibit recurrent maladaptive strategies in their interpersonal relationships, they may be markedly dissatisfied with the impact of their behavior on others and with their inability to function effectively. The resulting distress is prevalent in personality disorders—contrary to earlier concepts, which asserted that these patients were free from distress. Anxiety and depression are especially common and may be the chief complaint.

Substantial evidence suggests that individuals with personality disorders—which by definition are longstanding and at times lifelong disturbances in functioning—are at greater risk for various other psychiatric disorders, with symptomatic flare-ups occurring during occupational or personal stresses or developmental milestones (adolescence, mid-life crisis, aging, etc).

DIFFERENTIATION BETWEEN PERSONALITY DISORDERS & OTHER PSYCHIATRIC DISORDERS

Differentiation From Neurotic Disorders

Because anxiety and depression are common both in personality disorders and in neurotic disorders, these symptoms cannot be used as differential diagnostic criteria; however, other factors are useful in making a differential diagnosis. Individuals with personality disorders have **alloplastic** defenses and react to stress by attempting to change the *external* environment. For example, such patients often deal with a potential disappointment by threatening to retaliate and in that way manipulate another person to gratify rather than disappoint them. In contrast, patients with neurotic disorders have **autoplastic** defenses and react to stress by changing their *internal* psychological processes. For example, neurotic patients might rationalize that a disappointment is of no great importance.

Another distinguishing factor is the difference in self-awareness manifested in patients with the two types of disorders. In patients with personality disorders, character deficits are frequently perceived by the patient as **ego-syntonic,** ie, acceptable, unobjectionable, and part of the self. For example, patients with such a disorder disavow personal responsibility for hurting another person, have difficulty in appreciating the pain they have inflicted on another, and attribute blame to another person. In contrast, personal shortcomings in individuals with neurotic disorders are perceived by the patient as **ego-dystonic,** ie, unacceptable, objectionable, and alien to the self. Patients with neurotic disorders blame and chastise themselves for disappointing or hurting a valued person through their shortcomings.

Differentiation From Psychotic Disorders

Although there may be severe disturbances in social and occupational functioning in individuals with personality disorders, persistent psychotic features such as formal thought disorder (as manifested by loosening of associations), delusions, and hallucinations are absent. Transient psychotic states, or "micropsychotic episodes," in people with severe borderline personality disorders are important exceptions (see below). The quality of the psychotic disturbance in borderline personality disorder is different from that in schizophreniform psychoses; episodes are short-lived, directly related to a given situation, and usually self-limited, and they normally do not require hospitalization or medication. (See Chapter 21 for discussion of brief reactive psychoses.)

Differentiation From Organic Mental Disorders

Individuals with uncomplicated personality disorders have a clear sensorium; are oriented as to time, place, and person; and show normal intellectual functioning, so that memory for recent or remote events, fund of general knowledge, ability to perform calculations, and so on are within normal limits. Individuals with personality disorders may of course develop organic mental syndromes later in life and in certain cases may be at greater risk for such disorders (eg, through sustained alcohol or substance abuse). Multiple diagnoses are warranted in such patients.

PARANOID PERSONALITY DISORDER

Symptoms & Signs

The diagnostic criteria for paranoid personality disorder are summarized in Table 26–1.

According to *DSM-III-R*, the essential features of paranoid personality disorder include "a pervasive and unwarranted tendency . . . to interpret the actions of people as deliberately demeaning or threatening. . . ." These symptoms and signs are characteristic of the patient's long-term functioning and are not episodic in character or limited to particular episodes of illness. They are also associated with significant impairment in work and personal relationships. Patients are hostile, stubborn, and defensive, and they avoid intimacy. They are rigid and uncompromising, interested primarily in inanimate objects rather than human relations, extremely sensitive to rank, and disinterested in the arts and aesthetics.

Natural History & Prognosis

Systematic data are not available.

Differential Diagnosis

In paranoid schizophrenia and paranoid disorders, there are persistent psychotic symptoms, including delusions and hallucinations, that are not features of paranoid personality disorder. Individuals with paranoid personality disorder may develop paranoid

Table 26–1. *DSM-III-R* diagnostic criteria for paranoid personality disorder (coded on axis II).

The diagnostic criteria for the personality disorder refer to behaviors or traits that are characteristic of the person's recent (past year) and long-term functioning (generally since adolescence or early adulthood). The constellation of behaviors or traits causes either significant impairment in social or occupational functioning or subjective distress. Behaviors or traits limited to episodes of illness are not considered in making a diagnosis of personality disorder.

A. A pervasive and unwarranted tendency, beginning by early adulthood and present in a variety of contexts, to interpret the actions of people as deliberately demeaning or threatening, as indicated by at least 4 of the following:
   (1) Expects, without sufficient basis, to be exploited or harmed by others.
   (2) Questions, without justification, the loyalty or trustworthiness of friends or associates.
   (3) Reads hidden demeaning or threatening meanings into benign remarks or events, eg, suspects that a neighbor put out trash early to cause annoyance.
   (4) Bears grudges or is unforgiving of insults or slights.
   (5) Is reluctant to confide in others because of unwarranted fear that the information will be used against him or her.
   (6) Is easily slighted and quick to react with anger or to counterattack.
   (7) Questions, without justification, fidelity of spouse or sexual partner.
B. Does not occur exclusively during the course of schizophrenia or a delusional disorder.

psychoses, however, at which time an additional diagnosis is justified.

Illustrative Case

A 52-year-old man was referred for psychiatric evaluation after a medical workup revealed no basis for his persistent headaches. The headaches had begun 6 months earlier, at about the same time that he became preoccupied with the possibility that his supervisor wanted to fire him. They had an argument about the vacation schedule, and he felt that he was being taken advantage of unfairly, since coworkers with less seniority had more favorable schedules. After the argument, he had seen his supervisor joking with one of the other mechanics and had assumed that he was the object of their derision.

Although emotionally distant, the patient had been a loyal, serious, hardworking, and productive employee and had stayed at the same company for the past 18 years. Although he could always be counted on to do a good job, he tended to be excluded by other workers, who found him unable to relax and make jokes. He had been married for 25 years to a school librarian and described his marriage as satisfactory: "She's always there, but she doesn't make a lot of demands on me." They had decided not to have children, because "they're disruptive, unpredictable, demanding, take whatever they can get out of you, and then go off on their own."

In the interview, the patient appeared tense and vigilant, and he seemed to search for verbal or nonverbal clues indicating that the interviewer did not have his best interests at heart. When the interviewer suggested that he might have provoked his supervisor, he snapped back irritably that the interviewer, like most people, misunderstood him. The patient was understandable and goal-directed in his thinking, and there was no evidence of well-formed delusions or hallucinatory experiences. He admitted that he might be overreacting to the altercation with his supervisor. He noted that this had happened several times before and that in each instance he had been later reassured that he was a valued employee.

Epidemiology

Paranoid personality disorder is more commonly diagnosed in men than in women. A familial pattern has been suggested (see below). The relationship of paranoid personality disorder to paranoid schizophrenia and paranoid disorder is uncertain.

Etiology & Pathogenesis

The specific causes of paranoid personality disorder are not known. However, genetic predisposition may play a role, and if a patient has paranoid personality disorder, the chances are good that someone in the family has a paranoid disorder. Early childhood deprivation or child abuse alone or in concert with genetic susceptibility may lead to a paranoid sense of mistrust.

Treatment

An honest, respectful attitude is important in psychotherapeutic treatment of the patient with paranoid personality disorder. The therapist must pay attention to the degree of closeness shown toward the patient, since too much intimacy, warmth, and empathy may be seen as an intrusive attempt at control. Deep psychological interpretations tend to increase feelings of suspicion rather than clarify conflicts about warded off feelings or intentions. The therapist can reduce the chances of being perceived as yet another enemy by insisting on prompt and repeated examination of the patient's distorted image of the therapist (reality testing) in a firm but noncritical way.

The therapist should readily acknowledge and confirm any errors, feeling of irritation, or lapse in consideration, because patients with paranoid personality disorder will interpret denials of such behavior as proof of covert persecutory intentions. A tactful and polite but not overly elaborate apology by the therapist can do much to restore the patient's trust.

Paranoid Personality Disorder in Medical Practice

The paranoid patient's underlying mistrust, hypersensitivity to slights, fear of dependency, and underlying sense of shame and vulnerability are heightened during illness or even with the threat of illness. A trusting relationship between the physician and the patient is essential to ensure compliance with surgical or pharmacological treatments. A low-key and friendly but not overly intimate attitude on the part of the physician effectively counters the paranoid patient's dual expectations of being disregarded as worthless on the one hand and being intruded upon on the other. In the first few visits, the therapist can ask the patient about previous doctor-patient relationships, especially about both the helpful and the irritating elements. It is worthwhile to inquire whether the patient has ever abruptly terminated treatment with another physician because of actual or fantasied injury or betrayal. Such an inquiry is valuable with any patient but may be particularly informative in establishing an effective working relationship with a paranoid patient, since the physician can avoid the pitfalls encountered in the patient's previous relationships with health care professionals.

A physician who is being berated by a paranoid patient and who can acknowledge—without being defensive or attacking or encouraging the patient's distorted view—that the patient's pain and fear aroused by aspects of the physician-patient relationship are real is creating an invaluable opportunity to provide an atmosphere in which the patient can feel safe in working toward clarification of past difficulties. For paranoid patients, the primary problem in the doctor-patient relationship is frequently not any actual failure in treatment but rather the patient's subjectively distorted image of the physician as an individual with malevolent intentions toward the patient, a fear that proves ''justified'' when difficulties occur in diagnosis or treatment.

In discussion of the hostile, suspicious, and recalcitrant patient in medical practice, Dennis Farrell offers the following case (personal communication) as an example of the need to provide clear explanations of all procedures undertaken by the medical staff in treating such patients.

Illustrative case. A 42-year-old man with paranoid personality disorder who had presented at a medical clinic for treatment had a history of changing doctors and of not complying with prescribed medical regimens. The patient scowled when he was handed a prescription for medication, and the medical student assigned to work with the patient noted the patient's reaction aloud. The patient muttered a comment about ''cheap medication,'' and the student asked him to explain the remark. It appeared that when the dosage of the patient's medication had recently been changed, the patient had not received an adequate explanation and had merely been told that he was receiving the same medication. The patient concluded that the doctors had decided to give him some cheap, second-rate medicine because he was a clinic patient. To the patient's way of thinking, there was no good reason why the same medication should look different except that it was in some way inferior. When the medical student expressed genuine interest in the patient and offered a clear explanation of why the dosage had been changed, the patient felt comfortable in taking the medication as prescribed.

SCHIZOID PERSONALITY DISORDER

Symptoms & Signs

The diagnostic criteria for schizoid personality disorder are presented in Table 26–2. According to *DSM-III-R*, the disorder is characterized by ''a pervasive pattern of indifference to social relationships and restricted range of emotional experience and expression. . . .'' Patients have difficulty in expressing hostility. They are excessively self-absorbed and detached, and they engage in daydreaming. Their work performance is generally better than their ability to participate in interpersonal relationships.

Natural History & Prognosis

Onset is in early childhood. Prospective studies indicate that the majority of shy children do not go on to develop schizoid personality disorder. However, once he pattern is established, it tends to be stable during adolescence and throughout adulthood.

Table 26–2. *DSM-III-R* diagnostic criteria for schizoid personality disorder (coded on axis II).

The diagnostic criteria for the personality disorders refer to behavioirs or traits that are characteristic of the person's recent (past year) and long-term functioning (generally since adolescence or early adulthood). The constellation of behaviors or traits causes either significant impairment in social or occupational functioning or subjective distress. Behaviors or traits limited to episodes of illness are not considered in making a diagnosis of personality disorder.

A. A pervasive pattern of indifference to social relationships and a restricted range of emotional experience and expression, beginning by early adulthood and present in a variety of contexts, as indicated by at least 4 of the following:
  (1) Neither desires nor enjoys close relationships, including being part of a family.
  (2) Almost always chooses solitary activities.
  (3) Rarely, if ever, claims or appears to experience strong emotions, such as anger and joy.
  (4) Indicates little if any desire to have sexual experiences with another person (age being taken into account).
  (5) Is indifferent to the praise and criticism of others.
  (6) Has no close friends or confidants (or only one) other than first-degree relatives.
  (7) Displays constricted affect, eg, is aloof, cold, rarely reciprocates gestures or facial expressions, such as smiles or nods.
B. Does not occur exclusively during the course of schizophrenia or a delusional disorder.

Differential Diagnosis

Schizoid personality disorder must be differentiated from schizotypal personality disorder, in which there are eccentricities of communication and behavior and in which a positive family history of schizophrenia occurs more frequently. Schizoid personality disorder must also be differentiated from avoidant personality disorder, in which there is social withdrawal despite a desire for acceptance; this withdrawal in the avoidant personality is due to an exquisite sensitivity to rejection. People with schizoid personality disorder do not directly experience or acknowledge a wish for closeness.

Illustrative Case

A 32-year-old assistant professor of philosophy presented for psychiatric evaluation, primarily to satisfy a request from his aging parents. They were worried about their son's impoverished social life and wanted to see him happily married so they could die in peace, knowing that their son would not be alone in the world. He was not overtly dissatisfied with his life and found gratification in his theoretical writings and occasional intellectual debates with colleagues. He did not seem to feel the loneliness that troubled his parents. He said that it was not a matter of wishing to be included in the company of others or feeling shy about forming an attachment but that he simply had no wish to be close to others.

When the patient was not working, he spent his

evenings and weekends refining a mathematically elaborate system for winning at blackjack. In testing this theory, he always visited the casinos alone. He said that as a child he had preferred to read about politics and religion rather than participate in sports or associate with other children, and he felt that he had been a loner all his life.

In the interview, the patient appeared timid. He was unable to sustain eye contact, and he provided circumscribed, emotionally barren responses to questions. He fidgeted and appeared to be counting the minutes until he could leave the room. When asked if he resented being asked to come to the interview to relieve his parents' anxieties, he answered in the affirmative, but without any apparent feeling. The interviewer found it difficult to empathize with the patient, since he seemed so remote and uninvolved in the discussion.

Epidemiology

There is little evidence linking schizoid personality disorder to schizophrenia, in contrast to schizotypal personality disorder, which is considered part of the spectrum of schizophrenic disorders. The prevalence of schizoid personality disorder has not been established.

Etiology & Pathogenesis

It is not clear whether there is a genetic predisposition to development of schizoid personality disorder. Important psychological factors include a cold, unempathic, emotionally impoverished childhood, as shown by retrospective (not prospective) studies.

Treatment

Long-term psychotherapy has been useful in selected cases. The course of therapy involves gradual development of trust. If this can be achieved, the patient may share long-standing fantasies of imaginary friendships and may reveal fears of depending on others. Patients are encouraged to examine the unrealistic nature of their fears and fantasies and to form actual relationships. Successful psychotherapy will produce gradual change.

Group psychotherapy may be helpful. A prolonged period of silent withdrawal may often be followed by gradual involvement in the group process. It is important for the group leader to protect the schizoid patient from criticism by other members for not participating verbally in the early affiliative phase of the group.

Schizoid Personality Disorder in Medical Practice

The person with schizoid personality disorder sustains a fragile emotional equilibrium by avoiding intimate personal contact and thereby minimizing conflict that is poorly tolerated. Illness is not only a threat to personal integrity but also requires that the patient seek treatment from a health care team made up of people who may seem to impose a demand for dependent involvement that is hard for this type of patient to accept. For this reason, the patient may delay seeking help until symptoms become severe. Once treatment has started, the patient frequently appears detached, as though unappreciative of the help being offered. Such individuals may dissociate the tolerable, technical aspects of treatment from its frightening interpersonal context.

The physician should appreciate the need for privacy in a person with schizoid personality disorder and should maintain a low-key approach that focuses on the technical elements of treatment. Such a focus will caring and know that caretakers will not press beyond comfortable limits. The patient should be encouraged to maintain daily routines so that a sense of "life as usual" can counteract the worry that illness will shatter the patient's efforts to remain detached and uninvolved. Knowledge of the patient's usual pattern of functioning will counteract any tendency on the part of the health care team to become personally overinvolved or be too zealously concerned with providing social supports for the patient.

SCHIZOTYPAL PERSONALITY DISORDER

Symptoms & Signs

The diagnostic criteria for schizotypal personality disorder are set forth in Table 26–3. According to *DSM-III-R,* the disorder is characterized by "deficits in interpersonal relatedness and peculiarities of ideation, appearance, and behavior. . . ." The patient suffers from anxiety, depression, and other dysphoric mood states. If features of borderline personality disorder are present, both diagnoses may be assigned. Reactive psychoses and eccentric convictions occur. The patient also demonstrates magical thinking, as illustrated by superstition and by a belief in clairvoyance and telepathy.

Natural History & Prognosis

Systematic data are not available.

Differential Diagnosis

The differential diagnosis should include schizoid personality disorder, in which behavioral and communicative oddities do not occur; and schizophrenia, in which formal thought disorder occurs.

Illustrative Case

A 34-year-old single woman presented at a community mental health center complaining of feelings of detachment and unreality. She said she felt cut off from her environment, as though she were looking out at the world through "semitransparent gauze." She also complained that when she was walking in

Table 26–3. *DSM-III-R* diagnostic criteria for schizotypal personality disorder (coded on axis II).

The diagnostic criteria for the personality disorders refer to behavior or traits that are characteristic of the person's recent (past year) and long-term functioning (generally since adolescence or early adulthood). The constellation of behaviors or traits causes either significant impairment in social or occupational functioning or subjective distress. Behaviors or traits limited to episodes of illness are not considered in making a diagnosis of personality disorder.

A. A pervasive pattern of deficits in interpersonal relatedness and peculiarities of ideation, appearance, and behavior, beginning by early adulthood and present in a variety of contexts, as indicated by at least 5 of the following:
  (1) Ideas of reference (excluding delusions of reference).
  (2) Excessive social anxiety, eg, extreme discomfort in social situations involving unfamiliar people.
  (3) Odd beliefs or magical thinking, influencing behavior and inconsistent with subcultural norms, eg, superstitiousness, belief in clairvoyance, telepathy, or "sixth sense," "others can feel my feelings" (in children and adolescents, bizarre fantasies or preoccupations).
  (4) Unusual perceptual experiences, eg, illusions, sensing the presence of a force or person not actually present (eg, "I felt as if my dead mother were in the room with me").
  (5) Odd or eccentric behavior or appearance, eg, unkempt, unusual mannerisms, talks to self.
  (6) No close friends or confidants (or only one) other than first-degree relatives.
  (7) Odd speech (without loosening of associations or incoherence), eg, speech that is impoverished, digressive, vague, or inappropriately abstract.
  (8) Inappropriate or constricted affect, eg, silly, aloof, rarely reciprocates gestures or facial expressions, such as smiles or nods.
  (9) Suspiciousness or paranoid ideation.
B. Does not occur exclusively during the course of schizophrenia or a pervasive developmental disorder.

the evening, moving shadows cast by the wind blowing through the trees created the frightening illusion of a potential assailant. She momentarily visualized a menacing figure, only to realize it was merely an illusion. This experience occurred repeatedly.

The patient had supported herself over the past few years by tea leaf and palm reading and other forms of fortune-telling. She said that this choice of occupation followed from her long-standing belief that she possessed special powers. During adolescence, she had claimed to be clairvoyant. She was regarded as either odd or fascinating by her acquaintances. She was deeply superstitious and preoccupied with numbers, colors, and dates. For example, she only traveled on airplanes when the day of the month, the flight number, and the scheduled arrival time were even numbers.

The patient's relationships usually involved superficial acquaintances, primarily people who shared her superstitious belief systems. She spent long periods daydreaming and fantasizing that she was a beautiful woman who would achieve great prominence by foretelling important world events. Such daydreams usually occurred after she experienced insults or slights.

At the interview, the patient was colorfully dressed in a juxtaposition of clashing, gypsy-like styles that gave her a patchwork, disheveled appearance. Although she showed no frank disorder of speech such as incoherence or gross loosening of associations, her language was stilted, and she used inappropriately formal and technical terms in a disjunctive fashion that made her speech difficult to follow. There was no evidence of delusions or hallucinations. When she was asked about a family history of mental disorder, she replied that an older sister had undergone several psychiatric hospitalizations and was currently receiving antipsychotic drugs.

Epidemiology

The incidence of schizophrenia is increased in first degree relatives of individuals with schizotypal personality disorder.

Etiology & Pathogenesis

Schizotypal personality disorder shares a genetic relationship with schizophrenia, as shown by family, twin, and adoption studies, which have demonstrated that these disorders occur more often in genetically related family members than in unrelated individuals.

Treatment

The physician must exercise tact when exploring idiosyncratic belief systems during psychotherapy. Antipsychotic medication is useful in patients with pronounced psychotic manifestations, particularly during stress.

Schizotypal Personality Disorder in Medical Practice

The problems encountered in management of the schizotypal patient and the management approaches are similar to those used for schizoid patients, as described above. The physician must also be able to help the patient with reality testing and differentiating fantasy from fact. In this respect, management techniques are similar to those used for patients with paranoid and borderline personality disorders and patients with psychotic disorders. Occasionally, the physician may consider the use of antipsychotic medications if the patient becomes frankly psychotic. If psychosis persists, the possibility of a coexisting mental disorder must be considered, and psychiatric consultation is indicated.

HISTRIONIC PERSONALITY DISORDER

Symptoms & Signs

Table 26–4 lists the diagnostic criteria for histrionic personality disorder. *DSM-III-R* states that the

Table 26–4. *DSM-III-R* diagnostic criteria for histrionic personality disorder (coded on axis II).

The diagnostic criteria for the personality disorders refer to behaviors or traits that are characteristic of the person's recent (past year) and long-term functioning (generally since adolescence or early adulthood). The constellation of behaviors or traits causes either significant impairment in social or occupational functioning or subjective distress. Behaviors or traits limited to episodes of illness are not considered in making a diagnosis of personality disorder.

A pervasive pattern of excessive emotionality and attention-seeking, beginning by early adulthood and present in a variety of contexts, as indicated by at least 4 of the following:

(1) Constantly seeks or demands reassurance, approval, or praise.

(2) Is inappropriately sexually seductive in appearance or behavior.

(3) Is overly concerned with physical attractiveness.

(4) Expresses emotion with inappropriate exaggeration, eg, embraces casual acquaintances with excessive ardor, uncontrollable sobbing on minor sentimental occasions, has temper tantrums.

(5) Is uncomfortable in situations in which he or she is not the center of attention.

(6) Displays rapidly shifting and shallow expression of emotions.

(7) Is self-centered, actions being directed toward obtaining immediate satisfaction; has no tolerance for the frustration of delayed gratification.

(8) Has a style of speech that is excessively impressionistic and lacking in detail, eg, when asked to describe mother, can be no more specific than, "She was a beautiful person."

essential feature of this disorder is "a pervasive pattern of excessive emotionality and attention seeking. . . ."

Patients with histrionic personality disorder experience reactive dysphoria in the face of loss or rejection as well as difficulty with linear, analytic thought, although they are often creative and imaginative. Patients are impressionable, suggestible, and intuitive; ie, they "play hunches" instead of thinking decisions through methodically. There is a tendency toward somatization, and homosexuality may be associated with this disorder in some cases.

Natural History & Prognosis

Systematic data are not available.

Differential Diagnosis

Histrionic personality disorder must be differentiated from somatization disorder, borderline personality disorder, and narcissistic personality disorder. These three disorders may coexist in some combination with histrionic personality disorder, in which case all relevant diagnoses may be assigned.

Illustrative Case

A 32-year-old single professional photographer sought psychiatric treatment because of repetitive disappointments in her love relationships. She had achieved considerable success in her career over the last few years but was unmotivated to work after the recent breakup of an affair with an older man, one of the teachers at an art institute she had attended. The affair had begun when he was unhappily married, and during the course of the relationship, he had left his wife. After the separation, the patient grew disenchanted as she began to note his unattractive character traits. Instead of becoming more available to her emotionally, he became preoccupied with work, and she felt left out. In her own words, "His work became his mistress, and I felt like the other woman, abandoned, except for diversionary relief when he needed some entertainment."

The patient went on to describe several other disappointing love relationships that had occurred over the past few years and seemed unaware that she repeatedly chose powerful and attractive but self-absorbed men. She was the youngest of three daughters. Her father was an architect and her mother an interior decorator. Her older sister had a congenital heart defect; in the patient's view, "She got all the attention. My achievements were taken for granted, but a big deal was made out of everything she could do."

At the interview, the patient appeared attractive and chic. Her manner of relating to the interviewer was dramatically intense as she gestured widely and maintained unwavering eye contact. She showed labile emotional shifts from sadness to shame to anger as she reviewed aspects of her love relationship. Her thinking was organized and coherent but vague and highly emotional, with sparse detail in her descriptions of the difficulties in her relationships.

Epidemiology

Histrionic personality disorder is more common in women than in men, and there is an increased familial incidence.

Etiology & Pathogenesis

The causes of histrionic personality disorder are mainly psychological; in better-functioning patients, these are typically unresolved oedipal problems. The more immature, dependent (so-called oral) hysteric has a history of disturbance early in life in attachments and separation.

Treatment

Long-term psychoanalytic psychotherapy is the treatment of choice and should focus on developing the patient's insight into the reasons for repetitive difficulties in sustaining love relationships and on promoting autonomous self-expression. The therapist should also help the patient think more clearly and systematically, so that information processing and decision making are not distorted by vagueness or failure to attend to relevant details.

Histrionic Personality Disorder in Medical Practice

For people with histrionic personalities, self-esteem is heavily centered in perception of their body image, with physical prowess and attractiveness being prized attributes. Men with histrionic personality disorder may, when physically ill, display hypermasculine ('macho') behavior to counteract their perception of themselves as weak. Such counterphobic behavior may worsen the course of illness. Such men may act in an overtly seductive fashion toward female physicians and other members of the health care team. Women with histrionic personality disorder may attempt to reaffirm their sense of self-worth by exhibiting dependent and coquettish behavior in an attempt to evoke reassuring admiration from their male physicians. Patients of both sexes may attempt to draw the physician into a rescuing, admiring role in order to ward off anxiety associated with the threat to self-esteem that is posed by the illness.

The physician must be able to provide maximal emotional support and interest in order to lessen the patient's anxiety but at the same time must avoid entering into a close personal relationship that might be misinterpreted as sexual. The physician must also avoid fostering magical expectations of cure. The physician should adopt a kindly but objective stance and should periodically provide a clear explanation of the disorder and plans for treatment so as to foster trust and firmly counteract the patient's denial of illness. Such patients tend to fluctuate between a state of overwhelming anxiety about the potential loss of capacities (intrusions or flooding of affect) and a state of numbing and apparent disregard (la belle indifférence). A flexible approach combining support or tactful confrontation as appropriate will help the patient gain a realistic understanding of the disorder and cooperate with treatment. The patient's capacity for overly dramatic expression and the shifting focus of somatic distress raise the risk that the physician will dismiss the complaints as those of a hypochondriac or even as the conscious manipulations of a malingerer. The histrionic patient will challenge the physician's diagnostic acumen, since serious illness, conversion symptoms, and dramatization of minor somatic disturbances may coexist or evolve sequentially within the same individual.

Leigh and Reiser (1980) illustrate the difficulty that a patient with histrionic personality disorder has in coping with physical illness.

Illustrative case. A 59-year-old married businessman had severe chest pain and was admitted to the intensive care unit after an electrocardiogram and serum enzyme determinations confirmed that he had suffered a massive myocardial infarction. Absolute bed rest was prescribed in order to minimize the threat of further myocardial damage. The patient prided himself on his physical prowess, and when his physician empathically commented on how frightening the attack must have been for him, the patient replied, "No. I didn't get frightened at nothing—nothing scares me. All I did was holler up to my wife. I've got a bull voice—you know what I mean: I can't help myself. You understand. I got a powerful chest, so it comes out strong."

The patient presented a problem in management, because in an effort to ward off the anxiety associated with his illness, he persuaded himself that a daily exercise program would hasten his rehabilitation, and despite the admonitions of the intensive care unit staff, he began repeatedly lifting up his bed in order to improve his circulation. He told one of the nurses, "My doctor thinks I had a heart attack. All I need is to get my strength back, which I lost from being in here too long." His denial and counterphobic behavior precipitated a burst of cardiac arrhythmias that required urgent medical treatment and subsequent psychiatric consultation.

Appropriate psychological management of this patient would include a review of the events leading up to his admission to the hospital, tactful confrontation of his defensive need to appear invincible, and step-by-step efforts to help him gradually accept his real vulnerabilities while countering his fear of being a "cardiac cripple." The physician's admiration of the patient's efforts to cope more adaptively would help restore the patient's sense of self-esteem and safety.

NARCISSISTIC PERSONALITY DISORDER

Symptoms & Signs

The diagnostic criteria for narcissistic personality disorder are listed in Table 26–5. The disorder is characterized by *DSM-III-R* as "a pervasive pattern of grandiosity . . . lack of empathy, and hypersensitivity to evaluation by others. . . ."

Brief reactive psychoses may occur; in psychodynamic theory, these represent fragmentation of a coherent sense of self under psychosocial stress. This fragmentation is experienced as a loss of the sense of continuity of oneself as worthwhile and lovable in the face of a current disappointment, criticism, or rejection. Depression is common, as is chronic intense envy. Defensive self-delusion or lying to oneself by distorting the facts so that a feeling of self-importance is preserved ('sliding of meanings') is also seen. The patient may pretend to have certain feelings in order to impress others.

Natural History & Prognosis

Systematic data are not available.

Illustrative Case

A 38-year-old recently divorced and infrequently

Table 26–5. *DSM-III-R* diagnostic criteria for narcissistic personality disorder (coded on axis II).

The diagnostic criteria for the personality disorders refer to behaviors or traits that are characteristic of the person's recent (past year) and long-term functioning (generally since adolescence or early adulthood). The constellation of behaviors or traits causes either significant impairment in social or occupational functioning or subjective distress. Behaviors or traits limited to episodes of illness are not considered in making a diagnosis of personality disorder.

A pervasive pattern of grandiosity (in fantasy or behavior), lack of empathy, and hypersensitivity to the evaluation of others, beginning by early adulthood and present in a variety of contexts, as indicated by at least 5 of the following:

(1) Reacts to criticism with feelings of rage, shame, or humiliation (even if not expressed).
(2) Is interpersonally exploitative: takes advantage of others to achieve his or her own ends.
(3) Has a grandiose sense of self-importance, eg, exaggerates achievements and talents, expects to be noticed as "special" without appropriate achievement.
(4) Believes that his or her problems are unique and can be understood only by other special people.
(5) Is preoccupied with fantasies of unlimited success, power, brilliance, beauty, or ideal love.
(6) Has a sense of entitlement: unreasonable expectation of especially favorable treatment, eg, assumes that he or she does not have to wait in line when others must do so.
(7) Requires constant attention and admiration, eg, keeps fishing for compliments.
(8) Lack of empathy: inability to recognize and experience how others feel, eg, annoyance and surpise when a friend who is seriously ill cancels a date.
(9) Is preoccupied with feelings of envy.

employed actor who was the father of an 8-month-old sought help because of depression. He had left his wife and son 6 weeks earlier because he could no longer tolerate his wife's "slavish devotion to our baby boy; I may as well not exist as far as she's concerned." He complained that since his wife had become pregnant she was disinclined to admire his acting abilities and less interested than before in sympathizing with his envy of actors who obtained better and more frequent employment.

The patient was the eldest child and only son of a materially successful but emotionally withholding punitive, and sniping father who, in the patient's view, magnified his son's slightest imperfections. The patient described his mother as an indulgent and admiring woman who frequently made excuses for him. His two younger sisters were competent in their professions, and their success was a source of shame and guilt for him.

The patient had experienced a rapid turnover in friendships, since he initially idealized people and then impulsively trashed the relationships when he was frustrated or disappointed. Before his marriage he had fancied himself as a Don Juan, saying, "I had women on a string, but after a while I couldn't stand their vanity and pettiness."

In the interview, the patient presented as an ex-pensively dressed, well-groomed, and handsome man who tried to project a smooth, self-assured facade. There was, however, a palpable undercurrent of insecurity, loneliness, and depression. His distraught feelings had a quality of caricature to them that was evident to the interviewer. He presented himself as though he were a colleague rather than a patient, and he provided his own formulations for his psychological difficulties in an effort to save face. Although there were no gross abnormalities of thinking or perception, he presented an apparently distorted account of his role in his marital and occupational difficulties and cast himself in a better light than was warranted. He found an external power to blame, which lent a quality of self-delusion to his version of his interpersonal difficulties.

Epidemiology

The prevalence of narcissistic personality disorder is unknown, although it is apparently common in out patient psychiatric and medical practice.

Etiology & Pathogenesis

In normal psychological development, all very young children have an exaggerated sense of their own importance as well as an idealized view of parental figures as protective, powerful, and immortal. These immature, idealized views of the self and others are modified as children learn to face gradual, tolerable disappointments with the empathic support of their caretakers. The result of this process is that healthy adults can accept their own realistic limitations, tolerate criticism and setbacks, and still maintain an overall positive self-regard. In contrast, the early life experiences of individuals with narcissistic personality disorder were described by Kohut (1971) as marked by premature, repeated, and intense injuries to self-esteem as well as by radical disillusionment in parental figures, rather than gradual and tolerable disappointments in themselves and important caretakers. The long-term sequelae in adulthood are characteristic disturbances in self-esteem, with alternating idealization and devaluation of others that is accompanied by alternating grandiose and inferior images of the self.

Treatment

Long-term psychoanalytic psychotherapy and psychoanalysis have been attempted with these patients, although their use has been controversial. The goal is to increase the patient's capacity to tolerate disappointments, to appreciate the needs of others, and to develop healthy self-esteem.

Narcissistic Personality Disorder in Medical Practice

Narcissistic patients try to sustain an image of perfection and personal invincibility for themselves and attempt to project that impression to others as well. Physical illness may shatter this illusion, and a patient may lose the feeling of safety inherent in a cohesive sense of self. This loss precipitates a panicky sensation feels a sense of personal fragmentation. The narcissistic individual shares with the histrionic personality a concern about loss of admiration and approval, but the person with narcissistic personality disorder shows a more disturbed response to illness. The histrionic patient's idealization of the physician stands in contrast to the narcissistic patient's frequent contemptuous disregard for the physician, who is denigrated in a defensive effort to maintain a sense of superiority and mastery over illness.

Health care professionals must convey a feeling of respect and acknowledge the patient's sense of self-importance so that the patient can reestablish a coherent sense of self, but they must at the same time avoid reinforcing either pathological grandiosity (which may contribute to denial of illness) or weakness (which frightens the patient). An initial approach of support followed by step-by-step confrontation of the patient's vulnerabilities may enable the patient to deal with the implications of illness with feelings of greater subjective strength. The increased self-confidence may reduce the patient's need to attack the health care team in a misguided effort at psychological self-preservation and eases the pressure to provide perfect care, since the patient's antagonistic feeling of entitlement (defined by *DSM-III-R* as an "unreasonable expectation of especially favorable treatment") is reduced.

The following case shows the difficulty encountered in medical management of the narcissistic personality.

Illustrative case. A partner in a prestigious law firm was admitted to the specialized endocrine service of a teaching hospital for investigation of inflammation of the thyroid gland. The patient had sought consultation with the chief of the endocrine service after seeing the endocrinologist's recent research findings reported on network television and characterized as a glamorous, high-technology innovation. The patient recalled thinking at the time, "Finally, here is a doctor who can understand the complexities of my illness!"

When the patient arrived at the endocrine service, he was greeted by the junior resident, who introduced himself and explained that he would be responsible for the patient's day-to-day care, while the chief of the service would consult on major diagnostic and treatment issues. The lawyer flew into a rage and shouted, "No damn wet-behind-the-ears student doctor is going to lay a hand on me!"

The resident attempted to calm the patient and agreed to ask the chief of the service to mediate the dispute. When the chief arrived and was informed of the situation, his previous experience in dealing with influential patients enabled him to grasp the nature of the lawyer's narcissistic rage, the underlying sense of entitlement and fear that motivated it, and the embarrassment of the resident who was the unwitting target of the tirade. He welcomed the patient and apologized for not being able to meet him at the time of admission. He introduced the resident as "one of our brightest young colleagues—we are expecting great things from him" and continued, "He and I will work closely together to get to the bottom of your problems."

The lawyer was reassured by this respectful apology and the statement of confidence in the junior resident. The chief of the service had in effect transferred his reputation for excellence to his younger colleague ('passed the baton') and had thereby imbued the resident with the charismatic healing qualities the narcissistic patient needed in order to feel the trust necessary for a successful therapeutic relationship with the health care team.

ANTISOCIAL PERSONALITY DISORDER

Symptoms & Signs

The diagnostic criteria for antisocial personality disorder are set forth in Table 26–6. *DSM-III-R* states that this disorder is characterized by a history of chronic antisocial behavior that begins before the age of 15 and "a pattern of irresponsible and antisocial behavior since the age of 15," as indicated by poor job performance, academic failure, participation in a wide variety of illegal activities, recklessness, and impulsive behavior.

The patient with antisocial personality disorder also experiences a feeling of subjective dysphoria, characterized by tension, depression, inability to tolerate boredom, and a feeling of being victimized. There is also a diminished capacity for intimacy.

Natural History & Prognosis

Antisocial personality disorder tends to remit with time. After 21 years of age, the remission rate is about 2% of all patients each year. As destructive social behavior diminishes, patients tend to develop hypochondriacal and depressive disorders.

Differential Diagnosis

If characteristic features of antisocial personality disorder are present but the person is younger than 18 years of age, a diagnosis of conduct disorder is appropriate. When criminal behavior is present without other features of antisocial personality disorder, the appropriate diagnosis is adult antisocial behavior, usually without the precursory signs seen in adolescents with conduct disorders.

Illustrative Case

A 21-year-old divorced independent trucker was

Table 26–6. *DSM-III-R* diagnostic criteria for antisocial personality disorder (coded on axis II).

The diagnostic criteria for the personality disorders refer to behaviors or traits that are characteristic of the person's recent (past year) and long-term functioning (generally since adolescence or early adulthood). The constellation of behaviors or traits causes either significant impairment in social or occupational functioning or subjective distress. Behaviors or traits limited to episodes of illness are not considered in making a diagnosis of personality disorder.

A. Current age at least 18.
B. Evidence of conduct disorder with onset before age 15, as indicated by a history of 3 or more of the following:
   (1) Was often truant.
   (2) Ran away from home overnight at least twice while living in parental or parental surrogate home (or once without returning).
   (3) Often initiated physical fights.
   (4) Used a weapon in more than one fight.
   (5) Forced someone into sexual activity with him or her.
   (6) Was physically cruel to animals.
   (7) Was physically cruel to other people.
   (8) Deliberately destroyed others' property (other than fire-setting).
   (9) Deliberately engaged in fire-setting.
   (10) Often lied (other than to avoid physical or sexual abuse).
   (11) Has stolen without confrontation of a victim on more than one occasion (including forgery).
   (12) Has stolen with confrontation of a victim (eg, mugging, purse-snatching, extortion, armed robbery).
C. A pattern of irresponsible and antisocial behavior since the age of 15, as indicated by at least 4 of the following:
   (1) Is unable to sustain consistent work behavior, as indicated by any of the following (including similar behavior in academic settings if the person is a student): (a) significant unemployment for 6 months or more within 5 years when expected to work and work was available; (b) repeated absences from work unexplained by illness in self or family; (c) abandonment of several jobs without realistic plans for others.
   (2) Fails to conform to social norms with respect to lawful behavior, as indicated by repeatedly performing antisocial acts that are grounds for arrest (whether arrested or not), eg, destroying property, harassing others, stealing, pursuing an illegal occupation.
   (3) Is irritable and aggressive, as indicated by repeated physical fights or assaults (not required by one's job or to defend someone or oneself), including spouse- or child-beating.
   (4) Repeatedly fails to honor financial obligations, as indicated by defaulting on debts or failing to provide child support for other dependents on a regular basis.
   (5) Fails to plan ahead, or is impulsive, as indicated by one or both of the following: (a) traveling from place to place without prearranged job or clear goal for the period of travel or clear idea about when the travel will terminate; (b) lack of a fixed address for 1 month or more.
   (6) Has no regard for the truth, as indicated by repeated lying, use of aliases, or "conning" others for personal profit or pleasure.
   (7) Is reckless regarding his or her own or others' personal safety, as indicated by driving while intoxicated or recurrent speeding.
   (8) If a parent or guardian, lacks ability to function as a responsible parent, as indicated by one or more of the following: (a) malnutrition of child; (b) child's illness resulting from lack of minimal hygiene; (c) failure to obtain medical care for a seriously ill child; (d) child's dependence on neighbors or nonresident relatives for food or shelter; (e) failure to arrange for a caretaker for young child when parent is away from home; (f) repeated squandering, on personal items, of money required for household necessities.
   (9) Has never sustained a totally monogamous relationship for more than 1 year.
   (10) Lacks remorse (feels justified in having hurt, mistreated, or stolen from another).
D. Antisocial behavior does not occur exclusively during the course of schizophrenia or manic episodes.

referred for pretrial psychiatric evaluation after being charged with interstate transportation of stolen property. He had a history of repeated criminal offenses, prison terms, and psychiatric disturbance during childhood and adolescence. He had been apprehended 4 weeks earlier when a random road inspection revealed stolen automobile parts hidden among cartons of groceries.

About 8 months before his latest arrest, the patient had suddenly abandoned his wife when he learned from an acquaintance that she sometimes flirted with customers at the sandwich shop where she worked.

The patient was the second in a family of four boys. His alcoholic father was episodically violent toward him when drunk, and his mother was absent long hours while she worked to support the family.

During childhood, the patient had been evaluated and briefly treated in a community mental health cen-

ter after he had been caught setting fire to an abandoned warehouse. During adolescence, he had received counseling from a school psychologist because of a consistent pattern of antisocial behavior, including car theft, joyriding, drunk driving, driving with a suspended license, truancy, and stealing money from his mother. While he was growing up, he had no close friendships, although he was a peripheral member of a hot-rod gang. Though sexually active from a young age and proud of his sexual prowess, he was mistrustful of women and became easily bored with the same partner.

In the interview, the patient appeared nonchalant and composed, with an apparent equanimity that was incongruent with the seriousness of his situation. He made eye contact with the interviewer but appeared to be looking through the interviewer rather than at him. There was an unspoken but clearly communicated disregard for the interviewer's authority. There were no major disturbances in thought, perception, or mood, with the exception of a lack of remorse or anxiety when he was confronted with his lifelong pattern of destructive behavior and the seriousness of the charges presently lodged against him.

Epidemiology

Onset of antisocial personality disorder is before age 15, frequently around puberty in girls and quite early in childhood for boys. The disorder is more prevalent in men, with incidence being about 3% for men and 1% for women. Prevalence is increased in lower socioeconomic groups. Family histories are often positive for antisocial personality disorder, with increased incidence in the fathers of both male and female patients with this disorder. Evidence suggests that this familial occurrence is due to both genetic and environmental causes; the relative contribution of each factor is unknown. Antisocial personality disorder may be diagnosed in as many as 75% of prison inmates.

Etiology & Pathogenesis

A. Genetic and Biological Factors: Robins (1966) found an increased incidence of sociopathic characteristics and alcoholism in the fathers of individuals with antisocial personality disorder. Schulsinger (1972) reported findings of twin studies and adoption studies that support the hypothesis of a genetic component in this disorder. In a retrospective disorder, Raine et al (1990) reported that indices of psychophysiological underarousal at age 15 were predictive of criminality at age 24 years. Criminals had significantly lower heart rates and skin conductance activity and more slow-frequency electroencephalographic activity than noncriminals.

B. Psychological Factors: Bowlby (1944) correlated antisocial personality disorder with maternal deprivation in the child's first 5 years of life. Glueck and Glueck (1968) reported that the mothers of children who developed this personality disorder show a lack of consistent discipline, lack of affection, and an increased incidence of alcoholism and impulsiveness. These qualities contribute to failure to create a cohesive home environment with consistent structure and behavioral boundaries. In the prospective study, children found to be at risk by age 6 frequently showed features of antisocial personality at 18 years.

Antisocial Personality Disorder in Medical Practice

The relationship between a physician and a patient with antisocial personality disorder is characterized by mutual feelings of suspicion and, at times, hostility. The antisocial person's mistrust of the physician stems from unwarranted generalizations about physicians that are based in part on early abusive experiences at the hands of parental caretakers, especially during the formative periods of childhood and adolescence. The physician's mistrust of the antisocial patient may well be grounded in unpleasant personal experience. Persons with antisocial personality disorder may feign physical symptoms in order to obtain narcotic analgesics for substance abuse. They may attempt to defraud third-party health care payment sources in seeking reimbursement for services not rendered or may be delinquent in payment for services they have actually received. Unfortunately, individuals with antisocial personalities are at least as vulnerable to physical illness as any other type of patient and are in fact at higher risk for illnesses associated with substance abuse and stress, because of their chronic unstable interpersonal and occupational adjustments. The physician is therefore challenged to find a way to create an effective therapeutic alliance. A firm, no-nonsense approach that is not punitive but conveys a streetwise awareness of the patient's potential for manipulation will encourage respect without aggravating the patient's hostility against authority.

Illustrative case. A 25-year-old man presented for an initial visit to a local general practitioner and complained of recurrent backache. He said that he had tried many analgesics in the past and found that they either were ineffective or caused intolerable side effects, with the exception of high doses of codeine. Physical examination revealed significant disease of the lumbosacral spine secondary to a congenital defect in the alignment of the vertebrae.

Alerted by the patient's specific request for a potentially addictive narcotic that also had high resale value in the illicit drug market, the physician inquired further into the patient's work and occupational history. A typical unstable pattern of impulsive and manipulative interpersonal relations was identified, including an irregular work history and other features characteristic of antisocial personality disorder. A respectful but appropriately tough tone of inquiry into the patient's previous use of analgesics revealed a history of morphine addiction following lower back surgery. Denial of the patient's request for codeine led to an angry outburst, with the patient declining alternative treatment. Several months later, however, the patient reappeared with legitimate complaints of upper respiratory tract infection. He told the physician, "I came back to see you again because I figure you're nobody's tool, but you're not going to lecture me about how I should live my life either."

BORDERLINE PERSONALITY DISORDER

Symptoms & Signs

Table 26–7 sets forth the diagnostic criteria for borderline personality disorder. As described by *DSM-III-R,* borderline personality disorder is characterized by "instability of mood, interpersonal relationships, and self-image. . . ."

Table 26–7. *DSM-III-R* diagnostic criteria for borderline personality disorder (coded on axis II).

The diagnostic criteria for the personality disorders refer to behaviors or traits that are characteristic of the person's recent (past year) and long-term functioning (generally since adolescence or early adulthood). The constellation of behaviors or traits causes either significant impairment in social or occupational functioning or subjective distress. Behaviors or traits limited to episodes of illness are not considered in making a diagnosis of personality disorder.

A pervasive pattern of instability of mood, interpersonal relationships, and self-image; beginning by early adulthood and present in a variety of contexts, as indicated by at least 5 of the following:

   (1) A pattern of unstable and intense interpersonal relationships characterized by alternating between extremes of overidealization and devaluation.

   (2) Impulsivity in at least 2 areas that are potentially self-damaging, eg, spending, sex, substance use, shoplifting, reckless driving, binge eating. (Do not include suicidal or self-mutilating behavior covered in criterion [5].)

   (3) Affective instability: marked shifts from baseline mood to depression, irritability, or anxiety, usually lasting a few hours and only rarely more than a few days.

   (4) Inappropriate, intense anger or lack of control of anger, eg, frequent displays of temper, constant anger, recurrent physical fights.

   (5) Recurrent suicidal threats, gestures, or behavior, or self-mutilating behavior.

   (6) Marked and persistent identity disturbance manifested by uncertainty about at least 2 of the following: self-image, sexual orientation, long-term goals or career choice, type of friends desired, preferred values.

   (7) Chronic feelings of emptiness or boredom.

   (8) Frantic efforts to avoid real or imagined abandonment. (Do not include suicidal or self-mutilating behavior covered in criterion [5].)

The patient with borderline personality disorder is vulnerable to development of transient reactive psychoses (micropsychotic episodes) and may be chronically depressed. The patient alternates between the wish for closeness and the need for distance. Borderline personality disorder may coexist with schizotypal, histrionic, narcissistic, or antisocial personality disorder.

Natural History & Prognosis

Follow-up studies by Werble (1970) and by Carpenter et al (1977) suggest that the clinical picture in patients with borderline personality disorder is chronically unstable but that the disorder does not deteriorate into schizophrenia. In both studies, symptoms were present over long periods, and patients experienced major disturbances in social functioning and enjoyed little satisfaction from their low quality of life. These individuals were unlikely to marry. The patients in the two studies were suffering from a severe form of the borderline disorder; the prognosis is better for individuals with higher levels of functioning.

Differential Diagnosis

If an individual with characteristics of borderline personality disorder is under 18 years of age, the appropriate diagnosis is identity disorder.

Borderline personality disorder must be differentiated from cyclothymic disorder, in which there are hypomanic periods.

Illustrative Case

A 25-year-old single graduate student was brought to a crisis clinic by her girlfriend, who had become worried after the patient expressed a wish to commit suicide. Two weeks earlier, the patient's boyfriend had left for a summer vacation trip to Europe. The vacation had initially been planned as a joint trip, but the patient had persuaded her boyfriend to go alone so they could have a period of independence from each other. She was worried that they were becoming psychologically enmeshed and "like Siamese twins," a view that threatened her chronically fragile sense of separateness and autonomy. In the 2 weeks since his departure, she had grown progressively more distraught and had felt a panicky sense of abandonment, emptiness, and loss of all positive feelings and memories of her relationship with her boyfriend, all of which contributed to a sense of unreality about her life. She considered taking an overdose of drugs, because "nothing else would numb the pain I feel." She had also harbored an increasing sense of rage at being left behind, because "he didn't understand that I was only testing his loyalty when I told him to go alone."

The patient's current relationship, like her previous love relationships, had been characterized by periods of intense intimate contact alternating with flights into independence. She felt she could not achieve a comfortable compromise that would enable her to feel close to another person yet preserve a sense of her own separateness. Although she was a gifted student, she had enrolled in three widely different graduate programs after having made abrupt shifts in her career training just when she was nearing completion of any one program. Her academic interests were scattered over the fine arts, social sciences, and business. She was by her own description a "chameleon" who had no strong preferences of her own. She was powerfully influenced by charismatic teachers whose value systems and career goals she would make her own in an effort to counter her inner sense of emptiness and lack of direction.

The patient was an only child whose mother became bedridden with rheumatoid arthritis when the patient was between 18 and 30 months of age. Her mother made a partial recovery but struggled with physical pain and depression during subsequent relapses. Her parents were divorced when the patient was 9 years of age, and her father subsequently maintained only a distant relationship with the family. After her parents' divorce, the patient felt even more responsible for the health and happiness of her mother than she had before. She was made to feel guilty for placing her own social and intellectual needs ahead of those of her mother. In her view, ''Every step I took toward becoming my own person was a step closer to destroying my mother.''

In the interview, she was presented as an appealing young woman who seemed distraught and somewhat disheveled and physically exhausted. In describing her separation from her boyfriend, she oscillated between uncontrollable sobbing and furious rage but was able to regain her composure in responding to the structuring and supportive remarks of the interviewer. There was no evidence of delusions or hallucinations. Her sensorium was clear, though she reported a subjective sense of disorientation and unreality that she attributed to the change in her world as a result of her boyfriend's absence.

Epidemiology

No direct studies of the prevalence of borderline personality disorder have been performed, though it is believed to be common. In the Stirling County (Nova Scotia) study, Leighton et al (1963) found that 1.7% of the sample met the diagnostic criteria for emotionally unstable personality, a diagnosis with criteria similar to those of borderline personality disorder. The same study noted that the diagnosis was made more frequently in women than in men by a 2:1 ratio.

Etiology & Pathogenesis

A. Genetic and Biological Factors: Kemberg (1975) and Klein (1977) have suggested that patients with borderline personality disorder have a ''constitutionally based'' inability to regulate affects, especially anger. There may be a relationship between borderline personality and depressive illness, which is prevalent in first-degree relatives of patients with borderline personality disorder.

B. Psychological Factors: Kernberg hypothesized an arrest in normal psychological development, with failure to integrate ambivalent feelings originally aroused against the primary caretaker but later occurring in other close relationships as well. The primitive defenses ordinarily relinquished in early childhood are prolonged into adulthood, and patients tend to have distorted appraisals of others, who are perceived as virtual caricatures that are either ''all-good'' or ''all bad.'' This all-or-nothing thinking extends to an exaggerated view of physical symptoms as well, so that the patient tends to feel that he or she is either completely well or deathly ill. The threat of physical illness is exaggerated to terrifying proportions.

Mahler (1971) and Masterson (1972) have hypothesized that borderline personality disorder results after a disturbance occurring in children between 16 and 25 months of age during the rapprochement subphase of separation-individuation. In this phase, the child practices independent behavior and returns to the primary caretaker for approval, admiration, and emotional ''refueling.'' The critical, rejecting parent or the suffocating, smothering parent interferes with optimal progression of attachment-separation sequences.

Treatment

A. Psychological Treatment Measures: Controversy exists about which of the two dominant psychological approaches is more effective in the treatment of borderline personality disorder. Long-term psychoanalytic psychotherapy with some supportive modifications tries to develop trust early in treatment and progresses to deeper exploration with time. The other approach is long-term, more reality-oriented supportive psychotherapy that does not focus on unconscious fantasies and attempts instead to provide structure and prevent the deterioration or overstimulation sometimes seen in more insight-oriented approaches.

B. Drug Treatment Measures: Klein (1977) advocates the use of monoamine oxidase inhibitors for patients with borderline personality disorder who are sensitive to rejection. These patients experience intensely unpleasant affects, particularly anxiety and depression, when they feel rejected. The use of other antidepressant and antianxiety agents may become necessary at certain times. During brief reactive psychoses, low doses of antipsychotic drugs may be useful, but they are usually not essential adjuncts to the treatment regimen, since such episodes are most often self-limiting and of short duration.

Borderline Personality Disorder in Medical Practice

Persons with borderline personality disorder have marked difficulty in differentiating reality from fantasy, so that a minor health problem may be perceived as a life-threatening event. Loss of perspective and miscommunication with the physician may occur as a result. Such patients frequently delay in presenting for medical treatment. They fear the worst with regard to the diagnosis, and they mistrust physicians because of their previous experiences with unreliable caretakers. Some patients may have a subconscious need to suffer in order to expiate guilty feelings. Once they have delivered themselves to the health care team, these patients ward off their catastrophic fear of being damaged by imperfect caretakers by imagining them as ''all-good.'' If any problems occur, patients switch abruptly to an ''all-bad'' image of medical personnel; the omnipotent rescuer becomes the persecutory invader. The patient may bolt from treatment and attempt to resurrect an idealized relationship with a new doctor, only to be painfully disillusioned later. Patients with borderline personality disorder may interpret any "intellectual" errors in diagnosis or treatment on the part of the health care team on an emotional level. They see themselves as having been rejected, callously disregarded, and abandoned to struggle with their illnesses alone because they are unworthy of the time and interest of their physicians.

The physician should provide clear, nontechnical answers to questions to counter any elaborate fantasies about the dangers of the illness or its treatment. Honest but not overly dramatic information should be provided about the course of the illness and potential side effects of treatment. The physician should be careful to avoid encouraging the patient to idealize the physician and should not be drawn into the patient's denigration of other physicians. More frequent periodic checkups may reassure the patient of the physician's empathy and interest and may provide closer monitoring of illness; they also reduce the chances that the patient will create a frightening mental scenario out of proportion to any genuine threat. Although the physician should offer reassurance, this should not be premature, since it may deprive the patient of an opportunity to spell out these fearful expectations about the illness and may deny the physician a chance to clarify the often idiosyncratic and unexpected nuances of the patient's beliefs about the illness. The physician's tolerance of the patient's episodic angry outbursts demonstrates to the patient that the physician cannot be destroyed by the patient's strong negative feelings and that the physician will not retaliate by leaving the patient to a self-fulfilling prophecy of abandonment.

Illustrative case. A 29-year-old man was admitted to the chest service of a community hospital for investigation of an undiagnosed lesion found during routine annual physical examination. The night before a scheduled biopsy, the patient had a nightmare in which he was lying on the operating table surrounded by medical personnel. The two surgeons who were attending him appeared kindly at first, but as the dream progressed, their expressions grew more threatening. He finally awoke when the surgeons were transformed into vampire-like creatures. When the nursing staff arrived at the patient's bedside after the nightmare, he was extremely agitated. He was hyperventilating, complained of a pounding headache, and shouted that he was going to die. After the nurses encouraged him to talk about his fears, he said that he was convinced he had lung cancer that had spread to his brain, and he felt that his severe headache supported this self-diagnosis. The nurses explained that he probably had a tension headache because of anxiety about the biopsy, and they showed him a relaxation exercise that relieved his headache and enabled him to gain a more realistic perspective on his situation. The biopsy revealed a benign fibrous cyst that was treated without complication.

AVOIDANT PERSONALITY DISORDER

Symptoms & Signs

Table 26–8 sets forth the diagnostic criteria for avoidant personality disorder. Features of the disorder, as outlined by *DSM-III-R*, include social discomfort, hypersensitivity to criticism and rejection, and timidity. The patient with avoidant personality disorder also experiences depression, anxiety, and anger for failing to develop social relations.

Natural History & Prognosis

The prognosis is unknown.

Differential Diagnosis

Avoidant personality disorder must be differentiated from schizoid personality disorder, social phobia, and avoidant disorder of childhood or adolescence (when the disorder occurs before age 18).

Illustrative Case

A 34-year-old single professional musician sought psychiatric treatment to deal with chronic feelings of insecurity, inferiority, and shyness. Although she was a gifted and sensitive musician, success in her career had not been matched by parallel gratifications in her social life. She came for treatment several weeks after a man in her orchestral group had moved to a different city. She was particularly fond of this

---

Table 26–8. *DSM-III-R* diagnostic criteria for avoidant personality disorder (coded on axis II).

The diagnostic criteria for the personality disorders refer to behaviors or traits that are characteristic of the person's recent (past year) and long-term functioning (generally since adolescence or early adulthood). The constellation of behaviors or traits causes either significant impairment in social or occupational functioning or subjective distress. Behaviors or traits limited to episodes of illness are not considered in making a diagnosis of personality disorder.

A pervasive pattern of social discomfort, fear of negative evaluation, and timidity, beginning by early adulthood and present in a variety of contexts, as indicated by at least 4 of the following:

(1) Is easily hurt by criticism or disapproval.

(2) Has no close friends or confidants (or only one) other than first-degree relatives.

(3) Is unwilling to get involved with people unless certain of being liked.

(4) Avoids social or occupational activities that involve significant interpersonal contact, eg, refuses a promotion that will increase social demands.

(5) Is reticent in social situations because of a fear of saying something inappropriate or foolish, or of being unable to answer a question.

(6) Fears being embarrassed by blushing, crying, or showing signs of anxiety in front of other people.

(7) Exaggerates the potential difficulties, physical dangers, or risks involved in doing something ordinary but outside his or her usual routine, eg, may cancel social plans because she anticipates being exhausted by the effort of getting there.

man though reticent about approaching him on other than a superficial, chatty basis. She had fantasized their falling in love and was disheartened when he moved away before a deeper relationship could develop.

The disappointment she experienced in this potential relationship was a recurring pattern for the patient. She very much wanted to fall in love and be married but felt that any attractive, intelligent, and caring man would reject her. She was an esteemed member of her musical group but was perceived as someone who kept to herself, lived on the periphery of the group, and gave the impression of being a loner—all despite her wish to be one of the "in" group.

The patient described herself as having been a shy, insecure child and adolescent. Her role among her peers at school had closely paralleled her present position in the social structure of the orchestra. She had always felt that she was on the outside looking in, wanting to become involved but frightened that she would not be accepted. She had often daydreamed about artistic and social successes.

In the interview, the patient appeared to be a soft-spoken, articulate woman who seemed embarrassed by her situation and gave a low-key presentation of herself. She displayed no oddities of speech or behavior. Her mood was sad when she talked about her disappointment in the fantasied love relationship, but signs of a major depressive disorder were absent.

Epidemiology

The prevalence of avoidant personality disorder is unknown, and there are no clear data available on the sex ratio and familial pattern.

Etiology & Pathogenesis

A complex interaction of early childhood environmental experiences and innate temperament plays a role in the occurrence of avoidant personality disorder, but definitive studies concerning the cause have not yet been conducted. Avoidant disorder of childhood and adolescence is said to predict avoidant personality disorder of adulthood.

Treatment

Psychoanalytic psychotherapy is useful in selected patients with avoidant personality disorder. The therapist must expend considerable effort in establishing an effective therapeutic alliance, since their exquisite sensitivity to rejection often causes these patients to abandon treatment abruptly. Assertiveness training and training in general social skills may also be helpful. Group therapy may desensitize the patient to the exaggerated threat of rejection.

Avoidant Personality Disorder in Medical Practice

When a person with avoidant personality disorder

falls ill, preexisting shyness and insecurity may intensify. Since the person is already sensitive to social rejection, he or she may feel further stigmatized by the illness and uncomfortable about asking for help and attention from the physician. Embarrassment about being scrutinized during physical examination may also contribute to downplay of symptoms and delay in seeking help.

Tact and timing—especially in history taking and physical examination—are of the utmost importance in establishing the gradual deepening of trust and rapport required to form a satisfactory working relationship with these patients. This approach encourages the patient with avoidant personality disorder to disclose physical symptoms frankly and without undue embarrassment. The physician needs to steer a middle course between inadvertently cooperating with the patient to minimize complaints and possibly missing the diagnosis on the one hand and adopting an overly intrusive approach that may threaten the patient's sense of privacy and modesty and perhaps contribute to noncompliance on the other. A low-key approach that emphasizes the physician's friendliness and availability and includes prompt return of phone calls, respect for punctuality at appointments, and periodic reassurance of the physician's personal interest and commitment will counter the patient's normal inclination to see himself or herself as unimportant or undeserving of the physician's attention.

Illustrative case. A 23-year-old woman sought consultation with a dermatologist because of an extensive reaction following exposure to poison oak. The patient had delayed seeking help by persuading herself that she was overreacting and using a variety of home remedies that failed to stop the spread of the rash. When she finally requested an appointment, the receptionist inquired about the urgency of the problem in order to appropriately schedule the appointment. The patient replied, "Well, uh, it's not that bad, but it's sort of uncomfortable; I also have a mild fever."

The alert receptionist recognized the tentative quality of this response and brought the physician to the telephone. After more detailed inquiry into the severity of symptoms, an immediate appointment was arranged, and examination revealed a moderately severe allergic reaction with superimposed bacterial infection. The dermatologist took the time to explore the patient's ambivalence about seeking consultation without at the same time making her feel that she was being criticized. He explained the necessity for close follow-up examination in a low-key, friendly manner devoid of arrogance or pretense. He appeared genuinely unhurried and not overly burdened by the pressures of his practice, and he gave an impression of accessibility that was conveyed more through nonverbal communication than in anything he said. His manner of relating to the patient contradicted her stereotype of the doctor as one of the busy professionals who have better things to do with their time than "pander to my self-indulgent concerns." This new view of physicians made it more comfortable for her to comply with the recommendations for follow-up visits and easier for her to think about seeking consultation for future problems.

DEPENDENT PERSONALITY DISORDER

Symptoms & Signs

The diagnostic criteria for dependent personality disorder are listed in Table 26–9. According to *DSM-III-R,* the disorder is characterized by "a pervasive pattern of dependent and submissive behavior. . . ."

The person with dependent personality disorder may be anxious and depressed and may experience intense discomfort when alone for more than a short time. The patient is often intensely preoccupied with the possibility of abandonment. Dependent personality disorder may coexist with another personality disorder such as schizotypal, histrionic, narcissistic, or avoidant personality disorder.

Natural History & Prognosis

The prognosis is unknown.

Differential Diagnosis

Dependent personality disorder must be differenti-

Table 26–9. *DSM-III-R* diagnostic criteria for dependent personality disorder (coded on axis II).

The diagnostic criteria for the personality disorders refer to behaviors or traits that are characteristic of the person's recent (past year) and long-term functioning (generally since adolescence or early adulthood). The constellation of behaviors or traits causes either significant impairment in social or occupational functioning or subjective distress. Behaviors or traits limited to episodes of illness are not considered in making a diagnosis of personality disorder.

A pervasive pattern of dependent and submissive behavior, beginning by early adulthood and present in a variety of contexts, as indicated by at least 5 of the following:

 (1) Is unable to make everyday decisions without an excessive amount of advice or reassurance from others.
 (2) Allows others to make most of his or her important decisions, eg, where to live, what job to take.
 (3) Agrees with people even when he or she believes they are wrong, because of fear of being rejected.
 (4) Has difficulty initiating projects or doing things on his or her own.
 (5) Volunteers to do things that are unpleasant or demeaning in order to get other people to like him or her.
 (6) Feels uncomfortable or helpless when alone, or goes to great lengths to avoid being alone.
 (7) Feels devastated or helpless when close relationships end.
 (8) Is frequently preoccupied with fears of being abandoned.
 (9) Is easily hurt by criticism or disapproval.

ated from histrionic and avoidant personality disorder as well as the more severe personality disorders, including narcissistic, borderline, and schizotypal personality disorder.

Illustrative Case

A 32-year-old married postal worker presented for psychiatric evaluation because she was considerably upset after receiving a job promotion. She had earlier refused several promotions because she had not wanted to assume the responsibility for supervising others. She was now being forced either to accept a promotion or to leave her position. She desperately wished to maintain her present rank, despite the fact that she had an excellent work record and was regarded by management as a good candidate for the supervisory position.

The patient's husband was an ambitious and domineering man who "ruled the roost" in the family, just as her father had done when she was growing up. She was aware that she suppressed her own needs in favor of meeting those of her husband, and though she was occasionally frustrated because of this, she admired his strength of character and felt relieved to know that someone was in control.

The patient was the youngest child in her family and had two older brothers who had enjoyed fussing over their baby sister and of whom she said, "To them I was a real live doll to play with." When she was growing up, she had been hesitant to compete academically and had felt socially stigmatized as the "square" in her peer group.

During the interview, the patient seemed to be quiet, passive, and deferential and appeared younger than her stated age. She cooperated enthusiastically during the interview and in fact seemed eager to anticipate the interviewer's questions in an effort to appear likable. There were no abnormalities of thought, perception, or sensorial functioning. Although she seemed mildly anxious, her symptoms did not meet the diagnostic criteria for anxiety disorder.

Epidemiology

In the Midtown Manhattan Study, Langner and Michael (1963) found that 2.5% of the patients in their sample had passive-dependent traits, such as those seen in dependent personality disorder. The diagnosis of passive-dependent personality disorder is made more frequently in women than in men, and it is more common in the youngest child of a family.

Etiology & Pathogenesis

A. Genetic Factors: Gottesman (1963) found that the presence of submissiveness or dominance was more highly correlated in identical twins than in fraternal twins, which supports the hypothesis that dependent personality disorder has a genetic component.

B. Psychological Factors: A disturbance at the oral stage of psychosexual development is believed to occur in patients who later develop dependent personality disorder; it takes the form of maternal deprivation rather than overgratification during early attachment (see Chapter 4).

Treatment

Long-term psychoanalytic psychotherapy is the treatment of choice and should focus on the patient's exaggerated fears of damaging others or oneself by pursuing autonomy and becoming one's own person.

Dependent Personality Disorder in Medical Practice

Patients with dependent personality disorder may make a dramatic appeal for caretaking, with urgent and inappropriate demands for immediate attention to their medical complaints, which have an exaggerated quality. If they fail to receive a prompt response, they may erupt in angry outbursts that threaten important emotional ties, including that with the physician. Since illness provides secondary gains in the form of caretaking and attention, such patients tend to be passive participants in the healing partnership rather than seeking active solutions. The well-known oral characteristics of dependent persons may be expressed in food, alcohol, and drug problems. The physician must be especially alert to the possibility of abuse of sedatives, hypnotics, tranquilizers, and analgesics. Patients with dependent personality disorder are overly compliant in their acceptance of medical treatment and may search for gratification of their unmet dependence needs by seeking unnecessary procedures while minimizing the associated hazards.

The physician should provide reassurance and convey an impression of being available and accessible to the patient but should be careful to explain clearly and firmly the realistic limits of such availability. The physician can provide help in other ways, eg, coordinating support services and instituting flexible appointment scheduling, in which the patient assumes some responsibility for establishing the timing of appointments. Physicians treating these patients must guard against "burnout" and the hostile rejection that may be aroused by these patients' strong dependence needs. The patient's exaggerated compliance with the treatment regimen may lead to overutilization of medical care systems and is another item that health care professionals need to be aware of. Others members of the health care team, including nurses and physical therapists, may play an important role in communicating the physician's interest and concern and in alleviating physical discomfort, so that the burden of meeting dependence needs is distributed throughout the team rather than being focused exclusively on any one member.

Illustrative case. A 45-year-old man was admitted to the hospital for surgical repair of damaged cartilage in his left knee. On the evening of admission, the resident on the surgical service completed the preoperative physical examination and noted the following in the chart: "Except for the damaged medial meniscus in the left knee, the patient is in remarkably good health. He does, however, present a psychological management problem. He has made frequent requests for analgesics and bristled with irritation when I was called away to the emergency room before I could complete the physical examination. When I returned, the nurse assigned to his care remarked that the patient acted as though this were a Hilton Hotel and that he regarded his pain and anxiety as the only concerns of the hospital staff."

The resident held a meeting with the nurse, the physical therapist, and other members of the health care team in order to prevent further development of hostile reactions on the part of the staff toward this patient and to develop a management strategy. They agreed to meet the patient's requests for attention within realistic limits but decided that the burden of care would be distributed across the entire team. They also decided that a premedical school student summer volunteer should be assigned to the patient. This decision proved mutually rewarding, since it alleviated the patient's anxiety about being alone at a time when he felt vulnerable and provided the student volunteer with a glimpse of the way patients may react to illness.

COMPULSIVE PERSONALITY DISORDER

Symptoms & Signs

Table 26–10 lists the diagnostic criteria for compulsive personality disorder. *DSM-III-R* states that the patient with this disorder shows a "pervasive pattern of perfectionism and inflexibility. . . ."

Patients with compulsive personality disorder experience distress associated with indecisiveness and difficulty in expressing tender feelings. They are generally depressed and feel suppressed anger about feeling controlled by others, and they demonstrate extreme sensitivity to social criticism and excessively conscientious, moralistic, scrupulous, and judgmental behavior.

Natural History & Prognosis

Full-blown axis I obsessive compulsive disturbances may break out periodically and remit. Kringlen (1965) noted the presence of characteristics of compulsive personality disorder in 72% of individuals who developed symptoms of obsessive compulsive disorder. Despite the compulsive individual's worry about the loss of impulse control, the incidence of sexual or aggressive behavior that is out of control is not higher in individuals with compulsive personality disorder than it is in the normal population. The

Table 26–10. *DSM-III-R* diagnostic criteria for compulsive personality disorder (coded on axis II).

The diagnostic criteria for the personality disorders refer to behaviors or traits that are characteristic of the person's recent (past year) and long-term functioning (generally since adolescence or early adulthood). The constellation of behaviors or traits causes either significant impairment in social or occupational functioning or subjective distress. Behaviors or traits limited to episodes of illness are not considered in making a diagnosis of personality disorder.

A pervasive pattern of perfectionism and inflexibility, beginning by early adulthood and present in a variety of contexts, as indicated by at least 5 of the following:

(1) Perfectionism that interferes with task completion, eg, inability to complete a project because own overly strict standards are not met.

(2) Preoccupation with details, rules, lists, order, organization, or schedules to the extent that the major point of the activity is lost.

(3) Unreasonable insistence that others submit to exactly his or her way of doing things, or unreasonable reluctance to allow others to do things because of the conviction that they will not do them correctly.

(4) Excessive devotion to work and productivity to the exclusion of leisure activities and friendships (not accounted for by obvious economic necessity).

(5) Indecisiveness: decision-making is either avoided, postponed, or protracted, eg, the person cannot get assignments done on time because of ruminating about priorities (do not include if indecisiveness is due to excessive need for advice or reassurance from others).

(6) Overconscientiousness, scrupulousness, and inflexibility about matters of morality, ethics, or values (not accounted for by cultural or religious identification).

(7) Restricted expression of affection.

(8) Lack of generosity in giving time, money, or gifts when no personal gain is likely to result.

(9) Inability to discard worn-out or worthless objects even when they have no sentimental value.

risk of major depressive episodes appears to be increased during mid-life crisis.

Differential Diagnosis

Compulsive personality disorder must be distinguished from obsessive compulsive disorder, in which the patient experiences obsessive thoughts (eg, intrusive, unwanted impulses to shout obscenities or handle feces in an ordinarily controlled, moralistic, and meticulous person) or compulsive behavior (eg, repeated checking and rechecking of door locks) (see Chapter 23). The two disorders may coexist, in which case both diagnoses are warranted. Compulsive personality disorder must also be differentiated from schizoid and paranoid personality disorders. Obsessive traits (often seen in persons successfully engaged in professional careers) must be distinguished from full-blown compulsive personality disorder (which is maladaptive and interferes with normal functioning).

Illustrative Case

A 43-year-old senior vice president in an accounting firm sought psychiatric treatment because of a chronic sense of personal dissatisfaction. He had risen rapidly to the highest management level in his firm, but he derived no internal sense of pride and satisfaction. Reporting on this chronic feeling of dissatisfaction, he said, "When I successfully complete a project, it is a reprieve from my fearful expectations; when I experience a setback, it confirms my worst fears."

The patient's wife was a caring and competent woman who was a special education teacher. They had two children. The wife was a lively, articulate, and emotionally spontaneous person who had complained in the past about her husband's emotional remoteness and lack of adventuresome spirit. He felt great affection for his wife and children but was afraid to commit himself emotionally to these relationships, saying, "What if I allow myself to give and receive the love that I crave, and then something happens to them? I would be devastated." The patient was the eldest son of two professional parents. While growing up, he had been extremely well provided for materially but had felt a lack of warmth and intimacy at home. His primary involvement with his family had centered around performance, and he felt pressured to succeed in school and sports. He felt that the family had placed little value on the quiet unstructured times of just enjoying one another's company. He had excelled in school but felt driven, and he had feared that his competitive strivings alienated him from his peers. In addition, he had felt stigmatized when he was left out of social activities during adolescence.

At the interview, the patient was dressed conservatively in somber tones and was meticulously groomed. He was reserved, emotionally distant from the interviewer, and provided a carefully detailed account of his unhappiness. His manner was that of a colleague consulting with another professional about a third person's difficulties rather than that of a patient visiting a doctor. There was no evidence of delusions, hallucinations, or disturbance in consciousness. His thinking was characterized by marked intellectualization and rationalization, a tendency to veer away from emotion-laden topics, and preoccupation with details to the exclusion of understanding the overall issues. Although he said that he felt a chronic sense of unhappiness in his life, he denied the presence of vegetative or other specific symptoms of depression.

Epidemiology

Although compulsive personality disorder is frequently diagnosed in men and is believed to be common, especially in the oldest children of a family, its prevalence is unknown.

Etiology & Pathogenesis

A. Genetic Factors: Twin and adoption studies have demonstrated that there is a genetic contribution to compulsive personality disorder.

B. Psychological Factors: According to Freud, compulsive personality disorder is caused by arrest at the anal level of psychosexual development that results in repetitive power struggles with authority figures, dominance-submission conflicts, and emotional withholding. According to Erikson, disturbance in the stage of development characterized by the issue of autonomy versus shame and self-doubt predisposes to development of compulsive personality disorder (see Chapter 4). Family life is characterized by constrained emotions, and members are often criticized and socially ostracized if they express anger.

Treatment

Insight-oriented psychoanalytic psychotherapy is the treatment of choice. The focus must be on feelings rather than thoughts and would emphasize the clarification of the defenses of isolation of affect (intellectualized distancing from emotions) and displacement of hostility.

Group and behavioral therapy may be helpful in developing skills in achieving intimacy.

Compulsive Personality Disorder in Medical practice

When they are confronted with physical illness, individuals with compulsive personality disorder are particularly troubled by the sense of loss of control over bodily functions. Feelings of shame and vulnerability for being in a weakened condition are typical. The patient also feels angry about the disruption of routines and is fearful of relinquishing control to the health care team. There may be exaggerated worries about submitting to authority figures. Under pressure from the many emotional aspects of the illness, the patient may be apprehensive about the possibility of giving way to emotional outbursts. The patient will attempt to ward off these anxieties by redoubling efforts at composure and presenting a precisely detailed, orderly account of progression of symptoms in an emotionally detached manner.

A scientific approach on the part of the physician—as conveyed in thorough history taking and careful diagnostic workups—is reassuring and fosters the trust necessary for an effective therapeutic alliance. A well articulated account of the disease process and treatment alternatives reassures the patient that someone is in control and that the doctor respects the patient's capacities to participate as an informed partner in the healing process. The reassurance provides a foundation upon which the patient can begin to reconstruct a sense of order in everyday life.

Patients with compulsive personality disorder are not reassured by vague impressionistic overviews of their prognosis. Patients feel most comfortable when the doctor provides documentary evidence in the form of specific laboratory test results, eg, electrocardiograms or x-rays, or cites actual reports from the literature when presenting statistics about risk factors.

The healing process may be promoted by harnessing patients' innate thoroughness through encouraging such self-monitoring activities as measurement of fluid intake and output and weight fluctuations and control of graduated exercise programs. When feasible, patients can take over management of more routine procedures, such as changing their surgical dressings. Meticulous adherence to treatment protocols will restore morale as patients regain a sense of mastery and dignity in taking charge of their lives. The physician must remain alert to the possibility that compulsive patients may wish to carry this self-healing process too far and cross the boundaries of their competence while stubbornly resisting the expertise offered by the health care team.

Illustrative case. A 47-year-old woman who was an executive in a large accounting firm developed symptoms of unexpected weight loss and dizziness. Measurement of fasting blood glucose levels and urinalysis confirmed the diagnosis of adult-onset diabetes. The patient reacted to this news by conducting an extensive search of the literature on diabetes and by requesting that her internist refer her to an endocrinologist for further evaluation. The internist, who had known the patient for a long time, was empathically aware of how emotionally out of control the patient felt and promptly referred the patient to an endocrinologist, who confirmed the diagnosis and provided a detailed description of the nature and expectable course of the illness and alternative treatment strategies. The patient was reassured by the consensus of opinion shown by the two trusted experts and agreed to work with her internist in developing a treatment plan.

Although the patient was initially jolted into a state of panicky confusion by what she termed the "internal rebellion of my body," she regained a sense of order and predictability as she became an active partner in the healing process. Through a program of strict dietary control, weight loss, and exercise (which the patient meticulously pursued), she was able to bring her metabolic status within normal limits and thus avoided the need for exogenous insulin. In a 1-year follow-up appointment with the endocrinologist, the patient was complimented on her courageously disciplined response to the illness. When she was asked what had been most helpful in assisting her to cope with the problem, she replied, "Both you and my regular doctor had faith in my capacity to understand the illness and make informed choices about treatment, and you both supported my resolve to fight back. When I first became ill, I felt like a rudderless ship tossed about in dangerous waters. You were like a safe harbor, but even more important, you helped me regain the confidence that I could sail again on my own power."

PASSIVE-AGGRESSIVE PERSONALITY DISORDER

Symptoms & Signs

Table 26-11 sets forth diagnostic criteria for passive-aggressive personality disorder. According to *DSM-III-R*, this disorder is characterized by "passive resistance to demands for adequate social and occupational performance. . . ."

People with passive-aggressive personality disorder may experience a feeling of dependence and lack of self-confidence as well as a chronic sense of pessimism. They often fail to connect their passive-resistant behavior with their feelings of resentfulness and hostility toward others.

Natural History & Prognosis

In a follow-up study of 100 inpatients with severe symptoms of passive-aggressive disorder, Small et al (1970) found that of the 73 former patients located, 12% were free of symptoms and 79% had persistent difficulties. At the time of follow-up, 44% were employed full-time. A number of patients attempted suicide, although only one person succeeded. About 38% of patients were later rehospitalized. The prognosis is much better for people with milder forms of this personality disorder, for whom outpatient rather than inpatient care is the treatment of choice.

Table 26–11. *DSM-III-R* diagnostic criteria for passive-aggressive personality disorder (coded on axis II).

The diagnostic criteria for the personality disorders refer to behaviors or traits that are characteristic of the person's recent (past year) and long-term functioning (generally since adolescence or early adulthood). The constellation of behaviors or traits causes either significant impairment in social or occupational functioning or subjective distress. Behaviors or traits limited to episodes of illness are not considered in making a diagnosis of personality disorder.

A pervasive pattern of passive resistance to demands for adequate social and occupational performance, beginning by early adulthood and present in a variety of contexts, as indicated by at least 5 of the following:

(1) Procrastinates, ie, puts off things that need to be done so that deadlines are not met.
(2) Becomes sulky, irritable, or argumentative when asked to do something he or she does not want to do.
(3) Seems to work deliberately slowly or to do a bad job on tasks that he or she really does not want to do.
(4) Protests, without justification, that others make unreasonable demands on him or her.
(5) Avoids obligations by claiming to have "forgotten."
(6) Believes that he or she is doing a much better job than others think he or she is doing.
(7) Resents useful suggestions from others concerning how he or she could be more productive.
(8) Obstructs the efforts of others by failing to do his or her share of the work.
(9) Unreasonably criticizes or scorns people in positions of authority.

Differential Diagnosis

The differential diagnosis of passive-aggressive personality disorder includes dependent and avoidant personality disorder. In some cases, the patient may meet the criteria for both compulsive and passive-aggressive personality disorder.

Illustrative Case

A 47-year-old man reluctantly sought psychiatric treatment when progressive financial and marital difficulties led to insomnia. Despite his reputation as a capable housing contractor, he had repeatedly been unable to meet his deadlines with both homeowners and subcontractors. He would often forget important appointments, drag his heels on commitments, and make excuses for being behind schedule, while inwardly feeling, "I'll do it in my own sweet time." His wife was threatening to leave him because she was unable to obtain his help around the house; she felt that she had to ask him ten times to do anything, and even when he complied, he made only a half-hearted effort.

The patient was the youngest son in his family and had two older brothers who, he recalled with some bitterness, had teased and bullied him. He described his father as "the head honcho of the house," who had been more interested in maintaining peace and quiet than in being emotionally close to his sons. He felt his mother had been more caring but overinvolved in his life: "She had to know about every nook and cranny of my life and couldn't tolerate my keeping any secrets from her." As an adolescent he had enjoyed sports but had been prone to outbursts of righteous indignation when he felt he was being treated unfairly. He had been a good student but had been episodically disruptive in the classroom, particularly with strict male teachers. As an adult he had several close friends, but these relationships were strained because of his stubborn refusal to compromise on social plans and his chronic tardiness.

The patient arrived 20 minutes late for the interview and said that traffic had been heavy across town, when in actuality he was familiar with the traffic patterns and simply had not allowed enough time to ensure his prompt arrival. He indicated that he made the appointment reluctantly and only because of his wife's nagging complaints about his uncooperativeness at home. He provided little spontaneous information during the interview, so that the psychiatrist had great difficulty in obtaining useful data. The patient denied that he was in any way "testing" the psychiatrist when the latter tactfully confronted him about his provocative, obstructionist style. Mental status examination revealed no disorder of sensorium, thought organization, or perception, and though the patient's mood was irritable, he did not demonstrate any features of a major affective disorder.

Epidemiology

In the Stirling County (Nova Scotia) study, Leighton et al (1963) found that in a community sample, about 1% of the total population showed passive-aggressive or passive-dependent behavior patterns. The sex ratio and familial pattern of passive-aggressive personality disorder are not known.

Etiology & Pathogenesis

Prospective studies of passive-aggressive personality disorder are lacking. Psychodynamic and learning theories both hypothesize a pattern of parental punishment of the child's assertion and aggression that results in a style of pseudopoliteness hiding resentment that can then only be covertly expressed.

Treatment

A study by Small et al (1970) found that supportive psychotherapy was effective. The treatment of choice in most patients in insight-oriented (expressive) psychotherapy with a goal of gradually converting passive-aggressive behavior to more successful assertive behavior. The insight-oriented approach involves examination of the patient's covert expressions of hostility, first in the context of current repeatedly maladaptive social and occupational relationships and then in the patient's relationship with the therapist. Drug treatment is rarely used. When it is indicated, it is used mainly during periods of severe anxiety and depression.

Passive-Aggressive Personality Disorder in Medical Practice

Individuals with passive-aggressive personality disorder may be a source of considerable irritation to physicians, since they tend to make a dramatic display of their suffering while at the same time only minimally acknowledging the actual help they are receiving and exaggerating their continuing discomfort. Such patients derive secondary gains from remaining ill; eg, they have a means of punishing the envied and resented authority figures in their life, including physicians. they may attempt to place the responsibility for getting well on the physician's shoulders while they themselves subtly fail to cooperate with the treatment procedures. Such patients tend to forget appointments and be late in paying their accounts, and the physician finds little reward in treating them. The physician may then feel a sense of resentfulness and guilty responsibility, since the patient seems neither to improve nor to cooperate with the help offered but still seems to require the physician's attention.

The physician should take the time to acknowledge and empathize with the suffering of these patients before steering the conversation toward specific treatment recommendations. Such patients will then feel understood rather than forced into giving up their suffering before they are prepared to do so. Information is often presented to the patient more effectively in the form of questions rather than statements, such as "What will happen to you if you don't take your medication?" or "What do you think would be a fair fee for this treatment?" This approach encourages the patient's cooperation rather than inviting rebelliousness. If physicians understand that these patients have an investment in illness as a means of passively gaining control, they in turn need not feel weak or guilty because patients do not seem to improve.

Physicians should be alert to subtle forms of noncompliance; eg, patients may deliberately ask for information about treatment procedures so that they may later blame the physician for difficulties in treatment. A nonpunitive but frank discussion about the ways in which patients subtly undermine their own well-being may prevent such passive-aggressive patterns.

SELF-DEFEATING PERSONALITY DISORDER

Symptoms & Signs

Table 26–12 lists the diagnostic criteria for self-defeating personality disorder. This disorder, which represents a new addition to the personality disorder section in *DSM-III-R*, is characterized by a pattern of recurrent self-defeating behavior in work and interpersonal relationships. Individuals with self-defeating personality disorder complain that others exploit, abuse, or otherwise take advantage of them and are often unaware of their own contribution to their misfortunes, which may include repeatedly choosing inappropriate friends, lovers, or colleagues or provoking others to mistreat them. Individuals with this disorder see themselves as self-sacrificing and complain bitterly when their needs are not met. However, the supportive nurturant overtures of others are often overtly or covertly rejected.

Because such individuals both wittingly and unwittingly choose situations likely to be unrewarding and sabotage more promising situations, they experience more failures than successes. When success is attained, it is frequently met with an attitude of exaggerated worry and skepticism and viewed as an aberration rather than as progress toward positive self-esteem or healthy optimism.

Natural History & Prognosis

Systematic data are not yet available on this disorder. There is, however, a strong clinical consensus that individuals with this disorder show stable long-term maladjustment patterns in work and interpersonal relationships. These self-defeating patterns have an inertial quality—setbacks feed upon themselves, and internal negative models of the self are validated by repeated disappointments in life experiences. Because of the predominance of failures over successes in

Table 26–12. *DSM-III-R* diagnostic criteria for defeating personality disorder (coded on axis II).

The diagnostic criteria for the personality disorders refer to behaviors or traits that are characteristic of the person's recent (past year) and long-term functioning (generally since adolescence or early adulthood). The constellation of behaviors or traits causes either significant impairment in social or occupational functioning or subjective distress. Behaviors or traits limited to episodes of illness are not considered in making a diagnosis of personality disorder.

A. A pervasive pattern of self-defeating behavior, beginning by early adulthood and present in a variety of contexts. The person may often avoid or undermine pleasurable experiences, be drawn to situations or relationships in which he or she will suffer, and prevent others from helping him or her, as indicated by at least 5 of the following:

  (1) Chooses people and situations that lead to disappointment, failure, or mistreatment even when better options are clearly available.

  (2) Rejects or renders ineffective the attempts of others to help.

  (3) Following positive personal events (eg, new achievement), responds with depression, guilt, or a behavior that produces pain (eg, an accident).

  (4) Incites angry or rejecting responses from others and then feels hurt, defeated, or humiliated (eg, makes fun of spouse in public, provoking an angry retort, then feels devastated).

  (5) Rejects opportunities for pleasure, or is reluctant to acknowledge enjoying himself or herself (despite having adequate social skills and the capacity for pleasure).

  (6) Fails to accomplish tasks crucial to his or her personal objectives despite demonstrated ability to do so, eg, helps fellow students write papers but is unable to write her own papers.

  (7) Is uninterested in or rejects people who consistently treat him or her well, eg, is unattracted to caring sexual partners.

  (8) Engages in excessive self-sacrifice that is unsolicited by the intended recipients of the sacrifice.

B. The behaviors in criterion A do not occur exclusively in response to, or in anticipation of, being physically, sexually, or psychologically abused.

C. The behaviors in criterion A do not occur only when the person is depressed.

the lives of these individuals, they are at increased risk for major depressive episodes.

Differential Diagnosis

The differential diagnosis of self-defeating personality disorder includes chronic dysthymia and major depressive episode in partial remission. Self-defeating personality disorder and affective disorders may coexist and require combined treatment strategies. Individuals with this personality disorder sometimes share overlapping features with narcissistic, borderline, and passive-aggressive personality disorders.

Illustrative Case

A 38-year-old man sought psychiatric treatment because of depression and loneliness following the breakup of a love relationship. He had been involved

for 8 months with an attractive, intelligent, and caring woman. The breakdown of this relationship was particularly painful to him because the woman, unlike most women with whom he had been involved, had been genuinely committed to deepening the relationship. His earlier pattern had been to involve himself with self-absorbed, emotionally aloof partners who "trashed him in favor of someone more interesting."

He initially portrayed his current disappointment as yet another confirmation of his view that the world would victimize him and was not aware of having provoked the separation by repeatedly frustrating his lover's efforts to show him affection.

In the interview, he presented himself as a down trodden victim who seemed impervious to help and who seemed convinced in advance that treatment would be of no value. The mental status examination revealed no disorder of sensorium, thought organization, or perception. Although his mood was both sad and irritable, he did not demonstrate the prototypical features of major depressive episode.

Epidemiology

The incidence and prevalence of this disorder are unknown, although it is assumed to be common.

Etiology & Pathogenesis

Psychodynamic theorists emphasize an unconscious need for self-punishment related to real or imagined transgressions against parental and sibling figures during childhood. Learning theorists emphasize the low frequency of rewarding life experiences. Cognitive theorists point out the importance of pathogenic schemas, ie, irrational, enduring beliefs about the self as a helpless victim unable to effect positive changes in one's life.

Treatment

Long-term multimodal treatments that combine identification of self-defeating patterns, alleviation of unconscious guilt, revision of pathological beliefs about the self, and formation of more rewarding interpersonal relationships gradually alter maladaptive patterns. Antidepressant drug treatment with tricyclics or monoamine oxidase inhibitors is indicated when a major depressive episode complicates the course of the disorder.

Self-Defeating Personality Disorder in Medical Practice

Patients with self-defeating personality disorder present a special treatment challenge for the physician. Such patients frequently have an unconscious need to defeat the physician's efforts to effect a cure. Often, they overreact to minor side effects of treatment, discontinue treatment against medical advice, or develop symptom substitution. It is difficult to recruit the patient's active cooperation. When treatment is successful, such individuals frequently place themselves at risk for relapse by neglecting nutritional and exercise needs, abusing alcohol and drugs, or not complying with rehabilitation programs.

When treating self-defeating patients, it is useful for the physician to maintain the perspective that the course will be long-term and often complicated. The physician should resist the patient's witting or unwitting invitation to perform miracles only to be defeated by the patient's compulsive need to undermine help when it is offered. The physician should also anticipate the patient's difficulty in cooperating with treatment. Referral for psychiatric treatment, although initially met with reluctance, may later be accepted as the patients gradually gain insight into their own role in self-defeating patterns.

PATIENTS WITH MIXED PERSONALITY DISORDERS

The descriptions provided above present the personality disorders as discrete diagnostic entities so as to point out the distinctive characteristics of each disorder and thereby provide some framework around which to organize clinical observations. As is also sometimes the case in medical patients, psychiatric patients may show features of more than one disorder simultaneously, so that careful management using a skillful synthesis of the approaches described for each separate disorder is imperative, eg, for a patient with mixed compulsive and narcissistic personality disorder or one with mixed histrionic and borderline personality disorder. The problem is analogous to that encountered in medical management of multisystem disease, eg, coexisting diabetes and hepatitis. In the case of combined personality disorders, the physician must avoid minimizing or overemphasizing any one element at the expense of a balanced "systems" approach.

MANAGEMENT OF THE "HATEFUL" PATIENT

A common theme in this chapter is the resentment that may be aroused in physicians and other caretakers by certain patients with personality disorder. Groves (1978) describes the four types of patients with personality disorder who are most likely to evoke an attitude of dislike or even hatred in their physicians: dependent clingers, entitled demanders, manipulative help rejectors, and self-destructive deniers. The similarity of these four diagnostic categories to specific personality disorders described in *DSM-III* is readily apparent. The dependent clinger corresponds to dependent personality disorder; the entitled demander is the same as narcissistic personality disorder; the manipulative help rejector equals passive-aggressive or borderline personality disorder; and the self-destructive denier corresponds to histrionic or borderline personality disorder.

Groves frankly acknowledges the dislike that physicians often feel for certain patients. Although conscious recognition and acceptance of negative feelings toward a patient run counter to the idea of the physician as an unfailingly kind and generous healer of the sick, the denial of such feelings when they really exist can only lead to further disturbances in management of the patient. Recognizing feelings of resentment is an important cornerstone in developing an appropriate management strategy that will create a strong working alliance between the physician and the patient in order to facilitate healing.

REFERENCES

Bowlby J: Forty-four juvenile thieves. Int J Psychoanal 1944;25:19.

Carpenter WT, Gunderson JG, Strauss JS: Considerations of the borderline syndrome: A longitudinal comparative study of borderline and schizophrenic patients. In: *Borderline Personality Disorders: The Concept, the Syndrome, the Patient.* Hartocollis P (editor). Internat Univ Press, 1977.

Freud S: Three essays on the theory of sexuality (1905). In: *Standard Edition of the Complete Psychological Works of Sigmund Freud.* Vol 7. Hogarth Press, 1964.

Glueck S, Glueck E: *Delinquents and Nondelinquents in Perspective.* Harvard Univ Press, 1968.

Gottesman II: Heritability of personality: A demonstration. Psychol Monogr 1963;77:1.

Groves JE: Taking care of the hateful patient. N Engl J Med 1978;298:883.

Horowitz MJ: Sliding meanings: A defense against threat in narcissistic personalities. Int J Psychoanal Psychother 1975;4:167.

Kahana R, Bibring G: Personality types in medical management. In: *Psychiatry and Medical Practice in the General Hospital.* Zinberg N (editor). Internat Univ Press, 1964.

Kemberg O: *Borderline Conditions and Pathological Narcissism.* Jason Aronson, 1975.

Klein D: Psychopharmacological treatment and delineation of borderline disorders. In: *Borderline Personality Disorders: The Concept, the Syndrome, the Patient.* Hartocollis P (editor). Internat Univ Press, 1977.

Kohut M: *The Analysis of the Self.* Internat Univ Press, 1971.

Kringlen E: Obsessional neurotics. Br J Psychiatry 1965;111:709.

Langner TS, Michael ST: *Life Stress and Mental Health.* Free Press, 1963.

Leigh H, Reiser MF: *The Patient: Biological, Psychological, and Social Dimensions of Medical Practice.* Plenum Press, 1980.

Leighton DC et al: Psychiatric findings of the Stirling County study. Am J Psychiatry 1963;119:1021.

Mahler MS: A study of the separation-individuation process and its possible application to borderline phenomena in the psychoanalytic situation. Psychoanal Study Child 1971;26:403.

Masterson JF: *Treatment of the Borderline Adolescent: A Developmental Approach.* Wiley, 1972.

Raine A, Venables PH, Williams M: Relationships between central and autonomic measures of arousal at age 15 years and criminality at age 24 years. Arch Gen Psychiatry 1990;47:1003.

Robins In: *Deviant Children Grown Up: A Sociological and Psychiatric Study of Sociopathic Personality.* Williams & Wilkins, 1966.

Schulsinger F: Psychopathy, heredity, and environment. Int J Ment Health 1972;1:190.

Small F et al: Passive-aggressive personality disorder: A search for a syndrome. Am J Psychiatry 1970;126:973.

Werble B: Second follow-up study of borderline patients. Arch Gen Psychiatry 1970;23:307.

27 Sexual Dysfunction, Gender Identity Disorders, & Paraphilias

Evalyn S. Gendel, MD, & Emmett J. Bonner, PhD

This chapter discusses sexual dysfunctions, gender identity disorders, and the paraphilias. Sexual dysfunctions are defined in *DSM-III-R* as follows: sexual desire disorders (including hypoactive sexual desire and sexual aversion); sexual arousal disorders (including female sexual arousal disorder and male erectile disorder); orgasm disorders (including inhibited female orgasm, inhibited male orgasm, and premature ejaculation); sexual pain disorders (including functional dyspareunia and functional vaginismus); and sexual dysfunction not otherwise specified.

The sexual dysfunctions are the most common of sexual disorders. Gender identity disorders, paraphilias, and other sexual disorders are also discussed.

SEXUAL DYSFUNCTIONS

Early Recognition of Sexual Dysfunction

Sexuality is an important component of physical, intellectual, psychological, and social well-being. The central role of sexuality is affected by health and illness and in turn affects our responses to fluctuations in health.

Physicians have the opportunity to assess sexual dysfunction in the course of a routine history and examination of patients. A simple sexual history taken at an appropriate time during the office visit signifies to the patient that sexuality is as important as any other physical or psychological function. By taking such a history as a routine matter, medical students and physicians can help prevent sexual dysfunction, become more aware of paraphilias, and find cases of gender identity disorders. Since most patients do not present with sexual complaints, the responsibility rests with the physician to elicit and identify complaints as primary unexpressed problems, as possible early clues to organic mental and physical disorders, and as complications of general medical conditions.

Students who become interested in sexual factors

in diagnosis and treatment need to be encouraged to sustain their interest. Other physicians on the medical service must provide guidelines about this significant factor of workup.

Many students and physicians are uncomfortable with patients' questions about sexuality and feel uneasy about broaching the subject themselves. In some cases, they feel that such questions are an intrusion on the patient's privacy, even though they realize that bowel patterns, sleep disturbances, drinking, drug habits, and reproductive status are also private matters. In other cases, they believe that the patient's sexual concerns are not of medical significance or that their own ability to treat such concerns is limited; thus, they ignore or dismiss the patient's concerns.

Physicians must recognize not only the role of sexuality in health and illness but also their own feelings about patients' sexual problems, since this is a first step in learning to be more effective in caring for patients with sexual complaints.

Patients expect their physicians to be authorities on sexual matters, but they frequently are unable to express their concerns to the physician for fear of being criticized or misunderstood. Although there are no longitudinal, controlled research studies of most sexual dysfunctions, it is estimated that 60–80% are psychogenic in origin. These data reflect the fact that medical causes of sexual dysfunction are now diagnosed more frequently because more reliable diagnostic procedures are available. Many of these dysfunctions are never identified unless the patient introduces the subject. Surveys of practicing physicians conducted over the past decade show that only 10% of patients will initiate a discussion of sexual problems if the physician does not; but over 50% will describe a sexual concern if the physician provides an opportunity for discussion. These concerns frequently provide the first clue to other diagnostic considerations or are recognized as the major problem in an otherwise elusive diagnosis.

An example of a common problem involves male patients with repeated though episodic inability to achieve or maintain an erection. He reports to his family physician that he has not "felt like himself" but does not describe any specific symptoms. Physical examination reveals no abnormalities, but a sexual history is not taken. The patient is reassured that he is "quite healthy and there are no physical problems." This reassurance is puzzling. If he is well, why is he having this difficulty? Eventually the family physician or a specialist may refer him for psychotherapy or for marriage or sexual counseling. By this time, however, the problem is usually more difficult to treat. The primary physician has a key role in early detection of sexual dysfunction and can often provide satisfactory initial treatment or appropriate referral (or both), which would implement early recovery and prevention of the more severe, less easily treated problems.

Sexual Response Cycle

A. Sexual Instincts and Learned Behavior: Procreation through sexual activity is an adaptive response developed through biological evolution that gives the species a high potential for survival. Sexual behavior, however, is learned behavior and is influenced by familial patterns, sociocultural factors (public media, community institutions, and the social milieu), and individual experiences and patterns of development as well as by choice. This is in contrast to sexual behavior in other mammalian species, which is under instinctual control with timing governed by the estrous cycle of the female.

Even though sexual behavior and attitudes toward sex vary greatly among individuals, the desire for sexual pleasure is thought to be strong in most men and women. Although there are no data from longitudinal group studies on the quality and intensity of sexual desire or on the quality of sexual activity, clinical experience indicates that the intensity of desire and the degree of satisfaction vary throughout an individual's life. The factors that influence these variations are dependent on the relationship to a particular sexual partner or to different partners; changing sexual fantasies at different periods of growth and development-youth to old age; emotional mood and physical and mental well-being; and varying influences on self-image and self-esteem.

B. Phases of the Sexual Response Cycle: The biophysiological events in the sexual response cycle have been described by Dickinson (1949), Masters and Johnson (1966), and Kaplan (1974), with elaborations by them and others. However, four basic phases are generally recognized:

1. Appetitive or desire phase-In this phase, one or more stimuli (eg, visual, olfactory, tactile, fantasied) engender a desire to engage in sexual activity.

2. Excitement or arousal phase-This phase includes the individual's feelings of sexual pleasure and accompanying physiological changes. The major change in both men and women is pelvic vasocongestion with accompanying myotonia. In men, this results in penile tumescence, stimulation of Cowper's gland, drawing of the scrotum and testicles closer to the body, and penile erection. In women, pelvic congestion and myotonia result in engorgement of the vessels of the external genitalia and the vaginal lining; sweating (transudate production) of the vagina, which produces lubrication; increased tension of the pubococcygeal muscle surrounding the vaginal orifice; development of the orgasmic platform; increased sensitivity and enlargement of the clitoris; and "ballooning" of the inner two-thirds of the vagina Breast tissue frequently engorges, with accompanying nipple erection and sensitivity.

3. Orgasmic phase-In both men and women, generalized muscle tension is followed by muscle contractions, resulting in involuntary pelvic thrusting and heightened sexual sensations. With the release of muscle tension, there are rhythmic contractions of the pelvic and perineal muscles. In women, contractions occur in the lower third of the vagina and in the uterus, which has been elevated in relation to the other pelvic structures (orgasmic platform). In men, contractions of the prostate, seminal vesicles, and urethra propel seminal and prostatic fluids to the exterior while the bladder sphincter closes.

4. Resolution phase-In both sexes, vasocongestion and myotonia become less intense, and there is general body relaxation. Men experience a physiological refractory period before erection and orgasm can occur again. Vasocongestion and myotonia subside less quickly in women, and the clitoral and perineal tissues are sensitive enough to respond almost immediately to continued stimulation.

Symptoms & Signs

Most sexual dysfunctions are related to disturbances in one or more phases of the sexual response cycle. The disturbance may be physiological or psychological. For example, a man who feels strong desire for a partner (psychological) may find that he is not being aroused, as evidenced by an absent or partial erection (physiological). Similarly, a woman who is sexually aroused by her partner and responding physiologically may be unable to reach orgasm as she begins to worry about losing control.

Diagnosis of sexual dysfunction requires that the dysfunction be the central factor in the clinical course, even though it may not be the chief complaint. The dysfunction is usually chronic and perceived by the patient as a change in the sense of sexual pleasure as well as in performance. It is rare for a patient to have symptoms of inhibition or lessening of pleasure without a dysfunction being present; it is also rare for a dysfunction to be present without the patient exhibiting distress. Symptoms may be lifelong or of recent onset; they may be constant or may be present only at certain times (eg, "facultative"—with one partner but not with others); and they may be manifested as complete or partial sexual disability.

Patients' concerns are often focused on fear of not pleasing a partner or inability to feel confident about their sexual "technique." Men and women often describe a sense of "not doing it right," which contributes to further concerns about their sexual capabilities. This "spectatoring" (self-monitoring) exacerbates the symptoms.

The major complications occur in relationships with partners and often affect relationships with others as well.

Patients without partners can be treated for dysfunction. With couples, successful involvement of the partner in treatment is important in conducting therapy and can help prevent further complications.

Natural History

The general course of these conditions is variable, depending on whether they are chronic or recently acquired; persistent, episodic, or partner-specific; and complicated by other forms of dysfunction. The following discussion of sexual dysfunction demonstrates that although psychogenic disorders may have similar origins, their manifestations and response to treatment differ.

Differential Diagnosis

Many patients are concerned about whether they are "sexually normal." Questions often asked are whether sexual intercourse is as spontaneous and natural or as frequent as it "should" be for persons of the same age and marital status. The physician who suspects that such questions may be a clue to a sexual problem that should be explored must use the sexual history to distinguish patients who need further investigation from those who only need sensible information about intimate matters.

When an organic disorder (eg, physical reaction to medication) may have contributed to the sexual dysfunction, both diagnoses should be used, with the organic disorder described on *DSM-III-R* axis III (see Chapter 16 for further information about *DSM-III-R* procedures).

When symptoms are due primarily to a mental disorder, the diagnosis of sexual dysfunction should be avoided; the axis I mental disorder classification should be used. However, if sexual dysfunction developed first and was the cause of the resulting mental disorder, the axis I diagnosis of sexual dysfunction should be used.

If a personality disorder coexists or is an etiological factor in sexual dysfunction, the sexual dysfunction should be diagnosed on axis I and the personality disorder on axis II. A V-code condition (eg, marital problem, interpersonal conflict, or life crisis) is frequently the featured cause of sexual dysfunction and should be noted as part of the axis I sexual dysfunction diagnosis (see Chapter 25).

When the clinician believes that there has been inadequate sexual stimulation—inadequate either in focus, intensity, or duration—the diagnosis of sexual dysfunction is not appropriate. The clinician is dependent on the patient's description of the details of sexual interactions. The physician's skill at open-ended, nonjudgmental history taking is paramount to this process.

Epidemiology

The overall incidence of sexual problems is fairly equal in men and women. At one time, it was believed that more women than men sought treatment, but this no longer appears to be the case, according to recent surveys.

Sexual dysfunction may have its onset at any time. The most common period appears to be from 20 to 40 years of age—the time when long-term relationships are usually established. However, current data show that increasing numbers of people in their 40s, 50s, and 60s are seeking treatment of sexual problems.

Etiology & Pathogenesis

In both men and women, the cause of sexual dysfunction is usually multifactorial. Some sexual problems have their basis in experiences and circumstances far removed from the patient's current life situation. Most problems, however, have more immediate causes and arise after an extended relatively satisfactory period of sexual function. Patients usually postpone seeking help for 3–12 years, believing that the problem will be resolved when changes occur in activities (work, studies), relationships (pregnancy, marriage), or other aspects of their lives. They often believe there must be a medical problem and are usually willing to submit to physical examinations and tests so that a cause may be found and a "cure" instituted. It is only after these avenues have been explored that the patient arrives at the conclusion that there is some other cause.

A. Sociocultural Factors: Family customs, traditions, and attitudes may be incongruent with the patient's present situation but nevertheless exert a strong influence on the patient's beliefs and behaviors.

1. Sexual attitudes and values–The attitudes formed in early life may interfere with the ability to enjoy current behavior. For example, parents may instill the attitude that "sex is dirty" by associating it with elimination of body wastes or by scolding or punishment for masturbation, which often produces guilt without modifying the behavior. The attitude that display of passion is "animalistic" and the family's reinforcement of the "double standard" of behavior for men and women are other common examples.

2. Religious beliefs–Some religious sects or denominations try to impose restrictions on sexual activity—eg, by preaching that sex is only for procreation and that pleasure is somehow wicked.

3. Trauma in early adolescence–Examples include sexual awkwardness due to ignorance about sexuality and lack of experience; hasty sexual encounters in anxiety-provoking situations during adolescence; and incest or sexual abuse or assault (more common than previously believed).

B. Intrapsychic Conflicts:

1. Anxiety–Anxiety is probably the most common etiological factor and, regardless of its source, interrupts feelings of pleasure accompanying the cycle of sexual response.

a. Performance anxiety–This form of anxiety is usually self-imposed, and expectations or standards of performance are often based on something the individual has heard, seen, or read, such as exaggerated accounts of what constitutes sexual adequacy from peers and in fiction, magazine articles, and movies. Sexual adequacy becomes equated with the partner's approval rather than with the personal attainment of joy, satisfaction, intimacy, and love.

b. Performance pressure–There may be pressure from either the male or the female partner to reach orgasm. This occurs both in heterosexual and in homosexual relationships. Men may feel an obligation to achieve and maintain erection almost on demand, or this "duty" may be self-imposed. Women may feel an obligation to reach orgasm during intercourse or to attain multiple orgasms.

2. "Spectatoring"–The following may erect barriers to erotic feelings: monitoring one's own sexual expertise or reactions to pleasure; intellectualizing the sexual experience; imagining how one appears to others during lovemaking (eg, to the partner, the parents, or the children); and imagining that one's lovemaking is being heard or observed by neighbors or other people. Some patients will say, "I was mentally critiquing my own lovemaking."

3. Fear–There may be fear of abandonment because of some sexual or personal flaw, fear of loss of self-control during sexual excitement or orgasm, fear of displeasing a partner, or fear of unwanted pregnancy or sexually transmitted disease (eg, AIDS). In couples being treated for infertility, there may be fear of missing opportunities for conception.

4. Guilt–Guilt can be related to enjoyment of activity, choice of partner, or engaging in "forbidden" or "sinful" sexual activity. The list of origins of guilt for patients is extensive.

5. Self-hatred–The individual may feel unworthy of being loved or of experiencing pleasure.

6. Depression–Depression focused on life situations or events (eg, job, increased home or office responsibilities, illness in the family) may interfere with sexual activity.

7. Denial–An individual engaging in sexual activity may refuse to consider the activity as sexual behavior.

C. Interpersonal or Relationship Factors: These factors frequently incorporate many other etiological factors.

1. Anger–Anger may be either passive or active. Hostility toward the partner can be expressed by creating pressure and tension before sexual activity; choosing an inappropriate time to initiate sexual activity (especially when the time is known to be irritating to the partner); making oneself physically or psychologically repulsive to the partner (eg, deliberate lack of cleanliness, avoidance of physical contact, verbal attacks on family members or on the partner in the presence of others); or finding excuses to frustrate the partner's sexual desires (eg, claiming exhaustion, feigning physical illness, preferring to watch television or finish a book).

2. Lack of trust–Partners may feel that something they do sexually or otherwise will be used against them. Lack of trust may also result from repeatedly being asked to engage in sexual activities known by one partner to be unpleasant to the other.

3. Power struggles–Many satisfactory relationships are marred by each partner wanting to be "in control." Passive resistance to partners' wishes occurs. Devices are used to gain or maintain power, including threats to withhold money, a vacation, etc, if sexual demands are not met; threats to end the relationship or marriage; and threats of suicide or violence to a partner.

4. Lack of communication with the partner about sex–Failure to communicate what is pleasurable is often the result of unrealistic expectations: "If you really cared about me, you would know what I like." Failure to disclose what is desired or preferred establishes an unsatisfying pattern of sexual activity, and this pattern can last for many years. This type of communication problem—labeled "mind reading" by many clinicians—is a habit many couples develop in other aspects of their lives. Fearful of being hurt or of wounding the other person's ego, each attempts to decide what the other partner wants.

5. Development of a "sex manual mentality"–This is the belief that there is a specific recipe for sexual behavior and that following it step-by-step will lead to sexual gratification. The partners are convinced that if their sex life is unsatisfactory it must be because they have failed to learn the "right way" to make love.

D. Educational and Cognitive Factors:

1. Early learning experiences–Sources of information about sexuality (parents, other adults, peers) may convey biased attitudes or misrepresent "facts." These early learning experiences appear to strongly influence later sexual behavior.

2. Sexual ignorance–For example, failure to engage in erotic stimulation may be due to ignorance of its role in mature sexual activity.

3. Belief in sexual myths–

a. Sex role expectations–Stereotypical assumptions are that men are the initiators of sexual activity, are more experienced, and are easily angered if not allowed to maintain full control of the situation; and that women are submissive, need not enjoy sexual activity in order to participate, and are solely responsible for contraception. These assumptions are widely held and are a frequent major problem leading to sexual dysfunction.

b. Myths about age and appearance—There is a myth that old, disabled, or unattractive people are incapable of or uninterested in sexual activity or cannot find partners. People who believe they fit any of these categories or people who meet and are attracted to others who fit the stereotype may avoid sexual activity for fear of being thought "abnormal."

c. Myths about proper sexual activity—People often have strong opinions about what constitutes improper sexual activity (eg, taboos against manual genital stimulation or sexual activity during menstruation).

d. Myths about sexual prowess—Examples include the belief that penile size (generally in the flaccid state) is indicative of sexual potency or prowess; the belief that women with small breasts lack femininity or are unable to nurse infants; and the belief that ejaculatory capacity will be diminished at some particular age. Myths about masturbation are that it impairs sexual competence, is indicative of homosexual tendencies, or causes mental illness, among others.

E. Iatrogenic Factors: Lief (1981) and others have reported several instances in which comments, jokes, and casual notice given to sexual problems by physicians were adverse factors in psychosexual dysfunction. For example, an internist's remark to a diabetic patient—that he should realize that 50% of diabetics become impotent—was not accompanied by explanation; the patient developed sexual problems as he tried to deal with this prediction. In other cases, a superficial solution to a complex problem is offered. For example, when a 25-year-old woman complained of failure to experience orgasm with her husband, the physician gave her a book about female masturbation and told her she would no longer be abnormal if she read it and practiced what it suggested.

Levels of Intervention & Treatment

Although approaches to treatment of sexual dysfunction vary widely among clinicians, some general principles are applicable.

Sex therapy is generally characterized as follows: (1) short-term, eg, 5–20 visits approximately 1–2 weeks apart; (2) focused on the sexual problem; (3) directed to present and future goals, ie, not requiring retrospective analysis except to the extent the therapy suggests its usefulness; (4) action-oriented, ie, involving the individual or couple in assignments to be carried out at home; and (5) incorporating behavioral and psychodynamic approaches. Therapy can be instituted with patients without partners, homosexual or heterosexual, but appears to be most effective when a partner also participates. The approaches discussed below involve therapy for couples; however, specific suggestions for home assignments can be adapted for treatment of patients without partners.

Sex therapy is not always indicated or necessary. The clinician may diagnose and treat dysfunction long before intensive sex therapy is needed.

A. Ruling Out Organic Disease: Many patients with sexual dysfunction have had a physical examination before they seek or are referred for therapy. There is usually a strong feeling on their part that some physical problem exists and can be readily "cured"; thus, they prefer to believe in an organic rather than a psychological cause.

The clinician must verify or repeat the physical examination. In some cases, a review of the patient's previous medical records will suffice. In patients of either sex, laboratory reports of blood glucose levels, thyroid and liver function, and hormone levels should be normal. A history of current alcohol or drug use—prescribed, over-the-counter, and recreational—should be elicited.

B. Assessing a Contributing Physical Illness: Occasionally, there is a preexisting chronic medical condition (eg, arthritis) or a postsurgical condition (eg, following appendectomy or radical mastectomy) that does not interfere with sexual response but may contribute to the current behavior. (The presence of a contributing physical condition should be recorded on *DSM-III-R* axis III.)

C. Eliciting Discussion and Educating the Patient: The clinician should assist the patient in understanding the relationship between physiological and psychological components of dysfunction. While the history is being taken, the physician can encourage the patient ("give permission") to talk openly about sex and can also give educational feedback in a nonjudgmental manner about the patient's fears, anxieties, or items of misinformation. For an individual or couple, this session is often the first step in the therapeutic process. For a few, it may be the only session required. Many patients have never had the opportunity to discuss with a health professional what they are experiencing sexually with their partner. Partners who hear each other's perceptions of their problem in these circumstances often develop enough confidence to continue to explore the problem on their own. If the barrier of silence is broken and anger is sufficiently reduced, patients may feel less anxious about the situation. By the end of the second session, many couples wonder aloud, "Why couldn't we have done this on our own when our problem first began?" Couples or individuals with this attitude generally require only a short course of therapy.

D. Setting the Parameters of Therapy: Once patients have described the problems and their goals, they need to know what therapy will be like. Negative images and sensational images of sex therapy abound. A forthright explanation should be made about their active participation in therapy sessions and home assignments or exercises. They should also be informed of the ground rules, which will often seem mechanical but at the same time will make them feel emotionally vulnerable. The therapist should provide an overview which can be expanded as necessary during therapy and which allows the patients to recognize and take responsibility for much of their treatment.

E. Suggesting Forms of Therapy: Making specific suggestions for "homework" consisting of verbalization of sexual needs and physical expression of closeness actively involves the patients in their own care.

1. Sensate focusing exercises–These are structured 1-hour exercises, with three or four sessions assigned between office visits. The purpose of the exercises is to help the couple recognize that sexual orgasmic activity is not limited to sexual intercourse and that "pleasuring"—ie, stimulating the partner, which gives pleasure to oneself as well as the partner, and receiving pleasurable sensations—can be enjoyable without being regarded as foreplay or a preliminary to intercourse.

Early assignments are devoted to stimulating nongenital parts of each other's bodies, with emphasis on "nondemand" pleasuring—ie, pleasuring to explore one's own tactile feelings about the experience rather than to please the partner. Later assignments incorporate caressing breasts and genitals, but sexual intercourse is prohibited for the period of the exercise. The partners should be told how they can sabotage the process by not arranging for sufficient time to carry out assignments and by going through the motions but evading the spirit of the assignment.

Sexual arousal and intercourse are not the goals of these exercises. The partners are instructed to refrain from intercourse even if aroused and to continue to enjoy the sensations and physiological awareness. Caresses should be used rather than massage or sexual stimulators such as vibrators. Explaining to the partners how touching produces physiological responses is useful to their understanding of the treatment process.

Some therapists prohibit intercourse during the early weeks of treatment, others only during assignments. Patients may be told that they can indulge in orgasmic experiences, including intercourse, at times other than their assignment if they mutually desire to do so. In cases in which erectile or orgasmic problems are due to performance anxiety, these nondemand pleasuring exercises relieve the pressure to "succeed" and allow patients to experience their own sensations without concentrating on pleasing the partner. Verbalization of sexual needs and physical expression of closeness actively involves the patients in their own care.

2. Systematic sensitization or desensitization–In cases of premature ejaculation, the patient is taught to recognize (through sensate focusing exercises) when orgasm or ejaculation is about to become inevitable. If he has a partner, he can show her how he stimulates himself by masturbation or she can provide manual stimulation to be stopped at a signal from him when orgasm becomes imminent. The process is then resumed, and in this way a start-stop sensitization cycle is established. When some degree of control has been gained, the partners should then try intravaginal containment, usually with the man supine. Rhythmic movements are gradually increased until the man gives the signal to stop. After a pause, the movements are resumed and stopped again, etc, as the partners learn how to prolong the pleasure of intercourse while containing the urge to ejaculate.

This start-stop technique has almost entirely replaced the older squeeze technique, which required learning one inhibiting mechanism and later learning natural control.

Similar desensitizing and sensitizing techniques can be used in treating orgasmic problems in women. With progressive stimulation of clitoral and other genital areas by a partner, arousal is experienced without demand or pressure for intercourse. Gradual sensitization occurs until the woman can guide the course of stimulation and penetration.

For women with problems in initiating sexual activity, a series of exercises can be assigned to help the woman feel more in control and help the male partner feel less responsible for all aspects of expressing sexual desire. Sex role expectations—which may have inhibited interpersonal as well as sexual communication—are most likely to be overcome in this manner.

3. Therapy sessions following homework assignments–Sexual dysfunctions usually affect and are affected by other aspects of the patient's lifestyle. Important life events often precipitate dysfunctions, while ongoing daily pressures, lack of interpersonal communication, and family and business pressures prolong and exacerbate them. Consequently, couples who have developed poor patterns of relating (either caused by sexual problems or exaggerated by them) are often angry, resentful, distrusting, and guilty about each other's behavior. The dysfunction is often seen as "her" or "his" problem or as only "my" problem. These perceptions must be explored early in therapy.

Individuals without partners often perceive themselves as abnormal, deviant, unattractive, or unworthy of love and affection, and they are determined to overcome their sexual problems before becoming involved with anyone again.

The couple or individual must make a good faith commitment of time and effort to the sex therapy process. Partners do not have to be permanently committed to each other but must be willing to cooperate in treatment. The therapist observes their style of relating to each other and assists them in interpreting their behavior. Home exercises or assignments become the behavioral vehicle for a progressive integration of the partners' ideas of their own sexual functioning, anatomy, and physiology. They learn to develop nonverbal and verbal ways of communicating about sexual matters and become more aware of their own sensuality. The goals are to reduce anxiety, to eliminate or modify destructive or other maladaptive styles of relating, and to make decisions about what they would like to change. "Not having time" for assignments is often a form of resistance. Patients may feel that they should cancel an appointment because they have not done their homework. But doing the homework will not "cure" the problem, and patients need to be reminded that homework is only one aspect of this combination of psychodynamic and behavioral treatment.

HYPOACTIVE SEXUAL DESIRE

Symptoms & Signs

Hypoactive sexual desire can occur in men and women at any age. As shown in Table 27–1, one of the *DSM-III-R* diagnostic criteria is the persistent absence or deficiency of sexual fantasies and desire. The current life situation of the patient—and, more significantly, the history of events preceding the patient's first awareness of lack of desire—must be reviewed. Age, general health, the quality and frequency of sexual activity in the past, and the partner's responses may contribute to the problem. The problem is seldom presented as a medical complaint unless the patient has reason to be concerned about the partner's distress.

Some patients (both men and women) indicate that they have always had low levels of sexual desire, but the absence of desire is perceived by them as a different and disturbing circumstance. Some men have had difficulty with erection or with premature ejaculation. In the course of trying to correct the symptom, usually with a partner, the condition becomes worse, so that sexual encounters tend to then be avoided.

Etiology

Hypoactive sexual desire may be due to a combination of any number of factors listed in the general section on etiology (see p 308). The most common causes, however, are relationship and interpersonal factors and life stresses affecting the partners.

There are often other contributory organic factors, as in the patient with myocardial infarction who receives only vague or no information from the cardiologist or family physician about sexual activity. Because of uncertainty about the amount of exertion associated with intercourse, such patients may avoid initiating sexual activity with their partners. The partner may have similar fears and thus avoid initiating intercourse or responding to sexual overtures. A pattern of fear, avoidance, frustration, anger, and lack of communication may develop and continue for months or years before one or both partners decide that something must be done. Since myocardial infarction as such has no adverse implications for sexual function, psy-

Table 27–1. *DSM-III-R* diagnostic criteria for hypoactive sexual desire.

A. Persistently or recurrently deficient or absent sexual fantasies and desire for sexual activity. The judgment of deficiency or absence is made by the clinician, taking into account factors that affect sexual functioning, such as age, sex, and the context of the person's life.
B. Does not occur exclusively during the course of another axis I disorder (other than a sexual dysfunction), such as major depression.

chogenic factors are the cause of inhibited sexual desire in patients who have recovered and are back to work.

Treatment

The treatment method is partially described on p 310 but must be tailored to the patients' particular problems and to their willingness to try the assignments even if they are not sure they fully accept them. The major objective of graduated behavioral treatment is to reestablish the patients' ability to become involved in sexual contact and, through increased verbal feedback, to begin to experience sexual excitement. Patients with inhibited sexual desire have not lost their capacity to become sexually excited. The desire phase of the sexual response cycle has been affected, but the potential for arousal has not.

The chances for successful therapy are reduced if there is little "glue" in the marriage—if pregnancy, for instance, is repugnant to the wife or if the partners have become hostile and combative or involved in affairs. If both partners still have a hope and need for realized gains from their investment in the relationship, the chances for success are good.

SEXUAL AVERSION DISORDER

Sexual aversion disorder is characterized by extreme avoidance of genital contact with a sexual partner over a long period of time. It must be differentiated (1) from the sexual aversion that may be associated with an axis I disorder such as obsessive compulsive disorder or a major depressive episode and (2) from hypoactive sexual desire, which is a common presenting sexual disorder (sexual aversion disorder is rare). The *DSM-III-R* diagnostic criteria for sexual aversion disorder are listed in Table 27–2.

Table 27–2. *DSM-III-R* diagnostic criteria for sexual aversion disorder.

A. Persistent or recurrent extreme aversion to, and avoidance of, all or almost all, genital sexual contact with a sexual partner.
B. Does not occur exclusively during the course of another axis I disorder (other than a sexual dysfunction), such as obsessive compulsive disorder or major depression.

Symptoms & Signs

Individuals with sexual aversion disorder experience uncontrollable, overwhelming anxiety at even the thought of sexual activity. There is a phobic nature to their reaction, which may be accompanied by sweating, palpitations, and nausea and other somatic paniclike responses, while in others, there may be no outward manifestation of their intense distress.

Sexual aversion does not imply that sexual dysfunction is also present. Both men and women with this diagnosis are capable of experiencing orgasm on the rare occasions when they grudgingly participate in sexual activity to preserve a relationship. However, the conflict that frequently develops between partners because of the disorder may cause so much distress that the patient may lose the ability to respond.

Distress occurs in anticipation of any gesture that may be interpreted as preliminary to a sexual encounter with a partner, such as holding hands, hugging, or touching. Simply undressing or being nude in the presence of a partner may be threatening. Patients are likely to want sexual intercourse or other orgasmic experience without any preliminary fondling or caressing. As in other phobias, the anxiety is just as intense when anticipating the feared activity as it is when actually participating in it. Self-stimulation without a partner present does not provoke the same level of anxiety; this indicates that the libido is relatively intact.

Patients frequently have a history of an earlier period in their lives when sexual activity was not associated with phobic responses. There may be brief periods of lessened anxiety (often associated with a celebration such as a birthday or anniversary).

Etiology

Masters and Johnson reported on 116 cases between 1972 and 1977 and attempted to categorize some etiological factors. These were much the same as those causing sexual dysfunction, eg, negative parental attitudes toward sexuality during the developing years; inadequate emotional support or insensitivity to sexual concerns of a child by the family; restrictive or punitive reactions to sexual behavior; and sexual abuse. Some early adolescent loss of self-esteem may be evident, but, overall, these patients are more frequently achievers on the job or in school.

Differential Diagnosis

The diagnosis requires a careful history taking. Consistency of the phobic reaction is a critical component for establishing the disorder. Both males and females may develop the disorder, but it is more frequent in females. The phobic reactions are not usually associated with other phobias or panic reactions. Sexual aversion in males is frequently associated with global lifelong anxiety about sexual identity or orientation. For example, men who consider themselves homosexual because they do not relate sexually to women but who have not had sexual contact with men (self-classification by exclusion) are often placed in this category.

Treatment

Treatment consists of desensitization to sexual panic and phobic reactions through modified nongenital sensate focusing exercises (see above). The partner's activity must be adapted to the pace at which the patient feels comfortable. Exercises that provoke the least anxiety must be chosen. For example, the first assignment might be to hold hands and then progress to touching arms and shoulders (rather than assigning nongenital touching or caressing of the entire body). If the patient experiences phobic reactions, the exercise should be stopped and should be resumed only after the patient has been reassured by the partner that sexual contact is not the goal. Within this structure, the patient guides the activity over several weeks to a level that does not precipitate panic symptoms. Partners frequently improve their ability to talk about sexual problems. The goal is to decrease the level of anxiety and use insights developed to lessen the phobic reactions.

SEXUAL AROUSAL DISORDERS

Symptoms & Signs

Sexual arousal disorders, formerly termed impotence in men and frigidity in women, can occur at any age. In the past, the problem was thought to be more prevalent in older couples, but clinical experience reported from many sex therapy centers does not bear this out.

Although patients have no change in their level of sexual desire, they report recurrent and persistent decrease or loss of sexual arousal during sexual activity. The interference with function is at the second phase of the sexual response cycle (see p 307). In men, this results in inability to attain or maintain an erection to completion of intercourse. In women, the complaint is inability to feel sexual sensation, with accompanying partial or complete lack of lubrication sufficient for satisfactory intercourse. The *DSM-III-R* diagnostic criteria are outlined in Table 27–3.

Two major patterns may develop: (1) The first occurrence of problems with erection or lubrication may be dismissed as a matter of no importance. The partners may decide to increase the intensity of sexual stimulation, talk more openly about their sexual needs, and, in general, be supportive and exploratory. If continued attempts to overcome the difficulty produce no results, either partner may worry that the other partner has simply lost interest. Couples who go to doctors with such problems are most likely to be referred for psychological counseling, because of their expressed desire to remain sexually active. (2) At the first occurrence of the problem, one or both

Table 27–3. *DSM-III-R* diagnostic criteria for sexual arousal disorders.

Female sexual arousal disorder:
A. Either (1) or (2):
  (1) Persistent or recurrent partial or complete failure in a female to attain or maintain the lubrication-swelling response of sexual excitement until completion of the sexual activity.
  (2) Persistent or recurrent lack of a subjective sense of sexual excitement and pleasure in a female during sexual activity.
B. Does not occur exclusively during the course of another axis I disorder (other than a sexual dysfunction), such as major depression.

Male erectile disorder:
A. Either (1) or (2):
  (1) Persistent or recurrent partial or complete failure in a male to attain or maintain erection until completion of the sexual activity.
  (2) Persistent or recurrent lack of a subjective sense of sexual excitement and pleasure in a male during sexual activity.
B. Does not occur during the course of another axis I disorder (other than a sexual dysfunction), such as major depression.

partners may respond with disappointment, anger, fear, and intense anxiety. All sexual activity may cease at this point, and there may be no attempt at increased stimulation. Communication about sexual concerns may also cease, for fear of causing further anger or rejection. The couple may avoid the problem for months or even years before seeking help.

Between these two major patterns, gradations of distress are commonly reported.

Etiology

One or more of the factors listed in the section on etiology (see p 308) are usually present. The most common cause is performance anxiety, precipitated sometimes by the first episode of "failure." In such cases, the woman often assumes that her partner finds her unattractive or has become involved with someone else. The man assumes that his partner believes he has lost his sex drive and regards him as foolish or weak. He is fearful of losing her and feels more pressure to "perform." The point at which the partners are unable to express their fears to each other is often the time when they decide to seek help.

Many men believe that sexual prowess begins to decline at a particular age. This notion is sometimes reinforced by physicians, especially if the patient is over 55. The same feelings occur in women who once were easily aroused but suddenly find themselves unresponsive though their desire level remains high. If they are postmenopausal, they may be told by a physician not to expect the same arousal levels they had in the past.

Illustrative Case

The patients, both in their late 50s, had been married 25 years and reported having had a fulfilling sex life. About a year before seeking treatment, the husband found that he did not respond to their lovemaking in his usual way. At first, he believed his inability to maintain an erection was due to simple fatigue. The next time they made love, he lost his erection at the moment of penetration. He proceeded to stimulate his wife manually and orally to orgasm, but he did not become aroused (as he once did) by her responsiveness. Her unsuccessful attempts to stimulate him genitally made him impatient and angry. He sometimes experienced an ejaculation with no erection or sensation of orgasm, and this bothered and embarrassed him even more. He became reluctant to make any sexual overtures for a few days, though he and his wife "cuddled" at night before going to sleep.

During the next few months, the husband's anxiety and fear increased. He still felt a strong desire for his wife, but he could not achieve arousal. When partial erection was achieved, he would immediately attempt intercourse and then lose the erection entirely. He became frustrated and depressed each time this happened and began to worry whether the next attempt would also be unsuccessful. A cycle of negative expectations exacerbated the condition. The wife was concerned about her husband's health and persuaded him to have a thorough checkup. The examination showed nothing abnormal, and her sincere concern then began to irritate him, so that he reproved her for meddling in "his" problem. She began to wait for him to initiate lovemaking and no longer tried to excite him. Their frequent quarreling affected their older children (aged 20 and 23). The husband became less attentive at work and believed that, at age 56, he was probably just "old before his time."

As the patients described their history to the therapist, they were able to perceive the cycle of anger and anxiety that over the years had finally caused them to feel hostile and alienated.

The therapist urged the patients to discuss the positive things they wanted for their future and to describe how they envisioned sexual activity as part of that picture. Both expressed a desire to reintroduce sexual satisfaction and personal closeness into their lives. The husband began to recognize that performance goals for attaining erection and penetration prevented him from relaxing and enjoying sexual play. Both expressed the feeling that sexual encounters had begun to seem like work, and the more they worked or tried for the results they wanted, the more difficult sexual contact became. The wife admitted that in the beginning, she felt she was being rejected but could not understand why. Later, when she was able to voice these fears, her husband assured her that they were unfounded and that the problem was his.

To help the patients interrupt the goal-oriented sexual performance cycle, the therapist suggested structured 1-hour pleasuring sessions at home. In these sessions, intercourse was prohibited, whether or not the husband had a partial or complete erection. The patients were also encouraged to explore each other's feelings, deliberately recall their best sexual experiences together, and talk to each other about their assignments. Later assignments included taking turns initiating sexual pleasuring and becoming reacquainted with their own and their partner's sensuality.

Treatment

Therapy is discussed in the illustrative case above. For further details, see the section beginning on p 310.

INHIBITED FEMALE ORGASM

Symptoms & Signs

As shown in Table 27–4, this disorder is characterized by recurrent or persistent inhibition of female orgasm after a normal sexual excitement phase during sexual activity. Since some women are able to experience orgasm during noncoital clitoral stimulation but not during coitus in the absence of manual clitoral stimulation, clinical judgments about whether this response represents a sexual dysfunction are based on a thorough description of sexual behavior patterns and often require a trial of therapy.

A more accurate diagnosis can be made if the problem is further classified as (1) **primary anorgasmia (preorgasmia),** in which the patient has never had an orgasm either through coitus or through autoerotic activity; or (2) **secondary (situational) anorgasmia,** in which the patient has reached orgasm but can no longer do so or can only experience orgasm in specific situations (eg, through autoerotic stimulation or with certain partners).

Etiology

Primary anorgasmia is most commonly due to sociocultural factors that result in misunderstandings about the body, such as being taught to believe that

Table 27–4. *DSM-III-R* diagnostic criteria for inhibited female orgasm.

A. Persistent or recurrent delay in, or absence of, orgasm in a female following a normal sexual excitement phase during sexual activity that the clinician judges to be adequate in focus, intensity, and duration. Some females are able to experience orgasm during noncoital clitoral stimulation but are unable to experience it during coitus in the absence of manual clitoral stimulation. In most of these females, this represents a normal variation of the female response and does not justify the diagnosis of inhibited female orgasm. However, in some of these females, this does represent a psychologic inhibition that justifies the diagnosis. This difficult judgment is assisted by a thorough sexual evaluation, which may even require a trial of treatment.

B. Does not occur exclusively during the course of another axis I disorder (other than a sexual dysfunction), such as major depression.

the genital area is "dirty" or that "sinful" sexual desires will occur if a girl touches or examines her genitals. In one case, a woman reported that her mother gave her a separate washcloth to use for washing herself "down there."

In both primary and secondary anorgasmia, psychic factors may be fear of loss of control if genital stimulation and sexual excitement are permitted or guilt feelings about sexual pleasure. There is often a combination of factors, including fear of pregnancy and problems in interpersonal relationships. Sexual abuse, assault, or incest in the early years is being recognized more frequently as a cause of inhibited female orgasm.

Treatment

Both partners should work together and attend therapy sessions together, since sexual dysfunction is usually not only one person's problem. Success depends on the partners' agreement to strive together to achieve the goal of pleasure and satisfaction for both.

Women without partners often want to learn to attain orgasm. They have never been able to reach orgasm through fantasy and usually have never masturbated to orgasm.

The therapeutic approach to **primary anorgasmia** includes (1) discussing the patient's feelings about sexual pleasure; (2) discussing any myths or unfounded beliefs she might have about sexual intercourse and other sexual activity; and (3) helping her to see herself as a sexual person through therapy sessions and home assignments in which she appraises her nude body and gradually initiates manual stimulation of the mons, clitoris, and other perineal structures. Therapy sessions must be continued in conjunction with these assignments, since they are important for obtaining an adequate sexual history, including early childhood sexual experiences, sources of sexual information, and the patient's assessment of these and other factors. Behavioral assignments should not be offered in the absence of such therapy sessions.

The goals of treatment for **secondary anorgasmia** are to reduce the fear of loss of control or of intimacy or closeness; to increase communication between the partners; and to utilize nondemand pleasuring exercises (see p 311) to improve stimulation and communication. If premature ejaculation is a problem for the male partner, it may be contributing to the overall dysfunction. Both issues should be addressed in therapy.

INHIBITED MALE ORGASM

Symptoms & Signs

Inhibition of orgasm is recurrent or persistent and is manifested by a delay in or absence of orgasm and ejaculation following an adequate phase of sexual

Table 27–5. *DSM-III-R* diagnostic criteria for inhibited male orgasm.

A. Persistent or recurrent delay in, or absence of, orgasm in a male following a normal sexual excitement phase during sexual activity that the clinician, taking into account the person's age, judges to be adequate in focus, intensity, and duration.

B. Does not occur exclusively during the course of another axis I disorder (other than a sexual dysfunction), such as major depression.

excitement. *DSM-III-R* diagnostic criteria are set forth in Table 27–5.

Etiology

There are few organic factors that affect orgasmic response to the point of inhibition; almost all cases of orgasmic inhibition in males are of psychogenic origin.

The most common etiological factors are authoritative family patterns and the antisex bias of religious orthodoxy (eg, parental regulation of dating and other sexual behavior; inculcation of attitudes that sex is sinful, the genitals unclean, and masturbation destructive and evil). Other causes include rejection of the partner or spouse, episodes of homosexual activity, fear of pregnancy, and a broad spectrum of psychosocial problems.

Treatment

Careful explanation to both partners about the likely causes of this dysfunction is required. After the sexual history is taken, factors that seem specifically applicable to the couple's situation should be discussed. For example, if the woman wants to have children but there has been no mutual agreement about that, she may see the dysfunction as the partner's way of preventing conception. It is important to help her understand that his inability to ejaculate intravaginally is not deliberate and is not a defect in his physical or sexual capacity. Since the woman frequently plays an important role in the treatment of this problem, helping the couple overcome initial hostilities is necessary early in treatment.

Since men with this disorder generally have no difficulty achieving or maintaining an erection for long periods during coitus, their partners may sometimes be asked why they perceive inhibited intravaginal ejaculation as a problem. The fact is that they do, and the clinician's attention should be directed toward the ejaculatory problem, which is usually primary—ie, the man has never been able to ejaculate intravaginally and has difficulty reaching orgasm through masturbation or partner stimulation. Many men with this dysfunction claim they have not masturbated since they were adolescents. Although the patient himself is distressed by his inability to achieve orgasm, the partner usually cannot help feeling that

he wishes to withhold part of himself and that she is being rejected.

Behavioral therapy consists of progressive stimulation, beginning with nondemand sensate focusing and pleasuring (see p 311) and is similar to that used in management of inhibited sexual desire (impotence). Therapy helps implement the man's awareness of his own tactile sensations and improves the communication between partners by removing the pressure to perform. The woman is asked to take the leading role in manually stimulating the penis, taking instructions from her partner about how to do it and how long to continue. The man then watches while ejaculation occurs close to her vaginal orifice. In subsequent attempts, the woman inserts the penis so that ejaculation occurs intravaginally. Once this has been accomplished, the partners generally become highly encouraged and gradually establish confidence that intravaginal intercourse and ejaculation will occur. A prominent feature of treatment is the emphasis on effective patterns of communication, both verbal and nonverbal. If the patients cannot respond to such consensual activity because of unresolved issues concerning intimacy, referral for in-depth individual psychotherapy may be beneficial.

PREMATURE EJACULATION

Symptoms & Signs

Premature ejaculation, which is one of the most common sexual dysfunctions in men, is difficult to define clinically. Generally, in addition to the *DSM-III-R* criteria set forth in Table 27–6, it is defined in terms of the couple's interaction: The ejaculation occurs before the man wishes it and before the woman has reached orgasm, If the woman reaches orgasm quickly, even with a man who considers that his ejaculation occurs too early, ejaculation is by definition not premature. The clearest cases are those in which ejaculation occurs before, during, or shortly after intromission.

Etiology

The cause of premature ejaculation is not known. Although ejaculation is a reflex phenomenon governed by the autonomic and central nervous systems and probably by changes in endocrine activity as well, it is assumed that the major element in control over

Table 27–6. *DSM-III-R* diagnostic criteria for premature ejaculation.

Persistent or recurrent ejaculation with minimal sexual stimulation or before, upon, or shortly after penetration and before the person wishes it. The clinician must take into account factors that affect duration of the excitement phase, such as age, novelty of the sexual partner or situation, and frequency of sexual activity.

ejaculation is learned behavior. The pattern of control is believed to be established early in life, beginning with the onset of masturbation, when ejaculation most often occurs quickly and in secrecy. This pattern may carry over into the first sexual experiences, in which the same conditions may exist. Some families or peer groups may foster the idea that it is ''manly'' to be able to ejaculate quickly, and such early learning experiences may result in a reflex pattern that is not easy to alter.

Illustrative Case

The patients were in their mid 40s and had been married for 18 years before seeking therapy for what they described as sexual problems throughout their married life. Despite these problems, they were an affectionate and loving couple who shared interests in each other's professional lives. They had two teenage children.

The wife explained that although she was not satisfied sexually during intercourse in the early years of their marriage, she had not wanted to discuss this with her husband for fear it would be damaging to his ego. She thought the problem would eventually correct itself. She reached orgasm by masturbating when her husband fell asleep after intercourse. She explained that later she had partial success in ''catching up''—ie, she learned to reach climax sooner but never before he did.

In the course of the therapeutic sessions, the wife admitted that part of her reason for withholding comments from her husband about their sexual life was that everything else was going so well, She feared that if she talked about ''sex,'' her spouse might become defensive or hurt and might leave her and the children. Before marriage, she had once been rejected by a lover, but she had not experienced serious feelings of abandonment, because she had support from family and friends.

Two years after the birth of their second child, the wife began to resent her silence about the problem, which she felt was a result of her husband's not stimulating her adequately either before or after his own quick orgasm. In their first direct confrontation about her frustration and anger, the husband responded explosively because he had not been told sooner. Anger at himself and his wife caused him to ejaculate even more rapidly, sometimes before penetration. He then began having difficulty having an erection. They began avoiding sexual contact altogether, concentrating on their work, social schedules, and children. They agreed to seek assistance but delayed doing so for over 2 years.

By the time help was sought, the sexual problem was beginning to interfere with other aspects of the relationship. However, during their discussion of the problem, the therapist noticed how they were often able to laugh together. They were given initial nondemand pleasuring assignments, progressing to the start-stop sensitization method (see p 311). During therapy sessions, each partner was able to define the series of attitudes and behavior that contributed to the problem: He had at first not realized that a problem existed, and she did not complain. He later realized she was less responsive but did not want to explore the issue. She had tired of dealing with ''his problem.'' Their confrontation had not been helpful. He had experienced severe anxiety that exaggerated the problem and more recently had begun to lose erections. Hearing about each other's experiences in the therapist's office helped them understand the communication problem caused by their defensive positions. They progressed rapidly in therapy, chiefly because of the relative lack of conflict in most of the other areas of their lives. Encouraged by the therapist, they used their ability to cooperate and eventually were successful in postponing ejaculation to the satisfaction of both.

Treatment

Although the above case was unusual in that the couple's general living pattern had endured despite the resentments surrounding their sexual unhappiness, their delay in seeking therapy was not unusual. Sexual activity is of low priority for some couples, and many believe premature ejaculation is an ''inborn'' response that cannot be changed.

The broad principles of sex therapy described for other conditions (see p 310) apply also to the management of premature ejaculation. The optimal approach is to work with both partners, since the problem also distresses the woman and can cause anxiety as well as sexual frustration. The common pattern is that the woman begins to feel resentful and hostile toward her partner over a perceived lack of true intimacy in their sexual relationship. The man is concerned about these same issues, which often lower his self-esteem or cause increased anxiety. Helping the couple understand that premature ejaculation is not deliberate ''selfishness'' on the man's part and not a ''sexual defect'' is a first step. Open discussion and education should encourage the partners to cooperate in nonthreatening ways to achieve mutual sexual satisfaction.

A common traditional method of treating men with this condition was to have them concentrate on nonsexual activities (multiplication tables, etc) during sexual intercourse. This had the adverse effect of distracting the patient's attention from pleasurable sensations and control and usually resulted in even quicker orgasm. This would reinforce the woman's belief that the man was not truly concerned about her sexual gratification. The current treatment of choice consists of the sensate focusing and start-stop behavioral approach (see p 311), combined with psychodynamic therapy. The couple should be told that during the beginning phases of treatment, premature ejaculation will frequently occur despite the man's best efforts to indicate when stimulation should be stopped. The partners should be allowed to feel they have not "failed" and that, over time, they will be able to accomplish these behavioral tasks.

Patients who attribute their inability to maintain long-term relationships to premature ejaculation are often determined to "cure" their condition before they enter into another relationship. Such a patient should be advised to determine by masturbation the "point of no return" before ejaculation, then stop manual stimulation, and proceed in somewhat the same way as with a partner. Achievement of more and more control will establish a feeling of confidence. The patient should be advised, however, that the condition may recur when a new relationship is established. Men who consider masturbation an adolescent activity or who have inhibitions about it for other reasons may be unwilling to cooperate in this form of therapy. The factors influencing these beliefs should at least be discussed (not necessarily altered), and with the help of films and reading materials, many patients come to understand their condition in ways that may help them as they begin new relationships.

FUNCTIONAL DYSPAREUNIA

Symptoms & Signs

DSM-III-R defines functional dyspareunia as coitus associated with recurrent and persistent genital pain in either sex (Table 27–7).

This sexual dysfunction is rare in men; although pain may occur episodically, especially at the point of intromission and at the time of ejaculation, it is usually not persistent and thus does not meet the *DSM-III-R* criteria. Our discussion here will address the problem as it relates to women.

Etiology

About 15% of cases of dyspareunia in women are caused by organic pelvic disorders. These should always be considered in the initial assessment of the patient before functional dyspareunia is diagnosed.

In most cases, a major etiological factor is inadequate vaginal lubrication, caused by anxiety and apprehension on the part of the woman; tension about her sexual "performance" during intercourse; anticipation of pain (a reaction to previous experiences); or fear, guilt, and anger (self-directed, centered on

Table 27–7. *DSM-III-R* diagnostic criteria for functional dyspareunia.

A. Recurrent or persistent genital pain in either a male or a female before, during, or after sexual intercourse.
B. The disturbance is not caused exclusively by lack of lubrication or by vaginismus.

the partner, or both). Penile insertion can often be accomplished comfortably in the early stages of excitement with the aid of an artificial lubricant. However, if the woman's anxiety or stress continues during penile thrusting, vaginal lubrication may cease, and continued thrusting causes pain.

Treatment

Many women who have had a gynecological examination and have been advised to seek therapy for a sexual problem will delay doing so until the interpersonal problems in their marriages become worse. A patient who has delayed seeking therapy may say that her physician did not show concern for her problem and indicated it was "all in her mind." Thus, when treatment is sought, it is often with a feeling of defensiveness at the start.

In addition to obtaining a detailed sexual history and describing the general process of treatment, the therapist should reassure the patient that her concern about the problem is justified. As part of the therapeutic plan, the couple and the therapist should examine what the patient thinks is happening at the time of sexual intercourse. Sensate focusing with nondemand pleasuring (see p 311) keeps the couple in close physical contact and increases their confidence. Although it is tempting to advise the use of artificial lubricants or saliva, such temporary symptomatic measures do not lead to spontaneous lubrication from the vaginal walls. Progression to partial penetration controlled by the woman is accomplished with mutual cooperation and concentration on increasing pleasure. Behavioral and relearning assignments must be accompanied by therapy sessions in which the partners describe their progress and the therapist continues to assess their general interaction.

FUNCTIONAL VAGINISMUS

Symptoms & Signs

Functional vaginismus is characterized by recurrent and persistent involuntary spasms of the muscles of the outer third of the vagina that interfere with coitus (Table 27–8). In primary vaginismus, the woman has never experienced genital sexual activity without vaginismus. In secondary vaginismus, which is more common, the involuntary spasms and pain develop after periods of problem-free genital sexual functioning.

Most young women experience minor spasms and moderate vaginal pain when they first attempt to insert a tampon at the time of menarche, but this experience seldom leads to chronic vaginismus. The condition may become established, however, if the initial discomfort upon inserting a tampon or on inserting a finger during masturbation is associated with a type of fear that some women describe as close to panic.

Table 27–8. *DSM-III-R* diagnostic criteria for functional vaginismus.

A. Recurrent or persistent involuntary spasm of the musculature of the outer third of the vagina that interferes with coitus.
B. The disturbance is not caused exclusively by a physical disorder and is not due to another axis I disorder.

The fear is associated with images of injury, harm, or irreparable damage to the internal organs. Some women report a history of difficulty with pelvic examinations even when a small speculum or one-finger examination is used; these women are most likely to experience recurrent vaginismus during sexual contact.

Etiology

Vaginismus is now recognized to be a conditioned response, but it was once considered to be a hysterical or conversion symptom due to a specific intrapsychic conflict. Such clinical formulations are in agreement with the psychoanalytic theory of sexual development, and there are other plausible psychodynamic hypotheses also, all of which emphasize the patient's unconscious hatred of men; but even though many patients have been treated by psychodynamic methods and marital therapy, successful treatment based on these concepts has not been reported.

Functional vaginismus may be caused by a wide variety of psychological and social factors, such as strict religious upbringing, the psychological effects of rape, and sexual myths and misinformation. There may be anticipation of pain, due to other conflicts associated with shame, guilt, and anxiety about sex. In most cases, there is no clear-cut traumatic or psychic conflict.

Since functional vaginismus is by definition not due to organic causes, it is often regarded as the least common female sexual dysfunction. The true incidence is not definitely known, however.

Treatment

Behavioral treatment at home is usually successful in functional vaginismus and consists of having the patient insert plastic or metal dilators of increasing size—or her own or her partner's fingers—into the introitus. The goal of therapy is to prevent the reflex reaction of vaginismus. As the patient learns about the perineal structures and begins to recognize that she can control her responses, she relaxes the pubococcygeal muscles and the surrounding pelvic musculature. The patient must understand that dilators are used to help relax muscles, not to stretch the vagina. This should be stressed to dispel the patient's fears that she has an abnormally small vagina. Use of Kegel exercises (alternating contraction and relaxation of the pubococcygeal muscles)

also helps teach voluntary control of responses during intercourse.

Some therapists prefer that the woman first use dilators without assistance from her partner and then demonstrate to him what she has learned. She and her partner may then progress to use of the penis, placed against the vaginal orifice without penetration. The amount of movement and depth of penetration are controlled by the woman.

The most successful approach to therapy is to engage the partner in the process from the outset, so that his reactions to the problem can also be discussed. Couples frequently develop mutual hostility and anger related to the unconsummated sexual act, and many are unable to achieve sufficient alternative genital stimulation and thus become increasingly resentful and accusatory. The man often feels rejected, angry, and guilty and may attribute the problem to the woman's desire to control the situation. Awareness of the involuntary nature of vaginismus and a better understanding of the problem help resolve these feelings. Interpersonal and intrapsychic factors should be dealt with as they arise during treatment, and the therapist should be flexible in the choices of therapeutic approach.

SEXUAL DYSFUNCTION NOT OTHERWISE SPECIFIED

Sexual dysfunctions that cannot be classified as one of the specific dysfunctions outlined in the above sections are considered in this category. Examples given in *DSM-III-R* are (1) the lack of erotic sensations or the presence of complete anesthesia despite normal physiological components of sexual excitement and orgasm; (2) a "female analogue of Premature Ejaculation'; and (3) genital pain during masturbation. Although the specific cause and pathogenetic mechanism of the second are not known, some combination of the factors discussed on p 308 is usually present. Postcoital headache is an uncommon dysfunction that not only causes physical discomfort but may also become a source of tension between sexual partners. The therapist must determine that the pain is genuine and has no organic cause. Genital pain during masturbation requires differential diagnosis to rule out Peyronie's disease, pelvic varicosities, and other medical disorders. A woman who has an orgasmic response almost immediately on penetration may find this response to be a problem if it is her only orgasm and if the man is disturbed to know that his partner is experiencing no further pleasure as he continues thrusting to orgasm. The physician can usually help the woman and her partner discuss and understand their own reactions and develop a system of communication that eliminates speculation about each other's feelings.

GENDER IDENTITY DISORDERS

Gender identity disorders are disturbances in the development of the individual's sense of masculinity or femininity. Certain characteristics of personality and behavior tend to cluster around the concept of masculinity or femininity as a result of parental and social approval of those characteristics as befitting members of a given sex.

Definitions

A. Biological Sex: The chromosomal factor of sex (genotype) and physical appearance of the genitals (sex phenotype). The latter is also called anatomic sex.

B. Core Gender Identity: The sense of being male or female. This identification generally occurs before age 18 months and is irreversibly established by age 3 years.

C. Gender Identity: Feelings of masculinity or femininity; the sense of knowing to which sex one belongs and defining oneself as male or female.

D. Gender Role: The expression of gender identity toward oneself and others. It may be further defined as "everything that one says and does, including sexual arousal, to indicate to others or to the self the degree to which one is male or female." Money and Ehrhardt (1972) have said that "gender identity is the private experience of gender role, and gender role is the public expression of gender identity."

Gender identity disorders occur when a person experiences an incongruity between anatomic sex and gender identity. The individual has a strong desire to be a member of the opposite sex, which is not the same as feeling inadequate in behaving appropriately for one's gender role. The main forces creating gender identity are a feeling that psychological gender agrees with anatomic gender and that gender is congruous with what culture defines as acceptable behavior for that gender. True gender disorders are rare. It is important to stress that congenital sexual anomalies should not be confused with gender identity disorders.

What distinguishes the congenital sexual anomalies from the gender identity disorders is that they are primarily physical rather than psychological.

Some infants with ambiguous genitals do not receive surgical management and are nurtured and reared as male or female according to what the parents think is proper. The child thus adopts characteristics of that sex. At puberty, if secondary sexual development is the opposite of the sex of rearing, it becomes apparent that a mistake has been made, and surgical correction may be necessary. Surgery at this point usually does not alter gender identification but may make patients feel more at ease about the difference between their biological sex and their gender identity.

TRANSSEXUALISM

Symptoms & Signs

DSM-III-R characterizes transsexualism as "a persistent discomfort and sense of inappropriateness about one's assigned sex in a person who has reached puberty. In addition, there is a persistent wish to be rid of one's genitals and live as a member of the other sex." Transsexualism may be further characterized as "asexual" when no sexual activity with a partner has been experienced; "homosexual" or "heterosexual" if sexual activity with a partner has occurred; or "unspecified" when the history provides no clear record of sexual activity with a partner.

Natural History

The onset of transsexualism often occurs during childhood, with the full syndrome becoming evident at adolescence. Onset may also occur in adulthood even after the individual has married and had children. Some clinicians feel that these different times of onset represent different types of transsexualism: primary and secondary. Transsexualism creates social and occupational problems, especially since the individual tries to live as a member of the other sex. Many patients suffer from depression, and suicide attempts are common because of confusion about sexual orientation, social isolation, and the experience of being labeled deviant.

Differential Diagnosis

Differential diagnosis stresses the *persistence* of the desire to be rid of the genitals and to be a member of the other sex. Transsexualism must be distinguished from effeminate homosexuality, in which the individual may look like a woman and affect feminine mannerisms but has no desire to *be* a woman. Transsexualism can be differentiated from physical intersexuality (characterized by abnormal sexual structures), since the genitals are normal for the biological sex of the transsexual. What continues to puzzle investigators is that although transsexuals are reared in congruence with their biological sex, dysphoria develops despite this consistency.

Atypical gender disorder must also be ruled out. In this condition, the person experiences transitory stress that may precipitate a wish to be the other sex; the desire disappears when the stress is relieved. For instance, men undergoing severe mid-life crisis may feel that they would be more effective as women and could in that way escape male responsibilities and sexual expectations, which they believe they have failed to meet.

In schizophrenia, there may be delusions of belonging to the other sex, but patients do not wish to become the other sex by alteration of their genital anatomy.

In transvestic fetishism, the desire for cross-dressing in women's clothes occurs, but the transvestite does not wish to be rid of the genitals and become a person of the other gender.

Prognosis

The course of transsexualism is chronic and unremitting. The ultimate desire is for surgical reassignment of sex, and this is frequently attained. The long-range effects of these procedures are currently under study. Patients and surgeons agree on the usefulness of surgery for those who achieve success in becoming a member of the opposite sex, and many centers consider the surgery to be essential for the patient's future effective functioning. Some patients live successfully as members of the opposite sex without surgery. Relationships are established in which both partners agree that a sex-change operation is not necessary.

A common (though infrequently reported) history for transsexuals includes severe depression, suicide attempts, and drug and alcohol abuse in the early years. Once they recognize that they must and can meet the stringent criteria for surgery, they usually stop such behavior. However, those who have had little supportive help or who have had to resort to prostitution or petty crimes to live become increasingly harassed and frustrated. Because they are a visible group to police and mental health authorities, they frequently are thought of as "typical" transsexuals.

Medical personnel will see transsexual patients more frequently as their numbers increase, and they should be aware of the need for empathy and understanding. Patients who are "women" in gender identity need to be protected, for example, from being hospitalized in men's wards. When such patients are on a women's ward, the staff must be careful to avoid subjecting them to unnecessary exposure. Humiliating and painful experiences in such situations often keep these patients from seeking needed medical care.

Epidemiology

Transsexualism is rare and is more common among men than women. Estimates of prevalence are one in 100,000 men and one in 130,000 women. Sex reassignment clinics in the USA report that the ratio of men to women seeking surgery ranges from 2:1 to 8:1, though the rate of requests for female-to-male reassignment is increasing. One recent estimate is that 30,000–60,000 people annually in the USA are requesting sex reassignment surgery.

Etiology & Pathogenesis

The cause of transsexualism is not known. Most investigators agree that some disturbance in the par-

ent-child relationship may exist, although no consistent pattern has been recognized. Some authorities propose that there may be prenatal estrogen and androgen levels which influence neurological changes (pituitary and other brain areas) that may favor the development of transsexualism. Others have suggested that chromosomal abnormalities may be involved. The information is inconclusive, however, because there have been no in-depth studies of either of these hypotheses.

Other theories propose that transsexualism is a severe defense mechanism against an early identity conflict or that unconscious parental reinforcement of cross-sexual behavior created the problem.

Treatment

Psychotherapy has not been successful in the management of transsexualism. Few individuals ask for it in any case. Transsexuals may have other psychological problems (eg, depression, guilt and low self-esteem, alcoholism, and suicidal ideation) that may be helped by psychotherapy.

Not all individuals who request sex reassignment surgery are suitable candidates. Most clinicians have established criteria that require a 2-year period of living as a member of the other sex. Patients must demonstrate that they can function successfully in social situations and at work, and they must develop a supportive network of friends. During this period, the individual may receive hormone therapy (estrogen or testosterone). The person must be told that some changes that occur with administration of hormones are irreversible and also that the nature of the changes cannot be predicted with certainty. Assessment of general psychological health, coping abilities, and social adjustment is made during the waiting period.

GENDER IDENTITY DISORDER OF CHILDHOOD

Symptoms & Signs

Gender identity disorder of childhood is characterized by *DSM-III-R* as "persistent and intense distress in a child about his or her anatomic sex and the desire to be, or insistence that he or she is, of the other sex." These children consistently repudiate their own anatomic attributes.

Gender identity disorder of childhood is not simply a failure to fit cultural stereotypes associated with a particular sex and is not associated with physical abnormalities of the sex organs. Onset is prepubertal. Girls express a desire to be a boy or insist that they are boys.

Natural History & Prognosis

As stated above, symptoms of gender conflict may occur as early as age 4 years. As children with gender identity disorder become older—and as peer pressure and ridicule increase—they may give up overt behavior of the other sex, but the identity conflict continues. During adolescence, some individuals discover that they have a homosexual orientation. For others, the childhood disorder may merge with transsexualism.

Epidemiology & Differential Diagnosis

Gender identity disorder of childhood is rare. No information is available on the sex ratio of occurrence. Gender identity disorder of childhood must be distinguished from childhood tomboyism in girls and effeminacy in boys, in which children make no references to changing their genital anatomy.

Etiology & Pathogenesis

The cause of gender identity disorder of childhood is unknown. Some authors suggest that in boys the condition results from intense, excessive, and prolonged physical and emotional closeness between the infant and the mother and relative absence of the father. In addition, all of the theories about adult transsexualism are applied to both genders in the childhood disorder.

Another theory suggests that unavailability of the mother to a daughter in early infancy may be a contributing cause of the disorder in girls.

Treatment

Treatment must involve the entire family, since the family may be the source of the problem. One or both parents may feel threatened about psychotherapy, deny that they could have contributed to the situation, and refuse to participate. Intensive psychotherapy with the child may be necessary, especially if the condition is a result of early intrapsychic conflict (eg, if the mother was unavailable to her daughter, who repudiates her mother by repudiating her sex). If the condition is a learned response (eg, if a mother subtly encourages feminine behavior in her son), group therapy and behavior modification techniques may be beneficial.

Because of the increasing acceptance of alternative patterns of living and the recognition of cultural biases in sex role stereotyping, patients must be carefully evaluated to determine if a true psychological disorder exists before therapy is begun.

GENDER IDENTITY DISORDER OF ADOLESCENCE & ADULTHOOD, NONTRANSSEXUAL TYPE

Symptoms & Signs

As in other gender identity disorders this condition is characterized by a "persistent or recurrent discomfort and sense of inappropriateness about one's assigned sex." It occurs in people who have attained puberty and is associated with persistent or recurrent cross-dressing.

Differential Diagnosis

This disorder can be distinguished from transvestic fetishism by the fact that cross-dressing in this disorder does not produce sexual excitement. Transsexualism should be ruled out by the lack of "persistent preoccupation (for at least 2 years)" with the wish to be rid of one's genitals and secondary sex characteristics and the wish to acquire those of the other sex.

Etiology

The cause of this gender identity disorder is unknown. The history of sexual orientation may include asexual, homosexual, or heterosexual behaviors and does not appear to be predictive of occurrence.

Epidemiology

This disorder is rare and no information about sex ratios is available.

Treatment

Clinicians do not agree on the appropriate method of treatment or whether therapy is desirable or effective.

ATYPICAL GENDER IDENTITY DISORDER

Some patients may have a gender identity dysfunction that is not classifiable as a specific gender identity disorder. These patients should not be confused with men and women who have mannerisms of the other sex (masculine women and feminine men) but have no doubt about their gender and do not want to change it. They are not said to have a gender identity disorder, and they do not need therapy. If they are sufficiently troubled or uncomfortable, they may seek training to develop gender-appropriate mannerisms, but this is not usual.

PARAPHILIAS

The concept of normality in human sexual behavior is impossible to define, since accurate statistics on the frequency of different types of sexual behavior are not available. In recognition of these difficulties, the pejorative labels "perversions," "deviations," and "aberrations" have been abandoned in favor of the term "paraphilias" (derived from Greek words meaning "along side of" and "love").

Symptoms & Signs

The paraphilias represent patterns of erotic arousal that are different from the typical pattern of mutual sexual arousal with a human partner of the opposite or same sex. The typical feature of the paraphilias, according to *DSM-III-R*, is "recurrent intense sexual urges and sexually arousing fantasies generally involving either (1) nonhuman objects, (2) the suffering or humiliation of oneself or one's partner (not merely simulated), or (3) children or other nonconsenting persons."

These behaviors also occur among the general population to some degree, and couples will occasionally describe their erotic activities as incorporating some of these features. The imagery and acts may range from "playful and harmless" with a consenting partner to "noxious and injurious" with a nonconsenting partner. Clothing fetishism is considered a minor problem, whereas sadistic lust murder is of course a most serious crime.

For the paraphiliac patient, the imagery is persistent, and the fantasies evoked are necessary for erotic arousal, for relief from nonerotic tension, and for sexual excitement and orgasm. The fantasies may or may not be acted upon, but they are distinguished by their consistency. The occasional employment of fantasy or objects in sexual activity between consenting partners is therefore excluded. An individual may incorporate several paraphilias at one time. A paraphilia may coexist with some other mental disorder and is not a symptom of the other disorder.

Many people with paraphilias feel no distress, whereas others admit to feelings of shame, guilt, and depression. Paraphilia represents an "impairment in the capacity for reciprocal affectionate sexual activity." It may produce sexual dysfunction, and social and sexual relationships may suffer. Personality disturbances are common, and behavior associated with paraphilia may take over an individual's life and completely disrupt it because of social condemnation and violations of the law.

Epidemiology

Paraphilias are rare. They occur mostly in men, with very few cases reported in women.

Etiology

Except for some cases of transvestic fetishism, most authorities agree that the cause of paraphilias is unknown.

Treatment

The treatment pattern is the same for all paraphilias. The general goals of therapy as described by Lief (1981) are to "increase heterosexual responsiveness and decrease paraphiliac behavior," "establish a rewarding sexual relationship," and "control undesirable sexual behavior." Several types of therapy have been successful in achieving these aims. Group ther-

apy and marital therapy have been used, but individual psychodynamic psychotherapy and behavior therapy are the most commonly used types of psychotherapy.

Abel et al (1980) published a list of treatment recommendations for paraphilias. Not all of the recommendations must be used in treating each patient. The authors stress use of follow-up to provide reinforcement after therapy is concluded.

Many patients with paraphilia are deficient in basic social skills. As they become more competent, their paraphiliac behavior tends to occur less frequently or may disappear. However, the person may sometimes need assistance in adapting to rather than changing the deviant behavior, because to try to change would cause the patient more intense psychological suffering than the deviant behavior. Whenever possible, therapy should involve the spouse or other committed partner to facilitate change or adaptation.

FETISHISM

Symptoms & Signs

Fetishism is defined by *DSM-III-R* as "recurrent, intense, sexual urges and sexually arousing fantasies, of at least 6 months' duration, involving the use of nonliving objects (fetishes)." These objects do not include female clothing used in cross-dressing or objects specifically designed to be sexually stimulating (eg, vibrators). Sexual arousal may involve the object alone or may be incorporated into activities involving a human partner. Most fetishes are articles of clothing.

Natural History & Prognosis

Fetishism may be considered a "safe" behavior by the individual, because it avoids the dangers of interacting with another person. The condition tends to be chronic, and relationship problems are common. As seen in the illustrative case discussed below, individuals with fetishes rarely present for treatment except to discuss interpersonal problems related to their paraphilia.

Differential Diagnosis

Many articles of clothing may be sexually arousing in certain circumstances, but a differential diagnosis of fetishism requires that nonhuman objects be "persistently preferred or required" to achieve sexual excitement. The occasional use of some object to enhance sexual enjoyment is not fetishism.

TRANSVESTIC FETISHISM

Symptoms & Signs

Transvestic fetishism is defined in *DSM-III-R* as "recurrent, intense, sexual urges and sexually arousing fantasies, of at least 6 months' duration, involving cross-dressing (in a heterosexual male).'' Cross-dressing usually involves more than one article of clothing and may involve being completely dressed as a woman. Intermittent incidents tend to become frequent or habitual.

Natural History & Prognosis

Transvestic fetishism usually begins in childhood or early adolescence. It tends to move from partial to complete cross-dressing and from occasional to frequent, habitual incidents. This pattern may produce anxiety, depression, or guilt feelings, and the depression may lead to suicide attempts. Married patients are frequently unable to maintain stable marital relationships, and divorce is common. The behavior begins as a secret and private activity and progresses to going out in public dressed as a woman. Such behavior may cause further marital or family distress as well as danger to a patient living in an area where going out in public dressed as a woman is against the law. The publicity or shame surrounding arrest may cause major emotional trauma and ultimately lead the individual to seek treatment. Some transvestites find that their condition has evolved to transsexualism or has disguised true transsexualism from the beginning. In such patients, an assessment of the problem and a possible new diagnosis must be considered.

Differential Diagnosis

Transvestic fetishism must be distinguished from transsexualism. Transsexuals wish to lose their genitals and live as members of the other sex; they receive no sexual excitement from dressing as a woman. Transvestites consider themselves to be basically male. They become sexually excited, at least at first, from cross-dressing. Transvestites report sexual frustration when there is interference with cross-dressing. Sexual arousal that is caused only by the female clothing used in cross-dressing rules out a diagnosis of fetishism.

Epidemiology

Although transvestic fetishism may occur among women, there are no reported cases of women who become sexually aroused by dressing as a man.

PEDOPHILIA

The essential feature of pedophilia (literally ''love of children'') is defined by *DSM-III-R* as ''recurrent, intense, sexual urges and sexually arousing fantasies, of at least 6 months' duration, involving sexual activity with a prepubescent child.'' The age difference between the parties has been established as at least 10 years unless the individual is in late adolescence, in which case it is the judgment of the clinician that

determines whether the behavior may be diagnosed as pedophilia or not.

EXHIBITIONISM

The essential feature of this disorder, as defined by *DSM-III-R*, is ''recurrent, intense, sexual urges and sexually arousing fantasies, of at least 6 months' duration, involving the exposure of one's genitals to a stranger.''

Exhibitionism has been thought to be a disorder only of men, with the victims being exclusively women. However, there have been isolated reports of female genital exhibitionism. The onset may be at any time from adolescence to middle age but most commonly occurs in the mid 20s.

The diagnosis of exhibitionism is made only if the individual achieves sexual excitement from the act of exposure but does not seek sexual activity with the stranger. Excitement may lead to masturbation, but commonly the person is unable to achieve an erection even by masturbation.

VOYEURISM

DSM-III-R states that voyeurism is the ''recurrent, intense, sexual urges and sexually arousing fantasies, of at least 6 months' duration, involving the act of observing unsuspecting people, usually strangers, who are either naked, in the act of disrobing, or engaging in sexual activity.'' During observation of others, the individual masturbates, but no sexual activity with the person or persons being observed is sought. Voyeurism usually begins in early adulthood and tends to be chronic.

SEXUAL MASOCHISM

The essential feature in making a *DSM-III-R* diagnosis of sexual masochism is ''recurrent, intense, sexual urges and sexually arousing fantasies, of at least 6 months' duration, involving the act (real, not simulated) of being humiliated, beaten, bound, or otherwise made to suffer.'' The person exclusively prefers to be ''humiliated, bound, beaten, or otherwise made to suffer'' for the purpose of sexual excitement. Masochistic individuals intentionally participate in acts that cause physical harm or may be life-threatening to them in order to produce sexual excitement. Masochistic fantasies may begin in childhood, but activities with partners usually begin in early adulthood.

A diagnosis of sexual masochism is made only if the individual engages in acts, not just fantasies. Masochistic fantasies are commonly verbalized for the purposes of sexual arousal by many individuals, but they are rarely acted on. True masochistic behavior is repetitive and intentional.

SEXUAL SADISM

As defined in *DSM-III-R*, sadism is "recurrent, intense, sexual urges and sexually arousing fantasies, of at least 6 months' duration, involving acts (real, not simulated) in which the psychological or physical suffering (including humiliation) of the victim is sexually exciting." The cause is not known. There are essentially three manifestations of sadistic behavior. If the partner is nonconsenting, it is the "repeated and intentionally inflicted psychological or physical suffering" that characterizes sexual sadism. If the partner is consenting, the essential feature is that the "repeatedly preferred or exclusive mode of achieving sexual excitement combines humiliation with simulated or mildly injurious bodily suffering." Also with a consenting partner, "bodily injury that is extensive, permanent, or possibly mortal is inflicted in order to achieve sexual excitement." Although sadistic fantasies may occur earlier, activities do not usually begin until young adulthood.

Sadism is sometimes combined with rape or lust murder. However, not all rapists are sadists, and some men cannot commit rape if they see signs of suffering in the victim. Rape is usually an act of hostile aggression and not a response to sexual excitement.

FROTTEURISM

"Touching or rubbing against a nonconsenting person" accompanied by "recurrent intense sexual urges and sexually arousing fantasies" over a period of at least 6 months is the diagnostic criterion for frotteurism. The rubbing generally involves movement of the penis against the buttocks of a woman when both people are fully clothed. This behavior occurs most commonly on crowded buses or subway trains. The female victim may not be aware of what is happening.

ATYPICAL PARAPHILIA

Atypical paraphilias are rare types of abnormal sexual behavior, including sexual excitement produced by feces (coprophilia), urinating on a sexual partner (urophilia), being urinated on or thinking about urine (urolagnia), self-administered enemas (klismaphilia), filthy surroundings (mysophilia), sexual activity with a corpse (necrophilia) or an animal (zoophilia), and obscene telephone calls (telephone scatologia).

There is little information on the prevalence of these paraphilias or on other behavioral characteristics of the individuals involved. Some of these activities are noted in patients with other kinds of paraphilias. Isolated case reports are the major source of data. Although obscene telephone calls are frequently reported, few of the people making the offensive calls are caught and made available for examination.

OTHER PSYCHOSEXUAL DISORDERS

Sexual disorders not elsewhere classified by *DSM-III-R* are those that cannot be classified in any of the specific categories. In rare instances, this category may be used concurrently with one of the specific diagnoses when both are necessary to explain or describe the clinical disturbance. Examples include "(1) marked feelings of inadequacy concerning body habitus, size and shape of sex organs, sexual performance, or other traits related to self-imposed standards of masculinity or femininity; (2) distress about a pattern of repeated sexual conquests or other forms of nonparaphilic sexual addiction involving a succession of people who exist only as things to be used; and (3) persistent and marked distress about one's sexual orientation."

These conditions are uncommon, but their true prevalence is unknown, since many people never seek treatment.

REFERENCES

Abel GG et al: Aggressive behavior and sex. Psychiatr Clin North Am 1980;3:133.

Bancroft J: *Human Sexuality and Its Problems*. Churchill Livingstone, 1983.

Chalkey AJ, Powell GE: The clinical description of 48 cases of sexual fetishism. Br J Psychiatry 1983;142:292.

Chesser E: *Human Aspects of Sexual Deviation*. Jerrolds Publishing, 1971.

Kaplan H: *Disorders of Sexual Desire*. Brunner/Mazel, 1979.

Kaplan H: *The New Sex Therapy: Active Treatment of Sexual Dysfunctions*. Brunner/Mazel, 1974.

Kolodny RC, Masters WH, Johnson VE: *Textbook of Sexual Medicine*. Little, Brown, 1979.

Lester D: *Unusual Sexual Behavior: The Standard Deviations*. Thomas, 1975.

Lieblum SR, Pervin LA (editors): *Principles and Practice of Sex Therapy*. Guilford Press, 1980.

Lief H (editor): *Sexual Problems in Medical Practice*. American Medical Association, 1981.

Masters WH, Johnson VE: *Human Sexual Inadequacy*. Little, Brown, 1970.

Masters WH, Johnson VE: *Human Sexual Response*. Little, Brown, 1966.

Money J, Ehrhardt A: *Man and Woman, Boy and Girl*. Johns Hopkins Univ Press, 1972.

Munjack DJ, Oziel LJ: *Sexual Medicine and Counseling in Office Practice*. Little, Brown, 1980.

Pariser SF, Levine SB, Gardner ML (editors): *Clinical Sexuality*. Marcel Dekker, 1983.

Pauly IB: Female transsexualism. Arch Sex Behav 1974;3:509.

Stoller RJ: *Perversion: The Erotic Form of Hatred*. Pantheon Books, 1975.

Stoller RJ: *Sex and Gender*. Vol 2: *The Transsexual Experiment*. Jason Aronson, 1976.

Tollison CD, Adams HE: *Sexual Disorders: Treatment, Theory and Research*. Gardner Press, 1979.

Weinberg G: *Society and the Healthy Homosexual*. Doubleday Anchor, 1973.

Woods NF: *Human Sexuality in Health and Illness*, 2nd ed. Mosby, 1979.

Eating Disorders

28

Kim Norman, MD

This chapter provides an overview of the major eating disorders: anorexia nervosa, bulimia, and obesity. In reading this review, one should keep in mind that eating disorders are not illnesses per se but behavioral syndromes that develop in individuals who manifest a broad spectrum of psychological, biological, and sociocultural characteristics.

ANOREXIA NERVOSA

Anorexia nervosa is a complex disorder manifested by physiological, behavioral, and psychological changes and characterized by morbid fear of fatness, gross distortion of body image, and unrelenting pursuit of thinness. The name is actually a misnomer, since true anorexia (loss of appetite) does not usually occur until late in the course. Although it typically begins in adolescence, the average age at onset is between 10 and 30 years.

Symptoms & Signs

Individuals with anorexia nervosa go to incredible extremes in order to lose weight. They begin by drastically reducing caloric intake, with virtually complete avoidance of high-carbohydrate and fat-containing foods. They exercise incessantly—walking, running, swimming, cycling, dancing, and performing calisthenics. Hyperactivity is dramatic and persists even when weight loss has resulted in cachexia. Some patients alternate fasting with bulimia—episodes of uncontrolled gorging without awareness of hunger or satiation. Such eating binges are often followed by self-induced vomiting. Huge quantities of laxatives are commonly consumed. Diet pills and diuretics may also be abused in the effort to lose weight.

The eating behaviors of anorexics are often peculiar and may be bizarre. The diet may be exceedingly monotonous or highly eccentric. They may hoard large quantities or hide small amounts of food around the house. Although they eat very little, they are obsessively preoccupied with food and cooking. Food portions are carefully measured, and small meals may be eaten over many hours. Food is usually stored, prepared, served, eaten, and disposed of in specific, ritualistic fashion. Indeed, almost all types of behavior in which the patient engages may be highly ritualized, with each step taken or not taken, each bite swallowed

or refused, each calisthenic completed or not as if it had profound consequences for the future well-being of the patient and those the patient cares most about. Patients with anorexia nervosa are usually highly secretive and often lie in order to protect the privacy of their eating behaviors. Kleptomania and stealing are sometimes associated with this disorder, especially among individuals who also have episodes of bulimia.

Although the features of anorexia nervosa described above can occur in individuals with a variety of premorbid personality structures and traits, a fairly consistent profile of emotional and psychological manifestations common to all patients with this disorder has been described. Clinicians generally agree that the unrelenting pursuit of thinness manifests an underlying psychological struggle to maintain a sense of personal autonomy and self-control. On the surface, patients are stubbornly defiant and fiercely independent. They insist they are happy, fully aware of their condition, and completely capable of taking care of themselves. But underneath they are stricken with a paralyzing sense of helplessness and ineffectiveness, with control over eating and body size the only mechanisms through which a sense of autonomy and mastery can be sustained. This important insight into the psychology of anorexia nervosa was first emphasized by Bruch (1962), who also described two other essential features of this disorder: a characteristic misperception of internal body cues, with inability to recognize manifestations of nutritional deprivation as the most pronounced example; and a disturbance of body image, so that patients may see themselves as fat even when exceedingly thin. These cognitive and perceptual distortions accentuate the sense of personal ineffectiveness and reinforce the need to continue the pursuit of thinness in order to maintain a sense of control.

The lack of confidence in basic self-control is compounded by feelings of personal mistrust. Patients fear they will give in to overwhelming impulses and, so far as eating is concerned, gorge themselves into obesity. Individuals with anorexia nervosa also tend to view themselves in terms of absolutes and polar opposites. Behavior is either all good or all bad; a decision is either completely right or completely wrong; and one is either absolutely in control or totally out of control. Thus, patients may respond to the gain of an ounce with the same horror as if they had gained 100 lb. Self-mistrust and the tendency to view the world in absolutes reinforce the exaggerated need to maintain rigid control over what is and is not eaten.

Patients with anorexia nervosa often express fear about becoming adults, since that would mean taking responsibility for interpersonal and sexual relationships. They are often frightened of sexuality and usually avoid sexual encounters. When they do engage in sexual activity, it is usually without enjoyment.

Depressive symptoms are commonly associated with anorexia nervosa. These include dysphoric mood, crying spells, sleep disturbances (ie, insomnia or hypersomnia), and, occasionally, suicidal behavior. Low self-esteem is also characteristic, with many individuals claiming that thinness and the ability to lose weight are the only things they like about themselves.

Other psychiatric symptoms frequently associated with anorexia nervosa include obsessive compulsive or histrionic traits, anxiety, perfectionism, and hypochondriasis.

Many of the symptoms observed in anorexia nervosa also occur in individuals subjected to enforced starvation, eg, prisoners of war, famine victims, and research subjects. Thus, the reversal of starvation is the necessary first step in the treatment of anorexia nervosa.

A weight loss of at least 15% of the baseline or ideal body weight is necessary to establish the diagnosis of anorexia nervosa. In addition to weight loss, a number of physical signs of anorexia nervosa can be attributed to weight loss, malnutrition, and generalized stress. Amenorrhea or oligomenorrhea, independent of weight loss and often preceding initial weight loss, is always present in women. Anorexia nervosa with premenarcheal onset often results in short stature and delayed breast development. Prolonged amenorrhea in women with anorexia nervosa may lead to the development of osteoporosis. Patients frequently complain of epigastric distress, and gastric emptying time is indeed prolonged. Vomiting, constipation, cold intolerance, headache, polyuria, and sleep disturbances are also commonly reported. Autophonia is sometimes noted. In addition to emaciation, physical findings may include edema, lanugo, low blood pressure, bradycardia, arrhythmias, diminished cardiac mass, and infantile uterus. Males with anorexia frequently have hemorrhoids and experience loss of libido. Low testosterone levels associated with emaciation often do not return to normal after weight gain (Brotman et al, 1985).

Laboratory findings include abnormalities of vasopressin secretion, prepubertal plasma levels of follicle-stimulating hormone and luteinizing hormone, and a diminished response to gonadotropin-releasing hormone. Estrogen is at postmenopausal levels. There is abolition or reversal of the normal circadian rhythm of plasma cortisol; the metabolic clearance rate of cortisol is reduced; and there is incomplete suppression of adrenocorticotropin and cortisol by dexamethasone. There is diminished growth hormone response to insulin-induced hypoglycemia, arginine stimulation, and levodopa. Glucose tolerance test curves may be flat. Plasma levels of triiodothyronine (T_3) are reduced, and levels of plasma (reverse T_3) may be elevated. In severe cases, the glomerular filtration rate may be reduced. Hematological abnormalities may include leukopenia with a relative lymphocytosis, thrombocytopenia, and anemia. Bone marrow aspiration reveals hypocellularity, with large amounts of gelatinous acid mucopolysaccharide. The erythrocyte sedimentation rate is low, and plasma fibrinogen levels are reduced. Hypercarotenemia and hypercholesterolemia are common findings. Self-induced vomiting may produce a metabolic hypokalemia alkalosis. Electroencephalographic patterns may be abnormal, and the electrocardiogram may show flat or inverted T waves, ST depression, and increased intervals.

Natural History

The onset of anorexia nervosa often follows new life situations in which the patient feels inadequate or unable to cope. Such changes may be biological, such as the onset of puberty; psychological, such as the stages of adolescence; or social, as in entering high school or college. The onset of anorexia nervosa may also follow the breakup of a relationship or the death of a relative or friend.

Typically, anorexia nervosa begins in individuals who are at normal weight or slightly to moderately overweight. Dieting is initially supported, even actively encouraged, by family and friends as well as in many cases by dance teachers and sports coaches. The patient is thus praised for the initial weight loss and takes pleasure in the achievement. Once the original weight reduction goal is attained, however, a new one is immediately set. Ostensibly, this is for "insurance" to offset future weight gains, but weight loss in the pursuit of thinness soon becomes an objective in itself.

Patients usually come to medical attention not because of weight loss but because of complaints such as amenorrhea, edema, constipation, or abdominal pain. They may complain of specific "food allergies" and ask for aids in dieting such as diet pills or diuretics. Patients may also present as medical emergencies, since the complications of dieting or vomiting, such as dehydration and fluid and electrolyte imbalance, may be severe. The patient may be brought in by the parents, who become worried when weight loss is extreme or are alarmed by bizarre eating habits and personality changes.

The course of anorexia nervosa is variable. There may be a single episode with complete recovery, or multiple episodes spanning many years. A single episode may also be chronic and unremitting. Complete or partial recovery may occur spontaneously in some cases or may follow treatment. Both single episodes and fluctuating courses may progress to death.

Differential Diagnosis

Anorexia nervosa must be distinguished from weight loss due to medical illnesses such as neoplasms, tuberculosis, hypothalamic disease, and primary endocrinopathies (anterior pituitary insufficiency, Addison's disease, hyperthyroidism, and diabetes mellitus). These can generally be diagnosed on the basis of thorough histories, physical examinations, and laboratory studies. Patients with these medical illnesses do not present with the dread of fatness, unrelenting pursuit of thinness, and hyperactivity that characterize anorexia nervosa.

Weight loss frequently occurs in patients with depressive disorders or certain schizophrenic disorders characterized by peculiar eating habits prompted by delusions about food. Patients with other disorders also lack preoccupations with caloric intake, obsessions with body shape and size, and hyperactivity. Patients with somatization disorder may manifest weight fluctuations, vomiting, and peculiar food habits, but weight loss is usually not severe, and amenorrhea for longer than 3 months is unusual.

In order to establish the diagnosis of anorexia nervosa, patients should satisfy the *DSM-III-R* diagnostic criteria listed in Table 28–1.

Prognosis

There is marked variability in the prognosis for patients with anorexia nervosa. About 40% are completely recovered at follow-up, and 30% are improved; but 20% remain unimproved or severely impaired. The mortality rate for this disorder is as high as 22% in some studies, with suicide reported in 2–5% of chronic cases.

The presence of nonanorexic psychiatric impairments such as depression, anxiety, and agoraphobia is common at follow-up.

Table 28–1. *DSM-III-R* diagnostic criteria for anorexia nervosa.

A. Refusal to maintain body weight over a minimal normal weight for age and height, eg, weight loss leading to maintenance of body weight 15% below that expected; or failure to make expected weight gain during period of growth, leading to body weight 15% below that expected.
B. Intense fear of gaining weight or becoming fat, even though underweight.
C. Disturbance in the way in which one's body weight, size, or shape is experienced, eg, the person claims to "feel fat" even when emaciated, believes that one area of the body is "too fat" even when obviously underweight.
D. In females, absence of at least 3 consecutive menstrual cycles when otherwise expected to occur (primary or secondary amenorrhea). (A woman is considered to have amenorrhea if her periods occur only following hormone, eg, estrogen, administration.)

Indicators of a favorable prognosis include a good premorbid level of psychosocial adjustment, early age at onset, less extreme weight loss, and less denial of illness at presentation. Unfavorable prognostic factors include poor premorbid level of psychosocial adjustment, low socioeconomic status, extreme weight loss, greater denial of illness, and the presence of bulimia, vomiting, and laxative abuse. These indicators are all relative, since no single feature or set of factors can reliably predict the prognosis for any given individual.

Complete recovery in less than 2 years is unusual. The recovery rate is positively correlated with length of time at follow-up, ie, the more time that passes before follow-up, the greater the likelihood of finding recovery. Thus, clinicians will do well to remember the words of William Gull (1874), who described anorexia nervosa and wrote as follows: "As regards prognosis, none of these cases, however exhausted, are really hopeless while life exists."

Illustrative Case

A 17-year-old high school senior began dieting to improve her appearance. Although her family initially encouraged her, the parents became alarmed as her weight dropped precipitously and she became cachectic. She was obsessed with food and exercise, avoided friends, and for the first time her straight As became Cs and Ds. Her parents reported a change in personality from sweet and compliant to argumentative and stubborn. Although everyone told her she was too thin, she saw herself as grotesquely obese. She resented her family's pressure to gain weight and perceived them as being controlling and manipulative. She wanted to continue dieting and reported that her only concerns were that she was cold all the time, had trouble sleeping, could not concentrate well ("I feel in a fog"), and could not keep still.

Despite her protests, she seemed relieved when hospitalized on a psychiatric unit. A behavior modification protocol was implemented and she began to eat normally again. Her baseline personality returned as her weight goal was achieved.

In individual psychotherapy, she revealed that she was terrified about graduating from high school and leaving home to go to college. She felt she lacked the ability to take care of herself and did not have confidence that she could make friends or succeed academically away from home. She also worried that her parents, who seemed to fight all the time, would break up when she left home. She felt powerless and out of control of her life, with dieting being the only thing she felt competent to do.

Although apprehensive at first, the patient seemed most responsive to family therapy. She was pleased by her parents' resolve to work out their marital problems and reported that for the first time in years she could imagine liking herself.

Individual and family therapy continued for 1 year

after discharge, during which time the patient was able to maintain a normal weight. She elected to remain in therapy during her freshman year of college and continued to thrive.

Epidemiology

The prevalence of anorexia nervosa among women in the USA and western Europe is between 0.7% and 2.1% of the population (Hsu, 1990).

Etiology & Pathogenesis

A. Biological Factors: The number of hormonal changes in anorexia nervosa, as outlined above, suggest a hypothalamic-endocrine origin. However, the changes all appear to be secondary to the effects of starvation, weight loss, malnutrition, and stress, and no evidence of primary hypothalamic dysfunction has been adduced in any of the cases.

Although there is an increased risk for the disorder in biological siblings of patients with anorexia nervosa, twin and adoptive sibling studies have demonstrated no clear pattern of genetic transmission. Concordant and discordant identical twin pairs have been reported in approximately equal numbers. In addition, the fact that anorexia nervosa tends to occur chiefly in individuals of the upper and middle socioeconomic classes tends to refute an exclusive biological origin. However, because the physiological changes in anorexia nervosa (primary or secondary) definitely contribute to its pathogenesis, one must view the clinical features as resulting from interacting biological and psychological factors.

There is a high incidence of depression among relatives of patients with anorexia nervosa and among the patients themselves, as revealed during follow-up interviews. These findings have led some authors to postulate that anorexia nervosa may represent a variant of biologically based, genetically transmitted affective illness (Swift et al, 1986).

B. Psychosocial Factors: Because anorexia nervosa occurs predominantly in middle- and upper-class families, it is hypothesized that the disorder represents an exaggeration or caricature of class values emphasizing achievement and a thin, youthful appearance as primary virtues.

A number of psychological theories have been proposed to account for anorexia nervosa. Classical psychoanalysts have emphasized the avoidance of sexuality. They view self-starvation as a rejection of the wish to be pregnant and refusal of food as a behavioral response to fantasies of oral impregnation. Amenorrhea has been viewed as a symbolic manifestation of the wish to be pregnant. More recently, theorists have stressed impairment in the mother-child relationship as the primary cause. Such theorists view the characteristic struggle for autonomy as a manifestation of the failure to master conflicts associated with the process of separation and individuation. (See Chapter 4 for a discussion of these conflicts.) The cognitive and perceptual deficits associated with anorexia nervosa, such as the distortion of body image, may also arise from impairments in early childhood development. For example, repeated invalidation of a child's perceptions by overly intrusive parents who "know too well" what a child thinks, feels, and needs can result in development of a sense of personal mistrust characteristic of patients with this disorder.

In recent years, family systems theorists have argued that anorexia nervosa is the result of dysfunctional family interactions. The child who develops anorexia nervosa is seen as serving the function of maintaining the status quo, allowing the family to remain enmeshed, overinvolved, rigid, overprotective, and unable to handle conflicts openly. The child's illness may also provide the vehicle with which parents are able to seek fulfillment of their own unresolved dependency needs. (See Chapter 37 for a discussion of family dynamics.)

The abundance of theories reflects the multidimensional nature of this disorder. No single theory offers a satisfactory explanation of the origin of anorexia nervosa. Each has contributed a valuable perspective on treating this puzzling and life-threatening disorder.

Treatment

The initial goal of treatment is to counteract the effects of starvation by promoting weight gain and restoring normal nutritional balance. In mild cases, this may be accomplished on an outpatient basis; in moderate to severe cases, an initial period of hospitalization is usually required.

Weight gain may be accomplished by hyperalimentation or total parenteral nutrition. However, because of the risks of intravenous feedings, most programs utilize behavior modification protocols based on the principles of operant conditioning. While behavior modification may be effective in promoting initial weight gain, most outcome studies have concluded that behavior modification alone is not sufficient treatment. Lasting recovery occurs only when such methods are used in conjunction with psychotherapy that addresses the underlying psychological conflicts. Clinicians should also be advised that too rapid weight gain may cause dangerous gastric dilatation or precipitate congestive heart failure.

Drug therapy may be useful in at least some cases. Some clinicians have considered the perceptual and body image disturbances characteristic of anorexia nervosa to be manifestations of psychosis, and chlorpromazine and similar drugs have facilitated weight gain in some patients. However, it is not clear whether the benefits of such medications are due to their antipsychotic or their sedative effects. Antidepressants have also helped some patients, thus supporting the argument that a subgroup of patients with anorexia nervosa may have a primary affective illness. Cyproheptadine, an appetite stimulator and serotonin antagonist, has proved helpful in the treatment of a subgroup of anorexic patients with especially severe symptoms and a history of birth trauma.

Although psychoanalysis has not been generally effective in the treatment of anorexia nervosa, psychodynamically oriented psychotherapies that provide support to the patient and focus on issues relating to the struggle for autonomy and personal control are often successful. Family therapies, which view the symptoms of anorexia nervosa in the context of family structure and dysfunction, are also effective, especially in the treatment of children, teenagers, and adults still living at home.

In order to effectively treat anorexia nervosa, the biological, psychological, and behavioral changes must all be addressed. Effective treatment programs should not be welded to any single approach. Clinicians should be familiar with various methods of treatment and use them singly or in combination as called for.

BULIMIA

Bulimia is the episodic, uncontrolled binge eating of large quantities of food over a short period of time. It was originally described in the late 1950s as a pattern of behavior in some obese individuals. In the 1960s and early 1970s, it was recognized as a commonly associated feature of anorexia nervosa. Recently, it has been identified as a distinct disorder that occurs in persons of normal weight who are not obese and do not have anorexia nervosa.

Symptoms & Signs

The essential feature of bulimia is the episodic, uncontrolled gorging of large quantities of food in short periods of time. Patients are aware of their disordered eating habits and distinguish eating binges from simple overeating. They are usually unaware of hunger during binges and do not stop eating when satiated. They express fear about not being able to stop eating voluntarily and report that binges end only when nausea or abdominal pain becomes severe, when they are interrupted or fall asleep, or when they induce vomiting.

Binges are usually preceded by depressive moods in which the patient feels sad, lonely, empty, and isolated; or by anxiety states with overwhelming tension. These feelings are usually relieved during the binges, but afterward patients typically report a return of depressive mood with disparaging self-criticism and guilt feelings.

Binges usually occur in secret. They may last from a few minutes to several hours, typically less than 2 hours, with a median reported time of about 1 hour. Most binges are spontaneous, but some may be planned, especially as the disorder progresses to chronicity. The frequency of binges ranges from occasional (two or three times a month) to many times

a day. The quantity of food consumed varies but is always large. Bulimics report consumption of 3–27 times the recommended daily allowance for calories on binge days, and some claim to spend as much as $100 a day on binge foods. The food consumed is usually high in carbohydrates and of a texture that is easily swallowed. Patients often report eating the "junk foods" they ordinarily deny themselves but often eat whatever is available. Though high-carbohydrate foods are most commonly consumed, the nutritional content of binge foods varies. Although it is uncommon, some bulimics may eat huge quantities of vegetables, such as 7 lb of carrots at a single sitting.

Self-induced vomiting is very common but is not essential for the diagnosis. Some patients maintain normal weight by alternating binges with long periods of fasting, and many exercise excessively. Those who do vomit may use emetics such as ipecac syrup or induce vomiting by activating the gag reflex. Lesions on the back of the hand may be evidence of this. Many report that they no longer need chemical or mechanical stimulants to induce emesis, as they can simply vomit at will. Laxative abuse is commonly associated with bulimia, the use of diuretics is not unusual, and rumination may occur.

Patients with bulimia are usually self-conscious about their behavior and often go to great lengths to conceal it. They are very concerned about their physical appearance, and they fear becoming fat. Sexual adjustment may be disturbed, with behavior ranging from promiscuity to restricted sexual activity. A number of other symptoms related to poor impulse control are commonly associated with bulimia, such as alcoholism, drug abuse, stealing, self-mutilation, and suicidal gestures and attempts.

Most patients experience weight fluctuations, with weight typically ranging from slightly underweight to slightly overweight. Other symptoms associated with bulimia include edema of hands and feet, headache, sore throat, painless or painful swelling of parotid and salivary glands, erosion of tooth enamel and severe caries, feelings of fullness, abdominal pain, and lethargy and fatigue. Light-headedness, dizziness, syncope, and seizures may occur if vomiting is severe. Menstrual irregularities are common, but amenorrhea is usually not sustained.

Bulimia is usually not incapacitating except in extreme cases, where binge vomiting is a virtual full-time preoccupation. When vomiting is excessive, dehydration and electrolyte imbalances can occur and may result in medical emergencies. Deaths from gastric dilatation and rupture have been reported.

Natural History

Bulimia typically begins in adolescence or young adulthood in individuals consciously trying to stay slim. Some report a history of anorexia nervosa; others, of obesity. The onset often follows changes in living situations such as leaving home, starting college, changing jobs, or becoming involved in new relationships.

The course is usually chronic, and patients often engage in such behavior for years before seeking treatment. The chronicity of the illness may be punctuated by brief remissions in which the behavior is absent or the frequency and severity of the symptoms are reduced. Many report experiencing periods of relative improvement and other periods of worsening symptoms.

The natural history of bulimia may be affected in those who induce vomiting by the mechanism they use. Chemical emetics such as ipecac may cause death from poisoning, and in one case ingestion of baking soda led to metabolic coma.

Diuretic and laxative use may exacerbate the hypokalemic alkalosis caused by excessive vomiting.

Differential Diagnosis

The *DSM-III-R* diagnostic criteria for bulimia are listed in Table 28–2.

If the patient also satisfies the diagnostic criteria for schizophrenia or anorexia nervosa, that should be the diagnosis. Severe weight loss does not occur in bulimia, and amenorrhea is unusual.

In diagnosing bulimia, it is necessary to rule out neurological disease, such as epileptic-equivalent seizures, central nervous system tumors, Klüver-Bucy-like syndromes, and Kleine-Levin syndrome. Klüver-Bucy syndrome includes visual agnosia, compulsive licking and biting, exploration of objects by mouth, inability to ignore any stimulus, placidity, hypersexuality, and hyperphagia. This syndrome is very rare and unlikely to present a problem in differential diagnosis. Kleine-Levin syndrome occurs chiefly in males and is characterized by hyperphagia and periods of hypersomnia lasting 2–3 weeks.

Prognosis

The prognosis for bulimia is unknown, as there have been few controlled studies of this disorder, However, there are reports of a variety of successful treatment regimens, and clinicians report anecdotally that most of their patients with bulimia improve or recover completely. A number of deaths have oc-

curred from dehydration and electrolyte imbalances caused by excessive vomiting, but the incidence is not known. There is an obvious need for controlled treatment and outcome studies for this disorder.

Illustrative Case

A 20-year-old woman sought outpatient treatment for her binge eating and vomiting behavior. Her symptoms began at age 17 when she was a college freshman. Although very bright and attractive, she worried about whether men would like her. Her weight was normal for height and age, but she decided to lose a few pounds in the spring in order to "be prepared for bathing suit season." She went on a diet together with her roommate, who suggested vomiting after meals.

The patient reported binging three or four times a week, usually in the evening and always when alone. She usually felt depressed and anxious when the urge to binge became overwhelming. She typically binged on breads and sweets. It was not unusual for her to eat a half-gallon of ice-cream, a box of cookies, and a loaf of bread during a binge, which typically lasted about 30–45 minutes. She felt relief from her depression and anxiety during binges and reported sensations of warmth, safety, security, and unconditional acceptance. She ended the binges when her stomach ached, at which time she induced vomiting mechanically. After vomiting, she felt guilty and angry at herself for giving in to her impulses and being out of control.

The patient was 5 feet 6 inches tall. Her weight had fluctuated between 110 and 150 lb since the onset of her bulimia. Although she weighed 122 lb at the start of treatment, she reported wishing she weighed 15–20 lb less. She took large doses of laxatives daily and occasionally used diuretics. She had taken amphetamines in the past and was worried about her increasing dependence on alcohol. She complained of spending up to $60 on a single binge and reported stealing food from grocery stores.

She described self-hatred as a result of her behavior and told of superficially cutting her wrists on two occasions that she characterized as "semisuicide attempts."

The patient decided to seek treatment after reading an article about the medical dangers of bulimia. She had been too embarrassed to discuss her symptoms and felt she might be the only person in the world with such a bizarre disorder. She was surprised by the article, which reported a high incidence of the disorder.

She entered individual psychotherapy and attended a support group for women with bulimia. Her symptoms improved during the first 6 months of treatment, with the frequency of binges dropping to once a week. After a year of therapy, she improved even further, with binges occurring only occasionally. She decided to continue in therapy, not only to better understand her eating disorder but also to work on long-standing

---

Table 28–2. *DSM-III-R* diagnostic criteria for bulimia.

A. Recurrent episodes of binge eating (rapid consumption of a large amount of food in a discrete period of time).
B. A feeling of lack of control over eating behavior during the eating binges.
C. The person regularly engages in either self-induced vomiting, use of laxatives or diuretics, strict dieting or fasting, or vigorous exercise in order to prevent weight gain.
D. A minimum average of 2 binge eating episodes a week for at least 3 months.
E. Persistent overconcern with body shape and weight.

problems related to low self-esteem and difficulty in social relationships.

Epidemiology

The prevalence of bulimia is unknown, and the few rigorous epidemiological studies that have been attempted are complicated by the secretiveness and guilt associated with this syndrome, which may hamper accurate self-reporting. The syndrome is most common among adolescent girls and young women. However, 10% of reported cases are in men. Various surveys have reported the incidence of bulimia to range from 3% to 20% in college populations (Hsu, 1990). Although these figures vary greatly and include mild as well as severe cases, bulimia is becoming recognized as a common condition with an increasing incidence.

No familial pattern has yet been conclusively demonstrated in this disorder.

Etiology & Pathogenesis

The cause is not known. The episodic, uncontrolled nature of the eating behaviors has led some investigators to suggest that bulimia may be a variant of complex partial seizure disorder. However, the few electroencephalographic abnormalities reported in patients studied during the testing of this hypothesis did not correlate with treatment response to phenytoin.

Psychodynamic theories emphasize the symbolic nature of eating binges as representing gratification of sexual and aggressive wishes. Self-deprecation and self-induced vomiting following binges may thus represent guilt-induced self-punishment for fantasized transgressions.

Psychologists have also noted that the binge-vomiting cycle may represent a ritual acceptance and taking in followed by a rejection of symbolic love objects. Bulimia may thus represent an attempt to control the external environment. Patients with bulimia are noted to have low self-esteem, and the vomiting may represent a symbolic purging of bad aspects of the self. Patients with bulimia tend to have an overinvestment in body image and often have impaired object relationships that are recapitulated in their eating behaviors.

As with anorexia nervosa, cultural emphasis on thin, youthful appearance as a symbol of privileged social class may contribute to the increasing incidence of this disorder.

Treatment

There have been few treatment and outcome studies of bulimia, though many case reports have been published of successful treatment by individual and support-group therapies as well as with a variety of behavior modification techniques. The latter have included positive reinforcement, informational feedback, and progressive desensitization focusing on the thoughts and feelings prior to an episode of binge eating. There is a need for further clinical studies of this disorder.

Significant success has been reported with the use of antidepressants, including tricyclics, MAO inhibitors, and fluoxetine.

PICA & RUMINATION DISORDER OF INFANCY

Pica is the persistent ingestion of nonnutritive substances after the age of 18 months. It most frequently occurs with children but may occur in pregnant women also. It may be caused by poor nutrition, mineral deficiencies, or psychosocial deprivation. The condition is very responsive to nutritional and psychosocial intervention.

Rumination is a rare syndrome of infancy in which swallowed food is repeatedly returned to the mouth, pleasurably sucked on or rechewed, and then swallowed again. Rumination disorder is apparently caused by severe physical and emotional neglect, since it readily responds to substitution of caretakers. The behavior may be the deprived infant's attempt at self-stimulation. Rumination behavior has also recently been reported in adults in association with bulimia.

OBESITY

Simple obesity is not included among the eating disorders in *DSM-III-R*. However, when there is evidence that psychological factors play a substantial etiological role in a specific case, this may be documented by noting "psychological factors affecting physical condition" in the diagnosis.

Symptoms & Signs

Despite the absence of clear-cut psychological and behavioral profiles associated with the development of obesity, there is a subgroup of obese individuals who manifest emotionally based patterns of overeating. About 10% of obese individuals, usually women, display a night-eating syndrome characterized by anorexia in the morning and hyperphagia with insomnia during evenings. Such behavior is apparently precipitated by life stresses and tends to persist until the stresses are relieved. A smaller group of obese individuals (about 5%) are episodic binge eaters (see above). Such episodes tend to follow emotional stresses and may represent reactions to them.

Obese individuals with concomitant mental disorders may have severe disparagement of body image. They feel that their bodies are grotesque and that others view them with hostility and contempt. Such feelings may be reinforced by social attitudes, since fat people are often discriminated against and viewed by others as lazy, weak, self-destructive, and responsible for their condition. They also manifest low self-esteem and a negative self-concept. Ordinarily, obese persons with no coexisting mental disorder do not manifest disturbances of body image or self-concept.

Although many obese individuals tend to eat in response to emotional cues such as feelings of anxiety, fear, loneliness, boredom, and anger, so do many persons of normal weight. Obese individuals tend to chew less and eat more rapidly than other people, but both groups are strongly influenced by the eating behaviors of those around them.

Obese adults are usually physically less active than others, but this may be a consequence rather than a cause of obesity. Obese children are not less active than their normal-weight peers.

Dieting itself can be a significant biological and psychosocial stress factor. Dieting may cause feelings of frustration, agitation, irritability, and heightened emotional reactivity in otherwise normal persons. Thus, some of the emotional features traditionally attributed to obese persons may be a consequence of attempts to lose weight by dieting rather than a cause of their condition. In contrast, the jovial image projected by some obese individuals may be a psychological defense to gain acceptance by others.

Excess weight may cause low back pain, aggravation of osteoarthritis (particularly of the knees and ankles), and huge calluses on the feet and heels. Obesity may be associated with amenorrhea and other menstrual disturbances. The lower ratio of body surface area to body mass leads to impaired heat loss and increased sweating. Intertrigo in tissue folds, itching, and skin disorders are common. There is often mild to moderate swelling of hands and feet.

In massively obese persons, pressure of fatty tissue on the thorax combined with pressure of intra-abdominal fat on the diaphragm may reduce respiratory capacity and produce dyspnea on exertion. This condition may progress to the so-called pickwickian syndrome, characterized by hypoventilation with hypercapnia, hypoxia, and somnolence.

Obesity is associated with hypertension, hyperlipidemia, diabetes mellitus, carbohydrate intolerance, and renal and pulmonary disorders. Obese patients are at increased risk during surgery and anesthesia and in pregnancy. Obesity is also associated with increased risk of cardiovascular disease; however, it is not clear whether it is an independent risk factor or one resulting from associated hypertension, hyperlipidemia, and diabetes. It has also been suggested that certain health risks associated with obesity may be influenced by the pattern of distribution, as well as the total volume, of fat. Greater risks of cardiac disease, for example, may be associated with excessive accumulation of abdominal fat.

Natural History

Obesity can begin in childhood, adolescence, or adulthood. Amounts of body fat also increase with age even when weight remains constant. Obesity is usually a chronic and progressive condition.

Differential Diagnosis

By convention, obesity is defined as weight at least 20% above ideal weight listed in standard height and weight tables. Many investigators include measures of body fat, such as those taken with skin-fold calipers, in the diagnosis of obesity.

In assessing obesity, the clinician must rule out medical illnesses such as hypothyroidism.

Prognosis

The prognosis for losing excess weight and keeping it off is poor. In the late 1950s, it was reported that fewer than 5% of obese persons lose 40 lb or more, and even fewer maintain the loss. Although the prognosis for short-term weight loss has improved with the advent of new dieting and exercise strategies and the development of behavior modification programs, the long-term outlook remains poor. It is estimated that if an obese child does not achieve nearly normal weight by the end of adolescence, the odds against doing so later are 28:1. Morbidity and mortality rates for obese individuals are proportionate to the degree of obesity and the presence of associated risk factors such as hypertension and diabetes mellitus. Whereas mild obesity (overweight, but less than 30% above ideal weight) is not associated with an increased mortality rate, severe obesity (weight more than 50% above ideal weight) may increase the mortality risk by 90% compared to that of individuals of normal weight.

Epidemiology

Estimates of the prevalence of obesity among adults in the USA range from 15% to 50%. The prevalence increases with age up to age 50, at which point it falls sharply in accordance with the increased mortality rate. Obesity is more common in women, especially after age 50, because of the higher mortality rate among obese men after that age. It has been estimated that about 25% of children are significantly overweight.

Social and cultural factors play a major role in the prevalence of obesity. Obesity is more common among ethnic groups during their first generation in this country. Gradually improving socioeconomic status reduces the prevalence from 24% to 5% between the first and fourth generations.

In general, the prevalence of obesity is higher among people of lower socioeconomic status.

Ethnic and religious factors may also contribute to the development of obesity. A greater than 40% prevalence of obesity was found among Hungarian and Czech groups. Women with British or Italian ethnic backgrounds also tend to be overweight. Some studies have found a higher prevalence of obesity among Jews, followed by Roman Catholics and then Protestants.

Family studies of obesity show that 40% of adolescents studied at age 15 who had one obese parent were obese, while 80% of those with two obese parents were obese. This compares to only a 10% incidence of obesity among adolescents whose parents are of normal weight. Studies of monozygotic and dizygotic twins suggest genetic factors, but environmental influences are also present. Adoption studies have shown conflicting evidence for genetic transmission. Evidence for the heritability of somatotypes is stronger than for obesity. This fact may be significant in that even a moderate degree of ectomorphic body habitus may protect against the development of obesity.

Etiology

Although there is great variability in weight among humans, individuals show remarkable consistency over time. Humans who agreed to increase their weights 20–25% for experimental purposes generally returned to their starting weights when allowed to eat freely. Such observations have led to the theory that there is a biological set point for body weight in humans. This is supported by animal studies in which lesions of the ventromedial hypothalamus cause hypo- and hyperphagia, respectively. To the extent that the "set point theory" is applicable to humans, many obese individuals may be dieting in opposition to biological factors that make dieting far more difficult than for other people.

Weight gain can occur by an increase in either the number or the size of fat cells. The fat cells of adults with juvenile-onset obesity may be of about the same size as those of normal-weight persons, but there may be up to five times as many. Persons with adult-onset obesity may have a normal number of larger than normal fat cells. In studies in which fat cell number and size were determined, individuals tended to stop losing weight when fat cell size returned to normal. Since fat cells once formed do not disappear, fat cell number may determine the lower limit of weight for persons who by dieting have worked to reduce cell size to normal. There are two periods of cellular proliferation in normal-weight children: birth to 2 years of age and 10–14 years of age. In obese children, the period may extend well past 2 years of age, with consequent hypercellularity of fat tissue early in life. Although this may be partly under genetic control, the cellular theory of obesity thus has important implications regarding nutritional practices and weight regulation for children.

The gene governing triglyceride metabolism has recently been identified and coded. Anomalies in this gene may result in some cases of obesity. It should also be noted that there are multiple central nervous system and peripheral chemical regulators of appetite, eg, neuropeptides and gastrointestinal hormones (bombesin, cholecystokinin, somatostatin, and substance P), and the endogenous opioids (serotonin, norepinephrine, and dopamine). (See Morley and Levine, 1985.)

Early psychoanalytic theories of obesity held that obese individuals had unresolved dependency needs and were fixated at the oral level of psychosexual development. The symptoms of obesity were viewed as depressive equivalents, attempts to regain "lost" or frustrated nurturance and care. Recent studies have failed to demonstrate an increased incidence of psychopathological disorders in obese compared to normal weight individuals. However, a subgroup of juvenile onset obese subjects have gross disturbances in body image—ie, they view their bodies as hideous and loathsome and feel that others view them with contempt. They have a negative self-concept, are very self-conscious, and have impaired social functioning. Such experiences may contribute to the development and maintenance of obesity. Furthermore, since obese individuals are often discriminated against socially and are perhaps less often the object of sexual desire than normal-weight individuals, the maintenance of obesity may in some cases reflect an unconscious wish to remain isolated in order to avoid conflicts relating to sexuality or emotional intimacy.

Although there is no specific family constellation that predisposes to obesity, members of families lacking in warmth and love may use food and overeating as a "substitute for love." The mothers in such families are often lonely individuals whose own childhoods were marked by social, economic, or emotional deprivation. Such mothers may unconsciously wish to have fat children. Identification with their "well-fed, well-cared for" children may compensate for earlier deprivation. Such families may also equate physical size and the state of being "well fed" with physical and emotional strength. Obese children in such families may thus actually fear weight loss by concretely interpreting it as a loss of physical strength and emotional well-being.

The higher incidence of obesity among lower socioeconomic classes and certain ethnic groups is noted above. In some societies where food is scarce, obesity may be valued as a symbol of prosperity. In affluent countries such as the USA, value is instead placed on thinness, perhaps because foods low in calories but of high nutritional value are more expensive and unaffordable to the poor.

The definition of obesity may itself be culturally determined (Ritenbaugh, 1982). Since 1943, revisions in standard height and weight charts have steadily lowered the ideal weights for women. The ideal weight for an average 5 ft 4 in woman in 1943 was approximately 130 lb; in 1980 charts, it was under 120 lb. Ideal weights for men have also been lowered, though not as weights for men have also been lowered, though not as much, and in 1974 the ideal weight for an average 5 ft 10 in man was actually higher than the corresponding standard in 1943. These revisions have not been based on morbidity or mortality statistics but on measurements of the heights and weights of 25-year-old graduate students. Such standards do not take into account the fact that the percentage of body fat increases with age but instead reflect the fashion trends of the youthful, affluent college populations. For women, the steady decline in ideal weight reflects the upper-class emphasis on fashion model thinness as the standard of beauty. For men, there is greater acceptance of a wider variety of body types. Attractive men may be thin, eg, long-distance runners and basketball players; or bulky, eg, weight lifters and football players. This broader range of acceptability may account for the less consistent downward trend in ideal weights for men listed in standard charts.

If one accepts the 1980 standards for ideal weights and if obesity is defined as at least 20% above ideal, then the average American woman is by definition obese and the average American man is on the verge of obesity.

Treatment

Surgical procedures, such as intestinal bypass operations and gastric stapling, are effective in producing weight loss and in improving psychosocial functioning. These surgical procedures may also produce biological change, perhaps by lowering the body weight set point (Stunkard et al, 1986). However, risks of surgery and anesthesia, which are greater in obese individuals, plus the possibility of postoperative complications such as malabsorption syndromes following bypass procedures should limit the indications for these interventions to the treatment of massive and morbid obesity that has not responded to conservative management. Wiring the jaws shut to prevent the intake of solid food may help some individuals, especially when used in preparation for surgery. The use of intragastric balloons, a recently introduced noninvasive method of gastric restriction, appears promising but is still experimental.

Amphetamines were once widely prescribed as anorexigenic agents in the treatment of obesity. However, the high potential for abuse of amphetamines should preclude their use as diet aids. Furthermore, tolerance develops easily. Anorexigenic drugs with low abuse potential include diethylpropion, fenfluramine, and mazindol. Their effectiveness and side effects are comparable. The use of appetite suppressants alone is not currently recommended, since weight lost as a result of their use is usually rapidly regained. It can be argued that for these reasons, appetite suppressants that work directly on the central nervous system will always be problematic. Hope for the future probably lies with new drugs that regulate the peripheral conversion of food into fat.

Exercise regimens are recommended as part of most treatment plans. Exercise is helpful not only because of the increase in caloric expenditure but because physical activity (in otherwise sedentary individuals) is associated with decreased appetite and increased basal metabolism. This latter effect may offset the estimated 15–30% decrease in basal metabolic rate that occurs with caloric restriction and weight loss from dieting. Exercise also increases the proportion of weight loss from fat as opposed to lean body tissue. Exercise combined with low-calorie diets will result in weight loss; the difficulty, of course, is in motivating patients to comply with a disciplined regimen.

Support groups such as Overeaters Anonymous and Weight Watchers may be helpful in motivating some individuals to lose weight.

In recent years, behavior modification programs have been shown to be effective in reducing the high dropout rate associated with most weight reduction programs, especially when deposits of money are required and sums refunded with regular attendance or weight loss. Behavioral programs have been shown to be effective in the short run, but weight tends to be regained.

Although psychoanalysis and psychoanalytically oriented psychotherapy have not traditionally been regarded as being effective in the treatment of obesity, some studies (eg, Rand and Stunkard, 1983) suggest a more optimistic outlook. Of 84 men and women treated by 72 psychoanalysts, 72 had weight losses comparable to what was achieved by other methods even though only about 6% of obese persons who entered treatment did so because of their obesity. Analysts also reported dramatic improvements in body image perceptions in their patients. Whereas 40% of obese patients showed marked body image disturbances at the start of treatment, only 14% continued to have such problems at termination. This study suggests that psychoanalytic psychotherapy may be effective in some cases, especially for patients with disturbances of body image and self-concept.

SUMMARY

Abnormal eating behavior may arise as an attempt to calm and soothe unpleasant emotions, as an effort to resolve intrapsychic conflicts around aggression, sexuality, and interpersonal relationships; or to act out issues on behalf of a dysfunctional family. Biological factors may play a role by directly affecting the physiology of fat accumulation or indirectly by predisposing to affective disorders (anxiety and depression) commonly associated with eating disorders. Cultural factors such as society's preoccupation with youth and thinness also play a major role. Eating disorders clearly provide a clinical paradigm for the biopsychosocial model.

REFERENCES

Bemis KM: Current approaches to the etiology and treatment of anorexia nervosa. Psychol Bull 1978;85:593.

Boskind-Lodahl M, Sirlin J: The gorging-purging syndrome. Psychol Today (March) 1977;10:50.

Brotman AW, Rigotti N, Herzog DB: Medical complications of eating disorders: Outpatient evaluation and management. Compr Psychiatry 1985;26:258.

Bruch H: *The Golden Cage*. Open Books, 1978.

Bruch H: Perceptual and conceptual disturbances in anorexia nervosa. Psychosom Med 1962;24:187.

Gamer DM, Garfinkel PE: *Anorexia Nervosa: A Multidimensional Perspective*. Brunner/Mazel, 1982.

Gull WW: Anorexia nervosa Trans Clin Soc (Lond) 1874;7:22.

Halmi KA: Psychosomatic illness review: Anorexia nervosa and bulimia. Psychosomatics 1983;24:111.

Herzog DB, Copeland PM: Eating disorders. JAMA 1985;313:295.

Hsu LKG: Experimental aspects of bulimia nervosa: Implications for cognitive behavioral therapy. Behav Modif 1990;14:50.

Lacey EP: Broadening the perspective of pica: Literature review. Public Health Rep 1990;105:29.

Minuchin S, Rosman BL, Baker L: *Psychosomatic Families: Anorexia Nervosa in Context*. Harvard Univ Press, 1978.

Mitchell JE, Hoberman H, Pyle RL: An overview of the treatment of bulimia nervosa. Psychiatr Med 1989;7:293.

Morley JE, Levine AS: Appetite regulation: Modern concepts offering food for thought. Postgrad Med 1985;77:42.

Rand CSW, Stunkard AJ: Obesity and psychoanalysis: Treatment and four-year follow-up. Am J Psychiatry 1983; 140:1983.

Ritenbaugh C: Obesity as a culture-bound syndrome. Cult Med Psychiatry 1982;6:347.

Stunkard AJ, Stinnett JL, Smoller JW: Psychological and social aspects of the surgical treatment of obesity. Am J Psychiatry 1986;143:417.

Swift WJ, Andrews D, Barklarge NE: The relationship between affective disorder and eating disorders: A review of the literature. Am J Psychiatry 1986;143:290.

29

Factitious Disorders

Stuart J. Eisendrath, MD

The term "factitious" means "willfully produced." Factitious disorders are those in which the individual does something to produce the signs or symptoms of illness. The illness may be manifested chiefly by physical symptoms or chiefly by psychological ones. The goal of illness production is to receive medical, surgical, or psychiatric care, though there may also be secondary motivations such as obtaining drugs or financial assistance.

Formal attention to these disorders in this century began with Asher, who in 1951 coined the term **Munchausen's syndrome** to denote the disorder observed in patients who traveled widely in England, presenting at hospitals and surgeries with plausible but dramatic stories of medical illness that resulted in numerous hospitalizations and operations. As the clinical history and diagnosis became clarified in these patients, it was discovered that they had sought and received medical care for its own sake rather than to be cured. Asher noted that the patients told elaborate tales, often in a quite entertaining manner, and therefore named the syndrome after Baron von Munchausen, an 18th century German soldier and raconteur known for his tall tales.

Patients with Munchausen's syndrome have a history of repeated hospitalizations extending over years, so that they seem to have adopted the role of patient as a career. Reich and coworkers have found that these patients appear to represent a minority of those with factitious disorder with physical symptoms. Most patients do not have the Munchausen characteristics of sociopathy, imposture, peregrination, and marked resistance to treatment. They usually have intermittent and mild physical illness (eg, factitious dermatitis). They generally do not seek invasive interventions and often have stable family and work roles. Their episodes of illness usually occur in reaction to a specific stressor.

Some patients display factitious psychological symptoms in order to obtain psychiatric care. Others may display both physical and psychological factitious symptoms, either alternately or concurrently.

FACTITIOUS DISORDER WITH PHYSICAL SYMPTOMS

Symptoms & Signs (Table 29–1)

Any organ system will serve as a site of pain or other symptom for a patient with factitious illness, and histories compatible with virtually every known disease have been described by these patients. Laboratory abnormalities have also been produced, including anemia, hypokalemia, hematuria, hypoglycemia, coagulopathies, and hyperamylasuria. The choice of organ system is limited only by the patient's creativity and available resources. The means by which patients produce evidence of illness may be startling to the unsuspecting medical practitioner. One patient produced an elevated rectal temperature at will by alternately relaxing and contracting the anal sphincter to generate heat. Another patient would spit saliva into his urine sample so that the salivary amylase would elevate urinary amylase readings, thus producing spurious evidence of pancreatitis. Patients have injected insulin to produce hypoglycemia, and the spurious source was only detected by peptide studies.

A patient with Munchausen's syndrome may present to the emergency room with a classic history of myocardial infarction, bleeding ulcer, pulmonary embolism, etc. Upon admission, these patients are often loudly demanding of attention from the medical staff and may request high doses of narcotic analgesics. They are usually familiar with medical terms and procedures and may even suggest additional diagnostic tests to the attending physician. An important recurring symptom pattern is that these patients frequently request invasive diagnostic or therapeutic procedures. They often ask for surgery, saying, "I know that's the only thing that will help me."

Munchausen patients frequently travel from hospital to hospital, often over wide distances. Patients with Munchausen's syndrome represent a subset of the broader category of chronic factitious illness. Typical patients with chronic factitious illness do not travel unless forced to do so by rejection by a local hospital or physician. When traveling, these patients will often exhibit certain sociopathic characteristics such as lying without showing any feelings of guilt.

Table 29–1. *DSM-III-R* diagnostic criteria for chronic factitious illness with physical symptoms.

A. Intentional production or feigning of physical (but not psychologic) symptoms.

B. A psychologic need to assume the sick role, as evidenced by the absence of external incentives for the behavior, such as economic gain, better care, or physical well-being.

C. Does not occur exclusively during the course of another axis I disorder, such as schizophrenia.

They often take on the role of impostor, assuming the identity of a war hero, a lawyer, or even a doctor. They often let fall clues to the imposture, since part of what they are trying to achieve is to show how they have duped their admirers. When the imposture is discovered, they move on to repeat the pattern before a new group in a new hospital or city. Characteristically, these patients abuse narcotic analgesics and are strident in their demands for them. If the staff is reluctant to comply with their requests, they become angry and arrogant. If confronted with damaging documentation of their overuse of drugs or the possibility that their disease is factitious, these patients typically threaten litigation and leave the hospital against medical advice.

Detection of false illness is not usually difficult once the suspicion arises. A patient with bacterial abscesses has them only in areas accessible to self-inoculation. Unusual bacterial flora are noted on culture of the abscesses and indicate oral or fecal contamination. The major clue to detection lies in examination of the patient's background. In almost all cases, patients with factitious illness have worked in the health care field. When a patient with such a background presents with a chronic medical problem not fully explained by normal pathophysiological mechanisms, one should consider the possibility of factitious disease.

The psychiatric symptoms of these patients are quite varied. Normal individuals, given sufficient emotional distress, might resort to factitious disease as a coping mechanism. Patients with borderline personality who tend to act impulsively and have difficulty tolerating anger or depression may briefly decompensate into psychosis. Borderline patients tend to view everybody, including the staff on the medical-surgical floor, as either "good people" or "bad people" and may struggle to escape from or defeat the "bad ones." There is often controversy among the staff, with some taking the role of advocate for the patient and others acting with retaliatory anger.

Patients with factitious illness can produce illness at three levels. Certain individuals give only a **fictitious history** consistent with a known diagnosis without any supporting physical evidence. The second level of enactment involves the **simulation of signs of illness.** An example would be the individual who pricks a finger with a pin and squeezes a few drops of blood into a urine sample to give the appearance of hematuria and support a factitious history of renal stone. The most dangerous level of enactment involves those patients who actually produce **abnormal pathophysiological states.** Individuals in this category take anticoagulants, thyroid, or insulin or inject themselves with foreign substances.

Natural History

Since only a few patients with chronic factitious illness with physical symptoms have had the benefit

of careful psychological study, the natural history of the disorder is unclear. Most patients have a deprived early childhood, and many have had hospitalizations during the first 5 years of life for some medical problem. Children who stay home from school feigning illness are at risk for this disorder. Clinically significant factitious illness usually develops in the teen or early adult years.

Differential Diagnosis

Factitious disorder is an example of an abnormal illness-affirming behavior. Individuals with this behavior originate or amplify the idea that they are ill in order to achieve unconscious goals. Other examples of illness-affirming behaviors include hypochondriasis, somatization disorder, conversion disorders, somatoform pain disorders (psychalgia), and malingering. All of these must be included in the differential diagnosis of factitious disorder. The most important differential diagnostic problem is the true medical illness that is difficult to diagnose. The clinician must remember that even people with clear histories of factitious disorder do develop true medical or surgical disorders that must always be suitably investigated. Patients who perform self-destructive acts requiring medical care must also be distinguished. For example, the schizophrenic patient who performs some act of self-mutilation as part of a delusional psychosis certainly has produced the physical illness, but this differs from factitious disorders in that the goal of that individual's behavior was to act in accordance with the delusion (eg, to escape persecutory voices) and not to obtain medical care. Other behavior, such as persistent substance abuse or suicide attempts, also may cause the patient to receive medical attention. The primary goal, however, is usually not medical attention.

As shown in Table 29–2, in patients with hypochondriasis, somatization disorder, conversion disorders, and somatoform pain disorders, the production of illness-affirming symptoms or signs is entirely unconscious, as are the motivations of that behavior. These patients are not aware that they are exaggerating or focusing on normal bodily sensations. They are also unaware of the motivations for this behavior. An observer who is aware of the environmental situation might make psychodynamic inferences about the

Table 29–2. Differential diagnosis of factitious disorder.

	Illness Production	Motivation
Hypochondriasis, somatization disorder, conversion reaction, somatoform pain disorder	Unconscious	Unconscious
Factitious disorder	Conscious	Unconscious
Malingering	Conscious	Conscious

goal of such behavior. An example would be hysterical paralysis serving to avoid family conflict.

The malingerer, however, is aware of the conscious production of the signs or symptoms of a disease state, and the motive is known to the patient. For example, a soldier who claims illness in order to avoid an unpleasant duty assignment would be aware of why he was producing the signs or symptoms of illness. An outside observer would also be able to recognize the malingerer's motivation without needing to make a psychological formulation.

The patient with factitious illness is aware that he or she produces the illness but does not know why. This is analogous to the phobic patient who consciously avoids the feared object but cannot explain why. Motivation for feigning illness is entirely unconscious, and an observer would be unaware of a reason for the behavior without resorting to some psychological inference.

Prognosis

The prognosis for factitious disease with physical symptoms varies considerably. For the majority of patients without Munchausen's syndrome, there is good potential for successful psychiatric treatment. For patients with the syndrome, however, the prognosis is dismal, since they appear to have patienthood as a sole career. Their lack of social supports, wandering, and sociopathy contribute to the refractory nature of their condition. It appears that the intermittency of illness production rather than the level of illness production is the best predictor of response to psychiatric intervention.

Illustrative Case No. 1

A 30-year-old woman who worked as an x-ray technician was evaluated for skin lesions—superficial excoriations surrounded by normal skin, occurring over the inner thigh and pubic mound. A gynecological assessment for spotty bleeding revealed similar vaginal lesions. Her symptoms had developed a few weeks after she underwent a total abdominal hysterectomy and bilateral salpingo-oophorectomy for a ruptured ectopic pregnancy—her first attempt at childbearing.

The dermatologist used skin patching to determine that the lesions were factitious and referred the patient for psychiatric consultation. The psychiatrist learned from the patient and her husband that she had suffered significant depressive symptoms since her surgery. She noted that she "no longer felt like a whole woman" and had lost interest in sex. Her lesions were seen as an attempt to solve her problem by believing that "something's wrong down there." The vaginal bleeding was an attempt to produce a semblance of menstruation. She was referred for ongoing psychotherapy to help her deal with her sense of "lost womanhood."

Illustrative Case No. 2

A 30-year-old divorced registered nurse with a history of abdominal pain, nausea and vomiting, and hematemesis was admitted to a general hospital for evaluation. At the admissions desk she said, "I think I'll need surgery." She reported a 10-year history of peptic ulcer disease, for which she had been treated surgically. She had also had a cholecystectomy and several laparotomies for possible bowel obstruction. She described several episodes of septic shock for which no originating locus of infection had been found. She had several surgery scars on her abdomen and numerous cutdown sites on her arms and legs. There was a tenderness to deep palpation in the epigastric region but no rebound tenderness. Stool was negative for occult blood. Endoscopy revealed modest gastric imitation, presumably secondary to bile reflux. Since one of her physicians felt there was a strong psychosocial component to her pain complaints, psychiatric consultation was obtained. The patient was at first angry about the consultation but agreed to participate. She complained to the psychiatrist that pain precluded intercourse with her boyfriend. In fact, the current pain had begun just when the relationship had become a sexual one.

The family history disclosed that she had been reared by a cold, distant, and competitive mother who frequently criticized and humiliated her. The patient's father had raped her, according to her report, on two occasions when she was 12 and 13 years old. The patient felt guilty for perhaps having "unconsciously encouraged" her father's advances.

The consultant suggested psychotherapy and doubted that surgery would affect her pain complaints, since they seemed to serve an important psychological function in relieving sexual guilt. Surgery was performed, however, and she did well until 6 days postoperatively, when she went into septic shock. One day prior to that event, the patient's boyfriend had brought in a diamond engagement ring for her. No cause was discovered for the patient's sepsis. Blood cultures yielded multiple organisms. In reviewing her earlier history of septic episodes and in exploring the similarity between the current episode of sepsis and the patient's previously reported episodes, the psychiatrist gently explored the possibility that she had felt guilty about the engagement. After several sessions, she admitted she had injected urine intravenously because she felt guilty about her boyfriend being too nice to her. The patient was then referred for ongoing outpatient psychotherapy.

In psychotherapy, she revealed an extensive history of medical and surgical treatment for a variety of somatic complaints. She admitted that many of her symptoms were factitious but could not fully understand why she had committed the acts. Psychotherapy also revealed that the patient had numerous psychological conflicts relating to her sexuality. She longed for a close sexual relationship with a man but felt guilty whenever the opportunity arose. This was directly linked to her interactions with her father. Encouraging her surgeons to operate was seen as an unconscious attempt to re-create her sexual relationship with her father, with the pain associated with surgery being her punishment. The sepsis was seen as a way of reducing guilt over the relationship with her boyfriend. This function had been performed by her pain symptoms upon admission. The injection of urine intravenously appeared to symbolize sexual penetration as well as an immediate punishment.

This patient may have been able to enter psychotherapy because she had not been specifically confronted about her factitious disorder. Establishing rapport and making the interpretation that her engagement precipitated her septicemia allowed her to admit her actions and enter psychotherapy.

Epidemiology

Only a few studies have investigated the prevalence of factitious disease. Because of the nature of the disorder, factitious illness may be incorrectly diagnosed or not identified. The difficulty in identifying cases of factitious illness is even greater when the patient resorts to factitious symptoms rarely and intermittently. Factitious illness may also occur in patients who have documented organic illness, in which case diagnosis may be even more difficult. On the other hand, some individuals tend to be overreported in the medical literature as they go from hospital to hospital. Maur (1973) has reported one patient who had over 420 documented hospital admissions.

The best epidemiological studies have been described in patients with fever of unknown origin. In a study at the National Institutes of Health, over 9% of such patients were diagnosed as having factitious fevers. A similar study at Stanford indicated factitious fever in 3% of such patients. It appears likely that factitious disorders are more often seen at tertiary care centers where complex diagnostic problems are referred for evaluation.

This disorder appears to occur with equal frequency in men and women in some reports, but in several studies, females far outnumber males. In all studies, the health care field was the usual occupation of patients with factitious illness: nurses, ward clerks, physical therapists, x-ray technicians, and (less often) physicians. There are also a few reports of factitious disease occurring across generational boundaries; a mother of two children obtained the children's admissions by falsifying the results of the children's laboratory tests. Examples of "Munchausen's by proxy" have been reported more frequently in recent years.

Etiology & Pathogenesis

The psychodynamic origin of adult factitious disorders is believed to lie in early childhood experiences. Emotional and sometimes physical deprivation in childhood is a common feature of the developmental history. Early deprivation leads to a disturbance of self-image in these patients. Many authors have noted that patients with factitious disorders often have borderline personality characteristics. The borderline patient has a developmental difficulty during the separation-individuation (toddler) phase of childhood. When separation is not successfully achieved, the individual enters adult life with a poor self-image, feeling "needy" and dependent on others but expecting that needs will continue to be frustrated by authority figures.

The history often includes a period of hospitalization during early childhood when the patient's needs were met adequately by nurses and doctors who provided care and kindly ministrations. In other instances, a childhood hospitalization (and perhaps operation) was extremely frightening to a helpless and vulnerable toddler. Thus, childhood hospitalization may serve as a positive reinforcing experience or a major traumatic event. In still other instances, a patient's sense of vulnerability and helplessness is produced by the loss of a parent who was hospitalized.

The developmental history may uncover several major themes in a patient with factitious illness. The first involves the patient's sense of needing to be taken care of. The hospital provides a socially sanctioned way in which one can receive bodily ministrations and be an object of concern to symbolic parental figures, mainly doctors and nurses. Because of past experiences, however, the patient's desire to be taken care of is often accompanied by expectations of disappointment. Thus, these patients frequently present with a veneer of eager compliance over a hostile and wary underlying attitude.

Masochism is a second major theme. Anger over past deprivations often makes these individuals anxious and guilty. Such patients attempt to diminish guilt by being "punished" with invasive operations and diagnostic procedures. These painful interventions relieve guilt feelings while at the same time replaying early childhood experiences when the parents provided care as well as pain. Doctors and nurses thus represent parental figures of early childhood. Occasionally, these patients also develop positive feelings toward people in their lives, including their doctors and nurses. These positive feelings may have sexual features that cause just as much discomfort as their anger and hostility. Invasive and painful procedures may then serve to assuage feelings of guilt about positive responses as well as negative ones. Certain behaviors may then function as punishment for those feelings or as symbolic representation of the wishes involved with them. For example, a female patient who feels guilty about sexual arousal may invite a male physician to operate on her, an act that has both sexual and punitive symbolism.

A third major theme is mastery of an early trauma. Hospitalized children may feel extremely vulnerable. When repeating the experience as adults, they may not as children. This theme is often observable when patients appear to be unconcerned about their clinical status while physicians feverishly perform diagnostic workups.

The patient with factitious illness may also utilize disease as a way of mastering a relationship with a parental figure. The feigned illness may provide retaliatory gratification. In effect, a patient can win victory over authority figures by showing that they are unable to control the symptoms. In accomplishing this, the patient ignores the fact that the victory is a Pyrrhic one. It is the patient who pays the price of disability and illness.

Patients with factitious illness commonly allow their fabrications and actions to be discovered. They may leave a syringe on the bedside table or let other patients see them performing their deceptive actions. By allowing themselves to be discovered, the patients show their contempt for the staff while at the same time provoking the staff to anger. The staff's first reaction may be to feel duped and deceived. When the staff does react angrily by confronting or immediately discharging the patient, the patient feels successful in having proved mistreatment by parental figures.

Treatment

There is growing evidence that patients with factitious disorders are responsive to psychiatric interventions. Although Munchausen syndrome patients are generally considered untreatable, the vast majority of factitious disorder patients do not fall in this category.

Treatment should begin with a psychiatric consultation after the factitious disorder has been identified by the primary physician. The consultant must allow the staff to ventilate their anger at having been deceived and duped by these patients. Since the physician treats the patient on the implicit foundation of honesty, it is natural for the physician to feel tricked when the factitious origin of the complaints is discovered. The psychiatric consultant can help inform the staff about the psychopathological features of the patient's illness. This is important to keep the staff from acting out their anger. Operations and invasive diagnostic procedures should be avoided unless clearly indicated. If the staff does not act out of anger, the first step toward treating the patient has been accomplished—recognizing that the factitious behavior is a psychopathological symptom, not merely a hostile attack on the physician.

Two broad approaches are usually taken by psychiatric consultants in dealing with these patients. A standard approach has been to have the primary physician confront the patient with the factitious disorder diagnosis in a nonpunitive manner: "We know you have been producing this disorder and we realize that you must be in great distress to have used this way of getting help. We'd like you to have a more appropriate form of help from our psychiatrist." The

psychiatrist, who is often present during the confrontation, then tries to assist the patient as an ally rather than as a prosecutor.

More recently, because confrontational approaches often produced few results except humiliating the patient and driving him or her to another hospital, nonconfrontational techniques have been used with more success (Eisendrath, 1989). These techniques involve interpreting the patient's behavior and feelings as affecting their physical condition without specifically telling the patient that their condition has been diagnosed as factitious (see Illustrative Case No. 2). This often helps these patients feel better understood and may lead to their entering psychotherapy and eventually admitting to the factitious nature of the disorder on their own.

Factitious disorder patients can be referred for ongoing psychiatric management once the medical condition permits discharge. Most choose outpatient rather than inpatient psychiatric treatment. It is often quite helpful to involve the family, since valuable information can sometimes be obtained from them. The family may also be helpful in setting behavioral limits once the patient leaves the hospital. Occasionally, antidepressants and, more rarely, antipsychotics have been utilized with success in patient who show evidence of underlying depression or psychosis.

Management of factitious disorder patients requires a psychotherapist familiar with acting-out patients. These patients need substantial assistance in learning to talk about their feelings rather than acting out their distress. Therapy is aimed at increasing the patient's autonomy and self-esteem while diminishing the sense of helplessness, vulnerability, and anger.

Another nonconfrontational approach is to offer the patient a face-saving way to relinquish the factitious symptom. For example, one might tell the patient that unless the condition improves with a new medical treatment (eg, a trial of medication, a final surgical procedure, relaxation training, or biofeedback training) the physician's suspicion of factitious disorder will be confirmed. This strategy allows the patient the option of recovering without necessarily admitting that the disorder was factitious.

FACTITIOUS DISORDER WITH PSYCHOLOGICAL SYMPTOMS

Symptoms & Signs (Table 29–3)

Patients with factitious disorder with psychological symptoms often present with manifestations a lay person would regard as typical of psychiatric illness. Recently there have been reports of individuals presenting to Veterans Administration hospitals with factitious complaints of posttraumatic stress disorder. On investigation, many of these patients are discovered

Table 29–3. *DSM-III-R* diagnostic criteria for factitious disorder with psychologic symptoms.

A. Intentional production or feigning of psychologic (but not physical) symptoms.
B. A psychologic need to assume the sick role, as evidenced by the absence of external incentives for the behavior, such as economic gain, better care, or physical well-being.
C. Does not occur exclusively during the course of another axis I disorder, such as schizophrenia.

never to have been in combat, never in Viet Nam, and sometimes never even in the military. Rigorous review of medical records often reveals the diagnosis. Group therapy with true veterans of Viet Nam combat also often leads to identification of these factitious patients by the veterans.

Patients with factitious psychiatric disorders may have some familiarity with psychiatric entities and present to psychiatric hospitals with plausible histories. The motive is the wish to assume the psychiatric patient's role. The unconscious motivations are similar to those of the patient with chronic factitious illness and physical symptoms. Gelenberg (1977) has described such a case. One difference when psychological disorders are compared to physical ones is that verification of the diagnosis rests with the patient: Unless the patient admits falsifying the psychiatric history or there is conclusive psychological diagnostic testing (requiring the patient's cooperation), it may be impossible to prove that the patient does not have a psychiatric disease. With factitious physical disorders, there is usually some objective evidence that does not rely on the patient's cooperation. The patient who feigns psychiatric factitious disorder often has a true psychiatric disorder (eg, borderline personality disorder) but not the one being feigned. It also appears that some patients can present with both factitious psychological and factitious physical disorders at the same time or in alternating fashion.

Differential Diagnosis

The major differential diagnostic problem is malingering. Malingerers know their motivation, whereas the motivation for illness in patients with factitious disorder is unconscious and can only be arrived at by inference. Other differential diagnoses to be considered include brief reactive psychosis, schizophrenia, and organic psychosis. Occasionally, patients with borderline personality disorder may decompensate into psychosis for brief periods and may be difficult to differentiate from those with factitious disorder. The environmental context as well as an adequate history corroborated by family or friends usually clarifies the diagnosis.

Prognosis, Epidemiology, Etiology, & Treatment

Little is known about the incidence of factitious psychological disorders. In one study (Pope et al,

1982), 6.4% of patients admitted to a psychosis research ward were found to have factitious disorder. The causes, psychodynamics, and treatment are probably similar to those of patients with chronic factitious illnesses of a physical nature. Patients with factitious psychological disorder typically come from emotionally depriving families. They are a bit closer to treatment, since they have presented themselves in a psychiatric setting to begin with. The only completed outcome study, however, suggests that patients with factitious psychological disorders have a poorer prognosis than if they had a true major mental disorder. As Pope et al (1982) have concluded, "It appears that acting crazy may bode more ill than being crazy." All of their patients had recurrent hospitalizations and poor social functioning.

Illustrative Case

A 40-year-old man presented to a psychiatric emergency service at a general hospital, complaining of severe depression. He described severe early morning awakening, loss of appetite, marked weight loss, and suicidal ideation. He was admitted to the inpatient psychiatric unit, where he told his attending psychiatrist that he had had similar episodes of depression in the past (in a distant state) that had responded to antidepressants and inpatient psychiatric treatment. He claimed he had no living relatives, that his wife had recently died of breast cancer, and that her death had precipitated the current episode of depression.

By chance, a new psychiatrist on the unit recognized the patient from another hospital in a nearby city. The psychiatrist told the staff that the patient was well known for feigning psychiatric illness. When not being observed by psychiatric staff, the patient showed no signs of clinical depression. The patient was known to have several brothers and sisters and had never been married. Confronted with this information, the patient's apparent mood abruptly shifted from depression to defensive anger. He threatened litigation and signed out against medical advice. Since the patient was already receiving a disability pension, no apparent motivation for his behavior was determined during the hospitalization.

FACTITIOUS DISORDER WITH PHYSICAL & PSYCHOLOGICAL SYMPTOMS

Merrin et al (1986) have noted that some patients with factitious disorder display both physical and psychological symptoms, either alternately or concurrently. Most commonly, these patients initially feign a physical disorder; when this is discovered, they then feign psychiatric symptoms. For example, a 34-year-old man was admitted to a coronary care unit to rule out myocardial infarction. When it became clear that he had had numerous similarly negative evaluations, he immediately claimed he was depressed because his wife and children had been killed in an automobile accident. Family members revealed that he had never been married. The treatment strategy for these individuals usually consists mostly of psychotherapy.

SUMMARY

Factitious disorders comprise a fascinating variety of self-destructive human behavior. The physician should regard such behavior as a sign of intrapsychic distress probably stemming from trauma or deprivation during childhood and should not react with anger or punitive rejection.

REFERENCES

Aduan RP et al: Factitious fever and self-induced infection. Ann Intern Med 1979;90:230.

Asher R: Munchausen's syndrome. Lancet 1951;1:339.

Bursten B: On Munchausen's syndrome. Arch Gen Psychiatry 1965;13:261.

Eisendrath SJ: Factitious illness: A clarification. Psychosomatics 1984;119.

Eisendrath SJ: Factitious physical disorders: Treatment without confrontation. Psychosomatics 1989;30:383.

Gavin H: *Feigned and Factitious Diseases*. Churchill, 1843.

Gelenberg AJ: Munchausen's syndrome with a psychiatric presentation. Dis Nerv System 1977;38:378.

Maur KV et al: Munchausen's syndrome: A thirty-year history of peregrination par excellence. South Med J 1973;66:629.

Merrin EL et al: Dual factitious disorder. Gen Hosp Psychiatry 1986;8:246.

Pankratz L: Continued appearance of factitious posttraumatic stress disorder. (Letter.) Am J Psychiatry 1990; 137:165.

Perry JC, Klerman GL: Clinical features of the borderline personality disorder. Am J Psychiatry 1980;137:165.

Pope H, Jonas JM, Jones B: Factitious psychosis: Phenomenology, family history, and long-term outcome of nine patients. Am J Psychiatry 1982;139:1480.

Reich P, Gottfried LA: Factitious disorders in a teaching hospital. Ann Intern Med 1983;99:240.

Shafer N, Shafer R: Factitious diseases including Munchausen's syndrome. NY State J Med 1980;80:594.

Childhood Mental Disorders

30

Louis M. Flohr, MD, & Irving Philips, MD

The clinical manifestations and course of mental disorders of childhood and adolescence are varied. Many disorders discussed in the previous chapters first appear during childhood or adolescence and persist in adulthood. Other disorders are specific to childhood or adolescence; ie, they occur and resolve during this period. Because of the breadth of this field of study, it is not possible in a text such as this to review in detail each of the mental disorders suffered by children and teenagers. Therefore, a general approach to assessment is offered, and illustrative cases of disorders are presented with a review of essential features (symptoms, signs, and natural history). Comments on prognosis and treatment are made where appropriate. For disorders that also occur in adulthood (schizophrenic disorders, gender identity disorders, eating disorders), the reader is referred to other chapters for more detailed discussions.

THE DIAGNOSTIC PROCESS IN CHILD PSYCHIATRY

The evaluation of a child with emotional problems involves assessment of the child's family as well. As outlined in Table 30–1, a complete family history, including details of developmental, educational, emotional, and medical problems, should be elicited. The level of function is determined by psychological, neurological, and educational testing and by physical examination (see Chapters 11–13). Other special tests (eg, audiometry) may be indicated for children who exhibit speech and language problems or other defects in development.

Regardless of the duration of the diagnostic process—whether it be for a few visits or many—the clinician should try to establish a relationship with the child that fosters trust and self-expression. It is sometimes possible even in a time-limited relationship to judge the child's capacity for forming relationships and to determine what he or she is looking for in a relationship with an adult.

During the diagnostic process, the following questions are explored: What are the forces that shaped the child's and the family's development? How have they coped with problems in the past? What are the child's strengths? Where has development been blocked (eg, in learning, socialization, relationships with siblings or parents, self-image)? What can be done to facilitate the child's continuing development at an optimal pace?

Illustrative Case No. 1

A. Problem for Assessment: Young child with school phobia (separation anxiety disorder).

B. Description: A 5-year-old boy who had been having tantrums and a "runny nose" every morning for 3 days was brought by his mother to the pediatric clinic, where he was first examined by a medical student. The patient had no fever or other signs of acute illness. The following developmental history was obtained: The boy was adopted at birth; developmental landmarks were normal; and immunizations were kept up to date. The parents were divorced 18 months before, and the father remarried a year later. The young boy spent every other weekend at his father's home with the father's new wife and 6- and 8-year-old stepdaughters.

Table 30–1. Outline for assessment and management of childhood and adolescent mental disorders.

1. Identifying data (age, sex, source of referral, etc).
2. Chief complaint as indicated by the child, parents, and source of referral.
3. Patient's history and family history:
   a. Current and past emotional and educational problems.
   b. Current and past physical problems.
   c. Developmental milestones.
   d. Significant life events.
4. Assessment of the child (and family, if indicated):
   a. Physical examination.
   b. Mental status examination.
   c. Psychologic and educational testing.
   d. Other tests as indicated.
5. Assessment of other available data (medical and school records, etc).
6. Diagnosis and formulation of the problem (including provisional diagnosis and differential diagnosis).
7. Treatment plan.
8. Follow-up.

The patient had started nursery school at age 4 and was now in kindergarten. Two weeks before the clinic visit, he began to be fearful about going to school. For the past three mornings, he had had tantrums and refused to board the school bus. His mother wondered whether this sudden change in behavior could be caused by a brain tumor or other serious medical problem, although she also realized that her divorce and later romantic involvement with another man might have something to do with the problem. In any case, she wanted a speedy resolution because she needed to return to her morning part-time job.

Since no abnormal results were found on physical and neurological examination, the attending physician suggested (1) a telephone call to the kindergarten teacher; (2) one or more diagnostic playroom sessions with the child, allowing him to express his feelings through play; and (3) a meeting with both the father and the mother.

The findings were as follows: (1) The kindergarten teacher was puzzled by the change in her student and could not identify any reasons for it at school. (2) Although the patient left his mother reluctantly, in the playroom he became busily engaged in doll play. Among other things, he depicted a child being thrown out of the house and told, "This is not your house! Go find your own mommy!" (3) In the meeting with both parents, the father stated that his son's visits with him were viewed with some jealousy by his stepdaughters. When they discovered that the boy was adopted, they began to tease him about it, explaining to him that his "real mommy" gave him away. The parents agreed that the boy was probably worried that this would happen to him in subsequent visits. They decided to talk with him together several times at home and then report back to the clinic 2 weeks later. Upon their return visit, they related that their son was now satisfied that adoption meant he had a permanent home, and he was back in school again. He understood that his father moved out by his own free choice—not because of anything the child had done. Since the stepdaughters had been without a father for a long time and found it difficult not to tease their new brother when he visited, the parents decided to have him spend only one weekend a month at his father's home; during another weekend each month, the father would take him on an afternoon outing. At the 6-month follow-up visit, things were going fairly smoothly for the boy and his family.

C. Notes: This case demonstrates several points about childhood disorders and their assessment:

1. Primary-care health personnel are usually the first people to be asked for help by the distressed family. If they have adequate basic training in child development, primary-care physicians can often help families without referring them to specialists in child psychiatry.

2. When problems are clarified and family members begin actively communicating about them, reso-

lution is often a natural result. In the above case, no advice was given by the practitioners. A plan of action grew out of the involvement of both parents in an attempt to understand their situation. There is always danger in giving premature advice: The advice may be "wrong" if given without complete understanding of the circumstances, as so often happens in rushed practice settings; and even if the advice is "right," there is little chance it will be accepted by parents who feel they have not been fully heard. In this boy's case, the parents were able to work out a solution after they understood the problem.

3. Children do not realize that they need psychological help and thus do not ask for help directly. They usually present with a behavior problem (such as school phobia) that serves several purposes: It is momentarily adaptive because it helps them cope with immediate tensions (eg, staying home from school helped this boy control his fear of being locked out of the house), and it serves as a distress signal to alert adults to the problem.

4. In many cases, the child is not the only member of the family who needs help. The child's "cry for help" may in fact be an attempt to obtain help for or cope with problems of other members of the family—eg, serious strife between parents or problems of a severely depressed parent or a disturbed older sibling. In the above case, the pediatrician's questions also brought out the serious lack of fathering suffered by the two girls in the father's new family.

5. Diagnostic playroom sessions facilitate the child's self-expression of the problem. Although only one session was needed to get an idea of this boy's fears, three or four sessions (at intervals of a few days to a week) are often necessary. A playroom separate from the examining room provides a relaxing atmosphere for the young child. If a separate room is not available, however, the following toys can be kept in the examining room to encourage self-expression by the child: dolls, a doll-house with furniture, hand puppets, stuffed animals, toy guns, and crayons and paper. Children can tell remarkable stories in a brief time with this limited number of toys. For example, an 8-year-old depressed boy asked to draw a picture of "a family" produced a drawing of his father and mother with his younger sister between them; when asked where he was, he pointed to a small speck in the corner. **Note: It is better to ask a child to draw "a" family rather than "his or her" family, since children sometimes refuse to proceed when they feel confronted.** Children in playroom sessions should be told that they can play with all of the toys and say anything they want, but they cannot break objects or try to hurt themselves or the physician. Children with destructive impulses will test clinicians, sometimes repeatedly, to see if they mean what they say. Through their behavior, they are asking to be protected from these destructive impulses. The next case illustrates this point.

Illustrative Case No. 2

A. Problem for Assessment: Adolescent with physical concerns and emotional problems.

B. Description: A 15-year-old boy was in the 11th month of his 1-year probationary period for joyriding. As a condition of probation, he was regularly seeing a child psychiatrist. On this particular afternoon, he turned up at the pediatric clinic and asked to be examined for venereal disease. He wanted assurances that his visit would be kept confidential from his mother and psychiatrist. During his examination, he mentioned to the pediatrician that his probation would soon be over and then he could stop seeing his "shrink." As he said this, there was something in his voice that prompted the pediatrician to ask him, "And then what?" The adolescent replied, "Oh, I'll probably go back to the same gang and have some more fun." Thus alerted, the pediatrician asked more about the patient's life. He found out that he was living with his widowed mother and that his father had died 3 months before the joyriding incident. His psychiatrist was currently on a 2-week vacation, and the patient appeared to be fearful of ending his therapy. The following conversation ensued. *Physician:* "Do you want to know what I think? My guess is that it's tough for you to tell your psychiatrist that seeing him is useful and that you feel funny about quitting." *Patient:* "Well, he's only seeing me because the judge made me go." *Physician:* "Is that what he told you, or is that your idea?" *Patient:* "My idea." *Physician:* "Why not ask him?" *Patient:* "Well, maybe."

The adolescent then hesitantly agreed to discuss his concerns about ending therapy with the psychiatrist; he was not ready to ask for his mother's help about anything. The conversation continued. *Physician:* "Before I examined you today, I agreed that your visit here would be confidential. But I think what we need is limited confidentiality. . . . I want your permission to call both your psychiatrist and your mother so I can recommend that you continue therapy even without being on probation. We don't have to tell them you came here because you were afraid you had VD." *Patient:* "That sounds OK to me."

C. Notes: Communication with adolescents requires sensitivity to their mixed sense of dependence and wish for independence. They may deny needing help, actively reject help, or seek help indirectly from their parents or other adults. Concerns about confidentiality are linked to their ideas of privacy and independence of thought and action. In this case, the pediatrician's unhurried manner and sensitivity allowed the adolescent boy, who had real doubts about his own effectiveness, to ask for backup help from a respected adult. By careful listening and questioning, the physician was also able to determine what the patient really wanted to remain confidential and what he wanted someone to communicate to his mother and psychia-

trist. The physician did not confront the patient ("You just want me to do your talking for you. Why don't you take the responsibility for yourself?") but instead proceeded on the assumption that the boy would not be indirectly asking for help if he could handle his predicament alone. Although the patient came for only a "medical" checkup, the pediatrician felt free to ask questions about other areas of the adolescent's life. Most patients expect physicians to ask questions (ie, they consider it to be an expression of professional concern rather than prying), and adolescents in particular rely on their physicians to help them discover or express their real concerns.

CHILDHOOD PSYCHOPATHOLOGY

Most of the mental disorders of childhood and adolescence are viewed by child psychiatrists from a developmental perspective. Certain disorders are thought to arise from unresolved psychological or family conflicts or unmastered tasks during specific stages in the process of growth and development, while others would result from the complex interplay of biological and environmental forces. Some disorders (eg, autism in infancy) result in lifelong impairment, while others may be characteristic only of a particular period (eg, identity crisis of adolescence). Chapter 4 reviews normal human development. A developmental perspective on psychopathology does not permit us to describe and categorize all of the mental disorders seen in children and adolescents. Thus, a broader classification system, employing both the descriptive criteria outlined in *DSM-III* (1980) and *DSM-III-R* (1987) and the developmental categories outlined by the Group for the Advancement of Psychiatry (GAP, 1974), is used in this section.

Examples of typical cases seen in medical and psychiatric office practice illustrate the essential features of specific disorders. For the sake of clarity of organization, these are presented approximately in order of increasing severity, following the outline proposed by GAP in *Psychopathological Disorders in Childhood.* Examples will include the *DSM-III-R* diagnostic classification.

ADAPTIVE RESPONSES

Adaptive responses are the temporary and moderate behavioral changes seen in normal children responding to the forms of stress associated with normal growth and development. A clinician evaluating a child's behavior should always consider whether the child is exhibiting age-appropriate adaptive responses to stress. If this is the case, treatment is rarely required. Examples of adaptive responses are the **tem-**

porary regressions of young children (eg, increased thumb-sucking at the time of weaning); the stranger anxiety of infants 6-12 months old (''8-month anxiety'' was once a popular term); the separation anxiety of the toddler; the ''normal phobias'' of preschool children; the compulsive ritualistic behaviors of school-age children learning to work by rules and attempting to master earlier anxieties; and the identity crisis of adolescence, well within the reach of our adult recollections. Since adaptive responses are not considered disorders, there are no *DSM-III* classifications. Disconcerted parents of children with such problems usually respond well to an educational approach based on adequate assessment of the child's behavior in relation to his or her stage of development.

REACTIVE DISORDERS

Reactive disorders in children or adolescents are characterized by significant changes in mood or behavior or by the presence of physical symptoms and signs that occur in response to external stress. Although children may be consciously aware of both the distress and the external event causing it, their ability to express awareness is limited by their stage of cognitive development. *DSM-III* does not use the term ''reactive disorders,'' but several disorders described in *DSM-III* as ''adjustment disorders'' fall into this category, as shown in the cases that follow.

Illustrative Case No. 3
A. Diagnosis:
1. GAP– Reactive depression with psychophysiological concomitants.
2. *DMS-III-R*–Axis I, adjustment disorder with depressed mood; functional encopresis. Axis III, insulin-dependent diabetes mellitus.
B. Description: A 7-year-old boy had been aware of his parents' deteriorating marriage for about a year when he was told they were planning a divorce. Within a week, he had to be hospitalized to regain control of his insulin-dependent diabetes mellitus. While in the hospital, the boy began to show changes in mood and behavior. He cried and asked for his father at night, and he began to soil himself regularly, despite having been fully toilet trained since age 3 years. Because the encopresis continued, his parents consulted a child psychiatrist.
C. Notes: This boy's depression was manifested in multiple ways: (1) a psychophysiological reaction, ie, the diabetes was exacerbated by emotional stress; (2) adjustment problems with depressive mood changes (see Chapter 25); and (3) regressive soiling. *DSM-III-R* diagnostic criteria for functional encopresis are set forth in Table 30–2.

Table 30–2. *DSM-III-R* diagnostic criteria for functional encopresis.

A. Repeated passage of feces into places not appropriate for that purpose (eg, clothing, floor), whether voluntary or involuntary. (The disorder may be overflow incontinence secondary to functional fecal retention.)
B. At least one such event a month for at least 6 months.
C. Chronologic and mental age of at least 4 years.
D. Not due to a physical disorder, such as aganglionic megacolon.

DEVELOPMENTAL DEVIATIONS

This category includes lags, unevenness, and precocities in development—ie, the degree of maturation is not what is expected for a given age or stage of development. Developmental deviations are not necessarily of a fixed nature. They may resolve with the passage of time or be corrected with help from parents or others. The psychological reaction of the child and others to the deviation may also influence the degree of impairment, as shown in some of the cases below. Sometimes the developmental deviation represents the premonitory stage of a specific long-term disorder that can be differentiated only on follow-up. Biological factors are thought to contribute to many developmental deviations, particularly the specific developmental disorders listed in Table 30–3.

Illustrative Case No. 4
A. Diagnosis:
1. GAP–Delayed mastery of separation from the mother.
2. *DMS-III-R*–Axis I, separation anxiety disorder.
B. Description: A 6-year-old boy in the first grade began to whine and cling to his mother in the mornings before school. This behavior increased, and eventually he cried bitterly every morning and begged to be allowed to stay home from school. Since his mother had no close friends and was ambivalent about sending him off for an entire school day, the behavior was reinforced. The father, who had to leave home

Table 30–3. *DSM-III-R* list of the specific developmental disorders (coded on axis II).

Academic skills disorders:
 Developmental arithmetic disorder
 Developmental expressive writing disorder
 Developmental reading disorder
Language and speech disorders:
 Developmental articulation disorder
 Developmental expressive language disorder
 Developmental receptive language disorder
 Cluttering
 Stuttering
Motor skills disorder:
 Developmental coordination disorder
Specific developmental disorder not otherwise specified
Developmental disorder not otherwise specified

Table 30–4. *DSM-III-R* diagnostic criteria for separation anxiety disorder.

A. Excessive anxiety concerning separation from those to whom the child is attached, as evidenced by at least 3 of the following:
   (1) Unrealistic and persistent worry about possible harm befalling major attachment figures or fear that they will leave and not return.
   (2) Unrealistic and persistent worry that an untoward calamitous event will separate the child from a major attachment figure, eg, the child will be lost, kidnapped, killed, or be the victim of an accident.
   (3) Persistent reluctance or refusal to go to school in order to stay with major attachment figures or at home.
   (4) Persistent reluctance or refusal to go to sleep without being near a major attachment figure or to go to sleep away from home.
   (5) Persistent avoidance of being alone, including "clinging" to and "shadowing" major attachment figures.
   (6) Repeated nightmares involving the theme of separation.
   (7) Complaints of physical symptoms, eg, headaches, stomachaches, nausea, or vomiting, on many school days or on other occasions when anticipating separation from major attachment figures.
   (8) Recurrent signs or complaints of excessive distress in anticipation of separation from home or major attachment figures, eg, temper tantrums or crying, pleading with parents not to leave.
   (9) Recurrent signs or complaints of excessive distress when separated from home or major attachment figures, eg, wants to return home, needs to call parents when they are absent or when child is away from home.
B. Duration of disturbance of at least 2 weeks.
C. Onset before the age of 18.
D. Does not occur exclusively during the course of a pervasive developmental disorder, schizophrenia, or any other psychotic disorder.

---

early each morning for work, was unable to help his wife see the child off to school.

C. Notes: *DSM-III-R* diagnostic criteria for separation anxiety disorder are outlined in Table 30–4.

Illustrative Case No. 5

A. Diagnosis:
1. **GAP**–Delayed toilet training.
2. **DMS-III-R**–Axis I, functional enuresis.

B. Description: A 6-year-old boy was brought to the clinic by his mother when the first-grade teacher urged her to find help for his lack of bladder control, which was making him an outcast in his class. The mother was only mildly disturbed by her son's primary enuresis, since her brother also had had occasional episodes of wetting until he was 8 years old.

C. Notes: See Table 30–5 for *DSM-III-R* criteria for functional enuresis.

PSYCHONEUROTIC DISORDERS

Psychoneurotic disorders are thought to originate from unconscious conflicts over the handling of sexual and aggressive impulses. Although these conflicts are removed from awareness by repression, they remain active and unresolved. This aspect of psychoneurotic disorders distinguishes them from reactive disorders, in which children consciously experience a conflict between the environment and their own needs. Widespread personality disorganization is not seen in psychoneurotic disorders, although the symptoms can be dramatic, cause serious inconvenience, or markedly interfere with functioning. The patient usually functions adequately in other areas of life and finds the symptoms troublesome (''ego-dystonic''). Illustrative adult case examples are presented in Chapters 23 and 24.

AFFECTIVE DISORDERS

DSM-III-R indicates that the mood (affective) disorders of childhood and adolescence have the same essential features as affective disorders in adults (see Chapter 22). For major depressive episode and dysthymia the *DSM-III-R* criteria include age-specific associated features found in children and adolescents. The predominant feature (presenting symptom) of depression in young children may be anxiety, while that in adolescents may be antisocial behavior. Suicidal ideation or suicidal behavior may be noted. The description of manic episode does not include age-specific associated features in children (reflecting the extremely low frequency of that diagnosis in childhood), but the diagnosis can be used for children, of course, when it applies. Treatment of affective disorders usually includes psychotherapy and drug therapy—antidepressant medications for depression and lithium carbonate or antipsychotics for mania (see Chapter 32).

Illustrative Case No. 6

A. *DMS-III-R* **Classification:** Axis I, major depression, single episode.

B. Description: A 5-year-old girl's mother was admitted to a psychiatric hospital for the third time in less than a year. During the two previous hospitalizations, which lasted only 2–3 days, the mother's sister came to the home to care for the little girl. The third hospitalization was expected to last longer, so the girl was taken to the aunt's home. Beginning about a week after her mother's hospitalization, the girl became progressively more apathetic. She lost

Table 30–5. *DSM-III-R* diagnostic criteria for functional enuresis.

A. Repeated voiding of urine during the day or night into bed or clothes, whether involuntary or intentional.
B. At least 2 such events per month for children between the ages of 5 and 6 and at least one event per month for older children.
C. Chronologic age at least 5 and mental age at least 4.
D. Not due to a physical disorder, such as diabetes, urinary tract infection, or a seizure disorder.

---

her appetite and desire to play and would sit in a corner for long periods, holding her doll and ignoring her aunt and uncle when they tried to interest her in food or play. She also slept more than usual. After 2 weeks of such behavior, the aunt took the child to her regular pediatrician. He noted that she had lost 3 lb and suspected a diagnosis of depression. She was referred to a child psychiatrist, who confirmed the diagnosis and treated her for major depression.

C. Notes: *DSM-III-R* diagnostic criteria for major depressive episode are listed in Table 22–1.

Illustrative Case No. 7

A. *DMS-III-R* Classification: Axis I, major depression, single episode.

B. Description: A 15-year-old boy was brought to the hospital emergency room by his mother and a classmate. He and his classmate had made a suicide pact, and the patient had fulfilled his part by trying to hang himself, as the rope burn on his neck attested. His frightened friend cut the rope and called the boy's mother.

When interviewed alone, the patient said he had been preoccupied for over a year with fears of becoming a homosexual, and he felt that he was "losing the battle against it." His mother remembered having noticed changes in her son's mood starting about a year before, but she and her husband tried to ignore his bad moods and "concentrate on the positive" (ie, enjoy his brief periods of being in a better mood). Behavioral changes they noted included the son's tendency to watch television late into the night; his "sitting and staring at his books" but falling behind in school work; and angry outbursts toward his parents, usually when he felt he was being "slighted" and his sister "favored." Yet because he managed to get by both in school and at home, he was able to hide his despair from caring adults. Psychiatric evaluation revealed major depression and no formal thought disorder.

C. Notes: In this case, early symptoms of depression were overt, but their severity was not detected by the parents. Although suicidal intent was discussed by the boy with his peers, there was no overtly suicidal or self-destructive behavior prior to the hanging incident. This is in contrast to the potentially self-destructive actions frequently seen in "masked" depression of childhood and adolescence (see below).

Illustrative Case No. 8

A. Diagnosis: "Masked" depression.

B. Description: A teenage girl was about to be dismissed from the third school in the past 2 years. Unless closely supervised, she skipped school whenever possible, got into mischief with friends, and was considered a "chronic liar." This time she had set a small fire at school.

The history revealed that her mother had had pulmo-

nary edema during pregnancy and had developed acute renal failure while in labor for 72 hours. The girl had been delivered by emergency cesarean section, and her mother had suffered from chronic renal disease since that time. A kidney transplant had been rejected, and the mother's health continued to deteriorate while she was receiving hemodialysis. The responsibilities for child care were assumed by the father, who already had his hands full with his wife's medical care. The girl realized he was doing his best and frequently told him, "Don't blame my problems on Mom's illness."

By the time of the second interview, the school administrators had made their decision to expel the girl. She was then enrolled in a psychiatric day treatment program for adolescents, where she received individual, group, and milieu therapy in addition to a complete educational program. Her parents also began therapy. The mother was able to openly express feelings of sadness and anger, since this "weakness" could be attributed to her illness. However, the father and daughter had tried to be "strong" and had not openly expressed their feelings for 14 years, so it took them about 3 months in therapy before they could let down their guard enough to cry together. They eventually came to realize that expressions of sadness were not a sign of weakness. When the girl could admit to her feelings and express them openly, she no longer resorted to acting-out behavior. She continued outpatient therapy for another year "to make sure I don't skip anything important," and she kept the therapist's card for future reference "because I can't be sure how my mother's death will affect me."

C. Notes: While masked depression is not a diagnostic term recognized by GAP or *DSM-III*, it has clear utility in child psychiatry. Young people with masked depression protect themselves against the pain of their feelings by acting out in what sometimes appears to be a self-destructive or delinquent manner. This behavior is described as "pseudodelinquent" because it is secondary to depression and not part of an ingrained personality disturbance.

Illustrative Case No. 9

A. *DMS-III-R* Classification: Axis I, dysthymia.

B. Description: A 12-year-old boy was brought for evaluation by his mother, who was concerned about distinct changes in the boy's mood and behavior during the past 14 months. Until then, the boy had been easygoing and lovable and had gladly helped around the house. His attitude and behavior started to change about a month after his mother separated from her husband. He began by openly protesting and pleading against his parents' impending divorce. When he was unable to prevent the breakup, he became weepy for a few weeks and then turned surly and withdrawn. He was easily angered by his mother and was fearful and avoidant of his father, who was beginning to think that his wife was turning his son against him. Although the boy had been getting good grades, his school performance was deteriorating rapidly. During his first psychiatric interview, he admitted to fantasies of suicide.

C. Notes: Table 22–1 outlines *DSM-III-R* criteria for dysthymia.

SUICIDAL IDEATION & BEHAVIOR

Depressed children often express suicidal thoughts, either consciously (verbally) or unconsciously (on projective testing). Although suicidal thoughts are reported frequently, especially in hospitalized children, suicidal behavior in children under age 12 is extremely rare. It is more common after that age, and suicide is one of the major causes of death in adolescents. Suicidal gestures (superficial attempts) are made more frequently by girls than by boys, whereas true suicide attempts are made more frequently by boys. Although the majority of suicidal adolescents are depressed, only about 25% of them meet the *DSM-III* diagnostic criteria for depressive illness; thus, the diagnosis of masked depression is useful for this age group.

PSYCHOTIC DISORDERS & PERVASIVE DEVELOPMENTAL DISORDERS

The child and adolescent section of *DSM-III-R* does not include classifications for schizophrenic disorders or other psychotic disorders. The various terms used to describe these disorders in children (eg, atypical ego development, childhood schizophrenia, infantile autism, disintegrative psychoses) caused much debate in the past, and these disorders are now categorized by *DSM-III-R* as pervasive developmental disorders. Those few preadolescents and the larger number of adolescents who develop full-blown adult-like schizophrenic disorders (with hallucinations, delusions, or both) are diagnosed on the basis of *DSM-III-R* criteria for adults. Table 30–6 outlines the classification of developmental disorders (which include pervasive developmental disorders).

Psychotic disorders in individuals of all ages produce a widespread disorganization of the personality, with loss of reality testing and ego functions. When they occur in children, they result in pervasive deviations from the behavior expected for the child's age. Findings may include aloofness and inability to develop emotional relationships with others; preoccupation with inanimate objects; speech impairment, de-

Table 30–6. Classification of developmental disorders.

A. Mental retardation (see Fig 30–1).
B. Pervasive developmental disorders (see Table 30–7).
C. Specific developmental disorders (see Table 30–3).

lay, absence, or loss (depending on age at onset); disturbances in sensory perception; bizarre or stereotyped behavior and movement patterns; marked resistance to change in environment or routine; unpredictable temper outbursts; panic attacks; seeming absence of a sense of personal identity; and blunted, uneven, or fragmented intellectual development. In some cases, intellectual function is unimpaired, with the disorder confined to areas of personality function.

The following two sections describe and discuss psychotic disturbances at different levels of development.

1. AUTISTIC DISORDER

Extensive efforts to date at phenomenological description and involving neurophysiological, biochemical, and psychodynamic research have not yielded easily distinguishable subgroups of the severe chronic psychoses of childhood currently subsumed under the heading of Pervasive Developmental Disorders. The classification shown in Table 30–7 reflects the variety of severe deviations that affect all areas of development. It is an operational classification, using descriptive terminology of observable events that should facilitate future research into this group of catastrophic illnesses.

Although the full-blown picture of autism may not appear until 2½ or 3 years of age, a detailed developmental history usually reveals that characteristic signs developed during the first year of life, such as absence of social smiling at the parent, lack of anticipatory posture on being picked up, or lack of bodily molding when being held by the parent. The classic picture of infantile autism was first described by Leo Kanner in 1943 (see reference for Kanner, 1973).

Illustrative Case No. 10

A. *DMS-III-R* Classification: Axis I, autistic disorder, infantile onset (tentative diagnosis).

B. Description: A 2½-year-old boy who had never spoken a word or tried to communicate verbally was brought to the pediatric clinic for evaluation. The parents thought the child might be deaf, mute, or mentally retarded and were concerned about his eyesight as well.

During the examination, lack of eye contact with all adults was noted. The parents reported that the child was preoccupied with watching spinning objects and spent many hours watching his own hand movements in the air. His behavior in the examination room indicated that he could visually discriminate small objects, such as a piece of candy on a nearby table and the light switch on the far wall of the room. He ran to turn the switch on and off every time he could.

The developmental history and observation of this boy revealed that in addition to his muteness, he

Table 30–7. *DSM-III-R* diagnostic criteria for pervasive developmental disorders (coded on axis II).

Autistic disorder:
At least 8 of the following 16 items are present, these to include at least 2 items from A, one from B, and one from C.

Note: Consider a criterion to be met *only* if the behavior is abnormal for the person's developmental level.

A. Qualitative impairment in reciprocal social interaction as manifested by the following:
(The examples within parentheses are arranged so that those first mentioned are more likely to apply to younger or more handicapped, and the later ones to older, or less handicapped, persons with this disorder.)
  (1) Marked lack of awareness of the existence or feelings of others (eg, treats a person as if he or she were a piece of furniture; does not notice another person's distress; apparently has no concept of the need of others for privacy).
  (2) No or abnormal seeking of comfort at times of distress (eg, does not come for comfort even when ill, hurt, or tired; seeks comfort in a stereotyped way, eg, says "cheese, cheese, cheese" whenever hurt).
  (3) No or impaired imitation (eg, does not wave bye-bye: does not copy mother's domestic activities; mechanical imitation of others' actions out of context).
  (4) No or abnormal social play (eg, does not actively participate in simple games; prefers solitary play activities; involves other children in play only as "mechanical aids").
  (5) Gross impairment in ability to make peer friendships (eg, no interest in making peer friendships; despite interest in making friends, demonstrates lack of understanding of conventions of social interaction, for example, reads phone book to uninterested peer).
B. Qualitative impairment in verbal and nonverbal communication, and in imaginative activity, as manifested by the following:
(The numbered items are arranged so that those first listed are more likely to apply to younger or more handicapped, and the later ones to older or less handicapped, persons with this disorder.)
  (1) No mode of communication, such as communicative babbling, facial expression, gesture, mime, or spoken language.
  (2) Markedly abnormal nonverbal communication, as in the use of eye-to-eye gaze, facial expression, body posture, or gestures to initiate or modulate social interaction (eg, does not anticipate being held, stiffens when held, does not look at the person or smile when making a social approach, does not greet parents or visitors, has a fixed stare in social situations).
  (3) Absence of imaginative activity, such as playacting of adult roles, fantasy characters, or animals; lack of interest in stories about imaginary events.

(4) Marked abnormalities in the production of speech, including volume, pitch, stress, rate, rhythm, and intonation (eg, monotonous tone, questionlike melody, or high pitch).
(5) Marked abnormalities in the form or content of speech, including stereotyped and repetitive use of speech (eg, immediate echolalia or mechanical repetition of television commercial); use of "you" when "I" is meant (eg, using "You want cookie?" to mean "I want cookie"); idiosyncratic use of words or phrases (eg, "Go on green riding" to mean "I want to go on the swing"); or frequent irrelevant remarks (eg, starts talking about train schedules during a conversation about sports).
(6) Marked impairment in the ability to initiate or sustain a conversation with others, despite adequate speech (eg, indulging in lengthy monologs on one subject regardless of interjections from others).
C. Markedly restricted repertoire of activities and interests, as manifested by the following:
  (1) Stereotyped body movements, eg, hand-flicking or -twisting, spinning, head-banging, complex whole-body movements.
  (2) Persistent preoccupation with parts of objects (eg, sniffing or smelling objects, repetitive feeling of texture of materials, spinning wheels of toy cars) or attachment to unusual objects (eg, insists on carrying around a piece of string).
  (3) Marked distress over changes in trivial aspects of environment, eg, when a vase is moved from usual position.
  (4) Unreasonable insistence on following routines in precise detail, eg, insisting that exactly the same route always be followed when shopping.
  (5) Markedly restricted range of interests and a preoccupation with one narrow interest, eg, interested only in lining up objects, in amassing facts about meteorology, or in pretending to be a fantasy character.
D. Onset during infancy or childhood.
Specify:
  Infantile onset (before 36 months of age).
  Childhood onset (after 36 months of age).
  Age at onset unknown or not otherwise specified.
Pervasive developmental disorder not otherwise specified:
The category should be used when there is a qualitative impairment in the development of reciprocal social interaction and of verbal and nonverbal communication skills, but the criteria for Autistic Disorders, Schizophrenia, Schizotypal, or Schizoid Personality Disorders are not met. Some persons with this diagnosis will exhibit a markedly restricted repertoire of activities and interests, but others will not.

---

exhibited no communicative intent, unlike deaf or aphasic children who try to communicate with gestures or sounds. Inadequate development of attachment behavior (lack of social smiling and lack of preference for parents over strangers) also supported the diagnosis of primary autism. However, since deafness may coexist with autism, the boy was referred to a pediatric audiologist for evaluation. Several sessions with the audiologist were needed because of difficulty in gaining the boy's cooperation, but it eventually became clear that hearing was normal. He was

then referred to a child psychiatric clinic for further diagnostic work and treatment planning.

C. Notes: After a relative decline between 3 and 6 years of age, the incidence of childhood-onset pervasive developmental disorders increases in children over age 6, although they are seen in younger children also. Onset is preceded by normal development and may be gradual, with nonpsychotic symptoms (eg, phobias or obsessions) appearing first, followed by an increasingly psychotic picture. The definition excludes delusions, hallucinations, incoherence, and marked loosening of associations. Antipsychotic medications are of little value, except in the treatment of specific symptoms (eg, psychotic agitation) for circumscribed periods of time.

Illustrative Case No. 11
A. DMS-III-R Classification: Axis I, autistic disorder (childhood onset).

B. Description: The developmental history of a 7-year-old girl brought to the pediatric clinic for evaluation of behavior problems indicated nothing unusual until age 5. She was considered shy but bright. Between 5 and 5½ years of age, she changed remarkably. Her speech became monotonous; she acted self-centered and frightened; and she began to have episodes of head banging and violent tantrums when routines were not followed. Her toilet habits, which consisted of occasional loss of bowel control, changed to frequent soiling and long periods of withholding feces. Retention of feces eventually resulted in megacolon.

The girl was admitted to a child psychiatric ward, and her parents began psychotherapy simultaneously. Although therapeutic trials of three different antipsychotic medications resulted in no improvement in the girl, she responded to psychotherapy. By age 8, she was attending regular first grade in a public school. Her speech still retained a sing-song quality, and she still occasionally soiled herself but no longer withheld feces.

2. ADOLESCENT SCHIZOPHRENIC DISORDERS

Although schizophrenic disorders often begin in adolescence and persist in adulthood, many adolescent psychotic episodes are of brief duration and respond well to antipsychotic medications. DSM-III-R diagnostic criteria for child and adolescent schizophrenic disorders are the same as those for adults (see Chapter 20). Schizophrenic disorders appear with increasing frequency after 9 years of age.

PSYCHOPHYSIOLOGIC DISORDERS

Psychophysiologic disorders are characterized by disturbances of *involuntary* body functions. The disturbances are precipitated or exacerbated by environmental and psychologic stress and may be mild or severe, transient or chronic. Any organ system may be involved, as shown in the following examples of disorders that may be psychophysiologic: ulcers, ulcerative colitis, arthritis, skin diseases, growth retardation, headaches, eating disorders, stereotyped movement disorders, stuttering, functional enuresis or encopresis, sleepwalking disorder, and sleep terror disorder. The target organ or organ system involved is thought to be determined by genetic factors.

In *DSM-III*, the term "psychophysiologic disorders" is not used. For some cases, the axis I classification is "psychological factors affecting physical condition," and the axis III classification is the physical condition. In other cases, a more specific diagnosis (eg, sleepwalking disorder) is used.

Psychophysiologic disorders should not be confused with conversion disorders, in which a *voluntarily* controlled body part becomes dysfunctional as a result of some psychological state, eg, paralysis of one arm following a frightening murderous impulse (see Chapter 24).

Illustrative Case No. 12
A. DMS-III-R Classification: Axis I, adjustment disorder with depressed mood; Tourette's disorder. Axis II, developmental reading disorder.

B. Description: The mother of a girl with a 2-year history of behavioral and emotional problems had delayed taking her child for evaluation and treatment. By the time she decided to consult a child psychiatrist, the girl was 9 years old. The mother was worried about the child's problems but was preoccupied by an acrimonious property settlement controversy with her estranged husband. The mother indicated that her daughter had very few friends and received poor marks in school. She had recently been told that the girl had learning disabilities. When the psychiatrist asked about the girl's abnormal neck and facial movements (tics), the mother indicated that these had developed over a 2-year period, that the movements sometimes involved the entire body, and that they were occasionally accompanied by squeaks and grunts (vocal tics). The mother stated that the tics began about the time the marriage problems reached a peak. On further questioning, she also indicated that the tics had started a few months after the girl was sexually molested by a 12-year-old boy. During the interview, the child expressed her anger and sadness over the problems she was experiencing.

C. Notes: This case demonstrates the interaction of biomedical and psychosocial factors in the development of a childhood disorder. In most cases, Gilles de la Tourette's syndrome occurs without obvious psychological stressors. Symptoms may wax and wane, and the involuntary grunting and barking vocal tics may be accompanied by coprolalia (explosively uttered vulgar language). The motor and vocal tics may be embarrassing or even socially incapacitating. Some ability to voluntarily suppress the tics for minutes to hours is considered a diagnostic sign of the disorder, as is the observation that psychological and family changes result in remissions and exacerbations. Haloperidol frequently is effective in treating this unusual disorder.

Illustrative Case No. 13
A. DMS-III-R Classification: Axis I, sleepwalking disorder.

B. Description: A 12-year-old boy was taken to a pediatrician because he had experienced four episodes of walking in his sleep over the past 6 months. He was completely unaware of the first three episodes. In the fourth episode, he awakened to find himself sleeping on the floor of his younger brother's room; he became frightened because he had no idea how he got there. His mother said these episodes always occurred during the first 3 hours after the boy was in deep sleep.

C. Notes: See comments to the following case.

Illustrative Case No. 14

A. *DMS-III-R* Classification: Axis I, sleep terror disorder.

B. Description: About once a month or less often during the past year, an 8-year-old girl woke up her family by screaming during the night. When the parents came in, they would find their daughter deeply asleep yet in a state of panic and anxiety—sweating, breathing fast, eyes staring with dilated pupils (but not seeing her parents), and fingers picking at her pillow. She did not respond to their efforts to comfort her and seemed unable to physically escape from her terror.

C. Notes: Both sleepwalking disorder and sleep terror disorder arise during slow-wave sleep stages 3 and 4 rather than during rapid eye movement (REM) sleep (see Chapter 5). Sleepwalking appears to be a dissociative episode with amnesia, whereas sleep terror is more similar to a state of agitation in a delirious patient, with relative motor paralysis compared to the free movement of the sleepwalker. In both disorders, the electroencephalographic findings are normal, and the episode is not recalled as a dream or a nightmare. Treatment includes use of medications such as diazepam or antidepressants, which alter sleep stages 3 and 4.

DISRUPTIVE BEHAVIOR DISORDERS

This group of disorders includes oppositional defiant disorder (Table 30–8), conduct disorder (Table 30–9), and attention-deficit hyperactivity disorder (Table 30–10).

Illustrative Case No. 15

A. *DMS-III-R* Classification: Axis I, oppositional defiant disorder.

B. Description: An 8-year-old boy who was previously well-behaved "just went on a rampage," according to his mother. She explained that during the past 6 months, he refused to do his household chores, "talked back," and had tantrums when he did not get his way. The only explanation his mother could find was that after seriously considering marriage, she broke off a 2-year relationship with her boyfriend. Her attempts to talk with her son about this met with

Table 30–8. *DSM-III-R* diagnostic criteria for oppositional defiant disorder.

Note: Consider a criterion met only if the behavior is considerably more frequent than that of most people of the same mental age.

A. A disturbance of at least 6 months during which at least 5 of the following are present:
 (1) Often loses temper.
 (2) Often argues with adults.
 (3) Often actively defies or refuses adult requests or rules, eg, refuses to do chores at home.
 (4) Often deliberately does things that annoy other people, eg, grabs other children's hats.
 (5) Often blames others for his or her own mistakes.
 (6) Is often touchy or easily annoyed by others.
 (7) Is often angry and resentful.
 (8) Is often spiteful or vindictive.
 (9) Often swears or uses obscene language.
 Note: The above items are listed in descending order of discriminating power based on data from a national field trial of the *DSM-III-R* criteria for disruptive behavior disorders.
B. Does not meet the criteria for conduct disorder and does not occur exclusively during the course of a psychotic disorder, dysthymia, or a major depressive, hypomanic, or manic episode.

failure. ("No, Mom, that's dumb—I don't want to talk about it!")

C. Notes: Oppositional defiant disorder does not include breaking the rules of social interaction or infringement on the rights of others. Conduct disorders, by definition, do include such behavior (see below).

Illustrative Case No. 16

A. *DMS-III-R* Classification: Axis I, conduct disorder, socialized, nonaggressive.

B. Description: A 15-year-old girl was picked up by the police when she decided to "go into business for myself." She had been engaged in prostitution (and had a "manager") for over a year. She had run away from home several times but always returned. Although her mother was upset and worried about her daughter, she was afraid to ask authorities for help and thus allowed the daughter to come and go as she wished. The girl had several friendships that had continued since childhood, and she was considered a good-hearted and generous friend.

Illustrative Case No. 17

A. *DMS-III-R* Classification: Axis I, attention deficit hyperactivity disorder.

B. Description: A 5-year-old boy was referred to a pediatrician by his teacher during his second week in kindergarten because he was difficult to control and showed signs of impulsivity and inattention: (1) He moved quickly from one activity to another, acted impulsively and sometimes too aggressively, was unable to wait his turn in games or group discussions, and generally needed a great deal of supervision. (2) He was easily distracted and had difficulty

Table 30–9. *DSM-III-R* diagnostic criteria for conduct disorder.

A. A disturbance of conduct lasting at least 6 months, during which at least 3 of the following have been present:
   (1) Has stolen without confrontation of a victim on more than one occasion (including forgery).
   (2) Has run away from home overnight at least twice while living in parental or parental surrogate home (or once without returning).
   (3) Often lies (other than to avoid physical or sexual abuse).
   (4) Has deliberately engaged in fire-setting.
   (5) Is often truant from school (for older person, absent from work).
   (6) Has broken into someone else's house, building, or car.
   (7) Has deliberately destroyed others' property (other than by fire-setting).
   (8) Has been physically cruel to animals.
   (9) Has forced someone into sexual activity with him or her.
   (10) Has used a weapon in more than one fight.
   (11) Often initiates physical fights.
   (12) Has stolen with confrontation of a victim (eg, mugging, purse-snatching, extortion, armed robbery).
   (13) Has been physically cruel to people.
Note: The above items are listed in descending order of discriminating power based on data from a national field trial of the *DSM-III-R* criteria for disruptive behavior disorders.
B. If 18 or older does not meet criteria for antisocial personality disorder.
Solitary aggressive type:
The essential feature is the predominance of aggressive physical behavior, usually toward both adults and peers, initiated by the person (not as a group activity).
Group type:
The essential feature is the predominance of conduct problems occurring mainly as a group activity with peers. Aggressive physical behavior may or may not be present.
Undifferentiated type:
This a subtype for children or adolescents with conduct disorder with a mixture of clinical features that cannot be classified as either solitary aggressive type or group type.

listening to what was being said to him or staying with school tasks or play activities.

Although dismayed by her son's behavior in kindergarten, the mother said she expected such a problem, since he had also had problems in the several nursery schools he had attended. "He was even hyper before he was born," she explained. "Sometimes I thought he was doing somersaults in there. After he was born, his engine was always running; he even squirmed a lot in his sleep."

C. Notes: Attention deficit disorder may or may not be accompanied by hyperactivity. In the past, the disorder was often termed minimal brain damage, minimal brain dysfunction, hyperkinetic syndrome, etc. Impulsivity and inattention are hallmarks of attention deficit disorder. The boy in this case also had hyperactivity, as described by his mother.

In children with this disorder, the peak age for referral is 8–10 years. The disorder is most observable in situations that require self-application, as in the classroom, and thus the teacher is often the one to

recommend evaluation. The parents may disagree with the teacher's report, since they may have fewer opportunities to see their child in this context. The clinician s observations of the child in a playroom diagnostic setting often do not correspond with the teacher's observations either. Results of structured psychological and educational testing may support the diagnosis. Diagnosis is more difficult in children without hyperactivity. Those with hyperactivity usually have characteristic developmental histories.

Adolescents or adults who once satisfied the diagnostic criteria of attention deficit hyperactivity disorder but have outgrown their hyperactivity often retain the impulsivity and inattention, and their occupational or social functioning is adversely affected.

Treatment of attention deficit disorder in childhood includes family education about the disorder, drug therapy with methylphenidate or dextroamphetamine, psychotherapy, and remediation of coexisting learning disorders. Contrary to earlier beliefs and concerns, use of stimulants for attention deficit disorder is not associated with later drug abuse. However, it is still

Table 30–10. *DSM-III-R* diagnostic criteria for attention deficit hyperactivity disorder.

Note: Consider a criterion met only if the behavior is considerably more frequent than that of most people of the same mental age.
A. A disturbance of at least 6 months during which at least 8 of the following are present:
   (1) Often fidgets with hands or feet or squirms in seat (in adolescents, may be limited to subjective feelings or restlessness).
   (2) Has difficulty remaining seated when required to do so.
   (3) Is easily distracted by extraneous stimuli.
   (4) Has difficulty awaiting turn in games or group situations.
   (5) Often blurts out answers to questions before they have been completed.
   (6) Has difficulty following through on instructions from others (not due to oppositional behavior or failure of comprehension), eg, fails to finish chores.
   (7) Has difficulty sustaining attention in tasks or play activities.
   (8) Often shifts from one uncompleted activity to another.
   (9) Has difficulty playing quietly.
   (10) Often talks excessively.
   (11) Often interrupts or intrudes on others, eg, butts into other children's games.
   (12) Often does not seem to listen to what is being said to him or her.
   (13) Often loses things necessary for tasks or activities at school or at home (eg, toys, pencils, books, assignments).
   (14) Often engages in physically dangerous activities without considering possible consequences (not for the purpose of thrill-seeking), eg, runs into street without looking.
Note: The above items are listed in descending order of discriminating power based on data from a national field trial of the *DSM-III-R* criteria for disruptive behavior disorders.
B. Onset before the age of 7.
C. Does not meet the criteria for a pervasive developmental disorder.

important to warn patients and their families of the side effects of stimulants and to institute periodic "drug holidays." Adolescents and adults who have "outgrown" their hyperactivity tend to retain attention deficit disorders and thus frequently benefit from the ongoing use of stimulant medication.

OTHER DISORDERS ORIGINATING IN CHILDHOOD

Illustrative Case No. 18

A. DMS-III-R Classification: Axis I, reactive attachment disorder of infancy.

B. Description: A 6-month-old boy was brought to the pediatric clinic by his grandmother. She was visiting from out of town and was shocked to find her grandson so scrawny, apathetic, and unresponsive. The history was reviewed and the neglected infant immediately hospitalized for diagnostic studies, including observing the effect of adequate care and nutrition. The admitting diagnosis was failure to thrive. Results of physical and laboratory examinations were normal except for low weight, mild anemia, and apathy.

A social worker who visited the boy's home found his mother depressed, ineffectual, and terrorized by her alcoholic husband. The mother explained that she had her hands full with her two older children and with the two or three other children she "took in" for baby-sitting. She thought her son was too skinny because he was not a "big eater," but she indicated that he was a good baby.

Within days after admission to the hospital, the boy began to brighten up and to smile and look at people. His weight soon returned to normal, and he became a playful and assertive infant within a month. His mother found little time to visit him and said she was considering putting him up for adoption.

C. Notes: Diagnostic criteria for reactive attachment disorder are shown in Table 30–11. Although infants with this disorder are considered physically and emotionally starved, their longitudinal growth remains normal. After infancy, children with psychological and family problems may fall behind their previous rate of growth in both height and weight. Some children with short stature also have abnormally low levels of growth hormone, apparently caused by significant emotional pressures. This disorder in childhood, called **psychosocial dwarfism,** is not listed in *DSM-III;* although mentioned in this section, psychosocial dwarfism could also be classified as a psychophysiological disorder. Children with this disorder resume their normal rate of growth (and their growth hormone levels normalize) when the psychosocial causes of growth delay are corrected.

Table 30–11. *DSM-III-R* diagnostic criteria for reactive attachment disorder.

A. Markedly disturbed social relatedness in most contexts, beginning before the age of 5, as evidenced by either (1) or (2):
  (1) Persistent failure to initiate or respond to most social interactions (eg, in infants, absence of visual tracking and reciprocal play, lack of vocal imitation or playfulness, apathy, little or no spontaneity; at later ages, lack of or little curiosity and social interest).
  (2) Indiscriminate sociability, eg, excessive familiarity with relative strangers by making requests and displaying affection.
B. The disturbance in A is not a symptom of either mental retardation or a pervasive developmental disorder, such as autistic disorder.
C. Grossly pathogenic care, as evidenced by at least one of the following:
  (1) Persistent disregard of the child's basic emotional needs for comfort, stimulation, and affection. *Examples:* Overly harsh punishment by caregiver; consistent neglect by caregiver.
  (2) Persistent disregard of the child's basic physical needs, including nutrition, adequate housing, and protection from physical danger and assault (including sexual abuse).
  (3) Repeated change of primary caregiver so that stable attachments are not possible, eg, frequent changes in foster parents.
D. There is a presumption that the care described in C is responsible for the disturbed behavior in A; this presumption is warranted if the disturbance in A began following the pathogenic care in C.
Note: If failure to thrive is present, code it on Axis III.

CHILD MALTREATMENT

The spectrum of maltreatment of children ranges from nonorganic failure to thrive through child neglect to emotional, physical, and sexual abuse. Families at high risk for childhood mental disorders also are at greater risk for child maltreatment. In 1981, the National Center on Child Abuse and Neglect documented a physical abuse rate of 3.4 cases per 1000 children per year, an emotional abuse rate of 2.2 per 1000, and a sexual abuse rate of 0.7 per 1000. The incidence of educational neglect was 2.9 per 1000; of physical neglect, 1.7 per 1000; and of emotional neglect, 1 per 1000. These are underestimates, since some diagnoses are inevitably missed and many cases go unreported—especially cases of emotional abuse and neglect and educational neglect.

Even when there is a clear history, child protective services with limited budgets are able to intervene only in the worst cases of physical or sexual abuse. And even when help for the child is provided after abuse has occurred, it is usually too late then to prevent continuing negative interactions in the family and further abuse in the future.

1. NONORGANIC FAILURE TO THRIVE

Nonorganic failure to thrive is called "reactive attachment disorder of infancy" in *DSM-III-R.* (See

Illustrative Case No. 18.) After exclusion of organic causes of height and weight retardation below the third percentile (head circumference is usually normal), the diagnosis is based on the family history and on observation of the child-parent relationship. Studies demonstrate a variety of maladaptive mother-child interactions—in most cases impaired mothering due to chronic depression, drug dependence, and poor day-to-day functioning. Fathers in these studies were often described as ineffectual with respect to the mother-child relationship.

The outcomes of hospitalization of infants with a diagnosis of nonorganic failure to thrive have been studied by Rutter (1985). The best results (ie, resumption of normal growth) are reported for infants whose mothers suffer from acute depression; 40% of infants with mothers suffering from chronic depression or chronic medical illnesses lost weight after discharge; and infants whose mothers were described as "extremely angry and hostile" had the worst outcomes. Long-term follow-up shows concordance between nonorganic failure to thrive and later child abuse and neglect, with 42% of children falling below the third percentile in height or weight.

Family involvement in treatment, or foster placement as needed, offers the best hope for a favorable long-term outcome.

2. CHILD NEGLECT

Inadequate or negligent parenting, which is to some extent culturally defined, implies indifference to a child's physical safety and well-being, schooling, or medical care, with concomitant emotional deprivation of the child. Even though about half of neglectful families studied live under conditions of poverty, one cannot equate low socioeconomic status with physical or emotional neglect, since most poor parents are properly attentive to their children's needs (Rutter, 1985). Neglectful parenting should be suspected when the mother or father of an emotionally disturbed child refuses to recognize that a problem exists or fails to seek help or take appropriate action to find a remedy. Many neglectful parents themselves grew up as deprived children, so that they never developed good judgment about the emotional needs of children,

Physical and emotional illnesses and drug and alcohol abuse are risk factors for child neglect.

3. PHYSICAL ABUSE

Ten percent of emergency room visits by children under 5 years of age are occasioned by physical abuse. The number of such incidents reported annually in the USA rose from 7000 in 1967 to over 200,000 in 1979 (Rudolph, 1982). The fatality rate resulting from physical abuse is variously estimated to be 5–

25%; the average age at death is under 3 years; and the duration of exposure to physical abuse before the fatal outcome is a heartrending 1–3 years.

Physical abuse of children was first described as a pediatric entity by Kempe in 1962 and called by him the "battered child syndrome." The incidence of abuse is estimated to be 10 cases per 1000 live births per year (Steinhauer and Rae-Grant, 1983). Boys and girls are equally at risk overall, though the risk is greater for boys before age 12 and for girls during the teen years.

Most fatalities and serious injuries occur in children under age 3. Poverty, family dysfunction, and discriminatory under-reporting have resulted in higher reported case rates among ethnic minority families, but child abuse occurs in all ethnic and socioeconomic groups. The under-reporting of abuse and neglect in middle-class families is related to the way these families seek help. Since they tend to be referred to private therapists, they elude statistical reporting by government agencies.

Characteristics of Abusive Parents & Their Child Victims

The work of Kempe and Helfer (1972), amplified by Steinhauer and Rae-Grant (1983), has made it possible to characterize the abusive parent and the child victim in recognizable ways that are of help in case-finding and management.

A. The Parents: The parents commonly give an inadequate history of the incident and tend to be hostile or evasive, unconcerned about the child, and eager to establish their own innocence of wrongdoing. There may be an unexplained or fancifully explained delay in seeking treatment for the child, or a history of application to different hospitals in prior similar episodes. The parent may refuse hospitalization or diagnostic procedures for the child or may abruptly leave the child in the hospital after admission or even during the emergency room examination. If the child is admitted for observation and treatment, the parent may visit only infrequently or not at all and may show unconcern or relate poorly to the child during visits, thus provoking staff criticism. Lastly, the abusive parent is characteristically hard to reach by phone, changes residence frequently, has an unstable marital relationship, and has few friends or social resources,

B. The Child: The abused child characteristically has no explanation for its injury or gives a history contradictory to the parents' explanation—or parrots the mother's or father's obviously incongruous account of what happened. During the initial contact the child seems fearful, or passive and withdrawn, or hyperalert to the environment, looking to others and not to the parents for clues to how to behave. It responds to other adults indiscriminately, exhibits appeasing, smiling behavior, and shows obvious apprehension when other children cry. The workup of the child discloses injuries not mentioned in the history taken from the parent, often including multiple old fractures shown on radiographs. Developmental delays in gross motor function and speech and language skills are commonly present. There is general evidence of inadequate care, including dehydration and malnutrition, and the child typically gains weight in the hospital. There may be a history of ingestion of inappropriate food, drink, or drugs. Upon questioning, the child denies previous abuse or problems in the family. The child is viewed as "different" or "bad" by the family.

Contributing Factors

Factors contributing to child abuse are parental inadequacy resulting in low self-esteem and a wish to be "taken care of" by the child (role reversal); some "difference" in the child such as temperament; prematurity; a physical defect (cleft lip or palate, etc); and situational crises that provoke violent outbursts directed at the child as resident victim. Child abuse—like child neglect—often occurs in familial distribution from one generation to the next. Material abundance does not preclude attitudes of self-disparagement leading to physical abuse of children.

Treatment

When physical abuse of a child is suspected, the physician or other involved professional is apt to respond either by identifying with the child and directing anger toward the parents or, contrariwise, by identifying with the parent—who usually tries to deny or explain away the child's injuries, in some cases persuasively—and therefore denying the possibility of abuse. However, child abuse reporting laws require health care professionals to report all cases of suspected child neglect or abuse to local police officials, juvenile court officials, or the child protective agency of the county department of social services. Immunity against civil reprisal for groundless complaints is provided, and nonreporting is a criminal offense. The doctrines of confidentiality and privilege do not apply to reportable conditions.

Child abuse, once begun, becomes habitual and very difficult to stop despite repeated expressions of regret and the resolve to do better. It is therefore necessary to remove the child from the abusive environment during the period of assessment. Hospitalization is usually required to evaluate the extent of physical injuries and to begin the multidisciplinary team evaluation of the child and its family. The team should include a social worker, child psychiatrist, pediatrician, someone from the child protective agency, and, when necessary, a police officer. During the initial assessment phase, the child's siblings should be examined for evidence of injuries or neglect (Rudolph, 1982). Any person who has inflicted severe injuries on a child may be psychotic or suicidal and require emergency psychiatric evaluation.

Because of the recurrent nature of child abuse,

"crisis intervention" is not the answer. There must be an individualized long-term therapeutic program coordinated by the child psychiatrist, child protective agency, or child guidance clinic. Depending on the outcome of the multidisciplinary evaluation, the child may be permanently placed in a foster or adoptive family; may be removed from the family not permanently but for at least several months until the parents have proved they can offer a safe home; or may be returned to the family after assessment because a satisfactory rehabilitation plan is in place and there is a reasonable chance for successful reunion.

Assessment of Home Safety

Steinhauer and Rae-Grant (1983) have adapted guidelines from Kempe and Helfer (1972) as an aid to assessment of home safety when pondering the decision whether to return a child to its home or place it in foster care. It is of course a favorable sign if the parents have shown their willingness to accept help for the child and for themselves when it is needed. It must be clear also that help really is available at all times and that obstacles to seeking help are removed—eg, that there is a telephone in the home. Practical difficulties such as housing, food, employment, and illness should be in acceptable stages of resolution. It is a good sign if counseling has enabled the parents to accept an improved self-image and if they have developed some interests outside the home. Each spouse must be able to recognize when the other needs help and be willing to take necessary steps to obtain it. The parents must find the child "pleasing," with acknowledged needs of its own, and not "bad" and not "different" in unattractive ways. The parents' expectations of the child must be realistic. It is a very good sign if the parents consistently keep follow-up appointments for the child and themselves.

The Forensic Context of Child Abuse

Child neglect and abuse proceedings take place in juvenile or family court settings, where the people's burden of proof is not "beyond a reasonable doubt," as in criminal cases, but according to the civil standard of "the preponderance of the evidence." Even so, such proceedings are adversarial, and the parents' interests may be vigorously defended. For that reason alone, the need for unassailable documentation throughout the management of every case—including photographs and even videotaped child assessment sessions if possible—should be obvious.

Prognosis & Prevention

The prognosis for permanent cessation of child abuse is poor, even with protracted treatment. In the Rutter study, one-third to one-half of families abused the child victim again. One-fourth to one-half of children who are returned home without treatment beyond medical attention to injuries become victims subject to permanent injury or death.

In an attempt to ameliorate this grim prospect, Steinhauer and Rae-Grant (1983) have developed recommendations for social changes and professional safeguards aimed at prevention of physical abuse of children. Cultural as well as legal sanctions against the use of violence or force in child-rearing or in the schools are of first importance—sparing the rod to save the child. Social programs to eliminate poverty will ultimately benefit all children and remove from the home at least that stimulus for acts born of hopeless desperation. Adequate health care, social services, housing, and cultural and recreational facilities should be available to all citizens without exception. Family planning programs should include availability of abortion when appropriate to reduce the number of unwanted and rejected children. The same purpose without abortion can be served by family life education programs for young people preparing for sexual activity and perhaps marriage and parenthood. In the obstetrics unit in the hospital, the staff should be alert for evidence of rejecting behavior both before and after delivery. Child welfare and protective agencies should be adequately funded by an informed legislature and executive at the insistence of a concerned electorate. Lastly, physicians and other involved professionals should improve their cooperation in an effort to identify children at risk and act appropriately to prevent violence against children.

4. SEXUAL ABUSE

Definitions of child sexual abuse reflect cultural values and the professional orientation of the diagnostician. Mrazek (Rutter, 1985) perceives four types of child sexual maltreatment: exposure, molestation, sexual intercourse, and rape. Exposure includes pornography, the viewing of sexual acts, and exhibitionism. Molestation refers to fondling the child's genitals or asking the child to fondle the genitals of an adult. Sexual intercourse includes nonassaultive, often chronic vaginal, oral, or rectal intercourse. Rape is defined as assaultive, forced sexual intercourse. More than one type may be present in a single case. Incest is defined as sexual involvement with a relative whom the victim could not legally marry as an adult. The sexual abuser is usually an older sibling or parental figure (foster or adoptive parent). In 50–80% of cases, the abuser is known to the child or family (Steinhauer and Rae-Grant, 1983). The National Center on Child Abuse and Neglect (1981) estimates the incidence of child sexual abuse at 100,000 cases per year.

Various studies (Rutter, 1985) reveal that as many as 40% of adult women report at least one episode of sexual abuse during childhood; up to 6% were reported to the police. Most studies report a 10:1 ratio of girls to boys as victims.

Sexual assault of a child by a stranger is unrelated to family dysfunction, though children who develop protracted sexual relationships with adults outside the family do so in an attempt to satisfy unfulfilled emotional needs.

The most frequently reported form of incest occurs between father and daughter. Several studies have demonstrated that "incest is a family affair" (Steinhauer and Rae-Grant, 1983) in which many types of dysfunction, as well as the disinhibitory effects of drugs and alcohol, play a role. The family history often discloses incest in previous generations. The mother has often been described as rejecting her sexual role as wife, rejecting her daughter, and passively colluding with the perpetrating father. The father is typically described as authoritarian, immature, and sexually estranged from his wife. The other children in the family are often aware of the incest and may themselves be involved in incestuous behavior.

Clinical Findings

While extrafamilial sexual abuse is more willingly revealed by children, families fear the trauma of repeated questioning and the stress and humiliation of court appearances and publicity. Intrafamilial sexual abuse may never be disclosed, or not for years.

The child may present with symptoms or signs of medical, emotional, behavioral, or learning problems. Medical signs may consist of vaginal bleeding from trauma, recurrent urinary tract infections, proctitis, vaginitis, sexually transmitted diseases, pregnancy, and rectal or vaginal foreign bodies. Emotional or behavioral signs include psychosomatic illness, depression, attempted suicide, pseudomaturity, dissociative disorders, conversion disorders, shyness and avoidance of peer relationships, compulsive masturbation, precocious sexual behavior, adolescent prostitution, drug abuse, and running away from home. School-related difficulties include academic failure, frequent absences, poor peer relationships and avoidance of extracurricular activities, fearful or seductive behavior toward male teachers, and refusal to undress for physical education classes. The more of the above signs identified, the higher the likelihood that sexual abuse has occurred or is occurring.

Treatment

In cases of extrafamilial sexual abuse, the reactions of the average family may include self-doubt and questioning as well as outrage toward the perpetrator and protectiveness toward the child victim. Blaming the child victim or indifference to the event indicates serious family dysfunction. The effects of extrafamilial abuse on the child may be minimal (eg, after a brief episode of exhibitionism), requiring family discussion and reassurance that the perpetrator and not the child is "responsible" for what happened. At the other extreme, serious posttraumatic stress disorders can result from long-term or forcible abuse. Such posttraumatic stress disorders can be manifested by a wide variety of reactive psychological symptoms superimposed on preexisting personality organization.

5. CONCLUSIONS

Child maltreatment brings into focus the multiple problems of dysfunctional families. Abusive or neglecting parental figures are suffering people who themselves need or deserve help, but they are also generators of misery. Dysfunctional families should be considered a high-priority public health problem. Measures that might prevent child maltreatment include training professionals to recognize and deal with real or suspected child abuse at least on a first-aid basis (Steinhauer and Rae-Grant, 1983); funding of child protection and victim assistance programs; systematic cooperation between medical, legal, child welfare, and law enforcement agencies; guidelines for interviewing and legal processing of abused children and families to reduce the sometimes catastrophic consequences of criminal court proceedings; and continuing education of professionals in related fields.

ORGANIC MENTAL DISORDERS

As in adults, organic mental disorders in children are characterized by (1) impairment of orientation, judgment, learning, memory, and other cognitive functions; and (2) lability of affect. Brain damage may be diffuse or focal and may result from trauma, tumor, metabolic abnormalities, drug toxicity, or other causes. Both acute and chronic brain syndromes are seen (see Chapter 17).

Illustrative Case No. 19
A. *DMS-III-R* Classification: Axis I, barbiturate intoxication. Axis III, seizure disorder of unknown origin.

B. Description: A 7-year-old girl was falling behind in the second grade. Mental retardation was suggested because she had major motor seizures since the age of 4, and this implied "brain damage" to the family. During her yearly physical examination, her family doctor thought he detected mild nystagmus, a sign of barbiturate overdose. Since she was taking phenytoin and phenobarbital for her seizures, he ordered a blood test to determine drug levels. When the phenobarbital level was found to be elevated (above the therapeutic level), he instructed the parents to give her half of the usual dose. Within 2 months, the child's level of functioning in school returned to normal.

Illustrative Case No. 20
A. Diagnosis:
1. GAP–Chronic brain syndrome caused by drowning accident.

2. *DMS-III-R*–Axis I, delirium, followed by dementia. Axis II, mild mental retardation. Axis III, brain damage secondary to drowning accident.

B. Description: A 3-year-old girl wandered away from her mother and fell into a swimming pool. She was revived and spent 4 days in the intensive care unit in a state of delirium. She was hallucinating and confused and exhibited both stuporous and agitated states. Her condition showed some improvement within 2 weeks, and she was discharged from the hospital. However, her memory for recent events remained impaired; she cried and laughed at the slightest provocation and had difficulty understanding statements and requests she once was able to understand. This evidence of persistent injury marked the onset of dementia.

At 5 years of age, the girl was enrolled in a special kindergarten class. She was impulsive and had difficulty attending to tasks long enough to learn to complete them. The parents were on the verge of divorce, as their depression and turmoil had continued since the child's accident. The family physician met with both parents twice and encouraged them to seek help for themselves and their daughter at a child psychiatric clinic. They accepted his advice, and at 6-month follow-up, the family physician noted a decrease in anxiety and better coping skills in all three family members. Although the child continued to require special class placement because of her mild chronic brain syndrome (dementia), her behavior was much improved at school and at home.

MENTAL RETARDATION

The American Association on Mental Deficiency (1977) defines mental retardation as "significantly subaverage intellectual functioning originating during the developmental period, accompanied by impairment in one or more of the following: maturation, learning, or social adjustment." The IQ test (see Chapter 13) is the standard measure of intelligence used, and mental retardation is defined by an IQ of less than 70 (ie, 2 standard deviations below the mean of 100). The classifications (mild, moderate, severe, and profound retardation) and IQ score distributions of mental retardation are shown in Figure 30–1.

The prevalence of mental retardation in the USA is estimated to be 3% of the general population. In 1983, there were 6 million mentally retarded people—twice the combined total of those who suffer from blindness, poliomyelitis, cerebral palsy, and rheumatic heart disease. The incidence of emotional disorders in mentally retarded individuals is also very high—ie, 3–5 times that in the general population. It is usually an emotional problem or a difficulty in adjustment that brings retarded people to the attention

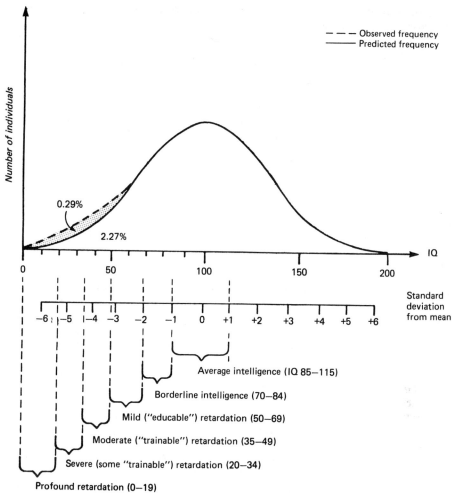

Figure 30–1. Distribution and classification of mental retardation. The shaded area denotes an increased incidence of 0.29% over the predicted frequency, resulting from organic causes of mental retardation. (Modified and reproduced, with permission, from Moser HW, Wolf PA: The nosology of mental retardation: Including the report of a survey of 1378 mentally retarded individuals at the Walter E. Fernald State School. In: *Nervous System.* Bergsma D [editor]. Part 6 of: The Second Conference on the Clinical Delineation of Birth Defects. Williams & Wilkins for the National Foundation–March of Dimes, Birth Defects Original Article Series 1971;7:117.)

of society. For the vast majority of these individuals (the 85% who are mildly retarded and educable), difficulties begin during the school years. With adequate instruction in a supportive environment, these people can function in the general population and find a suitable vocation.

This section will present several illustrative cases, discuss some misconceptions about mental retardation, and outline causes and characteristics of mental retardation syndromes.

Illustrative Case No. 21

A. DMS-III-R Classification: Axis II, mild mental retardation.

B. Description: When a 10-year-old well-ad-

justed boy was noted by his teacher to be a slow learner, she requested evaluation and consultation from the school psychologist. Testing indicated that he had an IQ in the range of 63–69. His teacher continued to give him individually paced instruction in her class. A similar approach, with individual tutoring as needed, was followed when he reached high school. The placid boy enjoyed participation on the track team and was accepted by his peers. His family encouraged his interest in fishing, and at age 16, he began to learn about commercial fishing at a local firm. When he was subsequently hired by the firm, he told his family, "I may never make it to manager, but I'll always make a decent living." He later married and had two children.

Illustrative Case No. 22

A. Diagnosis:

1. GAP–Anxiety reaction in an adolescent with moderate mental retardation.

2. DMS-III-R–Axis I, moderate mental retardation. Axis III, microcephaly.

B. Description: The neighbors of a moderately mentally retarded teenager (age 14) complained that he frightened their young daughter by asking her questions at the bus stop. The boy's parents were afraid that the next time this happened the police would be called and their son would be sent to a state institution for the retarded. They sought help from a child psychiatrist.

The history revealed that the boy was born with microcephaly after 8 months of gestation. He required assistance with breathing for 2 weeks in the neonatal intensive care unit. During infancy, he had multiple hospitalizations for respiratory problems. Between the ages of 2½ and 8 years, he attended a day school for retarded children. From there, he went to public school and attended special classes for the trainable retarded. He was still enrolled in school at the time of evaluation.

Initial assessment showed a moderately retarded boy with odd-sounding nasal speech. When he felt anxious, he touched people's faces and clothes, asked many questions, and fidgeted. When he relaxed, he could sit still for longer periods. The parents reported that his anxiety level and inappropriate behavior had increased since puberty. They expressed their own worries about his sexual maturity and immature coping abilities: "What if he masturbates in public? What if he tries to kiss a little girl? How can we explain to him what he should and should not do?"

The parents agreed to counseling for themselves and their son to help them cope with this new period of adjustment. The boy continued in school and lived at home until he was 19 years old. He then moved to a group home for retarded young adults in a suburb of his hometown.

Misconceptions About Mental Retardation

Societal attitudes toward mentally retarded people have in the past varied—from reverence and awe to disdain and fear to unconcern and neglect. When state mental hospitals and state institutions for the retarded were built in the late 19th and early 20th centuries, large numbers of retarded people were institutionalized. Such isolation and labeling furthered the stereotyped view of the mentally retarded as a homogeneous group of subhuman, dangerous individuals who would commit crimes of all types, especially sex crimes, if allowed to roam free in the community. Another commonly held fear was that the retarded would have an abnormally high reproductive rate, thereby "polluting the genetic pool of society." This reflected the mistaken belief that mental retardation is uniformly inherited (when in fact only a small proportion of mentally retarded individuals have retarded parents). In California, these fears were kept alive by the Human Betterment Foundation of Pasadena, which was so active in the eugenics movement that by 1943 California could claim responsibility for 40% of all sterilizations performed in the USA. Large numbers of state hospital patients were sterilized, including delinquents and retarded and epileptic patients.

As scientific data accumulated, public opinion began to shift. Studies showed that the mentally retarded have no greater propensity to commit crimes than the general population and that their reproduction rate is actually somewhat lower than the general rate. Other common misconceptions still abound, including the idea that mentally retarded people are all alike. As the illustrative cases above demonstrate, retarded people are individuals with diverse characteristics. Although their chronic and frequently stigmatizing handicap imposes greater stress and thereby predisposes them and their families to a greater frequency of emotional difficulties, most of these difficulties are similar to those encountered by others. And, contrary to another popular misconception, many of these problems can be alleviated, with resulting improvement in social functioning.

Many aspects of mental retardation are currently under study, and advances have been made in the prevention of retardation (eg, through genetic counseling, amniocentesis, special diets for children with phenylketonuria) and in early detection and management of the disorder. In addition, the range of community services, facilities, and special programs has been expanded. Many adults with moderate retardation who would previously have been institutionalized are now able to live in group homes in the community with varying degrees of assistance, and many are able to work at simple jobs.

Classification of Mental Retardation Syndromes

Mental retardation syndromes are commonly classified on the basis of prenatal, perinatal, and postnatal causes.

A. Prenatal Causes: Prenatal causes have traditionally been categorized as chromosomal (sex chromosome abnormalities and autosomal anomalies), biochemical (metabolic abnormalities), environmental (acquired prenatal conditions), and of unknown origin. However, there is some overlap in these categories.

1. Sex chromosome abnormalities–These abnormalities, which range from the absence of a sex chromosome (XO) to the presence of multiple sex chromosomes (eg, XXXXY), are often accompanied by mental retardation. In Turner's syndrome (45,XO karyotype), findings include sterility and, occasionally, retardation. Klinefelter's syndrome (XXY) occurs in one in 1100 male births and is characterized by sterility, gynecomastia, and neurodevelopmental abnormalities. Findings in the XYY chromosome complement syndrome are controversial; some researchers have reported an increased incidence of retardation, tall stature, and delinquency, but these data have not been validated.

2. Autosomal anomalies–

a. Down's syndrome–The most frequent genetic disorder causing mental retardation is Down's syndrome, first described as "mongolism" in 1866. The incidence is one in 650 births, and about 10% of institutionalized retarded patients have Down's syndrome.

Three distinct chromosomal types of Down's syndrome have been identified: (1) The best-known type, **trisomy 21** (nearly 95% of cases), results when nondisjunction of chromosomes 21 occurs during meiosis. The complete descendant cell line has three chromosomes 21, or a total of 47 chromosomes in each cell of the body. The incidence is directly related to maternal age (and according to some research, paternal age). The risk of giving birth to an infant with trisomy 21 is less than 0.2% in women under 35 years of age; about 0.9% in those 35–40 years; 1.4% in those 40–45 years; and 2.5% in those over 45. (2) The second major form, the **translocation type,** is caused by fusion of two chromosomes, usually 21 and 15. The total number of chromosomes is 46 because the extra chromosome (or part of one) is fused to another. The abnormal chromosome can be found in an otherwise unaffected father, mother, or sibling. This type occurs at any maternal age; it is heritable; and, once present, subsequent pregnancies of the same parents are theoretically at an increased risk of about 33%, although empirically the risk is approximately 20%. For this reason, the parents of any child with Down's syndrome should be given genetic counseling. (3) **Mosaicism,** the least frequent type of Down's syndrome, is caused by nondisjunction of chromosome 21 after fertilization during any of the early mitoses, which results in a "mosaic" of both normal and trisomic cell lines.

Down's syndrome has been extensively studied. Mental retardation, its cardinal feature, can be present to any degree—from profound retardation (IQ below 20) to borderline normal intelligence (IQ of 71–84). When the IQ scores of patients with Down's syndrome are plotted on a graph, the scores form a normal distribution curve (gaussian curve) between 0 and 100, with the mean at the high end of the moderately retarded range (IQ of 35–49). Thus, while the characteristic clinical features of the syndrome (see below) make it easily diagnosable at birth, the future intellectual and social functioning cannot be predicted with certainty at that time. Appropriate medical support and immediate enrollment of the parents and child in an infant development program are recommended to ensure optimal early development.

Although the full syndrome description includes over a hundred features and numerous medical complications, it should be emphasized that only some of the features will be seen in any one individual and that the physician's approach to a given family must strike a properly informed note—neither too pessimistic nor too optimistic. Besides the chromosome findings and some degree of retardation, characteristic features include epicanthal folds, oblique palpebral fissures, high cheekbones (hence the term "mongolism"), a large and protruding tongue, microcephaly, anteroposterior flattening of the skull, broad and thick hands, shortened and rounded small ears, and hypotonic musculature. Many patients have a single transverse palmar ("simian") crease that was originally thought to be pathognomonic of the syndrome but is seen in many other retardation syndromes and in nonretarded people as well. Biochemical studies have revealed abnormal blood platelet levels of sodium and potassium, of the enzyme adenosine triphosphatase, and of the content and rate of uptake of serotonin into platelets. Patients with Down's syndrome are more susceptible to infections in childhood, have a 30–50% incidence of congenital heart defects, and have an increased incidence of cataracts, diabetes mellitus, seizures, thyroid disorders, and acute lymphocytic leukemia.

b. The Fragile X syndrome is the most common inherited form of mental retardation (1 in every 1500 male births and one in every 2500 female births). It is caused by an abnormal segment of DNA and the tip of the X chromosome tends to break off in those affected. About one third of affected females suffer mild to severe mental retardation and about one half are normal except for learning difficulties. About 20% of males born with the abnormal X chromosome segment are normal, the other 80% can exhibit severe mental retardation or behavior problems such as violent outbursts, hyperactivity, hand biting, and poor eye contact.

c. Trisomy 18 and trisomy 13–The incidence of trisomy 18 is one in 5000 live births, while that of trisomy 13 is one in 5000–10,000 live births. These retardation syndromes occur by the same genetic mechanisms as trisomy 21 but are associated with higher death rates both pre-and postnatally. Subsequent offspring of parents of children with these syndromes have an estimated 1% risk of having the syndrome.

d. Other genetic disorders–Many other disorders that can result in retardation are caused by an autosomal dominant gene: tuberous sclerosis and neurofibromatosis; skull abnormalities (craniosynotosis, hypertelorism); connective tissue disorders (Marfan's syndrome); kidney disorders (nephrogenic diabetes insipidus); etc.

About a third of the population carry an **autosomal recessive gene** for severe mental retardation; it is estimated that there are 114 such gene loci. Several maldevelopments of the skull and brain result from these: **anencephaly,** an absence of parts of the brain and skull, which is usually fatal; **hydranencephaly,** a disorder in which the cranium is filled with fluid instead of brain tissue; **porencephaly,** the presence of cavities or large fluid-filled cysts in the brain; **microcephaly,** abnormal smallness of the head; and **hydrocephalus,** a disorder in which an excess of cerebrospinal fluid causes increased intracranial pressure, destruction of brain tissue, and resulting neurological problems. The latter two disorders may be due to a variety of different causes.

3. Metabolic abnormalities–These are caused primarily by endocrine disorders or by recessive gene abnormalities. Although the inborn errors of metabolism represent fewer than 10% of all known hereditary defects, they provide highly useful models for research into diagnosis, treatment, and prevention. The first described retardation syndrome due to a metabolic abnormality was **goitrous cretinism.** All forms of mental retardation were called cretinism until other syndromes began to be identified in the 19th century. Today the term refers to **hypothyroidism** and the resulting mental dullness, caused by various hypofunctions of the thyroid gland due to faulty hormone synthesis. Maternal hypothyroidism due to iodine deficiency in certain regions (endemic goiter) also results in hypothyroidism in infants.

a. Disorders of amino acid metabolism–The best-known example of the inborn metabolic errors is phenylketonuria, which has an incidence of one in 15,000. The disorder is due to a deficiency or defect in the liver enzyme phenylalanine hydroxylase, which gives rise to a series of biochemical abnormalities starting with accumulation of ingested phenylalanine (an essential amino acid) in the body. Most patients have severe mental retardation (some have normal intelligence), a small head and body, coarse features, and light complexion. Children with phenylketonuria exhibit the full range of disturbed behaviors associated with severe brain damage. Early diagnosis is essential, since brain damage can be prevented if a diet low in phenylalanine is started before 6 months of age; near normal intelligence is preserved if dietary treatment is begun by 3 months of age. Since phenylalanine is an essential amino acid, use of the special diet must be accompanied by regular follow-up evaluations. Many patients continue without mental impairment if the diet is stopped at 6 years of age, but some must remain on the diet for life. Women with phenylketonuria, regardless of their mental status, must take a low-phenylalanine diet if they intend to carry a pregnancy to term. Newborn testing for phenylketonuria is now required by law in most states.

Lesch-Nyhan syndrome is a rare disorder characterized by severe retardation and self-mutilation of the lips and fingers by biting. It is transmitted as an X-linked recessive trait, resulting in deficiency of the enzyme hypoxanthine-guanine phosphoribosyltransferase. This deficiency produces a 20-fold increase in serum uric acid levels (five times higher than in patients with gout). Thus, patients with Lesch-Nyhan syndrome also have gout and its complications (renal calculi, tophi) in addition to cerebral palsy, choreoathetosis, mental retardation, and the self-destructive biting that can only be partially controlled with firm physical restraints. Treatment for gout has no effect on the cerebral manifestations of this disorder.

b. Disorders of fat metabolism–These disorders include several genetically determined lipidoses. **Tay-Sachs disease** begins at age 4–8 months and results in death by 2–4 years. The *late infantile* form, called **Bielschowsky-Jansky disease,** starts at 2–4 years of age and results in progressive dementia, with death in a few years. The *juvenile* form, **Spielmeyer-Vogt disease,** usually begins with visual impairment at 5 or 6 years of age, progressing to blindness and mental deterioration over 10–15 years. The *late juvenile* form, **Kufs' disease,** is the rarest; it occurs after age 15. Although there is no treatment for Tay-Sachs disease, its occurrence is preventable by screening (through blood tests) for carriers of the recessive gene, which is found in about 4% of Eastern Europeans of Jewish ancestry. Two other types of cerebromacular degeneration, both of autosomal recessive origin, occur primarily in Jewish children: **Niemann-Pick disease** and **Gaucher's disease.**

c. Disorders of carbohydrate metabolism include **galactosemia** and several types of **glycogen storage disease.**

4. Acquired prenatal conditions–Mental retardation may result from exposure of the fetus to (1) **toxic agents** (teratogenic medications; maternal drug abuse, including alcohol intake even in moderation); (2) **infectious diseases** such as rubella (preventable with immunization), toxoplasmosis, and cytomegalovirus inclusion disease (the most frequent viral cause of retardation) as well as other maternal diseases; and (3) maternal **malnutrition.**

B. Perinatal Causes: Causes of mental retardation associated with the birth process include prematurity; anoxia due to birth injuries or hemorrhage; brain damage from mechanical trauma; and infections (eg, herpes simplex) acquired by the infant during passage through the birth canal.

C. Postnatal Causes: This very large category includes traumatic, metabolic, infectious, toxic, and other causes of brain damage, including accidents.

Genetic Counseling & Prenatal Diagnosis

According to Rudolph (1982), "Genetic counseling is a multifaceted technique with medical, genetic, and psychological components and has as one of its principal objectives informed decision-making by patients . . . and families." The professional's goal is not to impose a policy of prevention of specific kinds of genetic disease on the parents but rather to provide them with information so they can understand their risks and make their own decisions.

In prenatal genetic diagnosis, techniques such as amniocentesis and ultrasonography are performed to determine whether the fetus is affected by genetic diseases for which it is thought to be at risk. In **amniocentesis,** about 15 mL of amniotic fluid is removed from the uterus after a local anesthetic is applied to the site of needle insertion. The procedure takes about 10 minutes. Most centers recommend that women under age 35 (some say under age 37) should not have amniocentesis unless a possibility of genetic disease is disclosed by genetic counseling. The procedure is performed between the 15th and 18th weeks of gestation, but results may not be available until up to 4 weeks later. Test results are negative in 95%

of women over age 35. About 100 biochemical disorders and a large number of chromosomal problems are detectable.

Fetal visualization and biopsy are becoming increasingly useful for the detection of fetal abnormalities that are not associated with biochemical or chromosomal disorders. During the past 15 years, **ultrasonography** has replaced roentgenography as a means of visualizing uterine contents. Ultrasonography makes it possible to detect physical anomalies and intrauterine growth problems and to determine gestational age. **Fetoscopy** allows for direct fetal visualization and also makes possible sampling of fetal blood to detect hemoglobinopathies. **Chorionic villus biopsy** is a promising new technique that allows testing of fetal cells (without harm to the fetus) during the first trimester of pregnancy.

REFERENCES

American Association on Mental Deficiency: *Manual on Terminology and Classification in Mental Retardation.* Grossman H (editor) American Association on Mental Deficiency, 1977.

American Psychiatric Association: *Diagnostic and Statistical Manual Disorders (DSM-III),* 3rd ed. American Psychiatric Association, 1980.

American Psychiatric Association: *Diagnostic and Statistical Manual of Mental Disorders (DSM-III-R),* 3rd ed (Revised). American Psychiatric Association, 1987.

Group for the Advancement of Psychiatry (GAP), Committee on Child Psychiatry: *Psychopathological Disorders in Childhood.* Jason Aronson, 1974.

Kanner L: *Childhood Psychosis: Initial Studies and New Insights.* Winston/Wiley, 1973.

Kempe CH, Helfer RE: *Helping the Battered Child and His Family.* Lippincott, 1972.

Kempe CH, et al: The battered child syndrome. JAMA 1962;181:17.

National Center on Child Abuse and Neglect: *Child Sexual Abuse: Incest, Assault, and Sexual Exploitation.* US Government Printing Office, Department of Health and Human Services Publication No. (OHDS) 81-30166, 1981.

Rudolph AM: *Pediatrics.* Appleton-Century-Crofts, 1982.

Rutter M et al: Isle of Wight studies, 1964–1974. Psychol Med 1976;6:313.

Steinhauer PD, Rae-Grant Q: *Psychological Problems of the Child in the Family.* Basic Books, 1983.

Section IV. Treatment of Modalities

31

Introduction to Psychiatric Treatment

Beth Goldman, MPH, MD, & Howard H. Goldman, MD, PhD

As the preceding chapters have attempted to show, a multifactorial approach is necessary to explain the etiology and pathogenesis of psychiatric illness. Similarly, the most useful treatment approaches are developed within the framework of the biopsychosocial model (see Chapters 1–3).

Psychiatric treatment may comprise one or many modalities and may be rendered in a number of settings depending on both the needs and the circumstances— physical, economic, geographic—of each individual patient. Weekly outpatient behavior modification treatment would be appropriate for an otherwise happy and successful advertising executive who wishes to be cured of fear of flying, whereas involuntary inpatient treatment along with pharmacotherapy and, later, social service interventions would be mandatory for the psychotic, assaultive mayor of Wino Park (Chapters 9 and 15). Furthermore, different treatment approaches may be useful at different times over the course of any individual patient's illness. For example, a young person undergoing a major depressive episode may not be able to respond to or tolerate psychotherapy without prior antidepressant drug therapy and supportive treatment. In this chapter, the settings in which mental illness may be treated are described as well as the individuals who deliver such treatment. In Chapters 32–43, the actual treatment techniques and their advantages and disadvantages are discussed.

SETTINGS IN WHICH MENTAL HEALTH CARE MAY BE OFFERED

Mental health services are delivered in hospitals, outpatient office settings, day treatment programs, and emergency rooms. In some cases, psychiatrists and other mental health professionals may work in cooperation with other agencies such as penal institutions, law courts, schools at all levels, and places of employment.

Individuals requiring or requesting treatment may present in a variety of ways at a number of different "entry points" into the mental health care delivery system. New patients may present at the private offices of general physicians or specialists, mental health professionals, community-based crisis intervention centers, community mental health centers, or hospital emergency rooms. Specially trained professionals at these sites evaluate the current status and needs of each individual patient and make recommendations or referrals for further treatment. When patients are dangerous to themselves or others or are unable to care for themselves and do not understand their need for treatment, such a recommendation may be made mandatory by court order.

Inpatient Settings

Psychiatric hospitalization may be necessary for a variety of patients who cannot be effectively or safely treated as outpatients. Some patients require specialized diagnostic procedures (eg, for close observation of symptoms, specialized endocrine or sleep studies) that can only be safely and properly performed in a hospital; others may require almost constant nursing attention (eg, physically ill patients who develop dangerous side effects to medications, agitated patients who require seclusion) that can only be provided on an inpatient basis. Psychiatric patients are also admitted for their own protection or the protection of others, as in the case of suicidal or homicidal patients or patients who are so disorganized, depressed, or demented that they cannot care for themselves. Such patients are observed closely, protected, restricted, and confined and are usually treated for the specific mental disorder underlying their behavior. In some cases, individuals accused of criminal activity are admitted to a hospital for forensic psychiatric evaluation of criminal responsibility or competence to stand trial (Chapter 42). Hospitals may also be used inappropriately and unnecessarily when less intensive services would suffice, and some patients may even "manipulate the system" to obtain admission (eg, the homeless individual who uses the hospital as a shelter or the individual with antisocial personality disorder who is in trouble on the streets and "escapes" into the psychiatric unit).

Hospital settings offer a wide variety of treatment

options, including medical treatment; group, individual, and family psychotherapy; social worker services; and occupational and recreational activity therapies. Ideally, the treatment plan is tailored to meet the medical, social, and psychological needs of each individual patient.

In the United States, inpatient psychiatric care may be delivered in state and county mental hospitals, private mental hospitals, general hospitals (often in specialized psychiatric units), Veterans Administration hospitals, and military hospitals. Improvements in the efficacy of somatic treatments (Chapter 32) that resulted in shortening the period of acute symptoms in many patients shifted the emphasis from long-term to short-term care and away from reliance on state and county hospital systems. Furthermore, since hospitalization can lead to stigmatization, loss of self-esteem, dependency, and regressed behavior, the trend is toward minimizing hospital stays and utilizing less restrictive treatment settings (eg, day treatment) in innovative and more intensive ways. Progress in this area is encouraged by governmental agencies (Medicaid and Medicare) and private third-party payers (eg, Blue Cross), who are reluctant to pay for inpatient services for any but the sickest of patients. The trend away from hospital admissions would be further encouraged if payers were willing to reimburse for less expensive services provided in lieu of hospital days.

Outpatient Care

Outpatient services are provided in freestanding clinics, clinics attached to hospitals, community mental health centers (CMHCs) and private offices. Almost unknown in the 19th and early 20th centuries, ambulatory psychiatric services have expanded dramatically since 1955, when they accounted for only 23% of all episodes of care. By 1977, outpatient services had expanded 12-fold and represented 72% of all psychiatric care in the organized mental health sector. Nearly 10 million people in the USA are estimated to have kept one or more outpatient mental health care appointments in 1980 (25% seeing psychiatrists, 25% psychologists, and the remainder other providers). The median number of visits was 2, and the mean was 8 (Taube et al, 1984).

Outpatient treatment is appropriate for patients with a wide variety of psychiatric illnesses varying from problems of living and adjustment disorders to those with psychotic and mood disorders. As alluded to above, the trend over the past 30–40 years has moved away from inpatient care toward outpatient treatment. Traditionally, outpatient care has consisted of seeing a therapist in group or individual treatment for no more than a few hours a week. Although many people who function well at home and at work benefit from such limited treatment, there are many others with more severe mental disorders who need a more intense level of care but who do not require 24-hour supervi-

sion as is provided in a traditional inpatient setting.

In the past—and to a great extent even now—most patients who could not function within the limited framework of traditional outpatient treatment were hospitalized anyway for a number of reasons: (1) it is often easier to hospitalize a patient than to provide the complex and time-consuming kind of support that an outpatient in crisis may require; (2) third-party payers often pay for inpatient care more readily than intense outpatient care; and (3) few resources have been developed to provide intermediate alternatives to the choice between traditional outpatient and costly and restrictive inpatient care.

However, as insurance companies limit payment for inpatient treatment to only the sickest patients, innovations in outpatient care are developing.

Partial Hospitalization

In partial hospitalization programs, patients receive much the same range of services as is provided in traditional inpatient settings but are in most cases allowed to go home at night. (Rarely, patients work or study by day but stay at the hospital at night.) Such care may be offered to hospitalized patients to help them readjust to life outside the hospital or to fairly ill patients who need supervision but who can safely be at home nights and weekends. This form of treatment is much less expensive than hospitalization around the clock but is not covered by many insurance companies out of concern that some patients who could be managed with less intensive outpatient treatment will be offered the more expensive treatment instead.

Chronically ill patients sometimes receive similar care in "day treatment" programs designed to provide structure, training in social skills, vocational training, and other treatment over longer periods of time.

Residential Treatment Programs

Residential treatment programs (often called three-quarter houses or halfway houses) offer treatment in structured nonhospital settings. Some offer graduated services ranging from completely supervised homes with around-the-clock supervision and a full range of structured activities and treatments to less supervised arrangements (eg, an apartment shared by two patients) in which patients combine treatment with other activities such as volunteer or paid work. Such facilities slowly move the patient in the direction of semi-independent or fully independent living.

Residential self-help communities are usually sponsored by nongovernmental agencies for the purpose of helping individuals with some specific difficulty, often chemical dependency. Examples include Synanon, Delancey Street (both created for persons with drug and alcohol problems), and the Salvation Army. Residents in these communities often maintain ties with the community after leaving the residence.

Substitute homes provide shelter and limited treatment to patients who either do not require or would not benefit from other kinds of residential treatment programs. Persons living in such homes often are unable to live alone and unsupervised and have no family support or have families who cannot continue to provide care (eg, because of disruptive behavior or burnout). Treatment is usually confined to supervision of activities of daily living, medication, informal counseling (usually provided by a layperson who manages the home) and sometimes transportation to therapists' offices or in-house medication management provided by a psychiatrist on contract to the home. Examples include adult foster care homes, board and care homes, family care homes, and mental hygiene homes.

Other examples of substitute housing include "crash pads" for people withdrawing from drugs or in crisis and in need of a safe place. Similarly, temporary shelters for abused women and even the homeless may be regarded as part of the mental health care system.

Emergency & Crisis Intervention

Crisis intervention services are offered by hospital and nonhospital facilities and provide episodic acute intervention in life-threatening or extreme circumstances involving patients with mental illness or others in crisis. In such settings, patients are evaluated—sometimes over several hours—and, when feasible, attempts are made to help resolve the crisis. In many cases, these facilities serve as entry points into the mental health system whereby patients may be referred for further inpatient or outpatient care. In some crisis intervention settings, a patient may be seen frequently (eg, daily) on a short-term basis until the crisis has subsided. Crisis intervention settings use medical and psychosocial techniques; specific treatment methods are discussed in Chapters 41 and 43.

Also important are such services as suicide and drug prevention "hotlines" that offer telephone support and refer patients in crisis.

Social Support Services

Social support services are offered by most mental health and community social service agencies to bolster the patient's natural support system (eg, family, church, neighborhood) or to provide a substitute system if natural supports are lacking. The effect of these services may be to alter the acute course of illness so as to prevent chronicity.

Nonresidential self-help organizations are the "outpatient" parallel to the residential self-help services described above and are often founded by individuals who have survived a problem and have banded together to help others who have had similar life experiences. Examples are Alcoholics Anonymous, Narcotics Anonymous, Schizophrenics Anonymous, colostomy clubs, the Epilepsy Society, and burn recovery groups.

Miscellaneous agencies provide services, counseling, and assistance to a variety of individuals in need. Although not formally part of the mental health care system, these organizations often provide enough psychosocial assistance to prevent or avert crises. Examples include the Visiting Nurse Association, Homemakers Services, Big Brothers, Planned Parenthood, Traveler's Aid, and consumer credit agencies.

MENTAL HEALTH PROFESSIONALS

Professional mental health care providers are of many different kinds. Most have certain skill in common and provide similar services (eg, psychotherapy). Some have areas of specialized training and practice.

Psychiatrists are physicians—doctors of medicine or osteopathy—who have completed a 4-year residency training program in general psychiatry. Psychiatrists are trained to apply both biomedical and psychosocial diagnostic and therapeutic skills to the management of patients with physical and mental disorders. They are trained in techniques of psychotherapy and are skilled at both diagnosis and psychosocial formulation (psychodynamic, behavioral, or both). They are the only members of the mental health care team trained and licensed to prescribe medication and (along with nurses) to perform complete physical examinations. Subspecialties in psychiatry are discussed in specific chapters (eg, psychoanalysis in Chapter 33, geriatric psychiatry in Chapter 40, hospital consultation psychiatry in Chapter 41, and forensic psychiatry in Chapter 42).

Clinical psychologists are mental health professionals with doctorates (PhD, EdD, PsyD, DMH) or master's degrees who may be licensed as independent practitioners in psychotherapy and psychological assessment; some master's-level professionals have licenses restricting their practice to marriage and family counseling. These professionals attend graduate schools and have clinical placements and internships in which they learn psychotherapy, diagnosis, and psychological testing under supervision. When licensed, they may diagnose and treat patients with mental disorders. Psychologists often have specialized training in administering psychological tests and performing behavior and cognitive therapies. They also have more extensive research training than most physicians. Like the services of physicians, those of psychologists are now being reimbursed by insurance. In addition, psychologists are beginning to gain admitting privileges to some hospital inpatient services, permitting them to admit a patient jointly with a physician.

Clinical Social Workers are doctoral (DSW, PhD) or (more frequently) master's-level (MSW, MSSW) psychotherapists, caseworkers, and marriage, family, and child therapists trained in accredited schools of social work and social welfare and accredited by the

National Association of Social Work as having completed a specified program of supervised clinical training. They are licensed by many states as independent practitioners, and increasingly they are being reimbursed by health insurance payers. Social workers are skilled at psychosocial therapies, are knowledgeable about community and social welfare resources, and have a special interest in families.

Clinical nurse specialists are registered nurses who may take special training in psychiatric nursing. They may be licensed as independent practitioners, but more often they work in organized ambulatory health care settings and in hospitals. Nurses have special skills in the biomedical as well as the psychosocial aspects of mental health care.

Occupational, activities, and recreational/expressive therapists are registered practitioners from a variety of educational backgrounds with specialized training in using art, music, dance, drama, play, and vocational activities to help patients express their feelings, thoughts, learn new behavior, and develop or recover emotionally and socially valuable skills.

Pastoral counselors are clergy with specialized training in counseling patients with emotional disorders.

Other mental health care providers include **clinical sociologists, clinical pharmacists,** and specialists in other related clinical disciplines who have developed clinical skills related to their core academic or professional training and apply them in clinical settings.

Psychoanalysts are graduates of psychoanalytic institutes, including freudian, neofreudian, and jungian training centers, who have completed a course of study, a personal analysis, and supervised training analyses (see Chapter 33). Although most are psychiatrists, other professionals have been trained as lay analysts. Training takes many years after completion of other professional mental health training.

Multidisciplinary teams of mental health professionals function in psychiatric and general hospital and ambulatory settings. The **inpatient team** has a traditional hierarchy and division of labor, with the psychiatrist leading the team; the nurse managing day-to-day ward activities and medication and patient monitoring duties; the psychologist performing psychological tests or leading patient therapy groups; the social worker finding a place for the patient to go upon discharge, arranging for the financing of hospital and posthospital care, and often performing family therapy; and the occupational therapist organizing activities for the patient during the hospital stay. This traditional organization is still the mode, though in some settings the inpatient team has evolved with less differentiated functions and roles—and a less hierarchical organization.

The **outpatient team** tends to be less hierarchical, though certain functions are still performed by different disciplines (eg, psychiatrists manage medication and psychologists give tests and conduct behavior treatments). The functions of members of the **consultation/liaison team** are partly differentiated, as described in Chapter 41.

REFERENCES

Frances A, Clarkin, Perry S: *Differential Therapeutics in Psychiatry.* Brunner/Mazel, 1984.

Glick I, Hargreaves WA: *Psychiatric Hospital Treatment for the 1980's.* Lexington Books 1979.

Group for Advancement of Psychiatry: *The Family, the Patient and the Psychiatric Hospital: Toward a New Model.* (GAP No 117). Brunner/Mazel, 1985.

Jones M: *The Therapeutic Community.* Basic Books, 1953.

Kirshner LA: Length of stay of psychiatric patients. J Nerv Ment Dis 1982;170:27

McGuire T: *Financing Psychotherapy.* Ballinger, 1981.

Regier DA, Goldberg ID, Taube CA: The de facto US mental health services system. Arch Gen Psychiatry 1978;35:685.

Taube CA, Kessler LA, Feuerberg M: Utilization and expenditures for ambulatory mental health care during 1980. In: *National Medical Care Utilization an Expenditure Survey,* Data Report No. 5. US Department of Health and Human Services Publication No. (PHS) 84–20000, 1984.

32 Somatic Therapies

Glenn C. Davis, MD, & Beth Goldman, MPH, MD

Before World War II, the somatic treatment of psychiatric disorders consisted largely of "tranquilization," ie, sedating patients or restraining their actions. During the 1950s and 1960s, tricyclic antidepressants, monoamine oxidase inhibitors, and phenothiazine antipsychotics were developed. These agents provided not mere tranquilization but specific relief of specific symptoms.

The sections on psychopharmacology below are organized according to the treatment of five groups of syndromes: depression, mania, psychosis, anxiety (including anxiety disorders), and insomnia. The chapter concludes with a general introduction to electroconvulsive therapy and some brief comments on psychosurgery.

I. PHARMACOLOGICAL THERAPIES

In the sections that follow, each group encompasses several *DSM-III-R* diagnostic entities, which vary in their response to somatic treatments. The pharmacological agents are reviewed, including indications and side effects. Clinical strategies, including drug selection, initiation of treatment, increasing dosage, determination of duration of treatment, and maintenance management are discussed. Illustrative cases are presented where that appears to be useful.

INTRODUCTION TO RATIONAL PHARMACOLOGICAL THERAPEUTICS

TARGET SYMPTOMS & DIAGNOSIS

A common reason for treatment failure in any field of medicine is that an inaccurate diagnosis is made and, as a result, an inappropriate treatment plan is devised. *DSM-III-R* lists the current **defining symptoms for psychiatric disorders** (the diagnostic crite-

ria). Defining symptoms are those that serve to identify distinct syndromes. The purpose of defining symptoms is **differential diagnosis.** When defining symptoms are effective in the differential diagnosis of a syndrome, the criteria are said to have **discriminant validity.** It is essential to learn the *DSM-III-R* syndromes, but it is equally essential to understand that defining symptoms do not specify all of the symptoms that may be part of a given syndrome.

Target symptoms are those that respond to treatment. Observation of improvement of target symptoms permits the clinician to monitor improvement. Many diagnostic entities have symptoms that do not remit with pharmacological treatment, and these must be recognized and addressed in the course of treatment.

After an agent has been chosen, it is essential to proceed by a series of steps to determine whether the drug has been effective. Drug therapy is commonly discontinued without adequate trial, either because the dose is too low or because not enough time has passed to determine if the drug has been effective.

Conversely, it is not uncommon for drug treatment to be initiated and then maintained for months or years with no conscious determination made about whether the medication is effective; clinical psychopharmacologists make a good living discontinuing medications that other physicians have started and maintained without demonstrable benefits. In fact, the drug may in some cases have contributed to the patient's symptoms, in which case the patient improves following its discontinuation.

When changing medications it is important also to do so in a rational, stepwise fashion, using only one at a time, so that it is possible to determine which drug may have led to improvement or worsening of symptoms or undesirable side effects.

COMPLIANCE, "THERAPEUTIC ALLIANCE," & INFORMED CONSENT

Even the most effective drug is worthless if the patient does not take it as prescribed. Whenever possible, the development of a caring doctor-patient relationship should precede the prescription of a drug. There must be an understanding that the doctor and the patient will work together to help relieve the patient's distress. The physician must be able to listen to and respect the patient, and the patient must be able to trust the physician. This is often called the "therapeutic alliance." Within the relationship, the physician must be able to address the patient's concerns and fears about having to take psychotropic medication (eg, becoming addicted, being a "weak person"). Before starting the medication, the patient must be informed about the side effects of the drug and should be given a realistic account of what to expect while taking it (eg, understanding that the drug will not "work" right away). A patient is less likely to discontinue a drug if forewarned about possible uncomfortable side effects. This procedure is part of the process of **informed consent,** in which the patient is told of the potential risks and benefits of taking the proposed medication as well as of alternative treatments. Informed consent must be obtained before prescribing any psychotropic drug and must be clearly documented. It is helpful to provide patients with a written description of the drug's side effects, potential benefits, and alternative treatments.

PHARMACOTHERAPY OF DEPRESSION

AGENTS & CLASSES OF AGENTS

Two classes of drugs are the mainstay of pharmacological treatment for depression: the heterocyclic antidepressants and the monoamine oxidase inhibitors. A heterocyclic antidepressant is any antidepressant with a ring structure, including the familiar tricyclics. Some antidepressants do not have ring structures and are not technically heterocyclics. Other agents, such as lithium, anticonvulsants, antipsychotics, and thyroid hormone, may be used alone or as adjuncts to antidepressants in patients who are refractory to treatment (see Table 32–1). The depressive syndromes vary in their response to these agents. The different antidepressant agents are generally equally effective in treating major depression; however, individual patients may respond better to one agent than to another. Depressive syndromes defined in *DSM-III-R* include major depressive disorder, dysthymic disorder, organic mood disorder (depressed), adjustment disorder (with depressed mood), bipolar disorder (depressed), and cyclothymic disorder. Although each of these diagnoses is an indication for antidepressant therapy and responds variably in different patients, the focus of pharmacotherapy of depression is on the target symptoms.

Table 32–1. Antidepressants.

	Usual Therapeutic Range (mg/d)
Heterocyclics	
Impiramine	150–300
Amitriptyline	150–300
Desipramine	150–300
Nortriptyline	50–150
Doxepin	150–300
Protriptyline	15–60
Trimipramine	150–300
Clomipramine	75–400
Maprotiline	150–200
Monoamine oxidase inhibitors	
Phenelzine	45–90
Isocarboxazid	30–60
Tranylcypromine	30–50
Miscellaneous	
Amoxapine	150–450
Trazodone	150–300
Bupropion	200–450
Fluoxetine	10–40
Mood stabilizers	
Carbamazepine	600–1200
Lithium carbonate	600–2400
Valproic acid	750–3000

INDICATIONS

1. TARGET SYMPTOMS & SYNDROMES

The target groupings for depressive disorders are neurovegetative, psychomotor, mood, cognitive, psychotic, and secondary symptoms associated with social impairment.

The neurovegetative symptoms of impaired sleep, appetite, sexual drive, and altered diurnal rhythm are among the first symptoms to respond to treatment—often within 10 days to 2 weeks, but at times not for 3–4 weeks. When sleep improves in the first few days of treatment, it is usually due to the concurrent use of sedatives or sedating antidepressants and should not be mistaken for improvement in sleep, which will occur due to specific antidepressant effects.

Psychomotor symptoms may be either increased (agitation) or decreased (retardation) in depression. Both behaviors will improve, and generally over the same interval as neurovegetative features—usually 3–4 weeks after starting treatment, or 7–14 days after achieving an appropriate dosage level. Social withdrawal is frequently mistaken for psychomotor retardation. As the patient improves clinically, psychomotor behavior will normalize, though the patient may remain withdrawn. Psychomotor behavior can be monitored in the clinical interview or by the nursing staff, observing the patient's facial and hand gestures and total activity level.

Ironically, mood improvement lags behind recovery of neurovegetative and psychomotor functions.

The first indication of mood improvement may be transition of the persistent or predominant mood to another mood state. A common occurrence is the shift from profound and pervasive depressive mood to irritability or anger. It is important to recognize that the diagnosis of depression does not require the presence of depressive mood; other mood states may predominate in depression, such as irritability, dysphoria, or anger.

Concentration, attention, memory, and learning are important cognitive skills that are impaired in depression. This group of target symptoms tends to improve with mood.

Depressed thought lags significantly behind other aspects of depression. Guilt, distorted cognition, and rumination persist long after mood has begun to improve. Depressive ideation is the expression in thought of the disturbance in drive and cognitive skills that comprise depression. Its recovery depends on social and individual factors as much as on improvement in the depressive process.

Psychotic symptoms in depression improve slowly, though when neuroleptics are used concurrently there is a prompt reduction in agitation. Depressive delusions and hallucinations improve over many weeks.

While social impairment is not a biological feature of depression, it is listed as a target symptom in order to maintain awareness that rehabilitation and improved morale should be part of the treatment plan.

2. SPECIFIC DISORDERS

Major Depressive Episodes

In uncomplicated depressive episodes meeting the criteria for major depression, antidepressants should bring about a remission in 65–75% of patients. "Uncomplicated" has the following implications: a first episode, a recurrent episode in a well-treated recurrent disorder, no comorbid conditions such as drug or alcohol dependence, and good compliance with treatment. The entire syndrome of a major depressive episode should remit with effective treatment over the course of several months. The primary symptoms of depression remit sooner. Social impairment and demoralization caused by the disorder often persist and appear as "residual symptoms."

Dysthymic Disorder

DSM-III-R defines dysthymic disorder as a chronic depressive syndrome, symptoms being present for the better part of 2 years. While the list of symptom criteria may have the appearance of being less rigid than major depression, patients with this syndrome are usually quite impaired. There are few studies documenting the percentage of patients with dysthymic disorder who respond to antidepressants, but there is general agreement that the recovery rate is much lower than with major depression. The study

of dysthymia is further complicated by the fact that many—perhaps most—patients with dysthymia have a lifetime history of major depressive episode. A trial of an antidepressant is standard practice.

Organic Mood Disorder

Depressive syndromes secondary to organic causes do not have a predictable response rate to antidepressants. Selected disorders such as hypothyroid-induced depressive states respond very well to treatment (eg, thyroid replacement and antidepressants), though they respond more readily to electroconvulsive therapy. Depressive syndromes associated with brain injury may also respond to medication.

Adjustment Disorder

Depressive symptoms associated with adjustment reactions do not respond to antidepressants. When depressive symptoms following a stressor meet the criteria for major depression, the diagnosis of major depression supersedes (hierarchically) the diagnosis of adjustment disorder with depressive mood, and standard antidepressant treatment should be initiated.

Bipolar Disorder

A depressive episode in a patient with bipolar disorder will respond to standard antidepressant treatment. Nevertheless, a clear understanding of the natural history of bipolar disorder and its treatment is necessary in order to treat a depressive episode and manage the underlying vulnerability to recurrent depressive and manic episodes. Furthermore, antidepressants have the potential for precipitating manic or hypomanic episodes in bipolar patients. The diagnosis of bipolar disorder, depressed episode, requires knowledge of the use of lithium in bipolar disorder and of the difficulties of treating depression in a patient taking lithium.

Cyclothymic Disorder

Cyclothymic disorder is an attenuated version of bipolar disorder and may be treated with lithium and antidepressants. Often no treatment is required because the episodes are brief and tolerable. Furthermore, cyclothymic individuals frequently reject treatment (as do people suffering from bipolar disorder) because lithium blocks the hypomanias (which are "liked" by the patient). Few cyclothymic patients seek treatment or accept it when offered. A patient with bipolar II (a designation reserved for patients with major depression and hypomania) will often seek treatment since the depressive episodes are disabling.

DRUG CHOICE

Following accurate diagnosis and identification of target symptoms in the depressed patient, the next step in rational pharmacotherapy is selection of the proper antidepressant. Table 32–1 lists antidepressants in common use. In the last several years, a number of antidepressants, such as fluoxetine, clomipramine, and bupropion, have been approved for use in the United States. These agents have been available in other countries for a number of years. The more commonly used daily dosage ranges for antidepressants are included in Table 32–1.

Several principles guide the choice of pharmacological agent. It is important to obtain a history of the patient's prior responses to specific agents—including both efficacy and adverse reactions. If a particular drug worked in a prior depressive episode and did not cause problems, it is wise to use it again. If a member of the patient's family had a positive response to a particular drug, that drug should be considered for the patient as well. If there is no prior history of treatment, one must match the patient's clinical condition with the drug and proceed somewhat empirically.

1. HETEROCYCLICS

Efficacy

No drug has been found to be more effective than the heterocyclic agents in the treatment of major depression. Most claims for differential efficacy are limited to alternative classifications of depression, such as "atypical depressions," which may respond better to monoamine oxidase inhibitors (see below).

Compliance

The major cause of failure in the treatment of depression is lack of compliance. Patients often do not take antidepressants because of a failure in patient education. The patient should understand the symptoms of depression, the expected side effects of medication, the risks of no treatment, and the expected time course for improvement. Lack of compliance is often due to failure of development of a therapeutic alliance.

Adverse Effects

Most patients experience adverse effects. The particular spectrum of adverse effects in one class of antidepressants may limit their use—eg, the risks of anticholinergic side effects limit the use of heterocyclics in asthma and closed-angle glaucoma. A common clinical problem is the treatment of depressed patients with cardiac arrhythmias or congestive heart failure. Fluoxetine and bupropion are thought to impose lower risks in patients with compromised cardiovascular systems.

Table 32–2 lists the common adverse effects of antidepressants. The antidepressants vary in their side effect profiles. It is important to consult textbooks on psychopharmacology—as well as package inserts—whenever there is a question of drug-drug inter-

Table 32–2. Adverse effects of antidepressants.

Anticholinergic effects	Dry mouth, blurred vision, constipation, urinary hesitancy, toxic-confusional states
Antihistaminic effects	Sedation
Serotonergic activation	Sedation, restlessness
Adrenergic activation	Tremor, excitement, palpitation, orthostatic hypotension, weight gain

action. One must listen carefully to patients' complaints. After years of prescribing drugs, it is easy to dismiss a new complaint as unrelated to the medication. For example, when a patient taking nortriptyline reports tinnitus, it is tempting to regard the complaint as hypochondriacal or as a somatic preoccupation. Tinnitus is, in fact, listed as an infrequent possible side effect of nortriptyline, and in the case presently in mind, the tinnitus was dose-related and disappeared following reduction of the dose.

The presence of concurrent medical illness also affects the choice of antidepressant. For example, liver disease may cause the clinician to select a drug excreted by the kidney or at least to initiate treatment at low doses and delay dosage increases.

Finally, one may take advantage of some of a drug's side effects when selecting the most appropriate agent. For example, one may wish to choose a sedating drug such as doxepin when treating a depressed patient with insomnia, because the patient may initially be motivated to take it for its hypnotic effect. In contrast, a patient with severe psychomotor retardation may do better on a more stimulating drug such as protriptyline.

2. MONOAMINE OXIDASE INHIBITORS

Efficacy

Monoamine oxidase inhibitors are most often used to treat "atypical depression," which is characterized by hypersomnia, hyperphagia, somatic complaints, and dysphoria. They are also used as a second-line drug when treatment has been started with heterocyclic drugs but has failed.

Compliance

Because these drugs may lead to serious consequences when combined with certain foods and pharmacological agents (see below), it is important to assess the patient's ability to understand and comply with dietary and other restrictions. They should not be used, for example, by alcoholic patients who cannot remain abstinent.

Adverse Effects

Monoamine oxidase inhibitors were probably underutilized in the 1970's because of clinicians' fears about the adverse effects. They share some adverse effects with heterocyclic antidepressants, including orthostatic hypotension, sedation, urinary hesitancy, constipation, dry mouth, and weight gain. Specific effects of monoamine oxidase inhibitors include insomnia and daytime stimulation, hypertensive crises (due to interactions with medications and selected foods), muscle cramps, myoclonic twitches, and hyperpyrexic reactions. The spectrum of foods to be definitely avoided is broad and includes beer and red wine, aged cheeses, fava beans, yeast, smoked meats, and liver. All sympathomimetic amines need to be avoided. Particularly apt to cause problems are over-the-counter cold remedies—such as pseudoephedrine—because the patient believes drugs that can be purchased without prescription are "weak" or harmless.

Other prescription drugs such as meperidine and fluoxetine (an antidepressant) have been implicated in patient fatalities when combined with monoamine oxidase inhibitors. Patients must be carefully educated about the risk of hypertensive crisis, which is potentially fatal, and given lists of foods and medications to avoid. Some clinicians suggest that patients receiving these drugs be instructed to wear "Medic-Alert" bracelets so that potentially fatal drug interactions can be avoided in unconscious patients.

3. OTHER DRUGS

The miscellaneous drugs listed in Table 32–1 are no more effective than heterocyclic antidepressants for treating major depression but may be used because of special properties related to side effects or clinical characteristics of the patient. For example, fluoxetine may be preferred in a depressed patient who previously experienced weight gain while taking heterocyclic antidepressants. Trazodone may be chosen because of its low incidence of anticholinergic side effects. The student is referred to books on psychopharmacology and package inserts for discussion of each drug.

Lithium and carbamazepine are listed under the heading "mood stabilizers." These drugs are not very effective when used alone to treat a depressed episode, but they may be used in combination with an antidepressant to potentiate its effects. They may also be used to prevent recurrent episodes of depression. They will be discussed in greater detail below in the section on mania.

THERAPEUTIC STRATEGIES

1. HETEROCYCLICS

Desipramine is used as a prototype of the heterocyclic antidepressants in order to illustrate an approach to treatment. The therapeutic strategy will remain the same for the use of most heterocyclic antidepressants, though the dosing schedules may not, since all heterocyclics are not equipotent.

Pretreatment Workup

Workup before initiating antidepressants is done mainly to rule out organic causes of depression. In patients over 45 years of age or with histories of cardiac disease, an ECG is recommended. Other baseline tests, such as complete blood counts or liver function tests, are not usually necessary.

Initiating Treatment

It is essential at the outset to educate the patient about the antidepressant being recommended. One should proceed to use a given drug only after it is clear that compliance can be anticipated. If the patient has never taken an antidepressant before, it is wise to give a test dose the first night. A healthy young patient may be given 25–50 mg of desipramine, while a geriatric patient might be given 10–25 mg. The patient should be told what to expect and to call if there are unexpected adverse effects or if additional questions need to be answered.

Dose Increments

While individual patients may improve on low doses of antidepressants, most will not improve unless a dose of at least 150 mg per day of desipramine is achieved. An initial goal, then, is to achieve a dosage of 150 mg daily as quickly and safely as possible without affecting compliance. There are many schedules for dose increases. For example, 25 mg every other day or 50 mg every 3 or 4 days may be well tolerated in young healthy patients. Once 150 mg per day is achieved, a 7- to 14-day period can be used to monitor target symptoms. If no improvement occurs, the dose may be increased (for example) by 50 mg a week. The upper limit of desipramine dosage is generally 300 mg a day unless serum levels still fall well below the upper limit of the therapeutic range at that dose. It is important to emphasize that the major skills to be mastered are not pharmacological ones but rather assisting the patient in tolerating benign side effects and inculcating appropriate expectations for improvement.

Duration

A key reason for failure in treatment is the failure to treat for an adequate length of time. A 7- to 14-day trial at each dosage increment is adequate. When one has achieved either the maximum dose (eg, 300 mg/d of desipramine) or a dose that cannot be raised further due to adverse effects, a 2- to 4-week period should elapse before terminating the antidepressant trial. When adverse effects are benign (eg, dry mouth), further education about treatment and drug side effects is necessary prior to abandoning the drug.

Blood Levels

While serum levels are measurable for all antidepressants at least on a research basis, tricyclic levels are commonly the only measures available in most hospitals. A number of problems exist in regard to serum levels of drugs. Few drugs have established therapeutic ranges. Antidepressants have many metabolites, several of which may have therapeutic effects. Among the tertiary tricyclic antidepressants (amitriptyline and imipramine), both the parent tertiary and the derivative secondary amine (nortriptyline and desipramine, respectively) are, by convention, added together to form one serum level. Even when there are established therapeutic ranges, the information has limited utility. For example, for desipramine, the therapeutic range is 150–300 ng/mL. If the serum level is below 150 ng/mL, it is clear that the dose should be raised. If the level is above 300 ng/mL, the dose should be decreased (toxic levels usually exceed 500 ng/mL). When the serum level lies within the therapeutic range and the patient has been on the antidepressant for 2–3 weeks without benefit, the dose should be increased. Thus, a dose within the therapeutic range that fails to produce an antidepressant effect does *not* indicate failure of the trial. The trial should proceed until the upper limits of dose (in this case, 300 mg/d) have been achieved or until the serum level exceeds the usual therapeutic levels. In general, serum levels are measured toward the end of a clinical trial when no improvement has occurred. They are obtained more frequently in high-risk individuals such as the aged.

Treatment Failure

We have already mentioned some common causes of treatment failure: compliance problems, the inability to achieve an adequate dose of medication, and failure to maintain the patient on an adequate dose for a long enough time. Sometimes the patient has improved but the physician or patient fails to recognize the improvement. The background character structure of the patient may be depressive. The depressed patient may be so socially impaired that his behavior and self-report fail to improve while the biological aspects of the depression remit. Furthermore, concurrent medical problems and psychiatric comorbidity may make assessment difficult. Patients suffering from a major depressive episode who also have borderline personality disorder are particularly difficult to assess since their volatile affects and acting out behavior continue.

Another reason for failure is that the depressed patient has actually failed to respond to an adequate therapeutic trial. This may occur in an uncomplicated first presentation of depression between 5% and 15% of the time. In recurrent depressive illness or in depression with psychiatric or medical comorbidity, treatment failure occurs more frequently. "Refractory depressions" are defined by failure to respond to two complete antidepressant trials. Since many of the antidepressants are thought to work through similar mechanisms, an agent that differs in its spectrum of neurotransmitter actions should be selected for the second trial. For example, if desipramine (a drug that affects noradrenergic systems) was used in the initial trial, a trial of fluoxetine (a serotonergic agent) might serve as the next drug. Electroconvulsive therapy is the most effective treatment (90% success rate) for major depressive disorder and should always be considered after failure of drug therapy. Other treatment strategies, such as giving combinations of agents, are beyond the scope of this chapter.

Failure of a trial of treatment should always cause the physician to reconsider the initial diagnosis.

Maintenance & Prophylaxis

It is generally held that treatment should continue for 6 months to 1 year, with the first 6 months on full treatment doses, tapering thereafter to a maintenance dose starting at about 6 months. However, recent reports suggest that full doses should be given for up to 12 months. While maintenance doses have never been established, most clinicians use maintenance doses that are about half the therapeutic levels.

There is debate about whether a patient should remain on antidepressants for more than 1 year. Antidepressants do prevent recurrences, and the decision to maintain a patient on antidepressants for longer than a year is usually made because the patient suffers frequent recurrences, or because the symptoms recur during the process of dose tapering, or because there are severe morbidity or mortality risks without treatment.

2. MONOAMINE OXIDASE INHIBITORS

The strategy for initiating and titrating dosage with monoamine oxidase inhibitors is similar to that of heterocyclic antidepressants, though dosage increments are usually smaller. The physician must check the patient for orthostatic hypotension and continually reinforce the need for maintaining the tyramine-free diet and drug restrictions (many patients begin to "cheat" after successfully negotiating a slice of pizza, for example).

A different approach is used for monitoring the "dose" of monoamine oxidase inhibitors, though few hospitals have the appropriate assay available, ie, measurement of "percent inhibition." Several studies have demonstrated that monoamine oxidase must be 85% inhibited in order to achieve therapeutic results. Platelets contain monoamine oxidase and can be used to assay inhibition. A baseline sample of blood is drawn and platelets separated and tested with a monoamine oxidase substrate to determine its converting activity. After the patient has been on the inhibitor, platelets are again obtained and tested for monoamine oxidase activity. This later activity is compared with baseline, producing the measure "percent inhibition" (the dose is raised if monoamine oxidase activity is less than 85% inhibited over baseline). A target dose of 1 mg/kg is commonly used.

3. OTHER ANTIDEPRESSANTS

In general, blood levels are not available for the other nonheterocyclic antidepressants. In the case of fluoxetine, most patients respond to a single 20-mg dose given in the morning. The student is referred to pharmacology texts for information about other nonheterocyclic antidepressants.

Lithium may be used either as an adjunct to antidepressants or, in cases of frequent recurrent depression or atypical bipolar disorder, to prevent recurrences.

CASE STUDY: MAJOR DEPRESSIVE EPISODE

Mr M was referred by his primary care physician for assessment and treatment of depression. He had recently been involved in a boating accident in which he was severely burned over his lower extremities. After discharge from the hospital, he began to flounder in his work as an attorney in solo practice. His physician was concerned that he had developed depression.

Assessment of the patient showed a clearly depressive mood, terminal insomnia, loss of concentration, decreased appetite and a 12-pound weight loss, inability to work productively, and ruminations about his accident. He had passing thoughts of suicide and feelings of being overwhelmed.

Mr M was divorced, and his teenage son lived in the home. Furthermore, he had a strong family history of depression and, to make matters worse, a gun collection.

The psychiatrist judged Mr M to be suffering from major depression and was able to identify target symptoms for the early phase of treatment (sleep and appetite disturbance and some psychomotor retardation). After discussion of the various treatment alternatives, his living at home, and his gun collection, Mr. M agreed to the following plan.
  (1) Initiate desipramine, 50 mg at bedtime, to be increased to 150 mg at bedtime within 1 week (1 week's prescription at a time to be given because of the suicidal ideation).
  (2) Mr M's son to stay with his mother.
  (3) Mr M to move in with his parents for a brief time.
  (4) Mr M's brother to padlock the gun locker and keep the key. (The doctor to contact the brother and secure his agreement.)
  (5) Mr M to return in 1 week for reevaluation and to call in several days about drug effects.

Mr M called 2 days later and reported dry mouth and no improvement. He was tolerating the desipramine well. On reevaluation in 1 week, he was still tolerating the medication, now at a dosage of 150 mg at bedtime. He was seen weekly for 5 weeks. In the third week, his sleep and appetite began to improve (the dose had been increased to 200 mg at bedtime in the second week). He began to be able to work at the office a few hours a day during the fourth week and returned to his home. By the sixth week, he recognized clear improvement in mood and energy and had his son return home. Mr M continued seeing the psychiatrist and taking desipramine for about a year after returning to work.

PHARMACOTHERAPY OF MANIA

AGENTS & CLASSES OF AGENTS

Lithium is the standard treatment for manic episodes and is usually the first-line agent unless there has been documented treatment failure of the drug or is medically contraindicated. It is over 95% effective in the management of acute mania. Anticonvulsants, especially carbamazepine and valproic acid, are also used. Calcium channel blockers have been tried experimentally with variable results. Other agents, such as benzodiazepines, may also be used early in treatment along with lithium to help manage the patient, as lithium's antimanic effects have a fairly slow onset (7–10 days).

Prior to the introduction of lithium in the United States in 1970, neuroleptics were used to control the symptoms of mania and are still used in combination with lithium in "psychotic" or "tertiary" mania. In this chapter, the discussion will focus on lithium.

INDICATIONS

1. TARGET SYMPTOMS & SYNDROMES

The symptoms of manias likely to respond first are increased psychomotor activity, pressured speech, and lack of sleep. One then sees improvement in the patient's expansive mood, grandiosity, and intrusiveness. In some patients, affective symptoms may include irritability and hostility in place of expansiveness, or mood may be labile and shift from day to day or from hour to hour. Symptoms relating to disorganization of the form of thought (eg, flight of ideas, loosening of association) are more likely to respond to lithium than delusional content, such as paranoia. Target symptoms often do not begin to abate until 1–2 weeks after initiating treatment and may diminish slowly over time. Lithium alone is often not effective in treating psychotic manic symptoms such as delusions and hallucinations.

2. SPECIFIC DISORDERS

Lithium may be used to treat an acute manic episode and to prevent recurrences of mania. As mentioned above, it is also used in some cases in the treatment and prevention of depression, especially when a patient is judged to have an "atypical" bipolar disorder with brief hypomanic episodes preceding depressive periods. Lithium may also be considered in treating patients with hypomanic or cyclothymic disorders. In these cases especially, the decision to treat must balance the socioeconomic risks of the illness with the side effects of the drug.

Compliance

Voluntary discontinuance of lithium is a common problem in patients suffering from manic depressive illness and is often a function of the presence of grandiose-euphoric manias. Patients have difficulty understanding that the "highs" are part of their illness, and even when they do they may not wish to "give up" the mania. Bipolar patients with a predominance of depressive over manic episodes or those that have dysphoric, irritable, and paranoid manias tend to be more compliant, since they have generally suffered adverse consequences of mania. Side effects may also limit patients' willingness to take lithium, particularly if tremor develops.

Adverse Effects

Adverse effects of lithium include dry mouth, thirst, urinary frequency, tremor, and gastrointestinal distress, which may include nausea, vomiting, and diarrhea. Nontoxic goiter can occur in patients receiving chronic lithium therapy. Hypothyroid states may develop during treatment as well. Rarely, nephrogenic diabetes insipidus may develop. Serious lithium toxicity usually occurs at serum levels over 1.5 meq/L and includes drowsiness, slurred speech, blurred vision, hyperactive deep tendon reflexes, ataxia, cardiac arrhythmias, and seizures.

Several medical conditions may make the management of bipolar disease difficult—especially hypertension requiring the use of diuretics, since patients require less lithium and must be followed more closely if treated with both lithium and diuretics. Other conditions or drugs that influence salt and water balance may also pose difficulties for management with lithium.

THERAPEUTIC STRATEGIES

Pretreatment Workup

The patient should have had a complete physical examination within 6 months before treatment is started. It is also customary to check renal function and serum electrolytes and to assess thyroid function as a baseline for subsequent monitoring of function during chronic treatment with lithium. The clinician should be certain that women of childbearing age are not pregnant, and they should be warned not to become pregnant. An ECG may be obtained to rule out arrhythmias that may be exacerbated by lithium treatment.

Initiating Treatment

Lithium carbonate may be initiated at a dosage of 300 mg 2 or 3 times daily in young healthy adults. Most patients will require between 900 and 1800 mg a day to achieve therapeutic lithium levels. Large patients or those who have more severe symptoms may require higher doses; frail elderly patients or those receiving diuretics or who have compromised renal function may need lower doses.

Dose Increments

Three to 5 days after initiating treatment, a lithium level should be obtained in the early morning prior to the first dose. The dose should be increased by 300 mg if below 0.8 meq/L. Lithium levels should be measured frequently early in the course of management and less often once stable therapeutic levels have been achieved. Generally, the therapeutic range for lithium is considered to be 0.8–1.2 meq/L, and achieving this level may require lithium doses up to 2400 mg/d.

Duration

It may take 3–5 days to achieve a steady state for any lithium dose. Once a therapeutic level has been achieved, it takes 1–2 weeks for improvement in target symptoms. If no improvement has occurred by that time, the dose can be increased as long as the lithium level does not exceed the therapeutic range.

Blood Levels

Blood levels are an important part of monitoring lithium treatment. The sample should always be drawn as close to 12 hours after a lithium dose as possible, which usually means before the morning dose. Once the patient has been stabilized on a therapeutic dose, patients being maintained on lithium should have their levels checked about every 4 months or whenever their water or electrolyte status changes (eg, when diuretics are initiated, when sweating more).

Treatment Failure

Few manic patients will fail to recover on therapeutic lithium trials. In the few treatment failures that do occur, neuroleptics or carbamazepine may be added to the regimen. Occasionally, the diagnosis of mania is incorrect. Early in the course of illness, intoxication (eg, with stimulants), disorganized anxious states, and psychosis may be mistaken for mania. Most of these conditions will improve over time without intervention. Chronic manic-like syndromes can be caused by metabolic or endocrinological disorders.

A key cause of treatment failure is rapid-cycling manic depressive illness. Rapid cycling (conventionally defined as three or more episodes per year) is difficult to treat and may be exacerbated by lithium and by heterocyclic antidepressants.

Maintenance & Prophylaxis

Once the manic episode has abated, the patient's lithium requirement often decreases. In most cases, patients should also be kept on a maintenance dose of lithium (sometimes requiring levels of only 0.5–0.7 meq/L) to prevent recurrences. This is especially true of patients whose manic episodes result in significant destructive behavior. There is recent evidence that patients who frequently discontinue their lithium may eventually fail to respond to it when they become manic.

Patients receiving maintenance doses of lithium should continue to have lithium levels, thyroid function, serum electrolytes, and renal function monitored periodically.

CASE STUDY

Please see the Mayor of Wino Park in Chapter 15 for a description of the treatment of a patient with "tertiary" mania.

PHARMACOTHERAPY OF PSYCHOSIS

AGENTS & CLASSES OF AGENTS
(Table 32–3)

Over the centuries, sedation has been virtually the only method of treatment of psychosis, anxiety, and depression. Alcohol, bromides, opium, or, in the earlier part of this century, barbiturates have all been used to "calm" psychotic patients. Wet packing, restraints, and other nonpharmacologic treatments have been routinely used as well.

In 1952, chlorpromazine was used to protect the body from its own autonomic compensatory reactions during surgery. It was soon discovered incidentally to have a beneficial effect on psychotic patients who happened to receive the drug and thus was extended from anesthesiology to psychiatry. This drug and oth-

Table 32–3. Neuroleptics.

	Chlorpromazine Equivalence	Common Usage Range (mg)
Phenothiazines		
Chlorpromazine	1	100–1000
Thioridazine	1	100–800
Mesoridazine	2	50–400
Trifluoperazine	36	5–60
Perphenazine	11	8–64
Fluphenazine	85	2–60
Thioxanthenes		
Thiothixene	19	2–120
Chlorprothixene	2	100–600
Butyrophenones		
Haloperidol	62	2–100
Dibenzoxazepines		
Loxapine	7	20–160
Clozapine	1–2	50–900
Dihydroindolone		
Molindone	10	20–200
Depot		
Fluphenazine decanoate		12.5–25/month
Haloperidol decanoate		50–100/month

ers like it were the first therapeutic agents to have a *specific* antipsychotic action (rather than merely sedating effects). They are known as neuroleptics, antipsychotic drugs, or sometimes, inappropriately, "major tranquilizers." Almost all effective neuroleptics act on dopamine neurotransmission, blocking dopamine receptors.

There are five main classes of neuroleptics: phenothiazines (including aliphatic, piperidine, and piperazine types), butyrophenones, thioxanthines, indoleamines, and dibenzazepines. All neuroleptics are theoretically equally effective antipsychotic agents, but patients who fail to respond to a drug from one class may respond to one from another.

INDICATIONS

Neuroleptics are effective in treating psychotic symptoms which may be seen in schizophrenia, brief reactive psychosis, schizophreniform disorder, affective illness (manic and depressed), and organic mental disorders. They are less effective in treating delusional disorders and have a limited place in the treatment of severe anxiety states.

1. TARGET SYMPTOMS & SYNDROMES

Neuroleptics have pharmacological effects that lead to remission of some psychotic symptoms and attenuation of other associated symptoms. Since the effects of neuroleptics are not "disorder-specific" but rather "symptom-specific," leading either to remission or attenuation of symptoms, knowledge of the target symptoms is essential. Psychotic disorders are associated with disturbances of arousal, affect, psychomotor activity, thought content (both formal thought disorder and content disorder), and social adjustment.

Symptoms of arousal include agitation, anxiety, confusion, disorientation, insomnia, excitement, and vigilance. These symptoms are the first to improve after initiation of neuroleptics—within hours at the earliest but routinely in 3–5 days.

Affective symptoms often overlap with arousal. Reduction in arousal secondarily reduces affects as well. Common affective symptoms associated with psychosis include aggressiveness, anxiety, depression, grandiosity, hostility, irritability, negativism, and suicidal tendencies. Affects improve—after the initial effect of reduced arousal—over 1–3 weeks of treatment. The depression, which is often secondary, is less likely to respond than some other affective symptoms.

Formal thought disorder may be divided into fluent disorders (loosening of associations, flight of ideas, pressure of speech and thought, and circumstantiality), and nonfluent or negative symptoms (poverty of content of thought, blocking, and uncommunicativeness). Fluent thought disorder often dramatically improves following reduction in arousal and affect—often leaving some residual speech or communicative problem. Nonfluent negative symptoms do not tend to improve as dramatically and are frequently present after the resolution of other target symptoms.

Disturbances in content of thought include delusions, hallucinations, feelings of unreality, and paranoid or bizarre ideation. Neuroleptics are effective when these symptoms are acute or subacute but less effective when chronic. In the case of an acute disturbance, reduction in paranoia and delusional content may be seen within a few days to a week.

General motor and psychomotor behaviors are altered in psychosis. Catatonia, waxy flexibility, retardation, and hyperactivity can be observed. Psychomotor symptoms include peculiar mannerisms and facial grimaces and stereotypical behavior. While these motor symptoms may improve slowly (over several weeks), increased motor behavior associated with agitation will respond more promptly. Since neuroleptics have profound extrapyramidal side effects, ongoing assessment of motor behavior is important in order to detect akathisia and pseudoparkinsonism. It is important not to mistake these extrapyramidal syndromes for a continuation of psychotic motor behaviors.

As with depression, many symptoms experienced by schizophrenic patients are not specifically treated with neuroleptics. Defective judgment, social withdrawal, and deterioration of social habits fall into this class of symptoms. Poor rapport, lack of insight, and inappropriateness of affect may be primary symptoms of schizophrenia but remain largely untreatable with medication.

2. SPECIFIC DISORDERS

Schizophrenia

Schizophrenia is subdivided into catatonic, disorganized, paranoid, undifferentiated, and residual types. Neuroleptics are effective in treating the acute exacerbations of any subtype of the schizophrenias. Acute symptoms such as fluent thought disorder (a component of formal thought disorder) and the thought content problems of hallucinations and delusions respond well. There are no drugs with a similar spectrum of therapeutic action. Neuroleptics are less effective in treating residual symptoms, particularly nonfluent formal thought disorder, poverty of speech, poverty of content of speech, blocking, and negativism (the so-called negative symptoms of schizophrenia).

Neuroleptics are effective in the prophylaxis of acute schizophrenic episodes. Placebo substitution studies clearly demonstrate more frequent recurrences in placebo groups.

Delusional Disorders

Neuroleptics are infrequently effective in delusional disorders. This disorder with onset in the middle years of life has no known effective pharmacotherapy, though most psychiatrists will conduct a treatment trial in hope of a response.

Brief Reactive Psychosis & Schizophreniform Disorder

Neuroleptics are usually quite effective in reducing the acute psychotic symptoms associated with either brief reactive psychosis or schizophreniform disorder. Many clinicians withhold pharmacotherapy for a few days to see if hospitalization and withdrawal from a stressful environment will ameliorate symptoms. When neuroleptics are used, their prompt withdrawal is usually accomplished days or weeks after recovery. Many individuals with schizophreniform disorders go on to develop schizophrenia, in which case guidelines for the management of schizophrenia are in order.

Affective Illness

The neuroleptics are used in depressive disorders in the management of psychosis. Treatment is often initiated first with a neuroleptic and followed with addition of an antidepressant, though some physicians initiate both concurrently. In either case, the neuroleptic should be withdrawn after weeks to months as long as psychotic symptoms have remitted. Psychotic symptoms in depression—particularly delusions of self-deprecation and self-accusation—may respond to antidepressants alone, but frank hallucinosis usually requires neuroleptics.

A similar case can be made for psychotic mania. Neuroleptics are used in combination with lithium for a brief period to reduce arousal and psychotic symptoms. Since no parenteral form of lithium is available, neuroleptics alone are often used until the patient is willing to take oral lithium.

Anxiety Disorders

Neuroleptics are rarely indicated in anxiety disorders, though psychoses may be misdiagnosed as anxiety. Occasionally, arousal is so uncontrolled (eg, in a severe chronic case of posttraumatic stress disorder) that anxiolytics are ineffective and a brief course of neuroleptics may be indicated. Occasionally, neuroleptics are used briefly to reduce arousal and affective intensity in patients with borderline personality disorder.

Organic Mental Disorders

Psychotic symptoms are often present in brain disorders. Inflammatory, allergic, endocrine, or infectious diseases of the brain and degenerative disorders such as Alzheimer's, Huntington's, or Parkinson's disease can present with psychotic symptoms. Endocrine disorders may also present with psychotic symptoms. Symptomatic improvement can often be achieved using low doses of neuroleptics in psychoses of organic origin. Consultation-liaison services in hospitals are heavy prescribers of low-dose neuroleptics in dementia and delirium presenting with psychotic symptoms and behavior management problems.

DRUG CHOICE

Efficacy

While neuroleptics have major potency differences, all neuroleptics appear to have equal efficacy. Fluphenazine and haloperidol are among the most potent neuroleptics; among the least potent (milligram for milligram) are chlorpromazine, thioridazine, and clozapine. As a general rule, the more potent drugs have fewer nonspecific adverse effects such as sedation, hypotension, and anticholinergic effects than the high-potency drugs. However, high-potency drugs cause more extrapyramidal side effects than low-potency ones. Unless other factors intervene, it is reasonable to select a high-potency neuroleptic.

Factors that might influence this decision include the need for sedating effects (chlorpromazine, thioridazine); sensitivity to extrapyramidal effects, requiring very low doses at initiation of treatment; and patient preferences based on prior experience with the drugs. In general, a history of good response to a particular neuroleptic should prompt the clinician to use that agent again for that patient.

Recent approval of clozapine by the FDA makes available an agent with a somewhat different spectrum of side effects and a potential for effectiveness in schizophrenia refractory to other treatment. The risk of agranulocytosis limits the use of clozapine to patients who have at lease twice failed to improve on standard neuroleptics. Since clozapine has little effect on the extrapyramidal system, it may have use in the treatment of psychotic schizophrenics with tardive dyskinesia.

Compliance

Failure to consistently take neuroleptics is the major reason for readmission of schizophrenic patients in acute episodes. Patients do not like neuroleptic medication because it slows thinking and affects motor performance—("It feels like a mental straitjacket"). (One young patient dissolved his medication in his parents' coffee in the morning "so they will know how it feels.") Uncomfortable subjective effects of neuroleptics are corroborated by normal volunteers. Education of the patient and family is essential.

Two long-acting parenteral neuroleptics are available in the USA: fluphenazine decanoate and haloperidol decanoate. Both drugs may be effective for 1–4 weeks after injection. Compliance is still necessary, since the patient must appear at a treatment facility to receive the next injection. There is some additional risk of **neuroleptic malignant syndrome** with long-acting agents, presumably because the drug cannot be promptly discontinued upon emergence of the syndrome.

Adverse Effects

See Table 32–4 for a list of common adverse effects.

A. Pharmacotherapy of Extrapyramidal Syndromes: With the use of high-potency neuroleptics, adverse effects consist largely of extrapyramidal syndromes, the most common of which are acute dystonia, akathisia, and pseudoparkinsonism. Anticholinergic agents (Table 32–5) are the most common means of treating these conditions.

Acute dystonic reactions associated with neuroleptics include muscle spasms in the neck, oral, facial, buccal, and lingual regions. A typical reaction may be torticollis. Acute dystonias usually occur within a day after starting therapy or after a dose increase. Acute dystonia is the only extrapyramidal syndrome with a higher incidence in the young than the old. Oral, intramuscular, and intravenous anticholinergic agents are effective in eliminating the symptoms. Intramuscular or intravenous therapy is recommended

Table 32–4. Adverse effects of neuroleptics.

Anticholinergic effects	Dry mouth, difficulty urinating, constipation, blurred vision, toxic-confusional states
Alpha-adrenergic blockade	Orthostatic hypotension, impotence, failure to ejaculate
Dopaminergic blockade	Extrapyramidal syndromes, galactorrhea, amenorrhea, impotence, tardive dyskinesia, weight gain
Antihistaminic effects	Sedation

Table 32–5. Anticholinergic agents.

	Dosage Ranges (mg/d)
Benztropine	1–6
Biperiden	2–8
Diphenhydramine	50–300
Trihexyphenidyl	4–15
Procyclidine	10–20

initially since the symptoms are extremely disturbing. Diphenhydramine, 50 mg intramuscularly or intravenously, is given, followed by 50 mg orally every 4 hours for several doses. Benztropine and biperiden may be used as well. When a dystonic reaction occurs, the patient usually wishes to discontinue the drug. Therefore, it is important to recognize the patient's vulnerability to dystonias so that therapy can be started with low doses and stepwise increases by small increments. If anticholinergics are continued for a few days and the neuroleptic is continued—or reduced in dose—dystonic symptoms rarely return. Some clinicians (controversially) start all young patients on a "prophylactic" dose of anticholinergic agent. It is common for patients to state that they are "allergic" to haloperidol (for instance) because they once had an acute dystonic reaction.

The extrapyramidal movement disorder called **akathisia** is composed of purposeless movements, usually of the lower extremities, and a subjective feeling of restlessness. The subjective restless feeling is quite uncomfortable, often worse than the motor restlessness. Akathisias are treated with anticholinergic agents. Both akathisias and pseudoparkinsonism usually occur after 2 weeks of neuroleptic treatment. The dose of neuroleptic must usually be decreased in addition to adding an anticholinergic.

Neuroleptic-induced **pseudoparkinsonian syndrome** closely resembles Parkinson's disease: cogwheeling movements, pill-rolling tremors, gait disturbances, and flat facies may all be present. Pseudoparkinsonism is usually treated by a 2-week course of anticholinergic medication. After discontinuing the anticholinergic drug, careful monitoring for the return of extrapyramidal symptoms is important. In general, symptoms do not return. Few clinicians support continuous treatment with anticholinergics unless repeated efforts to discontinue the drug have resulted in resurgence of unwanted side effects.

The development of extrapyramidal side effects may be an indication that the patient is at increased risk of developing **tardive dyskinesia** later in life, or this syndrome may develop as a side effect of ongoing therapy. Tardive dyskinesia is an involuntary movement disorder that consists of irregular choreiform or athetoid movements (or both). Patients taking neuroleptics develop the disorder at a rate of 2–4% per year over the first 7 years of exposure. Elderly women are at greater risk. Dystonias range from darting tongue movements and mouth puckerings to trunk twisting, pelvic thrusting, and grunting. Needless to say, the disorder can be quite crippling socially.

Details of the treatment of tardive dyskinesia are beyond the scope of this chapter. Early recognition is essential, since drug discontinuation will lead to disappearance of symptoms in one-third of patients and attenuation of symptoms in another third. Unfortunately, there is no effective or standard treatment for tardive dyskinesia, though vitamin E, calcium channel blockers, and benzodiazepines have been used with minimal success. Patients may be switched to clozapine. The presence of tardive dyskinesia in patients with repeated acute psychotic episodes is a major clinical challenge.

B. Concurrent Medical Illness: Few medical conditions act as contraindications to neuroleptics in the treatment of psychosis. A number of illnesses (eg, liver disease) may affect the selection of drug dose and the frequency of visits and medical monitoring. Elderly patients should be treated with high-potency neuroleptics in low doses and should be monitored carefully for hypotension and anticholinergic symptoms, including delirium.

THERAPEUTIC STRATEGIES

The major use of neuroleptics is for control of acute psychotic symptoms. Clinical guidelines for their use in conditions other than schizophrenia are not described and should not be assumed to be identical. In particular, in other conditions such as psychotic depression or mania, the neuroleptic dose is often much lower and the duration of use briefer than in the treatment of psychotic exacerbations of schizophrenia.

Initiating Therapy

The first step before initiating therapy in an acute psychotic episode is a review of prior treatment. Successful treated of a previous episode serves as guideline for the choice of neuroleptic and its ideal dose. The goal of pharmacotherapy with neuroleptics is to use the lowest effective dose. Since the dosage range is broad, prior experience with the patient's requirement will shorten the acute treatment course. For illustrative purposes, initiation of haloperidol will be described. Other neuroleptics are used similarly, with dosages adjusted to account for potency differences.

In a first psychotic episode, 5 mg of haloperidol twice daily may not only initiate treatment but may be an adequate maintenance dose. Most psychotic patients will respond to a total daily dose of 5–15 mg haloperidol or its equivalent in another neuroleptic.

Dose Increments

If after 2–5 days the patient shows no improvement in symptoms of arousal, such as excitement, increase the dose by 2 mg. (If "prn" dosage has been prescribed, add an amount equal to the average such dose employed.)

Duration

There is a great temptation to increase the dose unnecessarily because of lack of patience. The effects of neuroleptics take time—even the effects on arousal may take a week, and hallucinations and delusions take much longer than that. Hallucinations may not be reported but may be elicited on specific inquiry for up to 2 or more weeks. Delusional material may take even longer to subside. Distorted thoughts may remain even after the persisting delusions have disappeared. Patience is essential. When treatment necessitates hospitalization, the use of high doses often serves a ward staff's need to achieve control on the unit rather than the patient's clinical need for treatment.

Blood Levels

In general, assays for neuroleptics are not available, and when they are available guidelines for their use in dosing patients are lacking in proof of validity.

Treatment Failure

Acute psychotic episodes usually respond to neuroleptics when the drug can be tolerated in appropriate doses. Chronic psychotic symptoms do not, in general, improve. Since both hallucinations and delusions may become chronic, it is often difficult to predict whether neuroleptics will be effective in a patient with chronic symptoms. One target symptom group that is useful in predicting treatment response is arousal (agitation, anxiety, confusion, disorientation, insomnia, excitement, and vigilance). When the presentation includes significantly increased arousal and the recent or subacute onset of hallucinations and delusions, there is a high probably of remission of all psychotic symptoms. When hallucinations and delusions have a long history or when little arousal is present, there is far less likelihood of improvement on neuroleptics.

The recent introduction of clozapine has provided a useful new drug for the treatment of refractory schizophrenia.

CASE STUDY: ACUTE PSYCHOTIC EPISODE

John S was brought to the emergency room in the morning by his father and mother. He had returned from college unexpectedly several days earlier. The family was angry at first, then puzzled and worried. John had been an A student in high school and been accepted at prestigious colleges but decided instead to attend a state university close to home. According to the parents, he had behaved in bizarre ways over the last several days. John himself reported that a number of people, including his college roommate, had a plan to kill him. He had been up all night and had become very upset when questioned by his parents about his ideas. With enormous effort, his father had convinced John to come with him to the hospital.

On examination by the emergency room physician, John was found to be in good health. A drug screen was negative for evidence of "street drugs" that might cause psychosis. The physician found John to be paranoid, hypervigilant, and delusional, his thinking confused and circumstantial, and observed behavior that he took to represent hearing voices. The physician determined that John's current symptoms had developed over about 6 weeks.

The psychiatrist on call confirmed the physician's findings, also determining that John had few friends in high school and a history of mild obsessive compulsive behaviors. The psychiatrist recommended hospitalization. John at first rejected the recommendation, but his father ultimately convinced him to enter the hospital voluntarily.

On admission, a diagnosis of presumed schizophreniform disorder was confirmed after careful evaluation for affective illness, such as mania. Haloperidol, 5 mg twice daily, was prescribed. John not only remained in his room most of the first 3 days but barricaded the door the first night. The nursing staff felt he was little improved by day 3, while the psychiatry staff felt he was slightly less aroused. Both felt his psychomotor behavior was reduced. John still demonstrated some speech interruption that appeared to be due to auditory hallucinations, though he denied hearing voices. His dose was increased to 5 mg 3 times a day on the evening of the third day.

John began to interact with the staff by the sixth day. He became less irritated and less seclusive. His speech was less circumstantial and rambling. At the end of the second week, John's psychomotor behavior increased, and he complained of restlessness—indeed, he could hardly sit still. An interview and physical examination suggested akathisia. One milligram of benztropine twice daily reduced his restlessness.

John was discharged to home care after 14 days. On discharge, he still had paranoid ideation, but it was less firmly held and subject to doubt. He was far less aroused and able to talk about school, career goals, and his hospitalization. He agreed to cooperate in a specialized day treatment program (described further in Chapter 31).

PHARMACOTHERAPY OF ANXIETY & ANXIETY DISORDERS

AGENTS & CLASSES OF AGENTS

The most popular class of anxiolytic compounds for the last several decades has been the benzodiazepines. These drugs have virtually replaced all other anxiolytics because of their specificity, potency, and safety. Buspirone, a recently introduced nonbenzodiazepine compound, has not found broad use as yet. Antihistaminics are still used as anxiolytics, though their effects are primarily sedative. Barbiturates and their congeners, anxiolytics of choice in past decades, have fallen into disfavor because they produce dependency and tolerance and are dangerous in overdosage. There is rarely any reason to depart from the use of benzodiazepines in the treatment of symptomatic anxiety. (See Table 32–6 for a list of drugs and their dosage ranges.)

INDICATIONS

1. TARGET SYMPTOMS & SYNDROMES

Anxiety may be manifested as an internal subjective experience characterized by apprehensive expectation or worry as well as in symptoms of motor tension, autonomic hyperactivity, and vigilance (ie, arousal). All anxiety-dependent symptoms respond to anxiolytics. When anxiolytics are effective, all symptoms improve over the same time course, and usually immediately. While diazepam and chlordiazepoxide were introduced for the treatment of anxiety in the 1960's, the use of anxiolytics to treat specific anxiety disorders had to await developments in the classification of disorders. Donald Klein and others in the early 1970's recommended separating panic and panic with agoraphobia from other anxiety conditions on the basis of their pharmacological responses to heterocyclic antidepressants and monoamine oxidase inhibitors. In 1980, *DSM-III* differentiated the neurotic disorders according to specific criteria. The new classification sorts anxiety disorders into groups that respond to specific forms of treatment.

2. SPECIFIC DISORDERS

Generalized Anxiety Disorder

Generalized anxiety disorder shares many features of dysthymic disorder, such as chronicity and comorbidity with major depression. This disorder may not hold up as a distinct illness in the next revision of *Diagnostic and Statistical Manual (DSM-IV)*. Patients meeting criteria for generalized anxiety disorder respond to benzodiazepine anxiolytics with a reduction in symptoms. Symptoms usually return when the drug is discontinued.

Panic Disorder

There are three approaches to the therapy of panic disorder, but data as yet fail to support one over the others. The major chemotherapeutic approaches to panic disorder include heterocyclics (eg, imipramine), monamine oxidase inhibitors (eg, phenelzine), and benzodiazepines (eg, alprazolam). Nonpharmacological approaches include behavior therapy (exposure) and cognitive therapy. With effective treatment, the frequency and intensity of panic episodes are reduced or eliminated. Anticipatory anxiety usually improves after effective treatment of panic. While there is controversy over whether agoraphobia exists in the absence of panic disorder, most psychopharmacologists believe that both groups of syndromes respond to appropriate treatment. Investigators have suggested recently that drug therapies are effective in treating the panic symptoms while behavior therapies are more effective in treating phobic avoidance and agoraphobia. While we emphasize the pharmacological treatment of panic in this chapter, attention to behavioral and cognitive therapy is warranted.

Target symptoms for panic attacks include the subjective inner experience ("I'm going to die," "I'm having a heart attack," "I'm going crazy") and symptoms of autonomic stimulation (tachycardia, tachypnea, tremor, shortness of breath, etc). Benzodiazepines such as alprazolam have the advantage of prompt reduction in anxiety (with panic attacks requiring several weeks to respond). Heterocyclics and monoamine oxidase inhibitors are both effective in reducing panic

Table 32–6. Anxiolytics.

	Dosage Range (mg/d)
Benzodiazepines	
Chlordiazepoxide	15–200
Diazepam	6–40
Chlorazepate	15–60
Halazepam	60–160
Prazepam	20–60
Lorazepam	1–6
Oxazepam	45–120
Alprazolam	1–6
Barbiturates	
Amobarbital	60–150
Pentobarbital	90–120
Phenobarbital	30–120
Beta-blockers	
Propranolol	60–240
Atenolol	50–100
Antihistamines	
Hydroxyzine	75–400
Diphenhydramine	50–300

attacks, but with these drugs there is a latency period of several weeks from the establishment of a therapeutic dose, and they have little to no effects on anticipatory anxiety. Alprazolam is usually effective in doses of 3–9 mg/d, while imipramine requires 100–250 mg/d and phenelzine 30–60 mg/d. Dose escalations of heterocyclics and monoamine oxidase inhibitors should follow the principles discussed in the depression section. However, it is thought that lower doses are required to treat panic disorder than to treat major depression. Furthermore, panic disorder patients are often prone to develop agitation and may need to be introduced to these drugs more slowly.

Simple & Social Phobia

The current treatment of choice for simple phobia is exposure, a form of behavior therapy. Some simple phobias may be ''agoraphobia-like,'' in which case the standard treatment for agoraphobia may be attempted.

Social phobia is a recent syndrome construct that has been the subject of few pharmacological treatment trials. When social phobias do not seem to be **performance-oriented** (the core feature of social phobia), they may really represent agoraphobia. The standard pharmacological approach to social phobias (such as ''stage fright'') has been the use of beta-blockers (eg, propranolol, 80–120 mg) to reduce autonomic arousal prior to social exposure such as a lecture.

Obsessive Compulsive Disorder

It appears clear that obsessive compulsive disorder is a distinct biological illness. The heterocyclic agent clomipramine has recently been approved for its treatment. Other heterocyclics and benzodiazepines have been of negligible benefit. Fluoxetine may be effective in obsessive compulsive disorder as well.

Both obsessional and compulsive symptoms improve with clomipramine treatment, usually after the first couple of weeks and continuing into the second month. About half of obsessive compulsive patients experience moderate to marked improvement. It is helpful to inventory compulsive behaviors (such as checking rituals) and collect baseline information on their frequency before starting clomipramine in order to titrate the dose. Clomipramine is a tricyclic antidepressant with potent serotonin agonist effects—adverse effects follow the pattern of other serotonergic drugs such as fluoxetine, including restlessness and impotence. The initial dose is often 50 mg daily, increasing (as with the heterocyclics) to 300 mg daily.

Posttraumatic Stress Disorder

There is no specific pharmacotherapy for posttraumatic stress disorder. Symptomatic approaches are frequently used, targeting anxiety (benzodiazepines), depression (heterocyclics), and sleep (again benzodiazepines). Heterocyclic agents appear to be useful only when the patient meets criteria for major depression. Anxiolytics frequently provide minimal benefit in high-arousal states. Patients often abuse alcohol or other substances to reduce arousal. Monoamine oxidase inhibitors may be of assistance in attenuating flashbacks, but this effect has not been proved.

Organic Mental Disorders

The response of organic mental disorders with associated anxiety to benzodiazepines is highly variable. Empirical trials are frequently recommended, but careful assessment is required to determine if improvement has occurred. Benzodiazepines may produce disinhibition in individuals with organic mental disorders.

DRUG CHOICE

1. BENZODIAZEPINES

Efficacy

The selection of a specific benzodiazepine is governed by its intended use. If the intent is to treat a brief episode of ''high anxiety,'' a short-acting rapidly absorbed agent is selected (such as alprazolam or lorazepam). For continuous coverage of anxiety or for prophylaxis of panic disorder, longer-acting potent benzodiazepines may be more desirable (diazepam is a reasonable choice, though clonazepam is receiving increased attention). One common problem is the prescription of short-acting benzodiazepines that ''wear off'' before the next dose, producing early abstinence or rebound anxiety and craving for the drug. This problem is alleviated by more frequent doses or by switching to a longer-acting benzodiazepine.

Compliance

For the most part, anxious patients ''like'' taking benzodiazepines, since the rapid anxiolytic action is quite reinforcing. In very anxious patients with only mild attenuation of symptoms, escalation of dose without the physician's knowledge may occur. Compliance with physician recommendations to discontinue benzodiazepine use can be a problem as well. Since physicians have very different approaches to the use of benzodiazepines, patients often feel trapped—eg, when referred to Dr Q, John S discovered that Q disapproved of Dr T's use of clorazepate. John also felt accused of being an ''addict.''

The ''prn'' use of anxiolytics may also provide difficulties in the management of anxiety. ''As needed'' use of benzodiazepines should be confined to individuals who require anxiolytics on a less than daily basis. For persistent anxiety states, daily ad hoc use may exacerbate anxiety through rebound anxiety or the failure to adequately manage the symptoms.

Adverse Effects

Benzodiazepines are safe and effective medications. Because sedation is the most common side effect, patients should be advised to be cautious (particularly initially) in tasks that require alertness (such as driving). Other less common side effects include dizziness, weakness, nausea, impaired performance of complex motor tasks, ataxia, and memory difficulties (anterograde amnesia).

While little tolerance develops to the therapeutic effects of benzodiazepines, physical dependence can become a problem. Patients should be withdrawn slowly (eg, 10% a day) if withdrawal symptoms are to be avoided. Common withdrawal symptoms include anxiety, tremor, palpitations, sweating, nausea, and confusion. Seizures can occur upon abrupt discontinuation of high doses of short-acting benzodiazepines.

2. OTHER DRUGS

Beta-blockers such as propranolol are successful in managing generalized anxiety in patients who are "tuned in to their bodies," eg, those who are particularly aware of their pulse rate. Since beta-blockers slow the heart rate, such individuals are reassured, and subjective anxiety may subside. For most anxious individuals, the internal subjective experience of anxiety is the central symptom, and for such patients beta-blockers are ineffective.

Antihistamines are often used in elderly patients or with chronic drug misuse or dependency problems. Unfortunately, they are more sedating than anxiolytic.

Neuroleptics are occasionally used to reduce "high anxiety" but do so less specifically through reducing arousal. Since neuroleptics have undesirable adverse effects, lack specificity, and are associated with long-term risks of tardive dyskinesia, they are uncommonly used even in severe anxiety.

Barbiturates are rarely used for the treatment of anxiety.

THERAPEUTIC STRATEGIES

1. BENZODIAZEPINES

Pretreatment Workup & Contraindications

There are few, if any, medical contraindications for benzodiazepines—they may be used safely in most medical conditions and in combination with most medications. Hypersensitivity to benzodiazepines or a history of paradoxical excitement are two of the rare contraindications. No routine laboratory studies are required prior to initiating treatment.

Initiating Treatment

The initial dose of an anxiolytic is often the therapeutic dose as well. There is little need to gradually increase the dose as is done with the antidepressants and neuroleptics. Only in panic disorder and agoraphobia is it necessary to systematically escalate the initial dose to achieve satisfactory therapeutic results.

Dose Increments

Initial daily doses are generally increased by 50–100% if the first dose is ineffective—eg, alprazolam, 0.25 mg 4 times daily, may be increased to 0.5 mg 4 times daily after 3–5 days and then, if necessary to 1 mg 4 times daily—a stiff dose for general symptoms of anxiety but still less than may be needed in panic disorder.

Duration

The duration of treatment is perhaps the major area of disagreement among physicians. Chronic management with benzodiazepines is generally accepted in specific disorders such as panic disorder and agoraphobia when discontinuance is followed by recurrence of symptoms. More controversial is the chronic use of benzodiazepines in the management of generalized anxiety disorder and "common anxiety." In cases where anxiety can be shown to disrupt occupational, social, or family functioning and if adequate functioning is restored with use of the drugs and discontinuance is followed by return of dysfunction, the chronic use of these agents seems justified.

Blood Levels

Therapeutic levels of benzodiazepines have been established in research settings but are not generally available. Even if they were, they would be cost-ineffective since appropriate doses can be determined quickly and safely.

Treatment Failure

Anxiolytics are highly effective in reducing anxiety but rarely eliminate all anxiety. Thus, "treatment failure" with benzodiazepines usually means absence of an *adequate* anxiolytic response. When high doses are not effective, careful reassessment of the diagnosis is called for. A masked psychotic state is commonly present and may require use of neuroleptics.

PHARMACOTHERAPY OF INSOMNIA

Insomnia has many causes. In this section, the term denotes the complaint of trouble falling asleep, sleep continuity interruption, poor sleep quality, or decreased total sleep time which has no cause that may be more specifically treated, eg, major depression. In *DSM-III-R*, primary insomnia is diagnosed when such disturbances occur more than three times a week for at least 1 month and result in daytime fatigue or impaired daytime functioning.

Insomnia is a common complaint in general medical practice. It is usually not due to a primary psychiatric disorder or other specific sleep disorder. "Ordinary" insomnia may be due to anxiety, stress at work or at home, or even poor "sleep hygiene," ie, bad sleep habits. The physician's first task is to determine whether there may be a specific psychiatric or medical cause for insomnia. In the absence of a primary cause, the decision must be made whether to prescribe hypnotics. Other management strategies may be more appropriate, such as behavioral instruction or even encouraging the patient to "live with the problem."

Agents & Classes of Agents

The most important class of sedative-hypnotics is the benzodiazepines (Table 32–7). As discussed in the section on pharmacotherapy of anxiety and anxiety disorders, any benzodiazepine may be used as a sedative-hypnotic in the proper dose. Nevertheless, pharmaceutical companies have marketed specific benzodiazepines as sedative-hypnotics and by their dosage formulations (milligrams of drug per tablet or capsule) have made them more convenient to use as hypnotics rather than anxiolytics, eg, flurazepam rather than diazepam for sleep.

INDICATIONS

Physicians differ widely in their opinions about use of sleep-inducing medications. Some guard

against abuse and dependency by rarely prescribing sedatives except in hospital settings, while others offer them liberally upon patient request, often over a period of years. Most physicians would agree that severe insomnia (eg, primary insomnia) which interferes with daily functioning and that can be anticipated to be of brief duration is a good indication for pharmacotherapy. Furthermore, most physicians would agree that the chronic prescription of sedative-hypnotics over months or years is not appropriate. In the prescription of anxiolytics and sedative-hypnotics, we are, as physicians, often at odds with the wishes of our patients. The best guide to appropriate prescription is (1) an understanding of the causes of insomnia, eg, in terms of acute stressors or personality factors; (2) good patient education about the risks and benefits of sedatives; and (3) monitoring, as objectively as possible, of improved functioning brought about by the use of sedatives. In most instances, daily use of sedative-hypnotics should not continue for longer than several weeks.

1. TARGET SYMPTOMS & SYNDROMES

The diagnosis and treatment of specific sleep disorders is beyond the scope of this chapter. Sleep symptoms (not associated with specific syndromes) are generally reported by patients as "trouble falling asleep," "wakefulness," or "not getting enough sleep." Identification of the specific sleep complaint is important, since "trouble falling asleep" (initial insomnia) may suggest the use of a short-acting benzodiazepine such as triazolam while a patient with "multiple awakenings" (sleep continuity disorder) may require a longer-acting sedative such as flurazepam.

DRUG CHOICE

1. BENZODIAZEPINES

Efficacy

All drugs in the benzodiazepine class appear to be equally effective as sedative-hypnotics if the proper dose is selected. The major differences lie in their pharmacokinetic properties. Selection of a specific benzodiazepine is usually based upon the type of insomnia (initial or terminal insomnia and continuity problems), the side effect profile, and patient preference.

Compliance

Compliance with the use of sedative-hypnotics is rarely a problem. Patients complaining of insomnia are generally seeking chemical assistance in producing or maintaining sleep. On the other hand, patients

Table 32–7. Sedative-hypnotics.

	Dosage Range (mg/d)
Benzodiazepines	
Flurazepam	15–30
Temazepam	15–30
Quazepam	0.125–0.5
Lorazepam	7.5–15
	2–4
Barbiturates	
Secobarbital	100
Phenobarbital	100–120
Pentobarbital	100
Amobarbital	160–200
Miscellaneous	
Chloral hydrate	500–1000
Ethchlorvynol	500–750
Antihistamines	
Diphenhydramine	50–150

may escalate the dose of sedative without the knowledge of the physician. Assisting a patient in giving up sedative-hypnotics is often a problem. The patient should understand that discontinuing medication will often result in rebound insomnia which is mistaken for ordinary insomnia. Return of insomnia may reinforce the patient's conviction that sedative-hypnotics are necessary for comfortable functioning during the day.

Adverse Effects

The adverse effects of benzodiazepines are discussed in the section on anxiolytics. Patients using sedatives most frequently complain of daytime grogginess. This can often be avoided by using a shorter-acting drug or by taking the nighttime dose earlier in the evening.

2. OTHER SEDATIVE-HYPNOTICS

Barbiturates and antihistamines are still commonly used for sedation—barbiturates in hospital settings and antihistamines for elderly persons or those with a history of substance abuse. Many physicians use sedating heterocyclic antidepressants. Since the second-choice drugs have other chemical and psychotropic effects, their use is discouraged.

THERAPEUTIC STRATEGIES

"Common insomnia" is generally reported as trouble falling asleep (long sleep latency) or multiple awakenings (sleep continuity disorder). In general, early morning awakening (terminal insomnia) is associated with major depression.

Pharmacological treatment of insomnia should be confined to several weeks. When symptoms persist and the patient appears to have reduced total sleep time even when taking a sedative-hypnotic such as flurazepam, referral to a sleep disorder center may be indicated. Attention to appropriate "sleep hygiene" is an important aspect of insomnia assessment and treatment. Does the patient nap during the day? Toss and turn in bed? Snack before bedtime? Patients are instructed not to nap, to get out of bed to work or read until sleepy, and to refrain from snacking. The more obvious approach of understanding and mastering anxiety and conflicts and life challenges that precipitate insomnia should not be overlooked. Patients need to understand the goals of the use of sedative-hypnotics—usually brief assistance with trouble falling asleep or awakening.

II. OTHER SOMATIC TREATMENTS

ELECTROCONVULSIVE THERAPY

Historical Overview

The historical origins of electroconvulsive therapy (ECT) date back to the late 19th and early 20th centuries, when scientists began to examine the phenomenology of mental disorders and to investigate the nature of brain dysfunction. Two important and unrelated ideas converged to result in ECT. During the 1920's, researchers counting heads in French "lunatic asylums" noted a low prevalence of epilepsy in schizophrenic patients. This finding led Marchand to hypothesize a biological antagonism between epilepsy and psychosis. The idea that one disease could be used to treat another was exemplified by von Jauregg, who treated tertiary syphilis by giving patients malaria. The confluence of these two ideas led von Meduna to induce seizures in schizophrenic patients (first by injecting oil of camphor and later with pentylenetetrazole). At about the same time, Sakel achieved a similar result by inducing insulin coma in psychotic patients, though the seizure resulting from the hypoglycemic state was at first considered to be an undesirable by-product of the procedure rather than its therapeutic basis.

In 1938, Cerletti and Bini performed the first procedure in which an electrical current was passed directly through the brain, resulting in a generalized tonic-clonic seizure. The patient, who was found wandering around the train station in Rome, recovered from his psychotic episode after 11 treatments and was discharged within a few months. After the success of this treatment was publicized, it rapidly replaced other forms of seizure induction because it is easier to control than seizures induced with injected substances and is demonstrably safer.

Initially, ECT was performed with the patient alert and awake. The procedure was both frightening and associated with complications resulting from the often violent tonic-clonic convulsions. In addition, the procedure was at first often used indiscriminately, since there were few alternatives for treating severely depressed psychotic or violent patients. The procedure has been portrayed as a tool used by sadistic psychiatrists to punish "difficult" patients (eg, *One Flew Over the Cuckoo's Nest*). Hence, the procedure fell into disfavor, particularly as effective antidepressant and neuroleptic medications were introduced.

Today, ECT is enjoying a resurgence of popularity. The technique has been greatly modified since the early days. The patient is paralyzed to prevent the peripheral manifestations of the seizure, and anesthesia (sleep) is induced so that the patient is not conscious of the frightening sensations of being paralyzed and having a seizure. Modern techniques have significantly reduced morbidity and mortality as well, allowing ECT to regain its place as a respected and legitimate method of treatment for selected patients with serious psychiatric disturbances.

Indications

ECT is used today as a first-line treatment for patients who need rapid resolution of life-threatening symptoms, who cannot tolerate the medical risks of other treatments, or who have a history of poor response to other treatments. It is considered to be effective treatment for major depression with or without psychotic features, bipolar illness (both depressed and manic phases), and catatonic schizophrenia. It should be considered also in cases of schizophrenia with strong affective symptomatology. It is not considered effective for other forms of schizophrenia, though it is sometimes used for this purpose in highly treatment-resistant patients.

There is controversy surrounding the use of ECT for some other conditions for which its efficacy is considered merely suggestive. These conditions include delirium, severe organic affective/psychotic syndromes that mimic functional syndromes, and several medical conditions, including Parkinson's disease and catatonia secondary to organic causes.

Efficacy

ECT is more effective than antidepressants alone for the treatment of major depression with psychotic features and is as effective as the combination of antidepressants and neuroleptics. In one study, ECT was effective in most cases in which drug treatment failed. As a rule, bilateral ECT is more effective than unilateral (80–85% versus 90–95%). However, since there is some evidence that bilateral ECT imposes a higher risk of memory impairment, bilateral ECT is usually reserved for patients who have failed unilateral ECT or for those in whom rapid resolution of symptoms is of paramount importance.

Contraindications

Although there are no absolute contraindications to ECT, the procedure is usually not undertaken in the presence of increased intracranial pressure. Patients with a recent history of myocardial infarction, recent intracerebral hemorrhage, bleeding or unstable vascular aneurysm, retinal detachment, pheochromocytoma, or untreated glaucoma and those who have an ASA (American Society of Anesthesiologists) anesthetic risk of 4 have been treated with ECT but require special care and expertise.

Adverse Effects

Many patients experience some degree of confusion following ECT, which is to be expected given the normal occurrence of confusion in the postictal state. In patients who remain confused for a day or two following each treatment, it is often advisable to give two rather than three treatments per week. ECT has also been associated with long-term memory deficits, which are usually characterized by little or no memory of the period of hospitalization and in some cases events just before and just after hospitalization. Fewer than 1% of patients complain of amnesia 6 months after the treatment.

Because both pulse and blood pressure rise significantly during the seizure, patients with cardiac dysfunction are at higher risk for untoward events such as ischemia or arrhythmia. The anesthesiologist often uses medications to control pulse and blood pressure during the procedure. Occasionally, a patient may experience a prolonged (usually defined as > 2 minutes) seizure or a "late" seizure (which may in fact simply be a prolonged seizure masked by the barbiturate the patient has received). An occasional patient may experience prolonged apnea or laryngospasm.

Other side effects include burns from poor contact with the electrode, loose or broken teeth, and peripheral nerve palsy. Most patients experience some anxiety and apprehension, especially early in the course of treatment. Headache, muscle aches, and a vague sense of confusion for a few hours after the treatment are common.

Morbidity & Mortality

Studies indicate that about one in 1300–1400 patients experience significant adverse effects from ECT. The risk of death is 4.5 per 100,000 treatments.

Mechanism

Although it is clear that central nervous system seizure discharge is required for ECT to be effective, we do not understand the underlying neurophysiological or neurochemical mechanisms. ECT has many central nervous systems effects, causing changes in the EEG, hypothalamic hormone secretion, calcium metabolism, biogenic amine levels, and receptor sensitivity. The amnesia precipitated by ECT may itself contribute to the improvement. Further research on the effects of ECT may clarify the neurochemical mechanisms that underlie affective disorders.

Technique

When ECT is being considered, it is important to be sure that both the patient and the patient's family understand its risks and benefits and concur with the decision to provide treatment in this way. It may be necessary to explain the procedure several times to the patient, who may have some cognitive impairment as a result of the illness. A thorough medical evaluation is then done to determine if the patient may need pretreatment of any kind or special care during the treatment. Of course, informed consent is required.

Treatments are commonly done in the morning, usually 3 times a week. The patient has nothing to eat or drink after midnight before each treatment. An intravenous line is started, and atropine or a similar agent is administered. The electrode sites are carefully cleaned, and once the electrodes are placed on the patient's scalp, the machine is tested to make certain that the circuit is complete. At this point, the patient is usually oxygenated with an Ambu bag and then given a short-acting barbiturate intravenously to induce light sleep. When the patient is asleep, a bite block is inserted to protect the teeth, and succinylcholine is administered. When paralysis is confirmed (eg, by testing with a nerve stimulator, looking for termination of fasciculations, or testing plantar response), the electrical stimulus is applied. During this process, the patient is carefully monitored. Pulse and blood pressure are checked before the procedure, after anesthesia, during the seizure, and periodically during and after recovery. Since many ECT machines have a built-in EEG monitor, the seizure itself may be directly monitored. If no EEG is available, seizure duration is monitored by inflating a blood pressure cuff on one leg (usually at the midcalf level) after the patient is asleep and before the succinylcholine is given. The seizure can then be timed by watching the tonic-clonic movements in the unparalyzed limb. If the clinician is satisfied that an adequate seizure has been obtained, the patient is monitored carefully until alert. If the seizure was not adequate, a second stimulus, usually of greater duration or intensity, may be delivered. After initial recovery (eg, in the recovery room or ECT suite), the patient's vital signs and cognitive status are monitored on the ward for several hours. It is also good practice to watch for persistent signs of organicity (eg, disorientation, confusion). When this occurs, the treatments are often administered less frequently or even discontinued. Most depressed patients receive between 9 and 12 treatments. Manic patients often respond to only one or two, while schizophrenic patients may receive 15 or more treatments. Some clinicians deliver several stimuli in one treatment session (multiple-monitored ECT). This procedure may lead to more severe cognitive impairment.

In most cases, patients start receiving antidepressant medication after the completion of treatment in order to prevent relapse. In some cases, periodic maintenance courses of one or two ECT treatments every several months, as indicated by the historical pattern of response, are recommended to prevent relapse.

PSYCHOSURGERY

Once a fairly common procedure, psychosurgery for mental disorders has declined precipitously over the last three decades to the point where the it is almost never used today. Most "psychosurgery" these days is done on patients with epilepsy and involves ablation of the presumed epileptic focus. Most remaining psychosurgery utilizes stereotactic techniques to localize small key areas of the brain. The anatomical target is chosen selectively based on symptoms. For example, cingulectomy has been used to treat patients with severe chronic pain, with depression and addiction, and internal capsulotomy has been shown to be effective in patients with severe obsessive compulsive disorder who have not responded to behavior therapy or pharmacotherapy. Severe chronic recurrent depressions have been treated with innominotomy, while posteromedial hypothalamotomy has been used in patients with restless, aggressive, and destructive behavior.

Unlike the psychosurgery done earlier in the century that involved larger and less selective areas of the brain—often leaving patients with extensive behavioral morbidity—modern techniques usually cause little or no personality change. However, clinicians recommending psychosurgery must scrupulously guard the rights of patients. Patients and their families should fully understand the risks and potential benefits.

REFERENCES

Abrams R: *Electroconvulsive Therapy*. Oxford Univ Press, 1988.

Akiskal HS: A proposed clinical approach to chronic and "resistant" depressions: Evaluation and treatment. J Clin Psychiatry 1985;46:32.

Anton R, Burch E: Amoxapine versus amitriptyline combined with perphenazine in the treatment of psychotic depression. Am J Psychiatry 1990;147:1203.

APA Task Force on ECT: The practice of ECT: Recommendation for treatment, training and privileging. Convulsive Therapy 1990;6:85.

Aronson T, Shukla SL: Long-term continuation antidepressant treatment: A comparison study. J Clin Psychiatry 1989;50:285.

ASA–American Society of Anesthesiologists: New classification of physical status. Anesthesiology 1963; 24:111.

Baldessarini RJ: *Chemotherapy in Psychiatry: Principles and Practices*. Harvard Univ Press, 1985.

Barchas JD et al (editors): *Psychopharmacology From Theory to Practice*. Oxford Univ Press, 1977.

Blume HW, Schomer DL: Surgical approaches to epilepsy. Ann Rev Med 1988:48.

Bouckoms AJ: Ethics of psychosurgery. Acta Neurochir 1988:44:173.

Boyer WF, Lake CR: Initial severity and diagnosis influence the relationship of tricyclic plasma levels to response: A statistical review. J Clin Psychopharmacol 1987;7:67.

Carpenter W, Heinrichs D: Early intervention, time-limited targeted pharmacotherapy of schizophrenia. Schizophr Bull 1983;9:533.

Chouinard G: Bupropion and amitriptyline in the treatment of depressed patients. J Clin Psychiatry 1983;44:121.

Cohen BM: The clinical utility of plasma neuroleptic levels. Pages 245–260 in: *Guidelines for the Use of Psychotropic Drugs.* Stancer H (editor). Spectrum, 1984.

Davidson J et al: A double-blind comparison of bupropion and amitriptyline in depressed inpatients. J Clin Psychiatry 1983;44:115.

Donaldson SR, Gelenberg AJ, Baldessarini RJ: The pharmacological treatment of schizophrenia: A progress report. Schizophrenia Bull 1983;9:504.

Endler NS: The origin of ECT. Convulsive Therapy 1988;4:5.

Feighner J et al: Double-blind comparison of doxepin versus bupropion in outpatients with a major depressive disorder. J Clin Psychopharmacol 1986;6:27.

Fink M: *Convulsive Therapy: Theory and Practice.* Raven Press, 1979.

Fink M (editor): ECT in the high risk patient. Convulsive Therapy 1989;5(1). [Entire issue.]

Fontaine R, Chouinard G: An open clinical trial of fluoxetine in the treatment of obsessive-compulsive disorder. J Clin Psychopharmacol 1986;6:98.

Frank E et al: Three-year outcomes for maintenance therapies in recurrent depression. Arch Gen Psychiatry 1990;47:1090.

Glenn M, Weiner RD: *Electroconvulsive Therapy. A Programmed Text.* American Psychiatric Press, 1985.

Goldberg HL: Buspirone hydrochloride: A unique new anxiolytic agent. Pharmacokinetics, clinical pharmacology, abuse potential, and clinical efficacy. Pharmacotherapy 1984;4:315.

Greenblatt DJ, Shader RI, Abernethy DR: Current status of benzodiazepine. (Part I.) New England J Med 1983;309:354.

Jefferson JW et al: *Lithium Encyclopedia for Clinical Practice,* 2nd ed. American Psychiatric Press, 1986.

Jenike M et al: Open trial of fluoxetine in obsessive-compulsive disorder. Am J Psychiatry 1989;146:909.

Keck P et al: Time course of antipsychotic effects of neuroleptic drugs. Am J Psychiatry 1989;146:1289.

Klein DF et al: *Diagnoses and Treatment of Psychiatric Disorders: Adults and Children.* Williams & Wilkins, 1980.

Latinen LV: Psychosurgery today. Acta Neurochir 1988;44(Suppl):158.

Lydiard RB et al: Recent advances in the psychopharmacology of anxiety disorders. Hosp Commun Psychiatry 1988;39:1157.

McCall WV: Physical treatments in psychiatry: Current and historical use in the southern United States. South Med J 1989;82:345.

McElvoy S et al: Valproate in the treatment of rapid-cycling bipolar disorder. J Clin Psychopharmacol 1988;8:275.

Mason AS, Granacher RPL: *Clinical Handbook of Antipsychotic Drug Therapy.* Brunner/Mazel, 1980.

Mavissakalian M, Perel J: Imipramine dose-response relationship in panic disorder with agoraphobia. Arch Gen Psychiatry 1989;46:127.

Meltzer HY (editor): *Psychopharmacology: The Third Generation of Progress.* Raven Press, 1987.

Mills MJ: Legal issues in psychiatric treatment. Psychiatr Med 1984;2:245.

National Institutes of Health: *ECT: Consensus Development Conference Statement,* vol 5, No. 11.

Perse T: Obsessive compulsive disorder: A treatment review. J Clin Psychiatry; 1988;49:48.

Pollack MH, Rosenbaum JF: Management of antidepressant-induced side effects: A practical guide for the clinician. J Clin Psychiatry 1987;48:3.

Poynton A et al: Psychosurgery in Britain now. Br J Neurosurg 1988;2:297.

Preskorn SH: Tricyclic antidepressants: The whys and hows of therapeutic drug monitoring. J Clin Psychiatry 1989;50:34.

Prien R, Gelenberg A: Alternatives to lithium for preventive treatment of bipolar disorder. Am J Psychiatry 1989;146:840.

Schatzberg AF, Cole JO: *Manual of Clinical Psychopharmacology.* American Psychiatric Press, 1986.

Schou M: Lithium prophylaxis: Myths and realities. Am J Psychiatry 1989;146:573.

Thase M et al: Treatment of imipramine-resistant recurrent depression: II. An open clinical trial of lithium augmentation. J Clin Psychiatry 1989;50:413.

Zak JP et al: The potential role of serotonin reuptake inhibitors in the treatment of obsessive-compulsive disorder. J. Clin Psychiatry 1988;49(Suppl):8.

Zitrin CM, Klein DF, Woerner MG: Treatment of phobias: I. Comparison of imipramine hydrochloride and placebo. Arch Gen Psychiatry 1983;40:125.

Psychoanalysis & Long-Term Dynamic Psychotherapy*

33

Robert S. Wallerstein, MD

Sigmund Freud said of psychoanalysis that it was three things:

(1) A theory of how the mind works. Psychoanalysis attempts to comprehend and explain the normal and the abnormal functioning of the human mind at all ages. Many of the central psychoanalytic concepts—the unconscious, psychic determinism, infantile sexuality and the theory of drives, the Oedipus complex, ambivalence, anxiety, the defense mechanisms, psychic conflict, the structure of the mind or of the psychic apparatus—form a body of scientific knowledge that has now become part of our intellectual heritage. (See Chapter 2.) In 1947, Ernst Kris summarized psychoanalysis as a theory of the mind most tersely: Psychoanalysis is "*nothing but* human behavior considered from the standpoint of conflict. It is the picture of the mind divided against itself with attendant anxiety and other dysphoric affects, with adaptive and maladaptive defensive and coping strategies, and with symptomatic behaviors when the defenses fail." However, psychoanalysis is more than a theory of the mind and behavior.

(2) An investigative or research method. The technique of free association by the patient (analysand) makes it possible for the analyst to gain access to the data and processes of mental life, conscious or otherwise and rational or not. The data thus retrieved are made coherent and intelligible according to the theory of psychoanalysis. As Otto Fenichel said in 1941, it is the phenomenal data of psychoanalysis that may be irrational; the method and the theory are rational.

(3) A specific form of therapy of mental illness. Psychoanalysis uses free association to obtain data in the form of thoughts, feelings, memories, fantasies, and dreams and then proceeds to order and comprehend them within the framework of psychoanalytic theory. Through interpretation of psychic data, leading to insight and "working through," the treatment process is carried progressively forward.

---

* This chapter is an edited version of a more comprehensive and detailed treatment of the subject matter prepared by Dr Wallerstein for publication elsewhere. The editor is grateful for permission to adapt it for *Review of General Psychiatry.* –HHG.

Dynamic psychotherapy—also called psychodynamic therapy, psychoanalytic psychotherapy, or psychoanalytically oriented psychotherapy—is intensive psychological therapy based on psychoanalytic theory but without the specific technique of free association. A variety of techniques are employed, including interpretation, to treat patients not considered suitable candidates for psychoanalysis.

Both psychoanalysis and the psychoanalytic psychotherapies described in this chapter are "open-ended," ie, protracted therapies that may continue for many years. At the start of therapy, a pact is made between the analyst, or therapist, and the analysand, or patient, to explore the patient's psychological problems for as long as necessary in order to achieve an acceptable result. This is in contrast to short-term or brief (time-limited) psychotherapy (described in Chapter 34), which usually consists of 12 or 20 weekly or twice-weekly sessions of 50 minutes each. The critical difference between psychoanalysis and short-term therapy is not only the difference in duration, important as that is, but also the fact that the patient in time-limited psychotherapy is conscious of the agreed termination date from the first session and knows that what is to be done must be achieved by that deadline. One consequence is that the patient may be tempted, consciously or not, to withhold painful areas from therapeutic scrutiny—to be "saved by the bell," as it were. If open-ended therapy is to be completed successfully, whatever is not talked about now or next week will come out later, because treatment continues until all of the relevant psychological issues and problems are explored and resolved to the extent that is possible however long it takes. Long-term and open-ended therapy is thus quite different in important ways from short-term (time-limited) therapy and not just the same kind of thing for more hours.

PSYCHOANALYSIS

Psychoanalysis is a process of examination in continuity of the internal working of the mind on a day-to-day basis. On each successive day, the analyst and the patient can pick up where they left off and go from there. Ideally, this process would go forward 7 days a week for an hour each day. (This became the "50-minute hour" to allow analysts time between patients in which to order their thoughts, make notes, and get ready for the next patient.) However, because analysts and their patients want weekends for other things, the analytic work week is the traditional 5 working days, and Freud often complained of the "Monday crust"—the sealing over of open mental surfaces during the weekend, so that the first task on Monday would be to reestablish the continuity of daily exploration. Because of the limited availability of qualified analysts and the need to accommodate more patients, analyses are now conducted 4 days a week in some settings. Most analysts do not consider fewer than 4 days a week proper psychoanalysis, because the vital element of continuity does not survive longer or more frequent interruptions. Ideally, each session is scheduled at the same time each day so that the analysis can blend into the rhythm of the patient's life.

In classical psychoanalysis, the patient is recumbent on a couch with the analyst behind and out of the patient's line of vision. Intrusions, such as telephone calls, are avoided except in emergencies. The patient expressly undertakes to try to say whatever comes to mind no matter how seemingly remote, irrelevant, trivial, repugnant, anxiety-provoking, or shameful (the "fundamental rule"). The patient agrees to refrain from motor activity so that all available energy can be channeled into the effort to verbalize mental content. The analyst decides when and how to interject questions and comments; no attempt is made to sustain a conversational dialogue. The analyst must unswervingly focus attention on the effort to track the shifting subject matter of the patient's discourse and keep personal concerns, prejudices, values, and judgments out of the analytic field. The purpose is to gain and maintain full access to the contents of the patient's mind, conscious and unconscious, now and in the remote past and even to infancy if that can be achieved. Dreams, fantasies, wishes, fears, thoughts, and feelings of all kinds are discussed in the analysis. What is experienced by people practicing or undergoing psychotherapy is that "one thing leads to another." The patient focuses on his or her mental processes and free associates in what is apparently a random manner. The analyst apprehends what the patient verbalizes by a counterpart process of "free-floating attention" without preconceptions about what is important or what the relationships are between various items of content.

It is within this "regressive" analytic process that the patient's mental life, including its conflictual matter, slowly begins to emerge around the figure of the analyst. Long-forgotten (repressed) feelings, traumas, and reaction patterns, along with active or discarded defensive or adaptive strategies, all eventually "come out again" in the interaction with the analyst, and what results is called the **transference.** The psychic past is reenacted in the analytic present. It is recognized and interpreted via the inappropriateness of the patient's present (transference) reactions and feelings to the reality of the ongoing interaction with the analyst. The complete revival of the past in the present is called the "regressive transference neurosis." Through the systematic interpretation of these complex transference phenomena, unresolved problems from the past are reworked, more adaptive solutions are found, and maladaptive, neurotic solutions are discarded. In the course of analysis, patients "rewrite" their autobiographies and along the way shed the neurotic symptoms and the problems that brought them to treatment in the first place.

Success in psychoanalysis relies essentially on skillful interpretation leading to enlarging insights. The analyst helps the patient see connections between unconscious wishes and beliefs and conscious speech and behavior. Slowly, patients begin to understand their own mental scheme of things. Symbolic meanings and mental connections begin to take on plausible configurations that "make sense." The insights gained are then "worked through" repeatedly as they reappear in other contexts as long as the analysis continues.

In a classic 1954 paper, Edward Bibring described five essential psychotherapeutic techniques: abreaction (catharsis), suggestion, manipulation, clarification, and interpretation. Different combinations of these techniques characterize the different psychoanalytically based psychotherapies. Within psychoanalysis proper, interpretation is the central technique, and the others are deployed only to enhance interpretation. There is a vast literature on the nature of interpretation: the issues of tact and timing in making interpretations; what makes interpretations "mutative" (ie, able to effect change); the special nature of interpretations of the transference relationship; interpretations in the here and now as opposed to reconstructive interpretations of past (including infantile) matter; and the role of interpretation and insight in relation to behavioral change. This essentially is what is involved in the proper conduct of psychoanalysis.

Indications & Contraindications

Psychoanalysis has been called the treatment of choice for that narrow middle band of patients who come for psychiatric evaluation who are sick enough to need it and well enough to tolerate it (Gill, 1951). Most psychiatric patients have symptoms or problems in living that can be resolved to their satisfaction with less intensive or less prolonged therapies than analysis (including expressive and supportive psychotherapies and crisis-oriented and brief dynamic therapies). Patients who do not need the thoroughgoing life and character reconstruction that psychoanalysis offers include those with acute reactive illnesses, situational maladjustments, and various circumscribed symptom-neurotic and character-neurotic states. There are also many psychiatric patients who come to psychotherapy—often needing psychoactive drug management also—whose illnesses are more severe and who cannot tolerate the anxiety-provoking stresses of psychoanalysis. For patients with fragile or vulnerable "ego strength" (including a tenuous hold on reality), an effort at psychoanalysis per se can be psychological disorganizing, with dangers of regressive, even psychotic swings, severe acting out, flight from treatment, or suicidal pressures. Such patients, who are deemed too ill for psychoanalysis and who need to be treated by other dynamic (more supportive) psychotherapies, include borderline and narcissistic patients, those with character disorders, addictive disorders, severe sexual disorders, those with character neuroses, and even some with severe and refractory symptom neuroses.

Of the patients who come for psychiatric evaluation and treatment, then, a narrow middle band are good candidates for analysis. There is controversy within the field between those who advocate "narrowing" versus those who advocate "widening" the scope of indications for psychoanalysis. From the perspective of a proponent of "narrowing," about 5% of those who come to psychiatric evaluation are suitable candidates for psychoanalysis. These are patients with classical symptom neuroses and moderate character neuroses set within the context of a "strong ego organization"—ie, they are not only amenable to psychoanalysis but able to tolerate it as well.

A. Benefits: Given the limited role of psychoanalysis in the treatment of neurotic disorders, it is proper to question both its social value and its scientific importance. Psychoanalysis is valuable and important in three areas: research, education, and treatment. As a research investigative technique, psychoanalysis affords access to the innermost workings of the mind and to knowledge of psychological development, character formation, and normal and abnormal mental processes. Knowledge about mental functioning derived from psychoanalytic research forms the basis of the theory of psychoanalysis as a comprehensive theory of the mind. Out of this theory have evolved the specific therapeutic applications of both psychoanalysis and the psychoanalytically based dynamic psychotherapies.

As an educational tool, the personal analysis of the therapist—required for those who seek certification as psychoanalytic practitioners and often sought by those who seek enhanced professional effectiveness as dynamic psychotherapists—is necessary to provide successive generations of clinicians best qualified to offer these therapeutic resources to patients who need them. As specific treatment for that small number of patients for whom it is indicated, psychoanalysis offers the best hope—not always realized—for the thoroughgoing resolution of neurotic problems and for fundamental character reconstruction. Since individuals in analysis are often in positions of responsibility, making decisions that affect others, the social value of the technique is apparent.

B. Limitations: Those who would widen the scope of indications for psychoanalysis feel that because the therapeutic goal of psychoanalysis is fundamental personality reorganization, the results when it succeeds are more complete and enduring than can be achieved with less ambitious forms of therapy. Over the years, psychoanalysis has therefore been extended and modified to treat broader categories of patients, including children and adolescents (Melanie Klein, Anna Freud)—an extension that has by now become the established discipline of child and adolescent analysis—groups (Henry Ezriel, S.R. Slavson), delinquents (August Aichhom), patients with psychosomatic disorders (Franz Alexander and many others), overtly psychotic patients (Harry Stack Sullivan, Frieda Fromm-Reichmann), narcissistic characters (Heinz Kohut and others), and patients with borderline personality disorders (Otto Kernberg). The movement to extend the indications for analysis to more kinds of mental disorders was reviewed by Leo Stone in 1954 in a widely cited article on the widening scope of psychoanalysis. Anna Freud (1954), in discussing that paper, undertook to spearhead the opposed trend toward narrowing the indications for analysis back to classically neurotic adults and children. Glover in 1954 divided patients for whom psychoanalysis might be the treatment of choice into three categories that he called the ideally suitable, the moderately suitable, and those for whom psychoanalysis was the last hope but a forlorn one. The patients in the third category had severe personality disorders and were to be offered analysis as a "heroic measure"—this was in the days before adjunctive pharmacotherapy was available. The concept of intensive psychoanalytic treatment for patients much sicker than those seen in the usual outpatient psychoanalytic practice was a major rationale for the psychoanalytic sanatorium (such as the Menninger Foundation), where treatment could be conducted in a protected milieu with total life management.

PSYCHODYNAMIC PSYCHOTHERAPY

The psychoanalytically based dynamic psychotherapies other than formal psychoanalysis have been divided conceptually into two types: expressive and supportive. These methods of treatment are available for that much larger population of psychiatric patients who are not candidates for psychoanalysis proper. Psychodynamic psychotherapy is a peculiarly American creation, now practiced worldwide. It was developed between World Wars I and II and refined as a coherent body of theory and technique in the decade after World War II when psychoanalytic theory became the dominant psychological perspective of American psychiatrists. The expressive and supportive dynamic psychotherapies arose in pragmatic response to the treatment needs of the vast majority of patients who were not suitable candidates for psychoanalysis proper.

The dynamic psychoanalytically based psychotherapies are of two types: (1) those whose treatment aim is **expressive,** ie, to uncover (or make conscious) psychological conflict through analyzing the patient's defenses and resistances and in this way to resolve conflict through interpretation, insight, and change motivated by insight; and (2) those whose aim is **supportive,** ie, to diminish the force of external (situational) or internal (instinctual, drive-related) pressures by a variety of ego-strengthening techniques. Supportive therapies thus increase the patient's capacity to suppress mentally painful conflict and its dysphoric or symptomatic expression, thereby effecting behavioral change and symptomatic relief through means other than interpretation and insight.

As useful as this expressive-supportive division is for heuristic, prescriptive, and prognostic purposes, it is also a misleading oversimplification. All psychiatric treatment that helps patients is supportive even when most uncompromisingly expressive, as in psychoanalysis. What could be more *supportive* than an open-ended psychoanalysis offered daily for as long as necessary, in which the patient is encouraged to express any kind or amount of verbal content and where the entire enterprise consists of two people whose energies and intellect are focused exclusively on the problems and concerns of the one? Or, as Herbert Schlesinger (1969) has reminded us, any treatment, no matter how supportive in the sense of strengthening defenses and suppressing unwanted conflict and symptom expression, must also be *expressive* of some aspect of the patient's concerns. The important question, according to Schlesinger, is not expressive versus supportive but rather *expressive of what?*—and when, and how, in regard to the patient's mental and emotional life—and *supportive of what?*—and when, and how, in regard to that same mental and emotional life. Indeed, in every therapeutic decision to foster the expression of some aspect of mental conflict and distress in whatever way, there is a tacit decision to avoid (ie, suppress) some other aspect of mental conflict and distress.

Whatever one thinks of these arguments, at the practical level of ongoing psychotherapy there has always been a useful distinction between therapeutic interventions that have a preponderantly expressive effect and those that have a preponderantly supportive effect. Paul Dewald in his 1964 book has presented in a systematic way every aspect of the psychotherapeutic process: (1) The beginning of the process and the establishment of the therapeutic situation and the "therapeutic contract." (2) The patient's role and activity and (3) the therapist's role and activity in the therapeutic process. (4) The handling of the transference. (5) The handling of manifestations of resistance, regression, and psychic conflict. (6) The role of insight and working through in bringing about change. (7) The emotional involvements of the therapist (the "counter-transference"). (8) The adjuvant role of psychoactive drugs. (9) The process of natural termination. All of the foregoing are discussed by Dewald from the contrasting perspectives of expressive and supportive psychotherapeutic approaches to each of these issues.

Techniques & Patient Selection

The dynamic psychotherapies, expressive or supportive, are quite similar to each other in procedural form and greatly different from the formal structure of the psychoanalytic interview. The patient sits in a chair facing the therapist, with the expectation of feedback and reciprocal exchange. Unlike psychoanalysis, where the burden is on the patient to keep saying whatever comes to mind while the analyst chooses when and how to intervene, in psychotherapy the format is more like a conversational exchange. The patient in psychotherapy has made no commitment to try to say everything that comes to mind without editorial revision or censorship. The patient has agreed only to present problems and distress for consideration as he or she feels able and willing to do, and no "fundamental rule" is violated by a decision to withhold specific items of mental content, either temporarily or permanently.

The frequency of weekly sessions with the therapist is more flexible in the case of psychotherapy, ranging from one to three or four sessions a week but most often once or twice a week. Unless some form of time-limited therapy is elected, the duration is open-ended, as with psychoanalysis. Although in practice psychotherapy is usually briefer in duration than psychoanalysis (1–2 years versus 3–5 years), it can continue for just as long and may even (unlike psychoanalysis) continue for the life of the patient. Such "therapeutic lifers" have consciously undertaken, out of need, to continue a supportive relationship with the therapist similar to the lifelong medical maintenance regimens required by diabetic patients, cardiac patients, and others with chronic and incurable but manageable disorders. In terms of total hours spent in therapy, the dynamic psychotherapies consume usually 50–200 hours as against, in analysis, 600–1000 hours. The treatment hour usually is 50 minutes, but in some sustained, essentially supportive psychotherapies, especially with schizoid and other individuals fearful of interpersonal intimacy, sessions are in some instances curtailed to no more than 30 minutes each. In both expressive and supportive therapies, at times of acute crisis or emergency, sessions may be extended as long as necessary—up to 2 hours or more. Occasionally in the psychotherapies, emergency weekend or evening sessions are held. Suppor tive treatment sessions may be scheduled less frequently than once a week, and the time may come—if the patient is seeing the therapist only once a month—when the sessions should be characterized as follow-up visits or "reporting in" rather than a continuing psychotherapeutic process.

In the psychotherapies (again in contrast to psychoanalysis), there is greater use of adjuvant drug management, coordination of care with the patient's family physician, telephone contacts, and involvement of third parties (family, employers, teachers, etc). All of these kinds of extra-session activities are more frequent the more supportive and the less expressive the particular psychotherapy is intended to be. Within this overall common structure, then, how do the technical interventions differ between the more expressive and the more supportive psychotherapies?

1. EXPRESSIVE PSYCHOTHERAPY

Essentially, in expressive psychotherapy, with the patient free to bring up problems and anxieties in his or her own way, the therapeutic emphasis is on interpretation and insight and the objective is to bring about beneficial change by resolution of as much psychic conflict as possible. This is accomplished by uncovering unconscious conflicts and, by understanding, achieving mastery. These are to some extent the techniques of psychoanalysis but without free association, dream analysis, or deep discovery of infantile sources of current pain.

Expressive psychotherapy is the treatment of choice for persons with enough ego strength, intelligence, and anxiety tolerance to participate in therapy and serious but relatively circumscribed neurotic conflicts and symptoms—ie, individuals who need help but not the greater commitment implied by a decision to enter analysis. If such patients will assume responsibility for their character traits and their problems in living and are willing to look introspectively at the irrational aspects of their interpersonal relationships, significant help and change can be effected without the full-scale reconstructive effort required to uncover the infantile developmental roots of the neurotic personality development. For example, the issue is whether a patient with severe marital problems can be helped to resolve the problems without the need to recreate the earlier prototype, the infantile conflicts with the mother, repressed behind the childhood amnesia. In psychoanalysis, the aim is to pursue conflicts back to their infantile roots so they can be carefully *analyzed;* the aim of analytically oriented expressive psychotherapy is to *recognize* (and only partially to analyze) those same conflicts and use that recognition in therapy. Insight is achieved but only to the "depth" of the problem being addressed—it never penetrates

to the unconscious infantile origins of the patient's original conflicts.

Expressive therapy is indicated for patients with problems similar to those treated in psychoanalysis—patients with classical symptom neuroses (dysthymic disorder, anxiety disorders) and the character neuroses (personality disorders). **Character neuroses** that cause problems in living (eg, rigidly compulsive or chronically depressive characters) and **symptom neuroses** (eg, characterized by irrational compulsions or bouts of depression) can at times blend into each other, or one may give way to the other.

The distinction between those who need psychoanalysis and those who can be treated by less intensive therapy is well illustrated by the example of psychotherapeutic work with a patient suffering from posttraumatic stress disorder (see Chapter 23). The therapeutic work would be limited to a defined sector of the individual's life and problems and directed toward the stresses precipitating the breakdown and enough of their underlying causes to permit resolution of the current conflict. Thus, in the case of the survivor of an accident, grief-stricken over his companion's death and feeling guilty because he himself luckily survived, the events surrounding the death, ambivalent (love? hate?) feelings about the companion, and perhaps even a parallel between the adult friendship and the conflictual sibling relationships of childhood might all come within the scope of the expressive therapeutic work. Therapy in this example probably would not explore earlier conflicts in the infantile relationship with the parents.

However, expressive psychotherapy need not be confined in this way to a specific area of difficulty. Expressive psychotherapy would include concern with characterological problems and symptoms and their maladaptive roles in the patient's life but with the object only of working at the level of the individual's willingness and capacity to assume responsibility for their modification in the present without the need for the concomitant uncovering of their infantile roots. Such treatment can be long-term and can undertake to explore and modify the entire range of the patient's life adjustments, attitudes, and reactions.

Conflict resolution and symptomatic relief in expressive psychotherapy are made possible by the relative "autonomy" of the conflict in the present from its earlier infantile prototype, though clearly a developmental line can be traced from the present-day neurotic problem to the original pathogenic conflict. Success depends on the ability of the patient and therapist to resolve the conflict in the "here and now," without needing to explore its roots in infancy or its development from earlier neurotic relationships. Such relative autonomy of conflict is common enough so that there is a very large population of psychoneurotic patients who can use expressive dynamic psychotherapy. Since it is received dogma among psychiatrists generally that expressive (uncovering, interpretive) treatment is "better" because it presumably leads to changes that are more stable and better able to with-stand adverse environmental pressures, the therapeutic tendency is fostered among practitioners of dynamic psychotherapy to—in the words of a popular training aphorism—"be as expressive as you can be and as supportive as you have to be."

2. SUPPORTIVE PSYCHOTHERAPY

It is easier to agree on and expound the indications for techniques of expressive psychotherapy than to explain when supportive psychotherapy is called for and how it should be managed. Expressive psychotherapy can be likened to a foreshortened analysis, and most interested people understand something about analysis even if they do not agree on when it should be used. Supportive psychotherapy, on the other hand, employs all manner of techniques and can be used in the management of all classes of patients not candidates for analysis or expressive psychotherapy.

In the early days of psychoanalysis, that method of treatment was acclaimed as the first successful scientific psychotherapy, in contrast to all preexisting therapies, which were viewed only as different types of suggestion therapy and therefore inherently unpredictable and unstable. Hypnosis was the prototype of such suggestive therapies. This view was expressed by Freud many times and was underlined forcefully by Edward Glover in 1931. As employed by nonanalytically trained practitioners, supportive psychotherapy is often conducted by giving heavy doses of common sense reassurance, to the extent that this too, along with suggestion, came to be considered a hallmark of the supportive approach. This perception is misleading and oversimplified. Explicit reassurance is seldom comforting to patients with problems severe enough to bring them to a therapist's consulting room in the first place. In such instances, the effort to give reassurance may only convince the patient that the therapist simply does not understand the nature of the difficulty or does not want to hear about it.

What, then, does supportive therapy actually consist of? One of the earliest efforts to explain supportive psychotherapy was that of Merton Gill (1951), who identified three kinds of interventions that he felt "strengthened the defenses," in contrast with expressive approaches that undertook to uncover and interpret defenses as a step toward eventual integration. These explicitly supportive interventions are (1) to consistently encourage adaptive (and discourage maladaptive) combinations of impulse and defense expression, both behaviorally and symptomatically; (2) to deliberately refrain from interpreting defenses and character configurations, no matter how rigid or maladaptive, that are deemed essential to maintain functioning; and (3) to partially uncover some aspect of

neurotic conflict (eg, within a troubled marriage or work situation) in order to reduce inner conflict that might be creating unwanted symptoms (eg, anxiety, depression, phobic avoidances). In this way the balance of psychic forces is altered, rendering repression of the core of neurotic conflict easier to accomplish. An example would be not exploring in detail the origin of a troubled marital or work situation in earlier ingrained patterns of interpersonal difficulty.

Bearing in mind the five therapeutic techniques listed by Bibring—abreaction, suggestion, manipulation, clarification, and interpretation—psychoanalysis could be described as utilizing mostly interpretation, with other techniques employed only when necessary to facilitate and enhance interpretation. Expressive psychotherapy could be described as depending to a large extent on interpretation but using clarification also and the other techniques as well. And supportive psychotherapy could be described as using all five techniques in whatever proportions seem to be called for by the specific needs of the patient, interpretation included.

Techniques of Supportive Psychotherapy

The principal common therapeutic ingredient of supportive psychotherapy is the evocation and firm establishment of a positive dependent emotional attachment to the therapist. Within this bond, the patient's emotional needs and wishes are allowed to achieve varying degrees of overt or covert (symbolic) gratification. In supportive therapy, the meanings and sources of the bond between the patient and the therapist are for the most part not interpreted or "analyzed."

This dependent emotional attachment seems, in turn, to be an essential precondition to the proper functioning of various other supportive mechanisms. It is also the basis of the so-called "transference cure," the willingness and capacity of the patient to reach therapeutic goals, change behavior and modes of living, and give up symptoms as something being done "for the therapist"—as the quid pro quo for the emotional gratifications received within the benevolent dependent attachment. Upon this base, then, other supportive devices are employed as indicated by the clinical needs of particular patients. If the dependent need for continued emotional gratification cannot be transferred (see below) or somehow either terminated or made therapeutically sustaining, it can be incorporated into a continuing and even unending therapeutic relationship.

These chronic maintenance supportive therapies may be employed over long periods in the management of vulnerable patients whose hold on reality is tenuous. Patients with comparable dependent tendencies but greater psychological resources (eg, a greater capacity to identify with the therapist) are often able to terminate treatment, perhaps after a period of "weaning" as first advocated by Alexander and French (1946). These are patients who can identify successfully with the therapist and the therapist's approach toward and mastery of conflict pressures and can thus learn to go forward on their own.

Intermediate between those patients who can be helped to achieve reasonable psychological autonomy by identification with the therapist and those for whom continued (perhaps lifelong) therapy is necessary are those whose attachments and the emotional gratifications derived therefrom can be "transferred" within the patient's now improved life situation. The transfer is usually made to the spouse, and the success of transfer depends not only on the effectiveness of the psychotherapeutic work within ongoing treatment but also on the capacity and willingness of the spouse to carry the transferred emotional burden indefinitely. Obviously, some patients will be more fortunate than others in the matter of availability of someone willing and able to accept such a burden.

Another useful supportive mechanism is to foster the displacement of the neurotic behavior into the therapeutic relationship so that its ill effects can be ameliorated in the "real life" of the patient. A typical example would be to encourage an unduly dependent and submissive patient to be more assertive outside treatment by allowing greater (covert) submissiveness to the therapist, which is experienced by the patient as requiring the altered (more assertive) external behaviors as the price of continuation of the dependent gratifications within the treatment. The success of this maneuver depends upon life circumstance, the reinforcing positive feedback, and enhanced self-esteem. Beneficial change stabilizes when the new behaviors bring real reward and gratification rather than neurotically anticipated disaster.

What has just been described are varieties of the "transference cure," whereby the patient "does what the therapist wants" in exchange for the satisfaction of emotional needs. The "antitransference cure" occurs when the patient makes changes not "for the therapist" but "against the therapist," ie, in the face of what are perceived as the therapist's contrary expectations, usually as an act of triumph over the therapist in the overt or covert treatment struggle. Such "cures," of course, must somehow be buttressed against their potential instability by enduring, beneficial real-life consequences.

The **"corrective emotional experience"** is a concept Alexander and French have invoked almost as the all-explanatory construct to elucidate the mechanism of action of supportive psychotherapy. Basically, this consists of deliberately responding to the patient's expressed emotional needs in a way that is different from what he or she has been led by accumulated life experiences to expect, with the effect of jarring entrenched patterns of neurotic (ultimately self-defeating) interactions. The concept can in a sense be applied to the entire range of supportive therapeutic techniques, since everything that goes on in psychotherapy is intended to function in one sense or another as a corrective emotional experience. However, the term is more useful if it is restricted to treatments whose central mechanism consists of interaction with a kindly, understanding, reality-oriented therapist able to absorb the patient's onslaughts and importunities in a spirit of benevolent neutrality without becoming entangled in the kind of interacting neurotic relationships the patient has used to maintain a life of suffering in the years before treatment was sought.

Reality testing and reeducation are related but differ in subtle ways from the corrective emotional experience in the conduct of supportive psychotherapy. Reality testing and reeducation consist of helping the patient who has difficulties in this area to distinguish internally derived expectations and fantasy from the external reality of the situation. Again, broadly speaking, they have a role in any type of psychotherapy, including psychoanalysis, but directly educational efforts by the therapist are more characteristic of psychotherapy when the therapeutic emphasis is in greater part supportive. The therapist gives advice, explains, and instructs the patient about what kinds of behavior are tolerable and expected in the community. The therapist must do all this in a way the patient perceives as nonjudgmental and, to the extent that the therapeutic intervention is coercive, as guided solely by the patient's well-being and best interests.

No purpose is served by trying to make a clear distinction between such educational activities and the steady provision of a corrective emotional experience. In both instances, the patient is taught the techniques of reality-oriented problem solving and reality-corrected emotional responses on the basis of the "borrowed strength" derived from psychological identification with the therapist in the role of helper and healer. Again, the stabilization of progress during and after treatment depends on positive reinforcement from the environment along with some measure of transfer of the attachments to the spouse or other stable life companion.

Another form of supportive psychotherapy involves the kind of life manipulation required by very ill patients who come to hospital, residential care, and day hospital settings—eg, the alcoholic, the drug addict, the acting-out or suicidal patient. In such cases, a major aspect of treatment involves the planned disengagement, temporarily or even at times permanently, from noxious life situations. For other patients, the opposite is true—ie, success can only be achieved if psychotherapy is conducted while contact with the patient's accustomed environment is maintained. With these patients, if the usual interacting life situation cannot be properly maintained, for whatever reason, the chances for an optimal result diminish, at times sharply.

Still another helping mechanism that can play a major role in supportive psychotherapy has been called the "collusive bargain." The "bargain" the therapist makes with the patient is to exempt specific problems, symptoms, and areas of personality malfunction from therapeutic scrutiny—leaving more or less consequential islands of maintained psychopathology—in return for the patient's willingness to make substantial changes in other areas. This is similar to the "transference cure," in the sense that the patient makes changes "for the therapist" in return for a specific reward—the shielding from therapeutic interference of a particularly tenacious or rewarding symptom or behavior. The success of such a maneuver depends on the value of the symptom or behavior to the patient as well as the patient's ability to detach the symptom or behavior from other problems or symptoms, which patient and therapist can then set about dealing with. For example, a homosexual patient with conflicts about professional achievement may decide with a therapist to discuss the professional life issues and to ignore or de-emphasize the lifestyle issues. Since the symptom or behavior "allowed" to the patient in this compromise solution is experienced as at least in some ways rewarding or gratifying, these particular therapeutic outcomes have a built-in stability.

Another technique available to patients who need supportive therapy is transfer of the attachment or dependency either to fortunate life circumstances (wealth, social or cultural advantage can play such a role) or to alternative psychological supports. These may be selected by the patients, sometimes with the concurrence of the therapist. Alcoholics Anonymous and similar self-help groups are examples. In turning to external material or alternative psychological supports for continuing emotional dependencies and gratifications, patients can sometimes save a failing or stalled therapeutic situation; ie, they can stabilize even if they cannot always enhance their level of psychological functioning.

It should be clear from the foregoing that there are many ways in which psychotherapy can support and maintain improved psychological functioning and additionally that ways can be built in to maintain such improvement in stable and enduring fashion. These techniques can be combined in various ways to meet the needs of specific patients—to form a basis for therapeutic "trades"; to replace maladaptive impulse-defense configurations with more adaptive (healthy) ones; to decide what to talk about and explore; and to decide specifically what *not* to talk about. Success in these endeavors may improve the patient's life situation; may help in the transfer of emotional attachments or in undertaking or disengaging from ongoing life context; and may provide positive reinforcements that result in enhanced self-esteem and more comfortable and rewarding life experiences.

Given this great variety of techniques available for supportive psychotherapy, it should be obvious that a high degree of skill and long experience are required supportive psychotherapy, it should be obvious that a high degree of skill and long experience are required by the therapist. This is contrary to the common misconception that more skill in psychodynamics is required to conduct expressive psychotherapy and that the supportive psychotherapists dispense mostly common sense, good will, and kindly reassurance. Actually, neither kind of psychotherapy involves less knowledge or skill than the other, though supportive psychotherapy calls for greater flexibility and permits or even requires a wider deployment of "extras" in regard to the 2-person treatment situation, such as the use of adjuvant psychoactive drug management, contacts with third parties (including other treating physicians), and telephone or other contacts with the patient outside of scheduled sessions.

Indications

Supportive psychotherapy is the treatment of choice for a more diverse range of patients than expressive psychotherapy. It is indicated for some patients "not sick enough" for analysis and for the great majority of very ill patients considered too sick for analysis or *any* intensive expressive approach. The first category includes many patients who may be caught up in disruptive responses (anxiety, depressed affect, rage) to traumatic or otherwise disturbing situations—some grief reactions, acute anxiety states, adjustment disorders, etc. In some cases, expressive-interpretive activity is also indicated, but often there may be just a need to slow up, to take stock, to reassess he clinical situation and the therapeutic options, and to reintegrate, over time, to the best of one's coping or mastery potential. Supportive therapy in such cases usually is of shorter duration than expressive psychotherapy or psychoanalysis.

A larger category of patients for whom supportive psychotherapy is indicated are those much sicker individuals who require sustaining psychotherapeutic relationships, perhaps for life, and who respond slowly to the therapist's best efforts. Stability of psychological functioning at the best achievable level is often the modest therapeutic goal, though at times the hope for cure should be pursued because greater success is sometimes possible. This group includes most patients with psychosis or severe personality disorders, severe addictions, alcoholism, sexual disorders, and acting out, delinquent, and antisocial characters. In almost all of these cases, some degree of expressive therapeutic work can usually be done, but with difficulty because these patients have poor impulse control and low tolerance for anxiety and are vulnerable to regressive (psychotic or suicidal) swings in psychological functioning and integrity. The eruption of a florid psychotic state is a potential danger that often cannot be ignored. Attempts at "widening the scope" of expressive therapy (including psychoanalysis) in an effort to do something for these much sicker patients (see p 393) have met with poor results.

OTHER SCHOOLS & PARADIGMS

The discussion of psychotherapies in this chapter has been within the framework of psychoanalytic (psychodynamic) theories of mental functioning. Other kinds of psychotherapies have been developed within different theoretic models of how the mind works, such as the behavioral model based on a learning theory paradigm and the existentialist-humanist model based on a phenomenological-existentialist view of mental life and function. The therapies that derive from these schools differ radically in concept and in practice from those described in this chapter, and they are discussed elsewhere in this book.

REFERENCES

Alexander F, French TM: *Psychoanalytic Therapy: Principles and Applications*. Ronald Press, 1946.

Bibring E: Psychoanalysis and the dynamic psychotherapies. J Am Psychoanal Assoc 1954;2:745.

Dewald PA: *Psychotherapy: A Dynamic Approach*. Basic Books, 1964.

Fenichel O: *Problems of Psychoanalytic Technique*. Psychoanalytic Quarterly, 1941.

Freud A: The widening scope of indications for psychoanalysis. (Discussion.) J Am Psychoanal Assoc 1954;2:607.

Freud S: Lines of advance in psychoanalytic therapy (1918). In: *Standard Edition of the Complete Psychological Works of Sigmund Freud*. Vol 17. Hogarth Press, 1955.

Gill MM: Ego psychology and psychotherapy. Psychoanal Q 1951;20:62.

Glover E: The indications for psychoanalysis. J Ment Sci 1954;100:393.

Glover E: The therapeutic effect of inexact interpretation: A contribution to the theory of suggestion. Int J Psychoanal 1931;12:397.

Kris E: The nature of psychoanalytic propositions and their validation. Pages 239–259 in: *Freedom and Experience: Essays Presented to Horace Kallen*. Hook S, Konvitz MR (editors). Cornell Univ Press, 1947.

Schlesinger HJ: Diagnosis and prescription for psychotherapy. Bull Menninger Clin 1969;33:269.

Stone L: The widening scope of indications for psychoanalysis. J Am Psychoanal Assoc 1954;2:567.

Wallerstein RS: 42 *Lives in Treatment: A Study of Psychoanalysis and Psychotherapy*. Guilford Press, 1987.

34

Time-Limited Psychotherapy

Charles R. Marmar, MD

HISTORICAL TRENDS & RATIONALE FOR BRIEF DYNAMIC PSYCHOTHERAPY

In the decades since Freud's original writings on the technique of psychoanalysis, the trend among practitioners working in the tradition of psychodynamic psychotherapy has been toward increasing length of treatment. Long-term treatments aim for both symptom resolution and fundamental changes in character structure such as capacities for intimacy and autonomy. Certain theoreticians have advocated briefer, more active, and more focused approaches to deal with carefully delineated areas of psychopathology. Ferenczi and Rank (1925) focused on the physical separation of the infant from the mother at the moment of birth and later the psychological emancipation of the child from the mother led to an emphasis on time-limited treatment, with a focus on the meanings of separation, a theoretical position reiterated in the contemporary work of James Mann (1973) (see below). Alexander and French developed new techniques for time-limited psychoanalysis. They emphasized the therapeutic potential of the **corrective emotional experience,** or the reexperiencing (under more favorable circumstances) of a traumatic emotional situation from the past. Alexander and French (1946) recommended that the therapist assume a particular role that might counteract the earlier trauma or interpersonal deficits. If, for example, a patient has repeatedly experienced painful relationships with critical, unappreciative, or abusive caretakers, the therapist might adopt a warm, empathic, and compassionate role to provide a compensatory experience.

Alexander's goal was to speed up the time course of psychoanalysis rather than to provide a specific set of technical guidelines for conducting brief, problem-focused dynamic psychotherapy. In contrast, contemporary schools of brief psychotherapy advocate a more restricted approach, with focus on a single problem or at most on several interrelated conflicts that have been purposely chosen to the exclusion of other possible issues. The theoretical writings of French are relevant in this regard. It was French (1958) who introduced the term **focal conflict,** which he defined as a wish or intention that conflicts with the person's enduring expectations and values. The conflict renders the person incapable of meeting his or her expectations, and the result is frustration, with use of various emotional defenses and compromises. For example, a person might wish to function as a more separate, independent person but fears that to pursue such autonomous aims would hurt other important people, who would be left out; the person would then compromise by resentfully stifling these strivings toward independence.

Choosing a specific focal conflict helps to organize the work in brief psychotherapy and focuses attention on an emotional problem of manageable proportions. Balint et al (1972) provide an excellent example of the technique for limiting the approach in brief treatment to a selected sector of the personality and guarding against diffusion of effort.

Features of Brief Dynamic Psychotherapy

A. Application of Psychoanalytic Principles: The principles of psychoanalytic psychotherapy are applied to the resolution of specific problems rather than to the entire range of personality functioning.

B. Selection Criteria: Specific selection criteria are designed to permit careful screening of prospective patients and selection of those for whom brief dynamic psychotherapy would be appropriate.

C. Primary Focus: A primary focus—typically a problem behavior or negative self-image that surfaces in the context of current difficulties in interpersonal relations—is chosen.

D. Therapeutic Alliance: Because of the time limits on brief psychotherapy, the therapist must actively seek ways to facilitate the rapid establishment of a therapeutic alliance. Such a partnership creates a safe environment in which the patient feels understood and views the therapist as empathic, respectful, and nonjudgmental, all of which help to deepen rapport. Within this alliance, patients ideally are willing to reveal thoughts and feelings, reflect on the nature of personal problems, and explore their own contributions to these problems.

E. Working Through: Treatment includes a phase of working through that concentrates on the resolution of the focal conflict. This phase usually includes an opportunity for the patient to express feelings and ideas about current stressful interpersonal experiences and to identify subjectively distorted meanings of these events. Distortion may take the form of exaggerated self-depreciation or identification of current negative feelings about the self with difficulties in earlier relationships. The patient's relationship with the therapist is clarified, and ways in which the patient repeats various aspects of the focal conflict in the relationship with the therapist are pointed out. When possible, the patient's distorted reactions to the therapist are linked to similar reactions in important current interpersonal relationships and to related patterns in earlier developmental sequences.

F. Termination: The meaning that termination of therapy holds for the patient is carefully considered in brief dynamic psychotherapy. Because of the short overall duration of treatment, the patient may perceive termination as an abrupt loss of a valued supportive relationship. Although both parties have agreed that treatment should be brief, the patient often feels rejected, and the same negative self-images that brought the patient into treatment in the first place may be transiently intensified during termination. The loss of the therapist at termination is therefore another opportunity for the patient to master general problems in the area of separation and attachment.

Summary of Rationale & Features of Brief Dynamic Psychotherapy

Brief dynamic psychotherapy is indicated when a specific emotional problem can be identified and when the patient can rapidly form a trusting relationship with the therapist and tolerate exploration of that problem in a brief time frame. The goals of work are focused and more narrowly defined, as opposed to the more thorough but more diffusely defined longerterm dynamic therapies. Common to all brief therapies is a limited or fixed number of sessions, usually between 12 and 20 but sometimes extending to 30, although some flexibility exists in different approaches. The rationale for brief therapy is practical: Treatment seeks to be cost-effective and accessible to a broader segment of the population, since many people cannot make the commitment of time, money, and emotional energy required for more protracted treatment.

CONTEMPORARY SCHOOLS OF BRIEF DYNAMIC PSYCHOTHERAPY

DAVID MALAN & THE BRITISH SCHOOL

Beginning with the ground-breaking work of Balint et al (1972) in the development of focal psychotherapy

and evolving further through the efforts of David Malan (1963, 1976) at the Tavistock Clinic in London, the British have made major contributions to the theory, practice, and research evaluation of time-limited dynamic psychotherapy. The technical guidelines advocated by Malan and his collaborators are discussed below.

Selection Criteria

For Malan, the initial selection process is a crucial first step. The pretreatment interview begins with a careful psychiatric history and mental status examination in order to exclude individuals with a current or past history of serious psychiatric disorders (eg, schizophrenia, mania, major depressive episodes), suicide attempts, severe childhood trauma, and longstanding complex family and marital problems. The second component of the evaluation is a psychodynamic history focused on current and past major interpersonal relationships, with a search for recurrent patterns of conflict. The patient's capacity to form an open, trusting relationship with the interviewer is evaluated as well as the patient's response to some initial tentative interpretations of recurring difficulties in interpersonal relationships. The extent to which the patient is motivated to engage in psychotherapy is also determined.

Duration & Focus of Treatment

Malan recommends that a fixed time limit be determined at the outset of treatment. Experienced therapists conduct treatments extending over an average of 18 sessions, whereas a time limit of 30 sessions is recommended for trainee therapists.

Malan emphasizes work on the focal conflict in the context of important recurrent maladaptive patterns in relationships and points to two specific triangular configurations to be used in working on the focal conflict. The first triangle consists of the patient's aim or intention, the subjectively perceived threat that makes expression of the aim dangerous, and the efforts to ward off anxiety through the use of specific defenses. For example, a patient may intend to be more open in expressing emotions in close relationships but feels that this would not gain the respect of others, who would feel that the patient was being too sentimental or emotionally out of control. The patient then tries to ward off the potential anxiety about others' reactions by being intellectual and distant rather than emotional.

The second triangle is a triangle of persons and involves the identification of recurrent patterns of relationships in three contexts: (1) the relationship with the therapist (the transference relationship); (2) the patient's relationships in current interpersonal situations outside of therapy; and (3) the real or imagined relationships (both past and present) with parental figures or siblings. To continue with the patient used in the example in the previous paragraph, the person who feels blocked in expression of emotion is likely to act in a controlled, intellectualized manner both with the therapist and in current emotional and occupational relationships; such a person is also likely to have originally developed this pattern in relating to parental figures.

Treatment

A. Order of Interpretive Work: Malan's technique consists of carefully timing the work to make the patient aware of the triangular structure of the recurrent relationship patterns. The technical competence of the therapist conducting brief dynamic psychotherapy is therefore in part determined by the ability to formulate such triangular patterns quickly and accurately and pace subsequent interpretations at a level of awareness that is tolerable for a specific patient. Malan's recommendations for the order of interpretive work in brief dynamic psychotherapy are as follows:

1. The nature of the focal conflict is communicated to the patient before extensive connections are made among past, current, and transference relationships.

2. In interpreting the focal conflict, the therapist discusses the patient's defensive avoidance of the expression of aims before undertaking in-depth exploration of the aims themselves. For example, a patient who wants to be more direct in expressing anger but fears harming others in the process may be quiet and withdrawn when angry with friends. The therapist might point out that the patient became withdrawn in the same way after the therapist made a certain comment, and the therapist would then invite the patient to examine this behavior before directly asserting that the patient must be angry with the therapist.

3. The repetitive pattern of maladaptive interpersonal behavior is interpreted in its past, current, and transference aspects. The way in which this is done varies and depends on the patient's capacities to appreciate this pattern in different relationship contexts. Once it is clearly developed, the manifestation of the focal conflict in the patient's relationship with the therapist receives primary emphasis.

4. The analysis of the links between the way in which the patient relates to the therapist and the similar way the patient related to parental figures in the past is termed the parent-transference linking interpretation. Malan stresses the importance of this interpretation above all other possible interpretations that can be made in brief psychotherapy.

B. Termination Phase: The loss of the therapist at the termination of brief psychotherapy has meanings for the patient that are explored for possible linkages to unresolved meanings of earlier losses, usually of parental figures. The focal conflict is frequently reactivated or intensified during the termination phase, so that there is yet another opportunity to work through the focal conflict.

PETER SIFNEOS: SHORT-TERM ANXIETY-PROVOKING PSYCHOTHERAPY

While Malan was formulating the technique of brief dynamic psychotherapy at the Tavistock Clinic, Peter Sifneos (1972) was articulating a similar approach based on his experience at Massachusetts General Hospital in Boston. Like Malan, Sifneos departed from the tradition of more supportive and anxiety-suppressive brief psychotherapies by advocating an exploratory, interpretive approach usually reserved for long-term psychoanalytic treatments. The objective of both theorists was to enable patients to make changes in their characters through resolution of certain key neurotic conflicts.

Selection Criteria

Sifneos's approach also emphasizes specific inclusion and exclusion criteria in order to select patients who can quickly engage in the therapeutic process and can tolerate the anxiety evoked by early and repeated interpretive work, in particular, frank examination of the transference reaction. Patients who are the most appropriate candidates for short-term anxiety-provoking psychotherapy have the following characteristics:

(1) Above-average intelligence, as determined by the capacity for new learning.

(2) A history of at least one mutual, give-and-take relationship, with implied shared intimacy, emotional involvement, trust, and the capacity for ambivalent feelings.

(3) Ability to acknowledge and express a range of emotions, as directly observed in the patient's interaction with the evaluating therapist.

(4) A circumscribed chief complaint related to a limited area of interpersonal functioning.

(5) Motivation for change, which Sifneos regards as a multifaceted characteristic that includes the capacity and willingness to look for personal contributions to one's difficulties, an ability to appreciate that symptoms are psychological in origin, the capacity to provide an open and honest account of feelings, a willingness to be actively involved in the therapeutic relationship, and a willingness to experiment with new ways of functioning. Sifneos stresses the importance of realistic rather than magical expectations about changes arising from therapy as well as the patient's willingness to make reasonable sacrifices with regard to schedule arrangements and payment of fees.

Treatment

Sifneos's approach incorporates five phases, as described below.

A. First Phase (Patient-Therapist Encounter): A therapeutic alliance is formed through mobilization of the patient's initial positive feelings toward the therapist as well as early exploration of the patient's apprehensions regarding treatment. In this phase, the therapist also arrives at a tentative psychodynamic hypothesis about the relationship of current symptomatic disturbances to long-standing character problems that cause conflicts in interpersonal relationships. The focus of treatment—an emotional problem which the patient is motivated to solve and which has relevance for both current interpersonal difficulties as well as basic (core) neurotic conflicts—is also determined during the first phase.

B. Second Phase (Early Treatment): The therapist is careful to differentiate realistic goals from the patient's more immature wishes to be totally gratified in disavowing adult responsibility for dealing with problems. The therapist tactfully confronts the patient's idealized versions of what treatment will accomplish in order to encourage active problem solving and discourage the development of an overly dependent relationship.

C. Third Phase (Height of Treatment): In the third phase, the therapist relates the patient's past unresolved difficulties in interpersonal relationships to current emotional problems. As these patterns of conflict are explored, the patient frequently experiences moments of resistance (**transference resistances**) to the deeper understanding of these patterns, in part because of fearful expectations of the therapist's reactions or attitudes toward the patient.

These impediments to treatment are discussed so that the patient is allowed to see the irrational basis for these fears and so that exploration can then return to bolder elaboration of the focus. A cycle of events then typically occurs: Progress in understanding leads to resistance, followed first by interpretation of the fears underlying the resistance and then by further deepening of the work. The therapist asks anxiety-provoking questions in order to help the patient observe how he or she evades painful feelings as well as to demonstrate the reasons underlying this avoidance. Such confrontations may trigger the patient's anger toward the therapist, a response that is made more acceptable to the patient because of the prior establishment of a therapeutic alliance.

Sifneos has likened this emotional problem solving to the completion of a complex mathematical puzzle. He cautions against an overly intellectualized approach, however, and emphasizes that it is a learning experience that occurs within the context of an emotional exchange between the patient and the therapist.

D. Fourth Phase (Evidence of Change): In the fourth phase, the therapist determines when sufficient mastery and resolution of the problem have occurred, so that termination may be considered. The criteria for resolution include less anxiety during treatment sessions; relief of symptoms such as sleeplessness, phobias, or self-defeating behavior; adaptive changes in the interpersonal behavior associated with the focus; and evidence that the patient can begin to relate what has been learned to new social contexts by making appropriate changes in behavior. For example, after

successful therapy, a patient who has stifled expression of independent wishes and actions in the presence of parental figures and who has sought treatment because this behavior has been carried over into the marital relationship will be able to define and assert needs not only with the spouse but also with important figures in the workplace or in social relationships.

E. Fifth Phase (Termination): Sifneos proposes that the exact termination date not be set until appropriate change has been demonstrated in the target behavior. At that point, the therapist addresses the natural ambivalence the patient feels at the thought of separating from the therapist. The disappointment of separating from a recently acquired helpful figure is set against the more realistic background of the gains achieved in treatment. The patient is encouraged to extrapolate this new knowledge to future challenges. The therapist in turn also experiences a resistance to termination that must be addressed, because as the therapist experiences growing concern for the patient, there will be a deepening curiosity about the origin of the patient's difficulties as well as anxiety and guilt in acknowledging that treatment is ending but has failed to address certain psychopathological problems (specifically, those not related to the central focus). Therapists may have to struggle with the temptation to extend treatment. Sifneos believes that separation at termination is facilitated by a progressive, active, problem-solving posture on the part of the patient rather than a more regressive dependent attachment.

HABIB DAVANLOO: BROAD-FOCUSED SHORT-TERM DYNAMIC PSYCHOTHERAPY

Habib Davanloo's (1979, 1980) work, which incorporates some theoretical concepts from both Malan and Sifneos, has broadened both the scope of problems that can be addressed in brief psychotherapy and the extent of the resolution hoped for in treatment.

Selection Criteria

In this approach, selection criteria in time-limited therapy have been expanded to include patients with long-standing severe characterological deficits (ie, personality disorders) that imply the existence of multiple interrelated conflicts that are not easily limited to a single focus. Davanloo considers neither severe problems nor long-standing difficulties as automatic criteria for excluding patients from treatment. Contrary to expectation, he reported some good outcomes in brief treatment of individuals with long-standing severe character problems and unexpected instances of poor outcome when mild character difficulties of more recent onset were the presenting complaint. Whereas Sifneos recommends his short-term anxiety-provoking psychotherapy for a rigorously selected

5–10% of psychiatric outpatients, Davanloo's broader selection criteria make it possible to treat about 30–35% of outpatients with psychiatric problems by broad-focused short-term therapy.

In 1979, Davanloo specified criteria for his approach to brief dynamic psychotherapy. These overlap the criteria of Malan and Sifneos (history of adequate interpersonal relationships, capacity to tolerate and express feelings, awareness that problems are psychological in origin, and response to the therapist's initial interpretations). Davanloo emphasizes the need to confront the patient's way of avoiding real feelings by including such defensive behavior as vagueness, passivity, denial, or withdrawal. Such repetitive confrontation is often irritating to patients, who are encouraged to express the frustration and resentment they feel about this process. The ability to express that anger and to begin recognizing the pattern of not expressing feelings under frustrating circumstances reflects qualities indicating that the patient is a suitable candidate for broad-focused short-term therapy.

Duration of Treatment

Davanloo recommends a flexible number of treatment sessions. For well-functioning patients with circumscribed problems, 5–15 face-to-face sessions lasting an hour each are usually sufficient to deal with the presenting problem. For adequately functioning patients with several presenting problems, 15–25 sessions are recommended; about 20–30 sessions are recommended for patients with long-standing severe personality problems.

Treatment

A. Early and Middle Phases: As in other brief dynamic psychotherapeutic approaches, the therapist assumes an active role and places high priority on the early and repeated interpretation of transference (ie, the ways in which the patient misperceives the therapist as a result of experiences in earlier relationships). For example, a patient with a harsh and critical mother was made to feel during her childhood that her anger toward her mother was not justified. The patient had therefore developed a pattern of suppressing her anger when frustrated and instead becoming moody and uncooperative, without clearly communicating what was upsetting her. Such a pattern is highly likely to recur during treatment, and when it does appear, the therapist will make the interpretation that the patient is feeling resentfully misunderstood, that she feels as though she is not justified in this anger, and that instead of expressing the feeling, she becomes moody and uncommunicative. After the pattern has been clarified, the therapist addresses the patient's unwarranted expectation that she will be punished for her behavior, and the patient gradually comes to trust more open expression of her frustration. This active, interpretive approach is recommended by Da-

vanloo both to accelerate the understanding and resolution of emotional problems and to prevent patients from becoming excessively dependent on the therapist. Instead, patients are encouraged to rely on their own coping capacities in preparation for the termination of treatment.

In treatments that are going well, the patient gains considerable understanding into these recurrent ways of avoiding the expression of emotions and usually begins to experiment with more open demonstration of feelings by about the eighth session. This increased communicativeness occurs not only in the treatment setting but also in the patient's relationships with other important persons in everyday life. At the same time, anxiety and depression are lessened, partly because the patient feels an upsurge in morale as a result of participating in a helpful treatment relationship and partly because the patient is able to negotiate more appropriately for satisfaction of needs in interpersonal conflicts. At this point, termination of therapy may be contemplated.

B. Termination Phase: Davanloo also recommends a flexible approach to the termination phase that takes into account the patient's level of functioning as well as the limited or extensive nature of the presenting problems. In well-functioning patients who are capable but hold themselves back in work and love relationships because of irrational fear of success, disengagement from treatment is uncomplicated, and patients do not ordinarily experience deep feelings of loss at termination. On the other hand, for those individuals who have sustained important losses in their lives, particularly during sensitive developmental periods in early childhood or adolescence, mourning the imminent departure of the therapist is an essential and helpful aspect of treatment. Because the patient knows when the relationship will end, there is an opportunity to explore the feelings about this loss, which stands in contrast to the more traumatic losses that occurred in earlier developmental periods. For patients with severe personality difficulties or those with multiple problems rather than a single focus, Davanloo recommends several additional sessions during the termination phase in order to help the patient negotiate a manageable separation.

JAMES MANN: TIME-LIMITED PSYCHOTHERAPY

James Mann's (1973) unique approach to brief dynamic psychotherapy places major theoretical and technical emphasis on the meaning of time—ie, the patient's difficulty in accepting the finiteness of time, in mastering separations, and in ultimately accepting his or her own mortality. As a result, the selection of patients, the development of the focus in brief treatment, the approach to working through emotional problems, and the handling of the termination phase are organized along a common theme that addresses the meanings of time for the patient. The termination phase assumes paramount importance, because it provides a living model of loss, separation, and the time-limited nature of attachments.

In his theoretical discussion, Mann differentiates two ways in which people experience time: (1) Categorical, or adult, time is governed by realistic understanding of the finite quality of time and is measured by the watch and the calendar; (2) existential, or child, time is governed by immature fantasies of timelessness and personal invincibility. Because the development of a mature appreciation of time is a challenge for everyone, particularly for people with a history of difficulty in early separation experiences (who are forever waiting for the loved one's return), a child's perception of time is never entirely set aside, even in the most mature adults. Both kinds of time may be used simultaneously to evaluate an experience. Stressful life events may alter a person's perception of time from a realistic, adult appreciation of its finiteness to a more childlike experience of time and functioning (regression with stress). Alternatively, the same individual may simultaneously reflect different levels of adaptation to the finiteness of time, as shown in successful time management in one sphere (being prompt for meetings) with an adherence to more immature perceptions of time in another area of functioning (failing to plan for retirement as a denial of aging).

Selection Criteria

Ideal candidates for Mann's brief dynamic psychotherapy are young adults in developmental transition, ie, those who are moving from the late stages of adolescence into young adulthood. The prototype is a college student struggling simultaneously to handle separation from parents and to establish autonomous social, occupational, and sexual identities. Mann's approach stresses that the patient must have the ability to tolerate the frustration of the time limits inherent in this type of therapy. Above-average intelligence, a criterion emphasized by Sifneos, is seen as helpful though not essential in Mann's approach. Mann has suggested that his approach, which is both short-term and fixed in duration, may be appropriate for those with limited economic resources and educational background. Long-term exploratory psychotherapies are frequently both too costly and too ambiguously defined to serve the interests of this group of patients.

The exclusion criteria for Mann's time-limited approach include past or current psychotic disorders, serious alcohol or drug abuse, and borderline personality disorder. Patients with strong passive longings to be cared for, who are frequently reluctant to give up these feelings in favor of more independent behavior, are also excluded. Individuals with these problems frequently require long-term dynamic psychotherapy.

Duration & Focus of Treatment

Mann specifies a 12-session, once-weekly, time-limited treatment. The focus emerges after a process of gradual clarification, which may require several sessions, and the 12-session limit begins only after a focus has been mutually defined. Once the focus has been established, the time limit is fixed, and the date of termination is set in advance. If no workable focus can be specified during the preliminary interviews, the patient is referred for an appropriate alternative treatment.

Mann describes four basic conflicts that are a frequent focus in treatment: dependence versus independence, passivity versus activity, diminished versus adequate self-esteem, and unresolved versus resolved grief. Mann emphasizes the paramount importance of the elements of separation and individuation as they relate to the four central issues. For example, while activity-passivity struggles may involve anxiety about surpassing a rival, anxiety about aggressively dominating another, or anxiety about separating from a caretaker, Mann considers the latter to be the most important theme.

Treatment

A. Early Phase: Mann describes an initial "honeymoon" phase characterized by the patient's relief in feeling understood, particularly when the therapist is tactful in defining the problem that is the focus. The recommendation for brief rather than longer-term treatment stimulates hope for a rapid resolution of difficulties. The patient is intellectually aware of the time limit; at an emotional level, however, the patient often longs for an open-ended and idealized reparative relationship with the therapist that will compensate for earlier disappointments and frustrations in formative relationships.

B. Middle Phase: The therapist's inevitable failure to meet all of the patient's expectations in the first few hours of treatment leads to disillusionment, which ushers in the middle phase of treatment, frequently at about the sixth session. The original presenting symptoms may intensify, as Mann (1973) explains:

> The characteristic feature of any middle point is that one more step, however small, signifies the point of no return. In the instance of time-limited psychotherapy, the patient must go on to a conclusion that he does not wish to confront. The confrontation that he needs to avoid and that he will actively seek to avoid is the same one that he suffered earlier in his life; namely, *separation without resolution from the meaningful, ambivalently experienced person.* Time sense and reality are coconspirators in repeating an existential trauma in the patient.

C. Termination Phase: With the inevitable approach of termination, a deepening sense of pessimism and disillusionment usually (not always) dominates the eighth through the tenth sessions. The patient is more or less aware of the threat of termination and struggles to guard against the emotional pain of the loss of a valued relationship only recently established. With surprising frequency, the patient seems to forget the termination date and believes there are more sessions left than are actually remaining. The therapist points out the patient's incorrect perceptions of time in the context of brief dynamic treatment. The patient's negative feelings toward the therapist at this stage frequently recapitulate negative feelings toward frustrating figures in earlier life. The important difference is that while facing an agreed upon termination date, the patient now has an opportunity to experience and master the emotions related to separation from the therapist. In so doing, the patient develops a capacity to function more independently and deal more adaptively with the imperfect and time-limited nature of human experience. Feelings of anger at being abandoned, guilt for having angry feelings toward frustrating figures, sadness at the loss of a valued figure, and wishes for reunion can be examined in this phase.

KLERMAN & WEISSMAN: SHORT-TERM INTERPERSONAL PSYCHOTHERAPY

Klerman and Weissman have described a time-limited psychotherapeutic method specifically tailored to treat individuals with depression. The focus of this approach is on interpersonal behaviors that contribute to depressive states (Weissman and Klerman, 1973; Neu et al, 1978). In contrast to the brief dynamic psychotherapies, little attention is directed toward the exploration of unconscious conflicts or the repetition of unresolved parent-child problems in the patient's relationship with the therapist (ie, there is minimal transference interpretation). Treatment is time-limited, averaging 14 sessions in one study. Weekly 50-minute sessions are provided for individuals with depression triggered and exacerbated by interpersonal problems.

Klerman and Weissman describe seven types of technical interventions. The first is **nonjudgmental exploration,** which is particularly relevant early in treatment and denotes the support and encouragement given to the patient to discuss problems openly. The therapist's availability, empathy, and nonjudgmental attitude are essential in facilitating the patient's self-disclosure.

Elicitation of material, a second technique, involves active probing for new information. Such probing is common during early treatment but may be indicated whenever a more complete understanding of past or current difficulties is indicated. Next is clarification, or rephrasing of the patient's comments to point out inconsistencies and make covert communications more overt.

Additional techniques include **direct advice,** in which the therapist guides the patient toward more adaptive interpersonal behavior to increase the chances that others will be warmly receptive of the patient rather than critical or distant. **Decision analysis** explores alternative courses of action in order to broaden the patient's understanding of short- and long-range consequences of behavior toward others. **Development of awareness** is used to facilitate insight into the patient's interpersonal behavioral patterns and clarify ways in which the patient attempts to disavow or ignore these patterns.

This brief treatment approach is noteworthy both for its careful specification of treatment approaches in published manuals as well as for the attention paid to research on the effectiveness of the recommendations. The approach may be of particular interest to general practitioners and other nonpsychiatrist physicians, since extensive training in psychodynamic theory and technique is not required.

EFFECTIVENESS OF BRIEF DYNAMIC PSYCHOTHERAPY

Despite the methodological difficulties encountered in assessing the outcome of various psychotherapies, major progress occurred in the 1970s. The most thorough research on the effectiveness of psychotherapy has been conducted by Smith et al (1980), who reviewed and analyzed 375 studies. Since the average duration of treatment was 17 sessions, this report mainly considers the outcome of brief psychotherapy. In general, the average patient who received treatment was better off than 75% of those who either received no treatment or were on waiting lists for treatment and were used as controls. Effectiveness of treatment was assessed by several criteria, including improvement in symptoms, patient satisfaction, and decreased reliance on medication. The study indicated that the many different schools of psychotherapy were about equally helpful. Brief dynamic psychotherapy—along with brief behavioral, interpersonal, cognitive, and other approaches—is a treatment with well-documented effectiveness in relieving various psychological symptoms, as described above.

The relative effectiveness of brief dynamic psychotherapy compared to long-term dynamic treatments has not been extensively studied. Although the general question of brief versus long-term treatment in the different approaches has been reviewed by Butcher and Kolotkin (1979) and by Luborsky et al (1975), the former failed to find a strong correlation between the efficacy of different therapies and the length of treatment. The negative finding may be due in part to currently limited abilities to reliably evaluate the types of personality changes that are more likely to occur in long-term treatment. Changes in psychological symptoms and social functioning, on the other hand, are more easily determined. Definitive evaluation of the merits of brief versus long-term treatment awaits development of improved methods of assessing characterological change.

Brief dynamic psychotherapy for outpatients with moderate to severe psychiatric conditions has been shown to be effective in alleviating symptoms and improving social functioning. Horowitz et al (1984) have found that brief therapy is effective in treating posttraumatic stress disorders. They have also discussed the modification of the techniques of brief dynamic psychotherapy for patients with different personality disorders. Weissman et al (1981) have studied the outcome of interpersonal psychotherapy and found that 14-session treatments have been effective in treating major depressive disorders. Very few negative effects of brief dynamic psychotherapy have been reported. Rather than becoming worse, patients for the most part either improve or (at worst) do not improve after brief dynamic psychotherapy. This method of treatment seems to be the most useful when a specific focus can be defined, when the problem is related to recent stressful life circumstances, and when the patient has the capacity to tolerate rapid engagement and confrontation, working through, and disengagement from the treatment process.

REFERENCES

Alexander F, French T: *Psychoanalytic Therapy: Principles and Applications*. Ronald Press, 1946.

Balint M, Ornstein PH, Balint E: *Focal Psychotherapy*. Lippincott, 1972.

Butcher NJ, Kolotkin RL: Evaluation of outcome in brief psychotherapy. Psychiatr Clin North Am 1979;2:157.

Davanloo H: Techniques of short-term psychotherapy. Psychiatr Clin North Am 1979;2:11.

Davanloo H (editor): *Short-Term Dynamic Therapy*. Vol I. Jason Aronson, 1980.

Ferenczi S, Rank O: *The Development of Psychoanalysis*. Nervous and Mental Disease Publication Co., 1925.

French TM: *The Integrations of Behavior*. Vol 3. Univ of Chicago Press, 1958.

Horowitz MJ et al: Brief psychotherapy of bereavement reactions: The relationship of process to outcome. Arch Gen Psychiatry 1984;41:438.

Horowitz MJ et al: *Personality Styles and Brief Psychotherapy*. Basic Books, 1984.

Luborsky L, Singer B, Luborsky L: *Comparative Studies of Psychotherapies*. Arch Gen Psychiatry 1975;32:995.

Malan DH: *Frontiers of Brief Psychotherapy*. Plenum Press, 1976.

Malan DH: *A Study of Brief Psychotherapy*. Plenum Press, 1963.

Mann J: *Time-Limited Psychotherapy*. Harvard Univ Press, 1973.

Neu C, Prusoff B, Klerman G: Measuring the interventions used in short-term interpersonal psychotherapy of depression. Am J Orthopsychiatry 1978;48:629.

Sifneos PE: *Short-Term Psychotherapy and Emotional Crisis*. Harvard Univ Press, 1972.

Smith ML, Glass GV, Miller TI: *The Benefits of Psychotherapy*. Johns Hopkins Univ Press, 1980.

Weissman M, Klerman G: Psychotherapy with depressed women: An empirical study of content themes and reflection. Br J Psychiatry 1973;123:55.

Weissman M et al: Depressed outpatients: Results one year after treatment with drugs and/or interpersonal psychotherapy. Arch Gen Psychiatry 1981;38:51.

35

Behavior Therapy & Cognitive Therapy

Hanna Levenson, PhD, & Kenneth S. Pope, PhD

Approach Shared by Behavior & Cognitive Therapies

Although there are many types of behavior and cognitive therapies, they have in common several elements that form an underlying core and theoretical rationale (see also Chapter 2), and the approach of the behavior or cognitive therapist involves an implicit five-step procedure:

(1) The individual is evaluated for "symptoms" of behavioral dysfunction, which may be noted by direct observation (eg, eating, stuttering, crying); by the individual's verbalization of thoughts and feelings (eg, suicidal thoughts, depression); and by clinical measurements (eg, blood pressure, heart rate). The behavioral-cognitive therapist does not conceptualize a problem in terms of a psychiatric diagnosis (eg, schizophrenia) but instead defines it in terms of **specific behaviors** that affect the individual's function (eg, hallucinating in public). Because it is not essential to use a "strictly medical" model in behavior or cognitive therapies, the individual seeking help is usually referred to as the client (not the patient).

(2) The therapist and client determine the goals of the treatment. These often focus on specific behaviors to be changed, ie, **target behaviors.**

(3) In addition to defining the problem in behavioral terms, the therapist assesses conditions that maintain or minimize these behaviors. Steps 1 and 3 are referred to as **behavioral analysis.** Careful documentation and quantification are of great importance in determining factors that influence or trigger the undesired behaviors and in evaluating the effectiveness of the interventions. Since clients are often unaware of sequences of events that lead to a specific type of behavior, direct observation of clients in their environments is sometimes a necessary part of behavioral analysis. Clients can often be trained in self-observation skills and in recording of events so that the behavioral analysis is more accurate. Data derived from the analysis are used by the therapist to formulate a clinical hypothesis about what stimulates (precedes) and what maintains (reinforces) the undesired actions, thoughts, feelings, or physiological changes.

(4) Using methods supported by theories and findings from the literature, the clinician tests the hypothesis of cause and effect by altering the behavior or the environment (or both) and observing the effects of the alternation on the client's dysfunctional actions, thoughts, and feelings.

(5) From systematic observation and documentation of behavioral changes, the clinician either revises the hypothesis or continues with treatment until the goals of therapy are reached, ie, the target behaviors are changed. It is important to stress that behavior therapy is based on a way of thinking about people and problems and is not a set of techniques. Testing one hypothesis often leads to the development of another hypothesis, which in turn must be tested.

Other Characteristics Shared by Behavior & Cognitive Therapies

In addition to sharing the empirical, scientific approach outlined above, behavior and cognitive therapies have other characteristics in common:

(1) Therapy involves action as well as discussion. It is often directive, structured, and brief or time-limited.

(2) The client must be a responsible participant in the therapy and capable of achieving personal change.

(3) The present (here and now) determinants of behavior are emphasized rather than the historic (then and there) determinants.

(4) It is assumed that human behavior follows natural laws.

(5) It is assumed that people's behavior reflects their adaptation to the environment and not necessarily underlying pathological disorders.

(6) It is assumed that behavior can be changed directly without changing personality dynamics.

(7) Paraprofessionals, lay people significant to the client, and even the clients themselves can carry out treatment.

(8) The treatment often involves "homework." Only in rare instances is treatment confined to 1 or 2 hours a week with the therapist. Exercise, rehearsal, practice, and other activities are generally carried out by the client between sessions.

Historical Context

In his experiments on learned and unlearned (conditioned and unconditioned) behavior, Ivan Pavlov

(1849–1936) trained dogs to salivate at the sound of a bell by repeatedly pairing a conditioned stimulus (bell) with an unconditioned stimulus (food powder) that naturally causes an unconditioned response (salivation). Similarly, John B. Watson (1878–1958) taught a 1-year-old boy to be afraid of a white rat by pairing the child's approach to the rat with a loud noise. The boy then generalized his fear to other white furry objects. This study suggested the process whereby phobias might develop and gave impetus to later work on aversive conditioning and counterconditioning.

For their research using **classical conditioning,** Pavlov and Watson are credited with beginning the systematic study of the effects of environment on behavior. However, it is **operant (instrumental) conditioning** that has had the major effect on behavioral theory as applied to clinical problems. In the 1950s, behavioral modification began to attract attention, largely because of the work of B.F. Skinner (1904–1990). Skinner used operant conditioning principles— which hold that behavior is a function of its consequences **(reinforcers)**—to change the behaviors of psychotic patients in the wards of state hospitals. Techniques such as extinction and positive reinforcement, as well as programmatic efforts such as token economies (all described in subsequent sections), are examples of applied operant conditioning principles.

Throughout the 1950s and 1960s, behavior modification focused on stimulus (S) and response (R), while factors mediating the S-R connection were largely ignored. However, with the accumulation of empirical clinical data, it soon became clear that the variance in how one responded to a situation would not always be predicted by the stimulus that preceded it or the consequence that followed it.

In order to improve their ability to understand, predict, and control behavior, therapists and researchers (eg, Albert Bandura, Julian Rotter) began exploring cognitive variables such as expectancy (predictions of future happenings), attributions (inferred characteristics of people or events), and mental images (ideas). While traditional behavior therapy focused on observable stimulus-response (S-R) connections, cognitive behavior therapy took into account the importance of mediating factors within the organism (S-O-R). As pointed out by Turner et al (1981) in the *Handbook of Clinical Behavior Therapy,* "the acceptance of the role of cognitive variables in behavior theory and therapy has been very slow and grudgingly given. From the very beginning of the behavior movement, cognitive behaviors and private events were viewed outside the realm of behaviors because they were not subject to direct observation, measurement, and manipulation." Since the 1970s, however, cognitive variables have been given a central role in the understanding of processes that influence behavior (eg, self-instruction, cognitive therapy for depression, imagery techniques).

Cognitive therapy—which is farther along on the continuum from behavior therapy to cognitive behaviorism—focuses more on the individual's interpretations of internal and external events and views them as crucial in understanding behavior. The purely cognitive view holds that dysfunctional thoughts may be influenced by dealing with the individual's thoughts directly.

Of recent interest to clinicians is the new field of behavioral medicine (see Chapter 38), which involves the use of behavioral and cognitive principles and techniques in the treatment of medical problems such as hypertension, weight reduction, obesity, and cancer.

TECHNIQUES

This section will briefly outline some of the many techniques that have been developed in the cognitive-behavioral area. Any attempt to classify these treatments into behavioral or cognitive categories is frustrating for all but the most naive, since the methods in the field have so intertwined behavioral and cognitive perspectives. We have, however, presented the techniques in a progression from those relying more on observable behavior to those relying more on private and subjective cognitions.

Positive Reinforcement & Extinction

Reinforcement and extinction are discussed first, since they represent an early attempt to apply behavioral principles to treatment of seriously disturbed patients. It is a well-known learning principle that the probability a specific behavior will occur is increased when the behavior is followed by certain pleasurable consequences (reinforcers). For example, in a now classic study, it was demonstrated that certain verbal responses of a patient would be increased by an approving "mm-hm" from the therapist. When a behavior is no longer reinforced and is ignored, the probability of its occurring is decreased. For example, ignoring a patient's request for special treatment should lead to the elimination of these requests.

A clinical example from the literature will illustrate not only the effectiveness of positive reinforcement but also the care with which behavioral data are used for determining improvement.

Illustrative Case

A 39-year-old woman with a diagnosis of schizophrenia exhibited self-destructive behaviors such as burning herself and her clothing with cigarettes at a baseline rate of once a day. Because she liked to smoke (ie, would frequently indulge in this behavior), hospital staff members were instructed to inspect the patient for burns every hour and to give the patient half of a cigarette (reinforcer) and praise her for her appearance (secondary social reinforcer) if she were found to be burn-free. If she burned herself during the hour, she received no further cigarettes that day. Burns decreased from one a day to one approximately every 4 days (0.24 burns a day), and during the last 2 weeks of her hospitalization she remained burn-free.

Among the learning theory concepts that are important in applying positive reinforcement and extinction are the concepts of shaping, prompting, and modeling. Since it may take some time for a specific behavior (eg, speech in a mute patient) to be elicited, the desired behavior must be **shaped** by the therapist's reinforcing successive approximations of the wanted behavior (eg, progressively rewarding lip movement, then vocalizations, then isolated words, and finally sentences). Desired behaviors may also be **prompted** (eg, shaping the lips of the patient) or **modeled** (eg, saying words in front of the patient).

In institutionalized settings such as inpatient psychiatric wards or prisons, behaviors can be reinforced indirectly by issuing tokens (secondary reinforcers) that can be "traded in" for primary reinforcers or for other reinforcers such as watching television. This **token economy** approach is based on the underlying premise that dysfunctional behavior exists because it has been reinforced. Even professional staff members inadvertently reinforce undesired behavior by attending to (and thereby reinforcing) unwanted behavior such as head banging or delusional speech. Token economies represent an effort to provide an environment that systematically reinforces the desired behavior and extinguishes self-defeating dysfunctional activities.

Tokens (such as poker chips or points) offer several advantages over direct reinforcers: (1) They are readily available and can be handed over immediately after the desired behavior. (2) Tokens may be saved and redeemed later when the desire arises for goods or services, so that satiation is not a problem. (3) The number of tokens issued for a specific behavior may be increased or decreased depending upon how consistently the new behaviors are evidenced.

The staff must be trained to recognize desired behavior, to administer tokens, and to ignore dysfunctional actions. They must consistently apply the reinforcement and extinction principles. One or two staff members who do not apply these principles reliably and readily can undermine the efforts of the others.

A study spanning a 6-year period including a post-institutionalization follow-up indicated that 89% of the patients in a token economy unit had improved while on the ward, whereas improvement was seen in only 46% of patients receiving milieu therapy alone. Eighteen months following discharge, 92% of patients treated in the token economy unit and 71% of those treated in the milieu therapy unit were living in the community. A little-emphasized but important result

of token economies is the improved morale and efficiency of the staff, who see progress and feel a sense of accomplishment with a difficult population.

Aversive Procedures

Much of our everyday behavior reflects avoidance of aversive consequences built into various components of our personal and institutional lives—disapproval from friends, failing grades, imprisonment, etc. The application of this principle to clinical problems is **aversive therapy.** Aversive procedures are useful clinically in two main sets of cases: when dysfunctional or inappropriate behavior is naturally reinforcing to the individual (eg, addictions, deviant sexual behavior) or when behavior is self-destructive and needs to be brought under control quickly.

There are three main aversive procedures: classical conditioning, punishment, and avoidance training. The aversive stimuli used clinically are numerous but usually involve electric shock, chemicals, or vivid descriptions of noxious scenes.

In **classical conditioning** procedures, the stimuli leading to unwanted behavior (eg, sight and smell of one's favorite alcoholic beverage) are paired with a noxious stimulus (eg, shock). After the unconditioned stimulus (shock) is repeatedly associated with the conditioned stimulus (alcohol), patients develop the same feeling toward the alcohol as they feel toward the shock (fear). Since learned responses are more generalizable in lifelike settings, clinicians have had barlike settings constructed in inpatient alcohol units. Here patients are exposed to the sights, sounds, and smells of a bar, but these stimuli are paired with shocks. The goal of such treatment is avoidance of bars by the patients once they have been discharged.

In **punishment** procedures, a specific behavior (eg, drinking alcohol) is followed by a noxious stimulus or punishment. In the bar setting just described, punishment was used as a component of the treatment. A patient who had poured a favorite alcoholic beverage received a strong electric shock to the little finger (punishment) when he or she started to take the drink, The shock continued until the patient spit out the alcohol (**negative reinforcement** or **escape conditioning**). Thus, the patient was punished for undesired behavior (drinking) and then reinforced for desired behavior (spitting out the alcohol).

In **avoidance training** procedures, patients can escape the noxious stimulus altogether if they avoid the undesired behavior. This is the theory behind the use of disulfiram (Antabuse). If the patient drinks even a small amount of alcohol while a dose of disulfiram is still in the body, severe nausea and vomiting will occur. The patient can avoid these unpleasant effects entirely by not drinking (see Chapter 19).

The effectiveness of aversive principles for the treatment of self-destructive behaviors is well documented. For example, Lovaas and Simmons (1969) reported a case in which a 16-year-old mentally retarded girl bit her hands (and had previously bitten them to the extent that one finger had to be amputated), ripped her nails out with her teeth, and severely banged her head. Five 1-second shocks following these behaviors eliminated the problem.

In general, aversive techniques are most effective when used in conjunction with other forms of treatment and with procedures that reinforce the patient for desired behavior. Aversive procedures have been shown to have little effect on patients who actively oppose treatment, because they do not generalize from the learning situation to the real world. However, regardless of the effectiveness of such techniques for voluntary, motivated subjects, one should consider ethical factors in using aversive techniques and keep in mind that aversive techniques are susceptible to greater and more harmful abuses than other procedures. Because of the potential for abuse, some states regulate the use of aversive procedures or even prohibit entirely their use with certain populations. For example, the District of Columbia prohibits the use of "aversive stimuli" for mentally retarded persons. The American Association on Mental Deficiency has recently issued a statement urging elimination of many of these techniques, including all which cause obvious physical pain and dehumanization (Rubenstein, personal communication, 1987). Similarly, some clinicians advocate that state licensing boards and professional societies approve and monitor the use of aversive techniques, especially in involuntarily institutionalized populations.

Systematic Desensitization

People may become "sensitized" to a stimulus, and this link leads to pathological, destructive, or unwanted behaviors. For example, the reaction of a very shy and insecure person to the "stimulus" of other people may be panic, and this reaction may lead the person to avoid other people as much as possible and become virtually incapacitated in the presence of others. A person who has grown up thinking sex is immoral, unclean, and forbidden may react to a sexual situation by becoming anxious and unable to function. A person who has been in a traumatic car accident may be overwhelmed with fear at the prospect of riding in a car again. In these cases, avoiding the stimuli (other people, sexual situations, and being in a car) can be positively reinforcing because it reduces panic, anxiety, and fear. The individuals are sensitized (in a defeating way) to the stimuli, and the problem is to help them become desensitized. To accomplish this goal, Wolpe (1958) developed a method of systematic desensitization.

In systematic desensitization, the strategy is to help the client create a state (ie, complete relaxation) that is incompatible with anxiety, fear, or tension and then to gradually introduce the stimulus. The incompatible state acts to inhibit the negative reactions. This part of the process is known as reciprocal inhibi-

tion. The connection between the stimulus and the anxiety is systematically weakened until complete desensitization occurs.

There are numerous ways to accomplish complete relaxation, but most are variations of the progressive relaxation procedure popularized by Jacobson (1938). Clients assume a comfortable, passive position in a quiet room. They are told to free their minds of all troublesome or anxiety-provoking thoughts and to become as comfortable as possible, beginning with relaxing their feet. First they tense all the foot muscles for several seconds (as is sometimes done in isometric exercises) and then let them go limp. This process not only helps them relax that part of the body but also helps them learn body signals relating to relaxation. They can feel the muscles release tension. They learn to identify the feeling of being without tension, which many people who are chronically tense have not experienced before. Once the feet are relaxed, the same process of tensing followed by relaxation is repeated for the calves and other parts of the body. This process may take some time to rehearse and learn. The next step is to begin desensitizing the stimulus, as illustrated below.

Illustrative Case

The client was afraid of parties, formal dinners, and similar social situations. He worked with his therapist to construct a hierarchy of cues (stimuli) associated with fear: Most terrifying to the client was actually being at such a gathering; slightly less frightening, driving to the gathering; still less intimidating, dressing for the occasion; and least intimidating though still a problem, receiving an invitation in the mail.

After he was thoroughly relaxed, the client began by imagining the least frightening stimulus in his hierarchy. When he became tense, he repeated the relaxation process. After he could contemplate receiving an invitation without having an increased heart rate, sweaty palms, and thoughts of panic, he progressed to thoughts about the next stimulus, dressing for the party. Several sessions, each focusing on one stage of the hierarchy, were required before the client could run through the stimuli in his imagination without experiencing overwhelming anxiety.

The client then began to repeat the process, starting with the least threatening aspect, in real rather than imagined situations. Slowly and systematically, he became desensitized to the stimuli. He was finally able to attend and enjoy social gatherings.

It is not clear why systematic desensitization is effective, although Wolpe believes that the process of reciprocal inhibition is responsible. (See the following section on exposure treatment for a different explanation.) What does seem clear is that the technique works for many clients in relatively few sessions.

Exposure Treatment

Recent work indicates that overcoming avoidance behavior (eg, phobias, obsessive compulsive behavior) may depend not upon relaxation paired with progressively more anxiety-provoking scenes, as Wolpe suggests, but actual exposure to the feared stimulus. Exposure treatment involves exposure of clients to the stimuli that evoke discomfort until they become accustomed to them. The types of procedures vary, ranging from those evoking little anxiety (as in the slow, graded, imagined process of desensitization described earlier) to those immersing the client in the feared situation (process of flooding).

Marks (1981) has done extensive work both in developing the theory and refining the clinical practice of exposure treatments. Based on past systematic research, he outlined the conditions most suitable for exposure therapy: agoraphobia, social phobias, illness phobias, simple ("specific") phobias, obsessive thoughts, compulsive rituals, and types of sexual dysfunction (see Chapters 23 and 27).

For treatment of agoraphobia, Marks suggests choosing to work on simple but important activities at first. Initially, a reassuring person should accompany the agoraphobic person into the feared situations (eg, driving on a freeway). Exposure can then be attempted alone but at less anxiety-provoking times (eg, not at rush hour). Prolonged exposures (1–2 hours) seem to be more effective than short exposures. The client is required to record behaviors in a diary. (See Marks's [1978] self-help book for clients, *Living With Fear*.)

Illustrative case. A married 40-year-old woman had been agoraphobic for 15 years. Lately, she had been unable to leave the house without her husband. She chose as her goal (target behavior) the ability to cross a busy street alone. Treatment began with crossing a street with the therapist. After they had done this several times, the therapist stood apart and then moved farther away as the client crossed the street. By the end of the first 1½-hour treatment session, the woman was able to cross the street alone. She felt pleased with her accomplishment and much calmer. She was given homework assignments consisting of crossing streets near her home. By the end of the eighth treatment, the woman was crossing streets and shopping alone without anxiety.

Self-Talk

It is common for children to repeat instructions to themselves as they attempt new tasks. For example, while crossing the street unaccompanied for the first time, a child may engage in a running monologue of the parents' instructions: "Stop at the corner. Wait for the light to change from red to green, and make sure the "walk" sign is on. Now look both ways to make sure no traffic is coming." These instructions may be repeated aloud, in a whisper, or silently. Adults too may attempt to learn new tasks in this way, eg, in taking up golf or tennis or assembling a bicycle.

People may be taught to use such self-talk—in the form of evaluative statements, suggestions, reminders of sequential steps, and encouragement—to help them relax, to improve performance of cognitive and physical activities, to increase motivation, and to become more aware and alert. Such self-talk is obviously related to the processes of covert modeling and cognitive therapy (see below).

Various techniques may be used for teaching self-talk in therapy, but the general approach is demonstrated by Meichenbaum's (1977) program of self-talk for children, which has been successful in treatment of problems related to hyperactivity, aggression, disruption, and cheating. There are five basic steps after the problem has been identified and the behavior to be learned has been defined: (1) The child observes as an adult model performs the behavior. While the child is watching, the model describes the behavior aloud. (2) The child performs the same task while the model gives instructions. (3) The child performs the task while giving instructions aloud. (4) The child whispers the instructions while performing the task. (5) The child performs the task without audible speech.

Cognitive Therapy

The underlying premise of cognitive therapy is that effect and behavior are largely functions of how people construe (structure) their world. According to one cognitive theory, everyone has "filters" through which the world is interpreted (eg, seeing the glass half-full versus seeing it half-empty). When these constructs become distorted and dysfunctional, clients often experience helplessness, anxiety, and depression (depressogenic schemas). Beck et al (1979) are the best-known investigators of cognitive therapy for depression. The goals of this cognitive therapy are (1) to make clients aware of their cognitive distortions through psychotherapy and (2) to effect change through correction of these distortions. Common distortions (errors in information processing) that make people depressed include selective abstractions (missing the significance of a total situation by selecting a detail out of context), arbitrary inferences (jumping to a conclusion with missing or contradictory evidence), over-generalizations (unjustified generalizations on the basis of one incident), and magnifications (exaggerating or elaborating on specifics). (See the writings of Beck et al [1979] for a detailed description of these common errors.)

The numerous strategies used in cognitive therapy are designed to help the client become aware of negative automatic thoughts (eg, "If I can't be perfect, then no one will love me"); to recognize connections between thoughts, affect, and behavior; and to replace distorted thoughts with more realistic and option-filled interpretations.

In a typical course of therapy for depression, clients are initially told how cognitive therapy works. They are then assigned "homework" such as keeping a schedule of activities to help them assess their present levels of functioning. In the next session, the relationship between thinking, behavior, and affect is demonstrated using specific experiences of the client. Later, the client is told how to recognize, monitor, and record emotions and situations associated with negative automatic thoughts (Table 35–1) and how to devise rational responses. These automatic thoughts and their underlying assumptions are then discussed in therapy and examined for logic, adaptiveness, and likelihood of promoting healthy behavior. The following discussions between patient and therapist are examples from Beck et al (1979):

P: The only way I could ever be happy is if I could be a great writer
T: What level of writing would you have to reach?
P: I would have to be as good as [a specific poet].
T: Did this poet achieve great happiness?
P: No, I guess not. She killed herself.

As the therapy progresses, the focus shifts to identifying recurrent or common themes and finally to uncovering major beliefs that make the person vulnerable to depression:

T: Your automatic thought was, "Your children shouldn't fight and act up." And because they do, "I must be a rotten mother." Why shouldn't your children act up?
P: They shouldn't act up because . . . I am so nice to them.
T: What do you mean?
P: Well, if you're nice, bad things shouldn't happen to you.
(At this point, the patient's eyes lit up.)

The course of treatment continues in this way for about 15–25 once-weekly sessions. In contrast to the more traditional psychotherapies, in cognitive therapy the clinician is active and directive and the focus is on "here and now" problems. In contrast to the more behavior-oriented therapies, cognitive therapy is concerned with altering the client's internal experiences (eg, thoughts, daydreams, feelings) rather than external behavior per se.

Beck (1985) summarized eight studies comparing the efficacy of cognitive therapy with that of antidepressant medication. Findings showed that: (1) cogni-

Table 35–1. Example of a daily record of dysfunctional thoughts*

Date	Situation	Emotion(s)	Automatic Thought(s)	Rational Response	Outcome
	1. Describe actual event leading to unpleasant emotion. **or** 2. Describe stream of thoughts, daydream, or recollection leading to unpleasant emotion.	1. Specify sad/ anxious, etc. 2. Rate degree of emotion, 1–100.	1. Write automatic thought that preceded emotion. 2. Rate belief in automatic thought, 0–100%.	1. Write rational response to automatic thought. 2. Rate belief in rational response, 0–100%.	1. Rerate belief in automatic thought, 0–100%. 2. Specify and rate subsequent emotion, 1–100.
9/8	Received a letter from friend who was recently married.	Guilty 60	"I should have gone to her wedding." 90%	It was inconvenient; she wouldn't be writing if she was angry about it. 95%	10% Guilty 20
9/9	Was thinking of all the things I wanted to get done over the weekend.	Anxious 40	"I'll never get all of this done. It's too much for me." 100%	I've done more than this before, and there is no law that says I have to get it all done. 80%	25% Anxious 20
9/11	Made a mistake ordering supplies.	Anxious 60	Pictured my boss yelling at me. 100%	There is no evidence my boss will be angry; even if he is, I don't have to be upset. 100%	0% Relieved 50
9/12	Pictured myself being depressed forever.	Sad/anxious 90	"I'll never get better."	I have gotten better in the past. Just because I think something is true doesn't make it true. 80%	40% Sad/anxious 60
9/13	My date called and said he couldn't go out with me because he had to work.	Sad 95	"He doesn't like me. NO ONE could ever like me." 90%	He asked me out for next weekend, so he must like me. He probably did have to work. Even if he didn't like me, it doesn't follow that "no one could ever like me." 90%	30% Sad 50

*Reproduced, with permission, from Beck AT et al: Page 288 in: *Cognitive Therapy of Depression.* Guilford Press, 1979.

tive therapy alone was as effective as three trials or more effective than two trials of antidepressant medication; (2) the combination of cognitive therapy and drug therapy was more effective than drug therapy alone; and (3) cognitive therapy alone appears to be as effective as drug therapy plus cognitive therapy. These studies indicate that cognitive therapy achieves good results in ameliorating symptoms of moderate unipolar depression in nonpsychotic outpatients.

In an important study sponsored by the National Institute of Mental Health (Elkin et al, 1986), cognitive therapy achieved results comparable to imipramine (antidepressant medication) in reducing the symptoms of depression and improving patients' functioning. Preliminary results indicate that symptoms were eliminated completely in 50–60% of patients who received cognitive, interpersonal (Chapter 34), or drug therapy and in 29% of those who received a placebo plus clinical management. Imipramine reduced symptoms more quickly, but in the last 4 weeks of the 16-week treatment period, both forms of psychotherapy were as effective as the drug. However, among the patients considered "severely depressed," cognitive therapy was the least effective treatment.

Most recently, Beck et al (1985, 1990) have applied the principles of cognitive therapy to the clinical problems of anxiety and personality disorders. Clinical and empirical studies in these areas are promising.

Positive Imagery

Singer (1974) pioneered the research, theory, and clinical applications of positive imagery. The idea is simple: Engaging in positive imagery tends to elevate one's moods and affects, tends to increase enjoyment, and can decrease the frequency and intensity of potentially debilitating and self-defeating thoughts and feelings. The key idea is that imagery need not be explicitly related to one's difficulties or embody modeled "answers"; it just needs to be pleasant. This approach has been effective in the treatment of pain, anxiety, severe depression, and phobic behavior.

Illustrative Case

The client presented for psychotherapy with the following pattern of severe anxiety and depression: On awakening each morning, she began to worry about her job, finances, and children. By the time she got to work, she was a "nervous wreck." She often returned home early because of "sickness," and more recently she began missing days of work. Though exhausted at the end of day, she had trouble falling asleep. Anxious about her situation and concerned and sad about the way things were going, she tossed and turned all night.

The treatment plan for modifying various aspects of the client's experiences, habits, and situation included the use of positive imagery: Four times a day (upon awakening and before lunch, dinner, and going to bed), the client spent at least 15 minutes with her eyes closed, thinking of the most pleasant scenes she could imagine. According to her reports during subsequent weeks of therapy, the imagery varied widely and included scenes of vacations she had taken or would like to take, funny scenes, and sexual fantasies. Some imagery was far from realistic (eg, she pictured herself floating high above the clouds). She found that these positive scenes were helpful in "setting the tone" for her days and nights; breaking the momentum generated by her depressive, anxious, and obsessive thoughts; relearning what it felt like to enjoy herself; and freeing her from the depression of what she described as "those days when my worries seemed to snowball and come down and crush me."

ISSUES & MISCONCEPTIONS ABOUT BEHAVIOR-ORIENTED THERAPY

Popular misconceptions and concerns about the use of behavior-oriented therapies, as expressed by numerous investigators and outlined in the American Psychiatric Association's *Task Force Report on Behavior Therapy* (1978), are listed and briefly described below:

(1) *Behavior therapy is coercive, manipulative, and controlling.* Because behavioral techniques are often powerful, direct approaches to changing behavior, they are criticized for controlling the individual's behavior. For this reason, behavior therapists have worked with both the American Psychological Association and the Association for the Advancement of Behavior Therapy to develop ethical guidelines for informed consent, use of aversive procedures, and protection of the client's rights.

(2) *Behavior therapy is superficial, and "symptom substitution" will occur.* Proponents of the theory that many undesired behaviors are symptoms of (or epiphenomena associated with) an underlying disease argue that if only symptoms are addressed, then new symptoms will appear at a later date because the underlying problem (ie, disease) has been left untreated. Although this theory of causation may be true, extensive empirical data from published reports fail to support any indication of new symptoms occurring after the target behaviors have been removed. In fact, effective treatment of specific target behaviors has often resulted in improvement in other aspects of the clients' lives.

(3) *Behavior therapists ignore feelings and thoughts and treat humans as robots.* Many of the techniques described in the previous sections are focused on the inner world of the individual (eg, images, thoughts, feelings). These private events are playing an increasingly important part in behavioral-cognitive therapies. The objectives of the behavior therapist, however, are to make the client's subjective experiences public by means of the client's self-report and self-observation and to define the experiences objec-

tively in terms of observable phenomena or physiological measurements. In this process, clients may become aware of their own feelings and thoughts for the first time and thus increase the likelihood of changing them.

Behavior therapy adheres to the principle of determinism, which holds that events have causes and that relationships between cause and effect follow orderly laws; however, the individual is not seen as a reflexive robot. In behavior therapy, the interaction between environment and behavior is viewed as a dynamic one. There is a reciprocal determinism that has relevance for issues such as responsibility and choice. The growing field of behavioral self-control and the increasing number of do-it-yourself strategies for control of weight, smoking, and stress indicate ways in which individuals can alter their external and internal environments. Such behavioral approaches often provide more options and actions for the individual and result in increased personal freedom and dignity.

(4) *Behavior therapy is limited to a narrow spectrum of disorders.* Disorders that seem particularly amenable to behavioral-cognitive psychotherapies include not only phobias but also obsessive compulsive disorders and other anxiety disorders, sexual disorders, adjustment disorder, marital problems, disorders of impulse control, unipolar depression, stammering, enuresis and hyperactivity in children, and the "habit" disorders (eg, obesity; tobacco, alcohol, and other drug dependence). In addition, the same therapeutic techniques may be used for improving social skills, assertiveness, basic self-care skills, and disruptive behaviors in severely disturbed patients.

(5) *Behavior therapy denies the importance of the therapeutic relationship.* To some extent this criticism is true, especially in regard to the manner in which behavior therapy was practiced in the 1950s and 1960s, when the focus was more on manipulation of environmental factors (see Historical Context, above). Today, factors affecting the outcome of therapy, such as the expectations for treatment success, the therapeutic alliance (successful working relationship between client and therapist), and the client's motivation, have become part of the therapist's concern. Persons and Burns (1985) investigated the nature and quality of the client-therapist relationship in addition to the technical cognitive interventions. They found that a reduction in the clients' negative mood was associated with a decrease in the clients' degree of belief in their automatic thoughts; moreover,

clients' good relationships with their therapists contributed additional positive changes.

(6) *Behavior therapy only works with nonverbal, unintelligent, severely disturbed people.* Current behavioral-cognitive approaches seem to be helpful in treating a broad spectrum of clients with a wide variety of backgrounds and personality traits. In fact, several cognitive approaches—eg, paradoxical intention, reframing (reconceptualizing problems), logical investigation of depressogenic assumptions—seem particularly effective in helping highly verbal, logical, intelligent individuals learn to recognize and control obsessional thoughts that interfere with social functioning.

(7) *Behavioral-cognitive techniques are practiced only by psychologists and paraprofessionals, not by psychiatrists.* This statement has some validity, although several of the well-known pioneers in these fields are psychiatrists. Behavioral techniques can often be implemented by paraprofessionals and the clients themselves. This is seem by many as an advantage, since professional time can be devoted to developing treatment strategies and performing thorough behavioral analyses. Unfortunately, most residency programs for psychiatrists do not include training in basic behavioral science, and few behavior therapists are directly involved in the programs. This is a regrettable situation, since research in behavioral science has led to a number of specific treatment programs and has provided a method of approaching problems that has great clinical value for the practice of psychiatry.

RECENT TRENDS IN BEHAVIOR & COGNITIVE THERAPIES

Two trends are clear: (1) Behavior therapy is becoming increasingly more cognitive in its approach. Perhaps the melding of the technology of behavior therapy with the clinical concerns of the cognitive therapists has prevented what Kelly (1963), an early cognitive theorist, called "the hardening of the categories." (2) Behavioral-cognitive approaches are being integrated with psychodynamic theory and practice. In general, the field of psychiatry is fortunately moving away from a "horse race" mentality, testing which "school" of therapy is best, to a more "process-oriented" approach, searching for which factors (eg, therapeutic alliance), regardless of the school, lead to better outcomes.

REFERENCES

American Psychiatric Association: *Task Force Report on Behavior Therapy.* American Psychiatric Association, 1978.

Bandura A: *Social Learning Theory.* Prentice-Hall, 1977.
Beck AT: Is behavior therapy on course? Behav Psychother 1985;13:83.

Beck AT et al: *Anxiety Disorders and Phobias: A Cognitive Perspective*. Basic Books, 1985.

Beck AT et al: *Cognitive Therapy of Depression*. Guilford Press, 1979.

Beck AT et al: *Cognitive Therapy of Personality Disorders*. Guilford Press, 1990.

Elkin I et al: Outcome findings of the NIMH collaborative research program. Presented at the National Convention of the American Psychiatric Association, May, 1986.

Gitlin B et al: Behavior therapy for panic disorder. J Nerve Ment Dis 1985;173:742.

Jacobson E: *Progressive Relaxation*. Univ Chicago Press, 1938.

Kelly GA: A *Theory of Personality: The Psychology of Personal Constructs*. Norton, 1963.

Kendall PC, Holloon S (editors): *Cognitive-Behavioral Interventions: Assessment Methods*. Academic Press, 1982.

Lanyon RI, Lanyon BP: *Behavior Therapy: A Clinical Introduction*. Addison-Wesley, 1978.

Lovaas OI, Simmons JQ: Manipulation of self-destruction in three retarded children. J Appl Behav Anal 1969;2: 143.

Mahoney MJ: *Cognition and Behavior Modification*. Ballinger, 1974.

Marks I: *Cure and Care of Neuroses*. Wiley, 1981.

Marks I: *Living With Fear*. McGraw-Hill, 1978.

Meichenbaum D: *Cognitive-Behavior Modification: An Integrative Approach*. Plenum Press, 1977.

Paul GL, Lentz RL: *Psychological Treatment of Chronic Mental Patients*. Harvard Univ Press, 1977.

Persons JB, Burns DD: Mechanisms of action of cognitive therapy: The relative contributions of technical and interpersonal interventions. Cognitive Ther Res 1985;9:539.

Singer JL: *Imagery and Daydream Methods in Psychotherapy and Behavior Modification*. Academic Press, 1974.

Sjoden PO, Bates S, Dockens WS: *Trends in Behavior Therapy*. Academic Press, 1974.

Thoresen CE: *The Behavioral Therapist*. Brooks/Cole, 1980.

Turner S, Calhoun KS, Adams HE: *Handbook of Clinical Behavior Therapy*. Wiley, 1981.

Wolpe J: *Psychotherapy by Reciprocal Inhibition*. Stanford Univ Press, 1958.

Group Psychotherapy

36

Nick Kanas, MD

Group psychotherapy is a form of treatment in which beneficial changes in emotionally disturbed patients occur as a result of their interactions with other patients and at least one trained professional therapist in a group setting. Therapeutic results include both relief of symptoms and resolution of intrapsychic and interpersonal problems. The therapist's tools are clinical experience and applied theories of individual psychodynamics and interpersonal systems.

HISTORY OF GROUP PSYCHOTHERAPY

The first psychotherapy group was described in 1907 by Joseph Pratt, a Boston internist, who developed a group method of educating and improving the morale of patients with tuberculosis. Around 1910, Jacob Moreno in Europe began using theatrical techniques to have patients "act out" problem situations in a group setting; this later became known as psychodrama. In the late 1920s and early 1930s, a number of psychiatrists began applying psychoanalytic theory to groups, emphasizing issues of transference, free association, and recapitulation of family problems.

During the late 1930s and early 1940s, Kurt Lewin began emphasizing the importance of group member interactions and introduced the notion of group dynamics, a phenomenon describing actions in a group as being more than the sum of individual interactions. The need to train more therapists in the theory of group dynamics became obvious after World War II, when large numbers of veterans requiring psychiatric assistance began to overburden the personnel resources of the mental health system. Programs to train therapists using Lewin's concepts were established at the National Training Laboratories in Maine and at the Tavistock Clinic in England, where the work of Bion and Ezriel led to the "group-as-a-whole" approach to treatment.

During the ensuing 30 years, numerous approaches to group psychotherapy were introduced, including transactional analysis, gestalt, interactional, existential, and behavioral approaches. Currently, techniques borrowed from a number of theoretical schools are being consolidated to devise new responses to the specific needs of patients.

EFFECTIVENESS OF GROUP PSYCHOTHERAPY

Clinical experience and anecdotal evidence support the view that group psychotherapy is effective treatment for properly selected categories of patients. Successes have been reported in both inpatient and outpatient settings with both psychotic and nonpsychotic patients. A number of theoretical approaches to group psychotherapy have been advocated.

Evidence from controlled studies also attests to the usefulness of group psychotherapy. Since 1975, a number of reviews have concluded that group psychotherapy is effective for patients with neurotic and personality disorders; schizophrenia; alcoholism; and medical illnesses, including asthma, myocardial infarction, obesity, chronic pain, and ulcers. Group psychotherapy has been found to be as effective as or even more effective than individual psychotherapy in studies directly comparing the two methods.

INDICATIONS & CONTRAINDICATIONS FOR GROUP PSYCHOTHERAPY

In organizing a psychotherapy group, the therapist must take into account both diagnostic and individual psychodynamic factors.

Diagnostic Factors

A. Indications for Psychotherapy in Heterogeneous Groups: Table 36–1 shows disorders for which treatment in a heterogeneous group (ie, consisting of a variety of psychiatric disorders) is most appropriate. In such groups, the diversity of problems and issues allows for maximal interaction and breadth of discussion. In getting the group together, the therapist should consider whether one patient will be perceived by the other as "too different," since this may result in scapegoating and rejection. For example, an elderly woman in a group of young adults might be rejected by the other members even though she is in the group to work on issues unrelated to aging. If at least two elderly patients were in the group, the tendency to scapegoat would be lessened.

Group psychotherapy with heterogeneous groups is particularly beneficial for patients with personality and neurotic disorders. Patients with personality disorders tend to blame others for their maladaptive interactions and lack insight into their own role in provoking interpersonal strife. Since they do not have significant degrees of anxiety or other symptoms, they are only weakly motivated to change and often come to treatment at the urging of a spouse, employer, or primary-care physician. The group psychotherapy setting is an environment in which such patients can display and then be confronted with their maladaptive interactions. At the same time, other group members can offer support and reinforcement for positive changes, and this "reward" encourages them to remain in treatment.

In contrast to patients with personality disorders, patients with neurotic disorders often have a number of symptoms, such as anxiety and depression, and perceive their difficulties as coming from within. For these reasons, neurotic patients do well in individual psychotherapy, although many also benefit from group psychotherapy. Such patients use the group to gain insight into the cause of their problems and to understand the effects their symptoms may have on other people.

Other patients benefiting from heterogeneous group psychotherapy include those with somatoform disorders or major depressive episodes. Such patients do well in supportive group settings where the impact of their illness on others can be explored. In some cases they may also gain insight into the causes of their problems.

B. Indications for Psychotherapy in Homogeneous Groups: Table 36–1 shows disorders for which a homogeneous group format is more appropriate. All of the patients have a similar problem, and the group is oriented toward addressing that problem. Homogeneous psychotherapy groups differ from support groups involving interaction with people who share some common problem in that the approach is more insight-oriented and the leader is professionally trained. A psychotherapy group made up of alcoholics differs from a meeting of Alcoholics Anonymous in that patients in psychotherapy not only gain support and encouragement for sobriety but also focus on problems related to their alcoholism, such as intrapsychic conflict and maladaptive interpersonal relationships. Although more limited in scope than their quickly become cohesive and allow for greater depth in exploring a particular set of problems.

Group psychotherapy in a homogeneous group is the treatment of choice for patients with substance use disorders such as alcoholism and drug dependency. By orienting these groups around the addiction problem, several issues that affect the patients in similar ways may be discussed. Such groups are particularly useful for confronting patients who deny having the diagnosed problem. Group psychotherapy of alcoholics should emphasize abstinence as the treatment goal and deal specifically with the members' denial. The predisposing causes of alcoholism should be ex-

plored only after its manifold sequelae are thoroughly discussed. At all times, confrontation and frank discussion should be tempered with support, advice, and reinforcement of positive changes.

Although a few stable schizophrenics can be treated in heterogeneous groups, most schizophrenics do better in homogeneous groups. In heterogeneous groups consisting of both psychotic and nonpsychotic patients, it is difficult to create a group environment meeting the needs of both populations. For example, the use of uncovering techniques may help a nonpsychotic patient, but self-disclosure may produce intolerable anxiety in a schizophrenic patient. Conversely, education and reality testing may help a psychotic patient but be experienced as unbearably boring by a less disturbed group member. Schizophrenics do well in homogeneous groups emphasizing controlled expression of emotions, reality testing, and socialization and contact with others.

Homogeneous groups are beneficial for patients suffering from chronic pain and illness such as asthma, myocardial infarction, and cancer. In such groups, themes involving disfigurement or loss of function, the responses of loved ones, and the fear of death can be raised and dealt with in a supportive, caring manner.

Patients with gender identity disorders also benefit from homogeneous group psychotherapy where sensi-

Table 36–1. Indications and contraindications for group psychotherapy, based on diagnostic considerations.

Indications
Most personality disorders*
Neurotic disorders*
Somatoform disorders*
Major depressive episode*
Substance use disorders†
Schizophrenic disorders†
Medical illness†
Gender identity disorders†
Posttraumatic stress disorders‡
Adjustment disorders‡
Contraindications
Acute manic episode
Antisocial personality disorder
Questionable§
Organic mental disorders*
Schizoid personality disorder*
Paranoid personality disorder*
Delusional disorders*
Dissociative disorders*
Factitious disorders*
Paraphilias‡
Sexual dysfunctions‡

*Therapy in heterogeneous groups (ie, groups of patients with different disorders) is recommended.
†Therapy in homogeneous groups (ie, groups of patients with same disorder) is recommended.
‡The type of group (heterogeneous or homogeneous) depends on the individual case.
§The decision about the appropriateness of group psychotherapy is based on such factors as the patient's degree of impairment and desire for treatment and on individual psychodynamic factors.

tive matters involving sexual themes can be openly discussed in a supportive, nonhostile environment. For treatment of some disorders, such as adjustment or posttraumatic stress disorders, either homogeneous or heterogeneous group psychotherapy may be indicated; the choice in specific cases depends on whether the patient needs help in dealing with the effects of a specific stressful event or the effects of stress in general on interpersonal functioning.

C. Contraindications to Group Psychotherapy: Group psychotherapy is not for everyone. Overstimulation in the group environment causes patients with acute manic episodes to become more hyperactive and pressured. Patients with severe antisocial personality disorders who are more interested in manipulating others than in improving their interpersonal relationships usually hinder group progress.

D. Questionable Indications for Group Psychotherapy: Table 36–1 lists several disorders for which group psychotherapy is "questionably" indicated. The decision about whether group psychotherapy is indicated depends on such factors as the degree of impairment, desire for treatment, and individual psychodynamic factors.

Individual Psychodynamic Factors

Along with general diagnostic considerations, individual psychodynamic factors must also be assessed in pondering referral for group psychotherapy. Since intrapsychic conflicts influence and are influenced by interpersonal relationships, it is helpful if patients can view their problems in terms of difficulties experienced in relationships with other. Some therapists view this capacity as a criterion of potential for gaining insight and making progress in group psychotherapy.

The process of uncovering unconscious conflicts can provoke strong feelings. For some patients, transference feelings evoked in a group setting are more intense than those that arise in individual therapy; for others, the group setting is more tolerable because transference feelings can be distributed among other group members in addition to the therapist. Patients with problems resulting from unconscious conflicts may benefit from group psychotherapy, particularly if they are unable to tolerate transference feelings evoked in individual psychotherapy.

Group psychotherapy is especially useful for patients whose psychodynamic problems lead to maladaptive interpersonal relationships, since these interactions can be observed and explored in the group. For example, authority or dependency conflicts may be observed in the way some group members relate to each other or to the group leader.

Extremely manipulative patients, inveterate malingerers, and those who are socially deviant or engage in extreme acting-out behavior do not do well in group psychotherapy except in controlled settings. Patients must have some ability to relate to others and tolerate individual differences. For this reason, patients with schizoid or paranoid personality disorder often do poorly in the group setting. Group psychotherapy patients need adequate impulse control so they can tolerate confrontation with other group members. Patients with severe organic mental disorders may become confused or anxious in group psychotherapy. Finally, a patient in acute distress and unable to tolerate the process of assimilation as a new member usually does better in individual psychotherapy, where his or her needs can be tended to more quickly and specifically.

PRACTICAL CONSIDERATIONS IN ESTABLISHING & LEADING THE GROUP

In setting up a psychotherapy group, the therapist should take into account its setting and purpose, the types of patients to be included, what their treatment goals will probably be, and whether they have complementary personality characteristics.

Numbers of Patients; Age Ranges

Most groups have 6–12 patients, and eight is often said to be the optimal number. Having four or fewer patients inhibits free expression because members are afraid to disagree lest someone drop out, which would mean that the sessions would have to be discontinued. With more than 12, there is too little time for each patient. Inpatient groups tend to be **open,** which means that new patients are admitted to the group as others are discharged. Outpatient groups may be open or closed. In **closed** groups, the makeup stays the same for long periods without addition of new members.

The age range of patients in most groups is 20–60 years, with adolescent and geriatric patients often being treated in homogeneous groups formed specifically for the purpose of dealing with the problems of people in those age groups. Some therapists advocate splitting up adults into groups of young (20–40 years) and middle-aged (40–60 years) patients.

Preparatory Sessions for Patients Entering the Group

Most therapists advocate preparatory sessions for prospective group members. A variety of formats for these sessions can be used, ranging from a brief one-to-one discussion with the therapist to participation in a minigroup in which patients sample the group experience by undergoing a number of structured exercises. Preparation reduces the patient's anxiety over what to expect, establishes a working alliance between therapist and patient, and allows the therapist to observe the patient's reactions in a structured interpersonal setting. Careful preparation significantly reduces the number of dropouts and improves attendance at the sessions. A combined factual-experiential approach is more effective than just giving factual information about "what group psychotherapy is all about."

Whether or not a patient goes through a preparatory phase, the therapist should have some idea beforehand of the patient's style of interacting with others. One way to find out is to ask about the patient's experience with other kinds of groups (at church, at the office, etc). A more direct approach would be to draw the patient's attention to the process of interaction during the interview. The patient's response—particularly the degree of defensiveness or interest in this novel way of looking at behavior—will serve as a clue to his or her later behavior in the group.

Ground Rules

Ground rules regarding timely attendance, payment of fees, notification of planned absences, and discussion of issues before making major life changes are important aspects of the group. Patients will sometimes violate these rules for psychodynamic and interpersonal reasons. The therapist should monitor such behavior and not hesitate to bring it up in the group for general discussion.

A patient who becomes threatening or disruptive may have to be temporarily excluded from the group. The reasons should be explained to the patient and discussed with the other members. When stable and in control again, the patient may reenter the group.

Frequency & Duration of Therapy

Most psychotherapy groups meet once or twice a week, although inpatient groups and psychodynamically oriented outpatient groups may meet three to five times a week. A typical session lasts 1–2 hours.

The duration of therapy in inpatient groups is influenced by the average length of hospitalization, which is 2–6 weeks in most acute care units. For this reason, inpatient groups are usually characterized by rapid turnover. Outpatient groups tend to be longer-term, with some patients remaining in the group months to years, depending on their problems and treatment goals. Briefer, time-limited outpatient groups (lasting 1–4 months) generally emphasize the establishment of realistic, limited treatment goals—eg, the resolution of current problems rather than the uncovering of unconscious conflicts—and the use of didactic and supportive techniques. In these groups, therapists tend to take an active role, encouraging patient responsibility and focusing on practical issues. Careful patient selection and pretraining are critical for the success of therapy in short-term groups.

Number of Therapists

Many group therapists prefer a **co-therapy model,** in which two therapists are present in the group. Both should have roughly equal training and experi-

ence so that one will not be perceived as " junior" and be scapegoated by the group. Since sessions may be disrupted or made ineffective by competition or by theoretic or technical differences of opinion between therapists, co-therapists should work to maintain a good relationship. Male-female co-therapy teams are effective in encouraging discussion of parental, gender, and sexual themes.

Advantages of co-therapy include enhanced objectivity in assessment of patients, resulting from discussion between the therapists after group sessions; the potential for increased transference feelings in the group; continuity of the group when one therapist goes on vacation or becomes ill; and better control of the group in times of crisis (eg, admission of a hostile, disruptive patient).

Combined Individual & Group Psychotherapy

Some patients undergo both individual and group psychotherapy at the same time. In some cases, the therapist is the same in both settings; in other cases, the patient has one therapist for group psychotherapy and a different one for individual psychotherapy. Most therapists prefer the former combination, since the patient can be managed without the need for time-consuming and perhaps conflictual communication with another therapist. Some group patients not receiving combined therapy resent another member's private access to the therapist; however, this competitive issue can usually be dealt with in the group.

Adding group psychotherapy for patients in individual psychotherapy is recommended if the patient does hot make adequate progress in the one-to-one situation and if it appears that the group setting would allow the patient to experiment with new ways of relating to others. The challenge and stimulation of group interaction can uncover problems in personality function while at the same time providing relief from a one-to-one treatment focus.

Adding individual psychotherapy for patients in group psychotherapy is recommended if the patient has difficulty sharing problems in a group setting; if the patient wants to intensify efforts to resolve a particular problem or conflict; or if it is felt that a sudden crisis or stressful event in the patient's life can be dealt with more quickly and effectively in individual treatment.

Problems of resistance or countertransference arising in one treatment setting should be dealt with in that setting; the issue should not be avoided by recommending both individual and group psychotherapy. If there is a danger that the dissonance resulting from two treatment approaches might overrun fragile defenses, combined treatment should not be used.

Format of Sessions

Most psychotherapy groups are **discussion-oriented.** Patients are expected to talk about problems and other significant aspects of their personal lives. They are encouraged to divulge feelings, be open and honest, and listen to issues involving other patients. Some issues directed toward the therapist may be referred back to the group, with the therapist asking what the members think about that issue. In order to stimulate discussion, the therapist may utilize a technique called "making the rounds," whereby each patient is asked in turn to express his or her thoughts about the issue at hand. In other group psychotherapy approaches, such as transactional analysis, a lecture format may be used, with interpersonal and intrapsychic issues diagrammed on a blackboard. Videotape playback is also used in some group settings to stimulate discussion.

Some psychotherapy groups are more **action-oriented.** In psychodrama, patients are asked to assume roles (spouses, parents, etc) in acting out a specific problem. In some behavioral approaches, patients practice techniques aimed at resolution of symptoms, such as systematic desensitization (see Chapter 35). In activity groups such as music or art therapy groups, patients meet to engage in activities that serve as a basis for intrapsychic and interpersonal learning.

GROUP DYNAMICS

When people come together in groups for any purpose, forces are set in motion that affect each member. Such forces are a feature of collective human behavior and go beyond the dynamics of dyadic (in pairs) interactions. For example, a normally nonviolent, law-abiding person may commit arson and other violent crimes in the context of a mob.

The therapist must be aware of the collective forces operating in a psychotherapy group at any given moment. Since the group environment exerts strong pressures on the members, the results may be negative as well as positive. The therapist's role is to maximize the therapeutic potential of the group environment for each individual. For example, in group settings where open and honest interactions occur, the members gradually learn the importance of free exchange of ideas and feelings and can apply these principles in their daily lives. If feelings are kept bottled up during group sessions and the therapist does not encourage their expression, group work will be unproductive and patients will be less inclined to express themselves openly in daily life.

Each individual in the group is affected by his or her perceptions of what other members think and feel about various issues. In psychotherapy groups, one often finds that many (perhaps all) patients have the same perception, which can be called a **group norm.** Group norms exert powerful predictive forces (pressure to conform) on the actions of individual members. If an individual's view of what is normative in a group is not in accord with reality, the discrepancy provides clues to psychodynamic and psychopatho-

logical factors affecting that member. For example, a withdrawn, paranoid patient might perceive the group setting as hostile and nonsupportive even though most of the other members see it as a place where they can express their concerns in a friendly environment. Such discrepancies alert the therapist to important issues of individual and group dynamics, issues that become "grist for the therapeutic mill."

The therapist may sometimes wish to point out a significant characteristic of the group, such as its avoidance of a specific topic. For example, following a suicidal gesture by a group member, it would not be unusual for this topic to be avoided in the next group session; the members might talk about emotionally bland or trivial matters or behave in a pressured, anxious manner. This resistance can be overcome by a simple comment: "Many of you seem anxious today. I wonder if John's overdose has something to do with that." In most instances, the patients will begin to discuss their feelings (anger, sadness, guilt) when the subject is raised. Such **process comments** are usually offered with the intention of providing opportunities for insight into psychodynamic or interpersonal issues or for the purpose of freeing up group resistance to a topic.

PHASES OF GROUP DEVELOPMENT

The group environment is affected by several factors, including the personalities of group members; the style and therapeutic stance of the therapist; the physical setting, ie, whether inpatient or outpatient; and, perhaps most importantly, the phase of group development. A developmental sequence of phases can be observed to occur in all groups but is most obvious in long-term, closed outpatient groups. Progress from one phase to another is dependent on successful resolution of issues involving the previous phase. Group development may cease to progress if this resolution does not occur.

Although numerous phases have been described (Beck [1981] identified nine phases), most conceptual models portray three main phases of group development. The **first phase** is characterized by hesitant participation and the establishment of initial group norms; the members depend on the therapist for guidance and approval. During this phase, the members should be able to perceive some common purpose in being there and declare their individual goals, while the therapist works in a quiet way to encourage the establishment of bonds between members. The **second phase** is characterized by conflict, dominance, and the establishment of a hierarchy ("pecking order") among the patients The therapist is often seen as an appropriate figure to be rebelled against, and fantasies may be entertained of excluding the therapist from the group. Several patients may band together to attack verbally or exclude a particular patient from their discussions, thereby identifying that patient as the group scapegoat. An important task of the leader is to help the group deal constructively with these aggressive tendencies. In the **third phase,** true group cohesiveness is established along with a sense of intimacy and mutual affection and need for each other. Overdependence on a rebellion against the therapist has been worked through, and the therapist is reintegrated with the group. A great deal of productive group work can be accomplished in the third phase.

THERAPEUTIC FACTORS

The benefits of group psychotherapy may be enhanced by the therapist's recognition of factors that contribute to improvement in a patient's condition. Bloch et al (1981) have reviewed the literature and discussed ten factors: self-disclosure, interaction, acceptance (cohesiveness), insight, catharsis, guidance, altruism, vicarious learning, instillation of hope, and existential factors. Yalom has described a method of studying some of these therapeutic factors, which he called curative factors. At the time of discharge, patients are given 60 statements describing 12 potentially helpful attributes of their experience in group psychotherapy and are asked to rank the statements from most helpful to least helpful. The ranking of statements is then used to create a similar ranking of the 12 curative factors. In one study (Yalom, 1975), psychiatric outpatients most valued their group experience for (1) giving them feedback on interpersonal behavior, (2) allowing them an opportunity to vent repressed feelings, (3) giving them a sense of acceptance by other people, and (4) helping them discover unconscious motivations for what they do. In contrast, psychiatric inpatients most valued their group experience for (1) giving them feelings of optimism through watching other patients improve and leave the hospital, (2) giving them a sense of acceptance by other people, (3) improving self-esteem through their ability

to help others, and (4) allowing them to feel less isolated (Maxmen, 1973). It is apparent that what is considered curative in a group may vary depending on the type of patient in the group, the group setting, and the length of stay. The therapist should keep these issues in mind and make appropriate use of the curative factors that are most suited to the patients' needs.

TYPES OF PSYCHOTHERAPY GROUPS

Psychotherapy groups can be categorized in a number of ways: inpatient versus outpatient, experiential versus didactic, supportive versus uncovering, affective versus cognitive, etc. Table 36–2 categorizes a number of psychotherapy groups in terms of their theoretical orientation. The therapeutic goals of most of these groups are relief of symptoms and resolution of intrapsychic and interpersonal problems. However, these goals are achieved in different ways. In some groups, the projection of unconscious conflicts onto the therapist is seen as crucial, and transference interpretations are viewed as major therapeutic interventions. In other groups, patient interactions are seen as prominent group activities, since they stimulate the discussion of interpersonal issues through which patients learn more about their behavior outside of the group. The focus of some groups is on activities that occur in the group itself **(here-and-now approach),** whereas other groups emphasize past events and activities that occurred outside the group **(there-and-then approach).** Many psychotherapy groups use a combination of theoretical principles borrowed from several of the schools represented in Table 36–2. When used in an appropriate and clinically relevant manner, this eclectic approach provides the therapist with a number of techniques to meet the patients needs.

Table 36–2. Types of psychotherapy groups.

Theoretical Orientation of Group	Major Goals	Importance of Patient-Therapist Transference Interpretations	Importance of Group Member Interactions	Importance of Here-and-Now Emphasis	Further Reading
Psychoanalytic	Resolution of intrapsychic problems	Extremely important	Moderately important	Moderately important	Day (1981)
Interactional	Resolution of intrapsychic and interpersonal problems	Minimally important	Extremely important	Extremely important	Yalom (1975)
Transactional analysis	Resolution of intrapsychic and interpersonal problems	Minimally important	Moderately important	Moderately important	Berne (1966)
Gestalt	Resolution of intrapsychic problems	Minimally important	Minimally important	Extremely important	Perls (1969)
Psychodrama	Resolution of intrapsychic and interpersonal problems	Minimally important	Moderately important	Extremely important	Moreno (1959, 1969, 1972)
Existential	Awareness of basic problems affecting existence	Minimally important	Extremely important	Extremely important	Miller (1978)
Behavioral	Resolution of symptoms	Minimally important	Minimally important	Moderately important	Harris (1979)

Issues and conflicts addressed in group psychotherapy may be categorized as affecting the entire group **(group-as-a-whole approach)** or affecting an individual or part of the group. Especially in early sessions of the group—when members may display similar affects, such as depression or helplessness, together with an attitude of dependency on the leader—the focus may be on issues and events that affect the group as a whole. As the group develops and as more differentiated and individualized responses and reactions occur, it may be necessary to intervene at the level of the individual or discuss interactions between several individuals. Theoretic approaches must be flexible enough to account for such developmental factors, and techniques should include both group and individual level interventions.

SUMMARY

Group psychotherapy is an established method of treatment in which patients may achieve relief of symptoms and resolution of intrapsychic and interpersonal problems as a result of interactions with other patients and the therapist, both in inpatient and in outpatient settings. Diagnostic considerations and individual psychodynamic factors should be taken into account in referring patients to a suitable group, and there are few absolute contraindications. Therapy groups may be heterogeneous (mixed disorders) or homogeneous (same disorder), open or closed. Adequate preparation of patients for group psychotherapy reduces the number of dropouts. Many groups use a cotherapist team approach, which offers several advantages over groups with just one therapist. Some patients benefit from being treated both individually and in a group during the same period.

Group therapists must be aware of issues involving individual psychodynamics, group dynamics, group development, and specific therapeutic factors relevant to the group. Most therapists use a combination of theoretic principles and techniques in constructing psychotherapy groups that best meet the needs of their patients.

REFERENCES

Beck AP: Developmental characteristics of the system-forming process. In: *Living Groups: Group Psychotherapy and General Systems Theory*. Durkin JE (editor). Brunner/Mazel, 1981.

Berne E: *Principles of Group Treatment*. Oxford Univ Press, 1966.

Bloch S, Crouch E, Reibstein J: Therapeutic factors in group psychotherapy. Arch Gen Psychiatry 1981;38:519.

Day M: Psychoanalytic group therapy in clinic and private practice. Am J Psychiatry 1981;138:64.

Grunebaum H, Kates W: Whom to refer for group psychotherapy. Am J Psychiatry 1977;134:130.

Harris FC: The behavioral approach to group therapy. Int J Group Psychother 1979;29:453.

Kanas N: Alcoholism and group psychotherapy. In: *Encyclopedic Handbook of Alcoholism*. Pattison EM, Kaufman E (editors). Gardner Press, 1982.

Kanas N: Group therapy with schizophrenics: A review of controlled studies. Int J Group Psychother 1986;36:339.

Maxmen JS: Group therapy as viewed by hospitalized patients. Arch Gen Psychiatry 1973;28:404.

Miller J: Attaining freedom in existential group therapy. Am J Psychoanal 1978;38:179.

Moreno JL: *Psychodrama*. Vol 1, 4th ed, 1972; Vol 2, 1959; Vol 3, 1969. Beacon House.

Perls FS: *Gestalt Therapy Verbatim*. Real People Press, 1969.

Vinogradov S, Yalom ID: *A Concise Guide to Group Psychotherapy*. American Psychiatric Press, 1989.

Yalom ID: *The Theory and Practice of Group Psychotherapy*, 2nd ed. Basic Books, 1975.

37

Family & Marital Therapy

Rodney J Shapiro, PhD

Contemporary family therapy offers an array of seemingly contradictory theories and practices, but some basic assumptions clearly distinguish family therapy from other psychotherapeutic approaches. A fundamental assumption common to all models of family therapy is that disturbed psychological functioning is not limited to a single individual but reflects disturbed interactions between persons who have significant relationships with each other. The family is the primary context in which important relationships develop and endure.

On the whole, family therapists are not much concerned with the origins of dysfunction, which are regarded as hypothetical matters and not amenable to change through psychotherapy. Rather, the emphasis is on the here and now and on the patterns of family interaction that currently act to sustain existing problems. The therapist can evaluate problems and design interventions on the basis of data provided by family members or observable in the treatment setting. The goal of family therapy is not to change the individual per se but rather to set right the system of relationships in which the individual is involved. Changing the interpersonal context of an individual may then result in beneficial change in one or more family members.

THE PRIMARY CONCEPTS OF FAMILY THERAPY

Research Contributions

Family therapy is a relatively recent development in the history of psychiatry The fundamental ideas and practices have emerged over the past 40 years, and the field is rapidly growing and diversifying.

The primary concepts grew out of the work of investigators exploring family factors related to schizophrenia in adolescents and young adults. Theodore Lidz (1972) and his group studied a large number of these families. The parents' relationships were frequently characterized by conflict or emotional distance, and Lidz discovered that in many cases the father exerted a negative influence on the child with schizophrenia. This recognition of the impact of the father's role represented a shift from the psychoanalytic preoccupation with the notion of the "bad mother" that was so prevalent in the 1940s and 1950s.

Murray Bowen (1966) is generally regarded as an originator and dominant figure in the history of family therapy. Beginning in 1954, he established a family research program at the National Institute of Mental Health to study schizophrenics and their families. A central premise that grew out of this work is that psychological dysfunction is directly related to level of ego differentiation. He viewed differentiation of self as necessary for change to occur, and his treatment approach was designed to facilitate such individuation. Another major component of Bowen's work was his multigenerational model of family dynamics. He noted that problems unresolved in one generation tend to be transmitted through succeeding generations.

Lyman Wynne succeeded Bowen as head of the Family Studies Section at NIMH. He and his coworkers generated a series of important studies on schizophrenia (Wynne et al, 1958; Singer, 1965). The term "pseudomutuality" was coined to describe the facade of unity and the prohibition of individual autonomy that is characteristic of schizophrenic families. Carefully designed research demonstrated an association between thought disorder in schizophrenics and patterns of deviant communication in their parents.

In the early 1950s, the anthropologist Gregory Bateson assembled a research group that included future leaders in the field of family therapy, such as Jay Haley, Don Jackson, and John Weakland. This creative group broke with existing models of psychopathology by basing their work on the assumption that all behavior (even symptoms) can be defined as communication. They explored patterns of communication in families, and their "double-bind" theory attracted considerable attention when it was first published (Bateson et al, 1956). The group postulated that schizophrenics are often beset by contradictory messages from parents that are impossible to ignore and yet cannot be responded to in any rational manner. The implication of this theory was that double-binding communication plays a role in the etiology of psychosis, but this idea was subsequently modified as it became evident that the double bind is not confined to schizophrenic family functioning. However, this group's studies on communication did greatly influence the concepts and practices of family therapy.

Don Jackson (1957, 1965) took the lead in formulating clinical applications of the group's communication studies, and his ideas continue to be fundamentally important for family therapists. He formulated the concept of "family homeostasis" to describe how interacting roles and behaviors tend toward maintaining the family system in a state of equilibrium. Patterned sequences of communication (feedback loops) ensure that parameters of permissible change are not breached. Dysfunctional families are particularly rigid and resistant to change. For example, freedom of expression may not be permitted even when it could be adaptive. Healthier families can tolerate greater degrees of change, sometimes even resulting in a new homeostatic system.If one parent is incapacitated, the rest of the family cooperates in modifying customary roles and filling in for the "missing" member, so that a new and successful pattern of family functioning is achieved.

Systems Theory & Cybernetics

The development of family therapy was strongly influenced by the emergence of general systems theory. Bertalanffy (1968) proposed a model of the human organism as an open system in constant interaction with the environment. A particular aspect of systems theory, known as the cybernetic model, explains the mechanics of self-regulating systems (such as homeostatic biological processes). This model was adopted by family therapists to explain how interactional patterns in families are regulated by communication transmitted through recurring feedback loops. The cybernetic principle demonstrates a fundamental tenet of family therapy known as circular causality. Traditional theories of psychology are based on linear causality, ie, a temporal sequence of cause leading to effect: $A - B$, $B - C$, $C - D$, etc. In order to understand a patient's current behavior, the therapist explores a chain of past events stemming from the original cause. The key assumption in family therapy is that problems or symptoms are maintained and reinforced by interactional patterns of communication. The past is deemphasized, and the focus is on the present for understanding and treatment of psychological problems.

CLINICAL INNOVATORS

The most notable clinician in the early history of family therapy was Nathan Ackerman (1966). He was trained as a child psychiatrist and psychoanalyst, but as early as 1937 he recognized the influence of family interactions on childhood disorders, and he departed from standard practice by treating the family as a unit. Nevertheless, his work continued to reflect a strongly psychoanalytic orientation. He was extremely adept at detecting nonverbal clues to underlying sexual and aggressive conflicts in family groups. Through active but gentle confrontation and incisive interpretation, he fostered personal disclosure and increased insight. His writings and considerable clinical

skills inspired many of the first generation of family therapists. In 1965, he established the Family Institute in New York City. Now known as the Ackerman Institute, it has earned international repute as a major center of family therapy training.

John Bell (1961) deserves mention as one of the first clinicians to develop family therapy techniques. His work with child disorders convinced him of the necessity for involving parents throughout the process of child therapy. He constructed a step-by-step approach for moving the focus of treatment from the identified patient (the child) to the parent-child interactions and finally to the parental relationship.

Virginia Satir became a legendary figure during her lifetime in part because of her charismatic personality and courage in challenging the mechanistic practices of conventional psychiatry. She had a pioneering role in developing family therapy. Her model of family therapy is still relevant and influential (Satir, 1964). She insisted that the therapist must offer direction and goals, facilitate a climate of personal safety and openness, and teach family members how to communicate. Implicit in this approach is the assumption that defensive distancing is the greatest impediment to psychological healing and enhanced self-esteem.

Among the first generation of family therapists, Carl Whitaker (1975, 1976) stands out as a uniquely innovative clinician. He abhors structured methods of treatments and insists that family therapy cannot be taught, yet his demonstrations and writings have inspired innumerable imitators. A point he emphasizes is the tendency for the therapist to become a target for family projections. To prevent this, the therapist must rely on subjective cues (warning signs) to avoid acting out the unconscious wishes of the family. For example, the therapist's subjective experience of intense anger may represent the projected rage of a seemingly compliant family member, or a subjective experience of nurturing may be a response to an unexpressed wish for protectiveness from a seemingly independent adult. Whitaker relies on such subjective signals to detect a core unconscious or concealed issue, and then he acts, often in unexpected or dramatic fashion, to unbalance defenses and spur increased disclosure. He strongly endorses cotherapy, so that one therapist can "risk" deep involvement in the maelstrom of family emotions while the other can play the role of reality check and rescuer. Whitaker's work is indispensable for the newcomer to family therapy. The originality and power of this clinician has been amply documented in a book by Napier and Whitaker (1978).

Salvador Minuchin (1967, 1974) devised his model of structural family therapy that broke from psychodynamic thinking. He conceptualized the family as a structure based on roles and boundaries. He emphasized an active role for the therapist and carefully planned strategies to achieve tangible treatment goals. As we shall see, structural therapy has come to be one of the dominant approaches in the field of family therapy.

CHARACTERISTICS OF FAMILY THERAPY

Despite obvious differences among practitioners of family therapy, there are principles of treatment to which most subscribe. In some basic respects, family therapy includes therapeutic practices that vary radically from those used by individual or group therapists.

Comparison With Individual & Group Therapy

For many years, individual therapy has been the principal mode in which psychotherapy is conducted, and the essential characteristics of individual therapy continue to reflect psychoanalytic tradition. The therapist works with one person who presents with a self-recognized problem or who is identified by others as having a problem. If deemed suitable for psychodynamic therapy, the patient is expected to freely verbalize thoughts and feelings. Significant events from the past are revived and reexamined. The therapist's role is that of listener endeavoring to understand the implications of these reports. The patient is guided toward greater self-awareness as a prerequisite to changes in behavior and symptoms.

These conditions rarely occur in family therapy, where participation by one or more family members is usually required. The therapist is interested in the objective reality of family relationships; individual dynamics, defenses, and symptoms are translated into interactional terms. Since family therapists are chiefly concerned with observable behavior, they are alert to nonverbal cues and communication sequences. Current functioning is the major focus in family therapy. The goal of individual therapy is to change the individual, whereas the family therapist strives to bring about change in the family's system of relationships.

On initial observation, family therapy may seem like group therapy applied to a group of family members. The only points of similarity, however, are that both group and family therapy require participation by more than one person, and both are concerned in varying degrees with interpersonal relationships. The distinction between the aims of individual therapy (changing the individual patient) and family therapy (changing the system of relationships) applies to the comparison of group therapy and family therapy as well. Group therapy is also designed to produce change in the individual patient. Interpersonal relationships among group members do provide significant material for group therapy but only in terms of highlighting the problems of individual participants.

There are other less apparent but highly significant differences between group and family therapy. The participants in group therapy are usually strangers to begin with; they may be urged not to see one another socially between sessions; and they may have no expectation of continuing contacts with one another beyond the life of the group. These conditions facilitate self-disclosure and confrontation, since there is no inhibiting concern that future relationships will be impaired. Furthermore, all members of the group admit to having problems; they are all ''in the same boat.'' Their shared identity as patients also provides assurance of acceptance and encourages self-revelation.

Families, on the other hand, are bound by historical continuity, and this creates a treatment situation radically different from that of group therapy. Family members are linked by a common past, have ongoing contact, and anticipate continuing involvement in the future. Concerns about impairing relationships may severely inhibit openness and confrontation. Family members are sometimes motivated to participate in therapy because they feel they can help the person who has been identified as the patient, while they themselves are simply glad they are not the ones who are ''sick''; they may deny or be unaware of the impact their own behavior or problems have on the identified patient. The relatives usually continue to resist being labeled as patients. These conditions make for greater resistance than is found in group therapy. A climate of support and acceptance is also less likely in family settings. Family members are all too aware of each other's faults, and criticism and even scapegoating are typical aspects of family life.

Families are generally more resistant to treatment at the outset than are patients seeking individual or group therapy This initial obstacle poses an immediate challenge to the family therapist. It may take considerable skill to neutralize resistance and establish positive relationships with family members so that therapy can proceed. On the other hand, family members are bound by deeply entrenched loyalties and obligations, and this common bond provides a powerful incentive for mutual involvement in therapy. In contrast, group therapy members experience transient relationships and less profound emotional involvement with one another.

Another difference between group and family therapy that has important clinical implications is that the therapist in the family group is literally outnumbered. Family members often share rigidly held beliefs and attitudes, and the therapist, as the representative of an alternative perspective, may not have sufficient power to influence the group. This situation is a special problem in psychotic families, which are characteristically impervious to messages from outside sources. Participants in group therapy—even if all of them are psychotic—do not share a history of common beliefs, and the group therapist often finds allies among the group members who may help influence the ideas and behavior of any one patient.

Indications & Contraindications for Family Therapy

Most family therapists maintain that instead of asking when family therapy should be used, clinicians should rephrase the question and ask when family therapy is *not* indicated. They contend that family therapy is indicated for all problems affecting family relationships unless practical obstacles prevent attendance of family members at meetings. Geographic distance can be a realistic obstacle; older patients may have outlived their families; and adult immigrants may have no family ties in their adopted country.

There are also some clinical conditions that make family therapy inadvisable. It may be unwise to initiate family therapy if one member is in the throes of a brief reactive psychosis. A paranoid individual may have such a hostile relationship with the family that attempts to bring all members together for meetings are doomed to failure. Family therapy is generally inadvisable when the irrevocable breakup of a family has already occurred; eg, if one spouse has decided on marital separation, it may simply postpone the painful process if both partners meet at the insistence of a therapist.

Obviously, the contraindications considered above apply to only a small percentage of the cases that typically come to the attention of practitioners of family therapy. For the great majority of patients, the inclusion of family members enriches the data source for a thorough assessment, and participation of the family can often expedite the treatment process. While family therapy is helpful for most problems, there are two problem areas for which family therapy is definitely the treatment of choice. Family therapists are unanimous in endorsing the value of their approach for problems of children and adolescents and for marital conflict. These areas deserve more detailed consideration.

FAMILY THERAPY FOR CHILDREN & ADOLESCENTS

In the case of children, there are two overwhelming arguments in favor of family therapy rather than individual therapy. First, it is assumed that problems of children always indicate family dysfunction; individual therapy for the child ignores the family's problems. Second, any therapeutic success from individual therapy with the child would be short-lived unless the dysfunctional family system were also treated. In fact, the family may well resist changes that seem incompatible with the needs of the parents and the other children. It is not uncommon for parents to undermine or terminate therapy at a point when the child is manifesting signs of healthier attitudes and behavior.

Some individual therapists object to family therapy for adolescents on the grounds that it impedes the adolescent's strivings for independence. They also argue that adolescents need confidentiality in order to talk freely about sex and other personal matters. Family therapists reply that adolescents with problems have failed to develop independence precisely because their families have difficulty in permitting or encouraging this phase of development. The therapist must help the entire family adjust to the increasing independence of one or more of its members. As the family learns to cope with the separation and individuation of the offspring, additional psychotherapy can be helpful for the adolescent who is now free to deal with problems in the world away from home. Usually, a combination of family therapy and individual or group therapy is most effective for adolescents.

Younger children should always be seen separately from their parents for at least one evaluation session. This ensures that they have the privacy and protection to report events and express feelings that might otherwise remain suppressed. In cases of known or suspected abuse, separate evaluation meetings for the child are essential. Children often do well with individual play and verbal therapy in addition to their involvement in family therapy.

The concept of triangulation has special relevance when working with problems of children. The difficult or symptomatic child is often that child who is most involved with the parents and thereby represents the third member of a triangle. The role may be identified with concern (the child as identified patient) or with negative attributions (the child as behavioral problem). How and why a particular child becomes involved in a triangle is an important question for the diagnostician, and attempting to modify or undo this dynamic is the task of the family therapist.

Illustrative Case

A couple requested help because their 7-year-old son, an only child, had developed school phobia. A thorough evaluation revealed that the child's presenting problem was an interpersonal relationship problem involving all family members. The mother, an extremely anxious and dependent woman, had always looked to her husband for direction and support. When they met, he himself was insecure, but he compensated by asserting strong control in the relationship, and he encouraged his wife's dependency. Over several years, however, the husband became increasingly successful in business, and as he developed greater self-confidence, he began to perceive his wife as undesirably weak and demanding. When the wife realized that her husband was becoming more distant emotionally, she became even more anxious and dependent. This caused the husband to become even more distant and preoccupied with work, so that the wife's anxiety in turn increased.

The birth of the child was welcomed by both parties. The wife looked to the child for the support her husband failed to provide. The husband hoped that his son would serve as his surrogate for his wife's attentions and thus free him from her demands and alleviate his guilt about his withdrawal from her. As the child grew, he learned to tolerate his father's lack of involvement, since it seemed to ensure the continuing attention of his doting mother.

This pattern of interaction stabilized over a number of years until an unavoidable developmental shift disrupted the family's equilibrium. At age 6 years, the son began to attend primary school. The start of formal schooling represented the first major separation for mother and son. The family had actively worked to minimize the son's earlier attendance at nursery school and kindergarten, but such avoidance was no longer possible. On most mornings before school, the child complained about various ailments and "upset" feelings. More often than not, the parents permitted him to stay home. Medical investigations ruled out any organic basis for the symptoms.

The parents grew increasingly distressed and felt great conflict about the situation. On the one hand, the child's symptoms helped to stabilize the marital relationship, and both parents now felt threatened by the possibility of a disruption of the status quo. On the other hand, the parents were genuinely concerned about the consequences of their son's missed days of school. Periodically, and with much ambivalence, they would urge the boy to go to school, but this simply heightened his anxiety and precipitated his symptoms. A conference with a pediatrician led to the referral for family therapy.

The goals of treatment were to facilitate a collaborative relationship between the parents, encourage a closer bond between father and son, help the mother achieve greater independence and autonomy, and firmly but benignly reinforce the son's school attendance as an important step toward appropriate separation from his parents. The family responded well to therapy, and these goals were realized to their satisfaction.

MARITAL & COUPLES THERAPY

The variety of family life-styles in our culture requires a broader focus than conventional marriage. Accordingly, in this chapter the term "marital therapy" is defined as the treatment of any unit of two adults who consider themselves a couple by reason of cohabitation or mutual commitment.

The conceptual basis of marital therapy is strongly identified with family systems theory. Marital therapy can best be distinguished from family therapy on the basis of the unit of treatment. It is confined to one generation (the adult dyad), whereas family therapy encompasses two generations (parents and children) and sometimes three (grandparents). All family therapists include marital therapy as part of their work, but not all marital therapists work with families.

Most therapists agree that marital therapy is indicated when presenting problems are primarily to do with the marital relationship. Treatment disposition is less clear-cut when the presenting problems are a mix of individual and marital concerns or when marital issues surface early in the course of individual therapy. The decision whether to implement couples therapy is usually determined by the therapist's assessment of the causes and the relative significance of each problem.

Most clinicians now recognize the effectiveness of involving the partner in cases of sexual dysfunction. There has been growing recognition that sexual dysfunction is best understood as one significant component of a complex interpersonal system. In practical terms, treatment of a sexual problem must take into consideration the couple's overall relationship. A knowledge of family systems theory and mastery of techniques of marital therapy are essential components of training for sex therapists. (See Chapter 27.)

Family and marital therapy have proved effective in the treatment of various forms of substance abuse. Several studies have produced important insights into the marital system of alcoholics and drug abusers. Shapiro (1982) and Steinglass (1981) have demonstrated how the spouse of the substance abuser may inadvertently play a role that reinforces addictive behaviors. No matter what treatment program is utilized, compliance with treatment and a successful outcome are extremely unlikely without involvement of the spouse in treatment.

A serious problem closely related to substance abuse is that of domestic violence. Conventional treatment methods have focused on the victims of abuse (women, children, the elderly). Male perpetrators are regarded as unmotivated to change and resistant to treatment, and the standard approach is to coerce them into treatment by means of court orders or the threat of legal recourse. Treatment for the male is usually individual therapy or participation in a group for male batterers. A different approach has been advocated by some clinicians who demonstrate that many of these men can be induced to enter treatment voluntarily and that couples therapy may be more successful in effecting cessation of violence (Shapiro, 1982).

The role of the therapist working with couples is more difficult and complex than that involved in working with individuals or entire families. When working with individuals, the therapist strives to achieve a working relationship with one person that is mutually positive. In work with families, there is always the chance that some members will dislike or attack the therapist occasionally, but there are also other members who will provide support and protection. With couples, however, the challenge is to establish a positive alliance with *each* partner within a context often marked by accusations, blaming, and attempts to manipulate the therapist into taking one side or the other.

A therapist who attempts to maintain strict neutrality (along the lines of traditional psychoanalytic psychotherapy) may lose the cooperation of both partners, since they are likely to ascribe the therapist's neutrality to a lack of interest or concern. The marital therapist must constantly change sides, but in a way that neither antagonizes one partner to the point of leaving nor establishes a one-sided alliance with the other. The goal is not to maintain neutrality but to be able to side with each partner individually at different points in the therapy.

The tendency to assume positions of right and wrong is most often seen in therapy with couples. The therapist must resist being drawn into arguments. A solid grounding in family systems theory is the therapist's best deterrent, since it is usually clear that there is neither a right nor a wrong answer when a couple's disputes are explored from an interactional point of view. Partners who adopt polarized positions are said to have become snared in a repetitive sequence of interactions and are unable to experience or choose alternative ways of responding. This is shown in the following illustrative case, which also demonstrates how a seemingly simple dispute can mask complex interpersonal dynamics.

Illustrative Case

A major source of conflict for the couple was the husband's apparent unwillingness to find secure employment. The wife came from a wealthy family and received a monthly allowance from her parents. The wife periodically became furious at her husband for his ''laziness'' in not finding ''significant work.'' He spent most of his time caring for their children at home and engaging in charity and volunteer work. He protested that they did not need the extra income and that he was unable to find suitable work in any case. The more the wife pressured him, the less the husband did to change the situation. At one point, the wife turned to the therapist in sheer exasperation and asked, ''Don't you think a grown man should have a steady job?''

The therapist's initial reaction was to agree with the wife that it was ''wrong'' for the husband to resist employment and that he was clearly sponging off her. The therapist refrained from expressing an opinion, however, and sought to understand more about the interactional dynamics of the dispute. It became clear that whenever the husband did make genuine efforts to find a job, tentative as these were, the wife did not support him and in fact put obstacles in his way; she was unconsciously resisting his possible employment. The dispute about work masked some underlying issues that could not easily be reduced to a matter of simple right or wrong. The wife had great difficulty expressing warmth and affection for either her husband or her children. The husband protected her from her deficiencies in parenting by taking care of the children during the day. One of the stabilizing influences in the marriage was the

wife's certainty that her husband would never abandon her. He was a dependent and rather masochistic partner and seemed to put up with a good deal of verbal abuse. His refusal to work also enabled his wife to remain dependent on her parents, who were sympathetic to her plight and provided emotional and financial support.

Avoiding employment served as a defense mechanism for the husband as well. He related to his wife as if she were a scolding mother. His dependency needs were met by knowing that his wife seemed to need him as much as he needed her. Despite their bitter arguments, he sensed that she actually tolerated his lack of employment. His immaturity and poor self-esteem made him feel safer with children than with adults, and he looked to his children for closeness and acceptance. Having always led a sheltered life, he had profound fears of testing himself in the everyday world and subconsciously protected his self-esteem by assuring himself that he was too good for most of the jobs that were available.

Attributes & Values of the Therapist

The personal attributes and values of the therapist can play a determining role in establishing a therapeutic relationship with couples and in effecting a successful outcome in treatment. The therapist's age, gender, sexual orientation, marital status, and cultural background may be significant in particular situations. A marked discrepancy in age is always a problem; couples may feel inhibited and awkward with therapists who are much younger or older than themselves, and therapists are more likely to experience countertransference reactions in such circumstances. Gender is also a significant consideration in couples therapy. If the therapist is male, the husband may see him as a competitor, while the wife may feel that he is incapable of understanding her. On the other hand, the wife may view a female therapist as a competitor, whereas the husband may believe that the therapist is biased against men. Racial and cultural differences between therapists and clients may also prove detrimental to treatment, particularly if these differences are unacknowledged or not discussed.

Nontraditional Couple Systems

Contemporary marital therapists cannot limit their work to couples who meet the legal definition of marriage. A high divorce rate and resistance to marriage are creating considerable numbers of single adults and parents, unmarried cohabitants, and people who marry more than once. Rapidly changing social and moral values are reflected in greater tolerance for alternative life-styles and confusion about what constitutes normal family functioning. The marital therapist must learn to work with unmarried couples, remarriage families, and gay or lesbian couples. Work with nontraditional couple systems is clinically challenging and requires an innovative and flexible approach to assessment and treatment.

Couples considering or going through separation often look to marital therapists for help. When one or both partners is considering separation, the marital therapist can provide a safe and productive environment for working through this difficult life event. If a separation has already been effected, it may be unwise to insist on conjoint treatment. Couples who are moving irrevocably toward permanent separation need to maintain appropriate distance not enforced closeness. One exception to this recommendation is the couple who mutually accepts the reality of separation and wishes to use couples therapy as an aid in working through the separation process. The term ''divorce therapy'' has been coined to describe this process of working through a dissolution of marriage. Therapy for couples contemplating or in the midst of separation and divorce may be especially helpful when children are involved.

CURRENT TRENDS IN FAMILY THERAPY

Many of the originators of family therapy were trained in psychoanalysis. Some retained their psychodynamic views, whereas others renounced psychoanalysis as incompatible with family therapy.

The initial schism in the field of family therapy occurred over the acceptance or rejection of psychoanalytic theory. The movement away from psychoanalysis has gathered momentum in recent years, and current trends reflect an almost complete break with psychodynamic theory and practice. Interpretation has little or no place in contemporary family therapy, and insight is regarded as irrelevant for change. The subjective states of client and therapist are largely ignored; the emphasis is on actual behavior and active treatment interventions.

Structural Family Therapy

In Salvador Minuchin's model of structural therapy (1974), the emphasis is on current functioning. The therapist initially explores the nature of the problem, translates this problem into interpersonal terms, and then devises a strategy for promoting change. Central to Minuchin's work is the concept of the family as a structural organization established by the hierarchical arrangement of relationships and the boundaries between family subgroups and members. In a well-functioning family, there is a clear hierarchical differentiation between the parents, who have executive functions, and the children, who have some input but much less power in decision making. The boundaries in a healthy family separate the parents from the children but allow sufficient interaction between the subgroups to maximize closeness and cooperation.

In dysfunctional families, there may be lopsided or chaotic hierarchical arrangements. For example,

a particular child may have inordinate power, with the result that the parental coalition is weak or nonexistent. Such families are likely to experience major problems in rearing and attempting to discipline their children. Another example of dysfunctional hierarchy is a family in which one parent has excessive power and the other parent is powerless. In dysfunctional families, boundaries between the subgroups tend to be either too rigid or too weak. When boundaries are extremely rigid—eg, between parents and children—a withdrawn quality is noted in relationships. These families do not offer closeness and a feeling of involvement, and the children are at risk of becoming delinquent or running away Families with weak boundaries between subgroups are said to be ''enmeshed.'' In these families, emotional dependency is so pervasive that family members may fail to achieve sufficient autonomy and differentiation to function successfully.

The goal of structural therapy is to modify the hierarchical relationships and boundaries so as to promote healthier functioning—eg, in a family in which the parental alliance is weak and one parent is overly involved with a child, treatment strategies are designed to form a parental subgroup that is separated from the child. The case of the 7-year-old child presented earlier demonstrates some of the principles of the structural approach to family therapy.

An impressive development resulted from the application of structural family therapy to the study and treatment of children suffering from diabetes, asthma, and anorexia nervosa. Minuchin et al (1978) distinguished between primary and secondary psychosomatic disorders. Primary psychosomatic disorders are those in which physiologic dysfunction is already present (eg, diabetes or allergic diathesis in patients with asthma). Existing physiologic symptoms are then exacerbated by emotional arousal due to stress. Secondary psychosomatic disorders are characterized by an absence of predisposing physiologic dysfunctions. In patients with these disorders (eg, anorexia nervosa), emotional conflicts are transformed directly into somatic symptoms.

Examination of the family systems of children with certain psychosomatic disorders reveals a characteristic pattern of personal dynamics: excessive emotional involvement of family members (enmeshment), overprotectiveness, rigidity of coping mechanisms, and ineffectiveness in resolving conflicts. A key finding is that children with certain psychosomatic illnesses are inappropriately involved with their parents' conflicts. A typical sequence of interactions recurs in these families. Conflict in the parental unit triggers stress and symptoms in the child; the child's symptoms become a focus of concern for the parents; and the conflict between the parents is temporarily diverted by the symptoms, which are both a reaction to stress and a temporary solution to stress. Family therapy is effective in breaking this cycle of interaction and bringing about improvement of symptoms. The Minuchin group used a rigorous protocol to confirm their results. For example, in their studies of diabetic patients, they drew blood samples during family meetings to look for rapid changes in free fatty acid levels. Increased free fatty acid levels are compatible with emotional arousal and signal the onset of diabetic ketoacidosis as well. This procedure furnished the group with exact data on emotional arousal associated with specific family interactions and also provided objective measurement of a positive outcome in treatment.

Strategic Family Therapy

The emphasis in strategic family therapy is on effective methods of promoting rapid change in families. The central idea of this approach is to define a problem and devise an appropriate strategy for solving that problem. Skillful methods of interviewing have been developed that rapidly and efficiently pinpoint key problem areas in families. Analysis should clarify the nature of interactions that reinforce and sustain the problem behaviors. A strategy is then designed to modify the interactional patterns and hence change the problem.

Although there are significant differences between the various models of strategic therapy, most focus on identifying current interactional patterns that keep a family "stuck" and on devising strategies to help the family change these patterns. The best-known approaches are the brief therapy methods of the Mental Research Institute group) Watzlawick et al, 1974, Weakland, 1974) and the brilliant problem-solving techniques of Jay Haley (1976, 1980) and Chloe Madanes (1981). Mara Selvini Palazzoli (1978) led a group of psychoanalysts in developing brief strategic methods of family therapy for anorexic and psychotic adolescents. The influence of this group has been far-reaching, both in terms of advancing our conceptual understanding of dysfunctional families and for developing interventions that are effective in overcoming resistance to change (Hoffman, 1981). The use of the therapy team was popularized by this group. While one or two therapists interview a family, several more therapists observe from behind a one-way mirror. The observing team may phone in suggestions or consult with the therapists during or after the session. The entire therapy team may confer following a session (while the family waits), and a written pronouncement or prescription is then read to the family. The statements are designed to unbalance family defenses by reformulating some basic assumptions. For example, a demanding wife might be described as "trying to help her husband improve himself"; a passive, compliant husband might be described as "sensitive and caring in not expressing angry feelings that could hurt his wife."

Treatment methods used in strategic family therapy often take the form of directives given to the family that require them to do something, either during the session or at home. An intervention may be directed at having only one family member make a minor change, since strategic therapists believe that a change in any one part of the system will result in a change in the whole system. These directives may be straightforward or paradoxical. If families appear to be reasonably compliant and likely to cooperate, the directives are usually straightforward. A simple example is that of a wife who was anxious about an impending job interview. The therapist realized that this anxiety was in part due to the wife's awareness of her husband's resistance to her taking a job outside the home. The directive given to this couple was for the husband to apply his considerable experience in the business world to the task of teaching his wife how to handle the job interview. This directive endorsed the power of the husband by putting him in charge of the symptom, and he successfully helped his wife prepare for and participate in the interview. This simple measure had in fact altered the relationship between the couple, so that the symptom was no longer "necessary."

When families are less compliant and oppose the therapist, paradoxical techniques are often successful. The idea of paradoxical therapy is based on the notion that resistant families have an interest in opposing change of any kind, from any source. The therapist therefore suggests a directive that if contradicted by the family would paradoxically lead to positive change. A common example of such an intervention is when a therapist, realizing that a new family case has defeated *all* previous therapists, patiently advises the family not to change, that in fact change might be harmful. In order to defeat this new therapist, the family must actually change. While this scenario seems simple, it actually requires a high order of therapeutic skill in implementation. The assessment of resistance must be accurate, the timing of the intervention is crucial, and the therapist must be perceived as sincere and empathic. If successful, the family is likely to prove the therapist wrong by making some small change. The therapist is careful not to respond enthusiastically to this development lest it quickly dissipate. Instead, the typical response would be to reiterate all the reasons why change may not be advisable. Should the process of change continue, the therapist then gradually accepts and supports the process; and with lessened resistance, the movement toward positive change becomes self-sustaining.

Strategic treatment methods may offer dramatic results, and therein lies both their strength and their weakness. When family systems are rigid and unyielding, sometimes only paradoxical methods can alter the entrenched equilibrium of the system. On the other hand, this dramatic type of intervention may hold a seductive fascination for therapists who are somewhat manipulative and impatient with the more difficult and time-consuming processes usually necessary in psychotherapy.

CURRENT STATUS OF FAMILY THERAPY

The current state of family therapy reveals a rift between traditional psychodynamically oriented family therapy and newer developments based on the interactional model. A few theorists continue to believe that integration of intrapsychic concepts and family therapy is possible.

They acknowledge that mainstream psychoanalysis is not compatible with family therapy, but object relations theory does hold some promise for bridging the gap between the individual and the family (Scharff & Scharff, 1987). Concepts such as introjection, splitting, and projective identification helps us understand more about the unconscious determinants of mate selection, and the process whereby one person in a system may be acting out the projections of other family members.

A theoretical synthesis of psychodynamic and systems theory has yet to be formulated, but this does not mean that the therapist cannot draw from both approaches in clinical work with families. The broad view is to regard psychodynamic theory and family systems theory as two different dimensions of the same phenomenon and that both yield data that contribute to an overall understanding of family dysfunction. The psychodynamic orientation permits in-depth examination of the motivation and subjective experience of each family member, while the interactional perspective provides information about the person's social context as a source of determining individual behavior. It is no coincidence that most of the master clinicians in family therapy have had extensive training and experience in psychodynamic therapies.

The practice of contemporary psychiatry reflects a movement away from long-term psychodynamic therapy and a greater concentration on brief methods of psychotherapy and medications. This shift toward pragmatic and focused treatment is compatible with the goals of family therapy and has resulted in increased cooperation between practitioners of individual-based therapy and family therapists. On the other hand, it is also important to recognize that family systems theory remains at odds with the dominant conceptual models of psychiatry and psychology. The interactional perspective is not congruent with linear causality as reflected in the emphasis on specific "causes" and diagnostic labeling that characterizes mainstream psychiatry. Although there is no theoretical synthesis that will accommodate these divergent paradigms, some movement toward this goal is already apparent.

Although family therapy is in a state of transition, it is clear that it is a valid type of psychotherapy whose clinical effectiveness has been amply documented in several reviews. The systems theory perspective has introduced a critical new dimension in revealing the interplay of family interaction and disturbed psychological processes. The development of new family therapy techniques is influencing the practice of psychotherapy as a whole. Recent studies also suggest that family therapy may be successfully used to treat psychotic and affective illnesses that do not respond to traditional psychotherapeutic approaches, eg, the management of patients with schizophrenia. Studies have shown that such patients living in stressful family situations are prone to frequent relapses despite carefully monitored drug therapy. Ensuring that the families of patients with schizophrenia are included in therapy significantly reduces the frequency of psychotic episodes and the need for rehospitalization.

Involvement of the family—particularly the spouse—has been shown to significantly increase treatment compliance in cases of serious or chronic medical illness. Evidence also suggests that family therapy is particularly effective in dealing with complex social and psychological problems such as substance abuse, domestic violence, sexual molestation, and delinquency.

The widespread applicability of family therapy has ensured that it is no longer regarded as simply an additional modality of therapy. Family systems theory has advanced our understanding of psychological dysfunction, and more and more therapists advocate family therapy as the preferred method of treatment for a host of clinical problems. Most training institutions in psychiatry, psychology, and social work include family therapy as an essential component of the curriculum.

REFERENCES

Ackerman NW: *Treating the Troubled Family*. Basic Books, 1966.

Bateson G et al: Toward a theory of schizophrenia. Behav Sci 1956;1:251.

Bell J: Family group therapy. Public Health Monograph No. 64, U.S. Department of Health, Education and Welfare, 1961.

Bertalanffy L von: *General Systems Theory*. George Braziller, 1968.

Bowen M: The use of family therapy in clinical practice. Compr Psychiatry 1966;7:345.

Erickson MH: The use of symptoms as an integral part of hypnotherapy. In: *Advanced Techniques of Hypnosis and Therapy: Selected Papers of Milton H. Erick-*

son, MD. Haley J (editor). Grune & Stratton, 1967.

Goldstein M (editor): *New Developments in Interventions With Families of Schizophrenics*. Jossey-Bass, 1981.

Gurman A, Rice D (editors): *Couples in Conflict*. Jason Aronson, 1975

1975 Haley J: The family of the schizophrenic: A model system. J Nerv Ment Dis 1959;129:357.

Haley J: *Leaving Home*. McGraw-Hill, 1980.

Haley J: *Problem Solving Therapy*. Jossey-Bass, 1976.

Haley J (editor): *Advanced Techniques of Hypnosis and Therapy: Selected Papers of Milton H. Erickson, MD*. Grune & Stratton, 1967.

Hoffman L: *Foundations of Family Therapy*. Basic Books, 1981.

Jackson DD. The question of family homeostasis. Psychiatr Q 1957;31(Suppl):79.

Jackson DD: The study of the family. Fam Process 1965;4:1.

Kaplan H: *Disorders of Sexual Desire*. Brunner/Mazel, 1979.

Kressel K, Deutsch M: Divorce therapy: An in-depth survey of therapists' views. Fam Process 1977,16,413.

Lidz T: The influence of family studies on the treatment of schizophrenia. In: *Progress in Group and Family Therapy*. Sager CJ, Kaplan HS (editors). Brunner/Mazel, 1972.

Madanes C: *Strategic Family Therapy*. Jossey-Bass, 1981.

Minuchin S: *Families and Family Therapy*. Harvard Univ Press, 1974.

Minuchin S, Rosman B, Baker L: *Psychosomatic Families*. Harvard Univ Press, 1978.

Minuchin S et al: *Families of the Slums: An Exploration of Their Structure and Treatment*. Basic Books, 1967.

Napier A, Whitaker C: *The Family Crucible*. Harper & Row, 1978. Paolino T, McCrady B: *Marriage and Marital Therapy. Psychoanalytic, Behavioral, and Systems Theory Perspectives*. Brunner/Mazel, 1978.

Palazzoli MS et al: *Paradox and Counterparadox*. Jason Aronson, 1978.

Satir V: *Conjoint Family Therapy*. Science & Behavior Books, 1964.

Scharff DE, Scharff J: *Object Relations Family Therapy*. Jason Aronson, 1978.

Shapiro RJ: Alcohol and family violence. In: *Clinical Approaches to Family Violence*. Barnhill L (editor). Aspen Systems, 1982.

Shapiro RJ: Psychodynamically oriented family therapy. In: *Treatment of Emotional Disorders in Children and Adolescents*. Sholevar GP, Benson R, Blinder B (editors). Spectrum, 1980.

Singer MT, Wynne LC: Thought disorder and family relations of schizophrenics: Results and implications. Arch Gen Psychiatry 1965;12:201.

Steinglass P: Family therapy with alcoholics:A review. In: *Family Therapy of Drug and Alcohol Abuse*. Kaufman E, Kaufman P (editors). Gardner Press, 1981.

Watzlawick P, Weakland J, Fisch R: *Change Principles of Problem Formation and Problem Resolution*. Norton, 1974

Weakland J et al: Brief therapy: Focused problem resolution. Fam Process 1974, 13:141.

Whitaker C: Psychotherapy of the absurd: With a special emphasis on the psychotherapy of aggression. Fam Process 1975;14:1.

Whitaker C: The hindrance of theory in clinical work. In: *Family Therapy: Theory and Practice*. Guerin P (editor), 1976.

Wynne LC et al: Pseudo-mutuality in the family relations of schizophrenics. Psychiatry 1958;21.205.

38

Behavioral Medicine Techniques

Daniel S. Weiss, PhD

Behavioral medicine is a broad field that deals with the application of behavioral science knowledge and techniques to problems related to *physical* health. Although the field was only defined formally in the 1970s, it includes topics once in the domain of psychosomatic medicine (see Chapter 3). What makes behavioral medicine different is its emphasis on modifying overt behavior contributing to physical (rather than mental) illness and its application of techniques of **directed attention** to manage both the somatic illness and the adverse effects of somatic treatments.

The principal techniques used in behavioral medicine are relaxation, imagery, hypnosis, and biofeedback. Relaxation is both a therapeutic technique in its own right and an important element of the others named. There is increasing awareness in several specialty areas (eg, cardiology) that the behavioral medicine techniques used in secondary and tertiary prevention may have an important role in primary prevention.

RELAXATION

Probably the most basic technique in behavioral medicine is the systematic induction of a state of relaxation. Psychologically, relaxation reduces arousal and tension, the almost universal concomitants of stress. Physiologically, the "relaxation response" (Benson, 1975) consists of slowing of the respiratory rate, reduction of blood pressure, and peripheral vasodilation.

Relaxation therapy has been used with documented success in the management of essential hypertension and headache. It is probably helpful in a wide variety of clinical conditions associated with stress, whether from threatening external events or pressures or from uncomfortable psychological or physiological state In addition, relaxation is used to enhance behavior therapy (see Chapter 35) and other behavioral medicine techniques.

Relaxation training, like any other complex learned behavior, calls for daily practice over a period of time. The beneficial effects of relaxation exercises are realized only through consistent and unswerving use of the techniques.

Audiotaped materials explaining the relaxation exercises and techniques are valuable teaching devices. Tapes are commercially available or may be prepared by the patient or therapist. A tape should include the four elements that Benson (1975) identifies as necessary to elicit the relaxation response: (1) a mental cue that is repeated several times silently during each exhalation; (2) a passive disregard for trying, succeeding, or being distracted, so that attention can be centered on the repetition of the cue; (3) a comfortable position that minimizes muscular activity and tension; and (4) a quiet environment with minimal distractions.

Relaxation can be facilitated by the creative use of words that connote passivity rather than activity and have positive rather than negative association; by proper timing—allowing the individual to move at his or her own pace; and by establishment of specific times and places for practice. Setting aside a special time for relaxation exercises and nothing else may be helpful in its own right. An example beginning induction follows:

> Close your eyes . . . Let your whole face become comfortably heavy and relaxed. . . . Now . . . slowly breathe in through your nose . . . and allow the air to fill the spaces in your lungs. . . . Feel your chest expand with air. Now . . . hold your breath. . . . Now . . . without pressure or force . . . slowly exhale through your mouth. Feel the air as it passes over your lips. Repeat the breathing cycle . . . inhale . . . hold . . . exhale and relax. Feel your body relaxing. . . . Feel the tension flow out and the calmness and warmth flow in., etc.

IMAGERY

Techniques involving the use of imagery are related to relaxation techniques, and the two are frequently used in conjunction. Visual imagery is most frequently used, but auditory, kinesthetic, olfactory, and gustatory imagery may be used also. Most of what is said here about visual imagery and visualization techniques applies to all.

The ability of some people to alter the depth, vividness, and intensity of mental imagery is well documented, and there is anecdotal evidence for a relationship between visualization techniques and creative activity, peak performance, and repair and restoration of physical and mental equilibrium. Like relaxation techniques, visualization techniques take practice. Samuels and Samuels (1975) present an interesting and optimistic account of the history and uses of visualization techniques with and without the use of mind-altering drugs. The Lamaze program for childbirth uses visual imagery to achieve relaxation and reduction of pain.

Some of the techniques used in visualization and other kinds of imagery overlap those used in relaxation and hypnosis. Relaxation is a prerequisite for visualization. Then, depending upon whether the imagery is to be guided by a clinician or taught to the patient for future use, the major activity is the intense focus of attention upon the image (eg, a warm beach—to promote relaxation—or a strong antibody—to promote healing). As with relaxation, the major obstacle is distraction. The trick is to let distractions enter and flow past rather than trying to resist and overcome them.

As with other behavioral medicine techniques, the use of visualization should be integrated into an overall treatment program that is acceptable to the patient. Although these techniques may only be of use as adjuncts to other treatments, they may be of use with some patients with medical or psychiatric disorders.

HYPNOSIS

In spite of some lingering antipathy toward the subject, there is no doubt that hypnotic phenomena, induction of trance states, and suggestion can play important roles in the treatment of some types of anxiety and phobias and may even serve the purpose of anesthesia in some individuals. The discussion below of the mechanism of hypnosis is still open to debate.

As is true also of many of the other behavioral medicine techniques available to the clinician, hypnosis can be used in the management of a variety of complaints. The technique is especially valuable for use in children, who are often remarkably responsive to suggestion in situations associated with actual or anticipated pain. Children who acquire a facility for entering the trance state can call upon the technique later in life in situations where hypnoanesthesia might be useful.

Hypnosis should not be offered casually. The patient should give a suitably detailed medical and psychological history, and the therapist should initiate a preinduction discussion during which any anxieties and misconceptions about hypnosis can be verbalized and dealt with. The aim of this phase of the hypnosis experience should be to establish rapport and raise positive expectations in the patient's mind. The thera-

pist may discuss such things as relaxation, attention, the need to trust the hypnotist, the importance of motivation for help, and hypnosis as an experience in itself. The therapist should listen for cues suggesting that certain induction techniques (arm levitation, arm lowering, coin technique) might be resisted. It is better to choose a technique that will be comfortable for the subject than one the therapist happens to prefer.

Once a choice of technique has been made, the therapist gently and progressively suggests that the phenomenon is occurring (eg, the arm is growing heavier, the subject is getting weary holding it up, etc). Instructions for induction are best communicated directly and experientially and are not presented here. However, if induction does not occur promptly, attention may be directed to the *opposite* of the suggestion in a subtle way. This change of direction may succeed because it now accords with the patient's actual experience (eg, the arm feels lighter, not heavier).

Once induction occurs, several techniques are available for deepening the trance state. All depend upon integration of the suggestion with what is already happening: ''You will feel your arms growing more relaxed with each breath you take.'' These deepening procedures allow the patient to become more fully attuned to internal rather than external stimuli and thus strengthen suggestions given during hypnosis.

Termination of the hypnotic session should be done in such a way that the subject gradually reorients awareness outward, notices external stimuli, and reengages with reality. The therapist's cue for signifying that the trance has ended should be chosen to suit the patient. The cues should be clear—many clinicians use a countdown procedure. Even though the therapist may have finished the hypnotic instructions and suggestions and given an instruction to reengage, it may take 10 minutes to fully reengage. During this time, the therapist may usefully review the experience with the patient, noting what was satisfactory and unsatisfactory.

BIOFEEDBACK

The most dramatic example of behavioral medicine techniques in the treatment of somatic complaints is biofeedback. Fuller (1977) has described biofeedback as

. . . the use of instrumentation to minor psychophysiological processes of which the individual is not normally aware and which may be brought under voluntary control. This means giving a person immediate information about his or her own biological conditions such as: muscle tension, skin surface temperature, brain wave activity, galvanic skin response, blood pressure, and heart rate. This feedback enables the individual to become an active participant in the process of health maintenance.

The process of electronic feedback includes instrumentation that will filter and amplify a psychophysiological signal that is then analyzed and transformed into another kind of signal capable of being "fed back" to the patient in a perceptible and comprehensible way. For example, the patient hears a tone get louder or sees a light flash more rapidly as muscle tension or heart rate increases. This ability to associate perceived bodily experiences with processes that are ordinarily outside of conscious awareness or experience is the presumed mechanism that initiates voluntary control of the processes.

Biofeedback as a technique for treatment began in 1968, when several lines of pure research led to the discovery that in monkeys and other animals as well as humans, physiological functions thought to be out of voluntary control were modifiable by appropriate monitoring techniques made perceptible to the subject.

Among the conditions that are now currently treated with biofeedback procedures are migraine headaches, insomnia, Raynaud's disease, enuresis, encopresis, chronic pain, hypertension, muscular tension, irritable bowel syndrome, peptic ulcer, esophageal spasm, fecal incontinence, and many neurological diseases and their sequelae.

Initiation of a biofeedback treatment regimen requires the same careful consideration of diagnosis, etiology, alternative treatments, role of the complaint in the patient's life, and the impact of treatment on the patient as is required for any other treatment decision. The patient should be given a clear explanation of the procedure and its rationale.

The basic elements of biofeedback treatment are an initial evaluation session; a baseline session that will introduce the concept of home practice; a goal-setting session that will introduce the feedback part of biofeedback; a series of treatment sessions; a phase of terminal treatment sessions; and a period of follow-up.

The type of instrumentation needed to produce biofeedback depends on the behavioral problem of the patient. The beginning practitioner must learn to identify artifacts in electrophysiological recordings and to distinguish specific physiological events, background levels, and spurious measurements.

The activities in a biofeedback session consist essentially of practice in control of involuntary physiological processes. For example, to teach relaxation of the face and neck muscles to a patient with tension headache, the therapist first attaches the electronic machinery and then develops, with the patient's help, a series of instructions to attain the goals that had been set for that session. Thus, the goal might be to keep a tone below a certain threshold for 15 seconds four distinct times. At the conclusion of each session, specific homework is given, with the results to be reviewed the following session.

SUMMARY

Behavioral medicine has been an outgrowth of a variety of applied and basic science efforts. The emphasis is on functional analysis of the behavioral aspects of somatic and psychological difficulties. The goal is to enable the patient to control bodily functions and psychological responses.

The practitioner should be aware of the growing scope of behavioral medicine. The techniques are safe and may well play an increasingly importantly role in the prevention and treatment of illness and in the promotion of healthy attitudes and behavior.

REFERENCES

Benson H: *The Relaxation Response*. William Morrow, 1975.
Boudewyns PA, Keefe FJ (editors): *Behavioral Medicine in General Medical Practice*. Addison-Wesley, 1982.
Clark CC: *Enhancing Wellness*. Springer, 1981.
Clarke JC, Jackson JA: *Hypnosis and Behavior Therapy*. Springer, 1983.

Fuller GD: *Biofeedback: Methods and Procedures in Clinical Practice*. Biofeedback Press, 1977.
Gaarder KR, Montgomery PS: *Clinical Biofeedback*. 2nd ed. Williams & Wilkins, 1981.
Samuels M, Samuels N: *Seeing With the Mind's Eye*. Random House, 1975.

Caring for the Chronically Ill & Dying Patient

39

Gary M. Rodin, MD

The aim of medical treatment is to improve the quality of life of sick patients. Although psychotherapy is specifically directed toward this goal, it is often overlooked as a form of treatment in general medicine. This is unfortunate, since psychological distress is common among medical patients, and psychological interventions not only may relieve emotional distress but also may alleviate physical symptoms.

This chapter will focus on psychotherapy in the management of patients with chronic or terminal medical disorders. Psychotherapy can be especially useful for such patients, whose suffering may extend over many years. A sensitive and informed physician can manage the emotional care of most patients with chronic illness. However, some patients may need or may request more specialized psychological treatment requiring referral to a psychiatrist or other mental health professional. This chapter reviews the indications and contraindications for psychotherapy of such patients. Consideration will be given to the referral process and to special issues in the psychotherapy of medical patients. These issues are relevant to the psychotherapeutic management of medical patients by both primary physicians and trained psychotherapists who are treating medically ill patients. The psychiatric treatment of patients with acute medical illness is described elsewhere. (See Chapters 38 and 41.)

CHARACTERISTICS OF SUPPORTIVE & EXPRESSIVE THERAPY

As described in Chapter 33, psychotherapy is usually divided into two major categories: supportive and expressive (or insight-oriented) psychotherapy. Both forms of therapy require that the therapist understand something of the emotional life of the patient. With the medically ill, this includes an appreciation of the meaning of the illness and of its intrapsychic, interpersonal, and environmental consequences. The traditional role of the medical practitioner in maintaining a consistent, reliable, empathic professional relationship with the patient is itself psychotherapeutic. The value of this relationship may be underestimated by physicians who feel that they must respond to a patient's emotional distress by "doing something"— prescribing medication, offering advice, ordering further laboratory tests, etc. In fact, a supportive relationship with a physician may lessen the need for analgesics or psychotropic drugs and reduce the problem of noncompliance with treatment regimens.

Although feeling "understood" can be a therapeutic feature of all psychodynamic therapy, unconscious motivations and defense mechanisms are not routinely interpreted in supportive psychotherapy. Indeed, it is important in such treatment to respect the adaptive value of coping mechanisms. For example, the capacity to deny the seriousness of an acute myocardial infarction may be associated, at least in the short term, with improved survival, although such denial may be maladaptive in the long term if it leads to noncompliance with treatment or unrealistic planning for the future.

Supportive psychotherapy is more structured, as a rule, than insight-oriented psychotherapy and is more likely to include such interventions as education, reality testing, reassurance, and advice. However, reassurance and advice are also commonly misused forms of supportive intervention. Reassurance is most helpful when it is based on a true appreciation of the patient's situation, including the affective component of symptoms. Premature or unrealistic reassurance is rarely comforting to the patient and may reduce the physician's credibility in harmful ways. Similarly, advice is helpful only when it is based on a realistic appraisal of the needs of the patient, particularly with regard to illness-related issues. Advice should be given sparingly in personal matters, especially since it is apt—coming from a physician— to be given undue weight. It is usually best to help patients make their own decisions rather than try to make decisions for them.

The overall aim in supportive psychotherapy is to bolster adaptive coping mechanisms, to minimize maladaptive ones, and to decrease adverse psychological reactions such as fear, shame, and reduced self-esteem. This treatment can often be provided most effectively by an interested primary care practitioner who has had an ongoing relationship with the patient. Expressive (insight-oriented) psychotherapy usually requires referral to a trained psychotherapist.

INDICATIONS & CONTRAINDICATIONS FOR PSYCHOTHERAPY IN PATIENTS WITH CHRONIC MEDICAL DISORDERS

Supportive psychotherapy may be indicated for patients with any chronic medical illness who are experiencing psychological distress but who do not need or want insight therapy or for whom insight therapy would be contraindicated. This applies to most medical patients, who want symptomatic relief from emotional suffering rather than insight into the origin of their difficulties. Supportive psychotherapy may also be most appropriate for patients who have difficulty in impulse control or who are unable to tolerate intense feelings. For most patients, supportive psychotherapy is indicated during acute exacerbations of chronic disease and in situations of overwhelming stress.

Expressive (insight-oriented) psychotherapy aims to promote self-understanding and intrapsychic change. Such change meliorates the patient's present life adjustment and may also diminish future vulnerability to stress. Insight-oriented therapy is indicated in a small proportion of patients. It is suitable for medical patients with identifiable psychological or interpersonal problems, the motivation for insight, the capacity to verbalize and to understand feelings, and the ability to form a relationship. The latter is important, because the relationship with the therapist is central to this form of treatment.

By disrupting the patient's psychological equilibrium, medical illness permits underlying conflicts and vulnerabilities to emerge. This state of temporary upheaval provides some opportunity for growth and change but may also precipitate feelings of anxiety and despair. Indeed, symptoms and signs of depression may be found in up to half of all medical patients and major affective disorders in over 10%. In addition to depression, other psychiatric disorders that may require referral for psychological treatment include anxiety, panic and dissociative disorders, alcohol dependence, and adjustment disorders precipitated by the stress of illness. Psychotherapy for such conditions does not preclude other treatment, including pharmacotherapy.

The psychological impact of illness is largely determined by the personality and perceptions of the patient. Lowering of self-esteem may follow the onset of a physical illness, particularly when it is serious, disabling, or visible to others. Bodily appearance and functioning are important determinants of identity and self-esteem throughout life. Disturbances in body image commonly result in feelings of weakness or personal inadequacy. Physical illness may also aggravate conflicts related to dependency and hostility. Patients who have denied feelings of dependency, either because of the need to demonstrate strength and self-sufficiency or because of difficulty trusting others, may be deeply troubled by the realistic need to depend on others when they are ill. Psychotherapy may help

such individuals accept appropriate support and deal with their fears. The sense of helplessness associated with an illness commonly stimulates feelings of anger and frustration. Patients may feel too indebted to or too dependent on those in their environment to express such feelings. Psychotherapy may provide an atmosphere of safety in which such feelings can be expressed and understood.

Some relative contraindications to insight-oriented psychotherapy of the medically ill include (1) conditions in which the emotional arousal associated with expressive therapy may be medically hazardous, eg, recent myocardial infarction; (2) medical crises or other stresses that limit the patient's capacity to tolerate anxiety or emotional disruption, which may occur during the course of insight-oriented therapy; and (3) organic brain syndromes due to cardiovascular, neurologic, metabolic, or other disorders that are associated either with cognitive impairment, which limits the capacity for verbal expression and understanding, or with emotional lability, which may be aggravated by expressive psychotherapy. Emotional exploration with such patients may be hazardous because it may precipitate a state of disorganization and distress. The cognitive and affective functions of all medical patients should be carefully assessed before insight-oriented psychotherapy is recommended.

REFERRAL FOR PSYCHOTHERAPY

Emotional disturbances are extremely common in the medically ill. Many such disturbances do not require specific treatment and are alleviated by supportive contact with the attending physician. The need to refer a patient for psychotherapy will depend on a variety of factors, including the severity of the patient's distress, the motivation for psychological assistance, and the capacity of the attending physician to deal with such matters. Referral for psychotherapy may be unnecessarily delayed or may occur prematurely. Premature referral without careful assessment of the patient's emotional state may result when the physician is uncomfortable with emotional issues. In such cases, speedy referral to a psychiatrist or other mental health practitioner may represent avoidance by the physician of the patient's distress. At the other extreme, physicians reluctant to acknowledge the limitations of their own therapeutic influence may hesitate to refer patients for psychological consultation or treatment. Referrals for psychotherapy may not occur because some physicians do not recognize that psychotherapy is a specific treatment modality that involves more than "chatting" with patients. Finally, physicians who are unaware of the indications for psychotherapy may feel frustrated and confused when patients who are referred do not benefit from or are not accepted into treatment.

In some cases, the physician is unaware of a patient's psychological disturbances. Up to 50% of psychiatric disorders in medical patients are unrecognized by nonpsychiatric physicians, in part because patients refrain from expressing feelings unless the physician indicates a readiness to listen. Some physicians underestimate the significance of emotional disturbances by assuming that it is "natural" for patients who are medically ill to be upset. Too often, when it is "understandable" that a patient should be depressed, specific treatments such as psychotherapy or pharmacotherapy are not offered. Physicians may recognize that symptoms such as depression are present without appreciating that treatment may be available. Such nonintervention may be particularly hazardous with patients who are suicidal. Most patients who commit suicide have been in contact with a physician from within a few hours to a few months before death. In many cases, the significance of symptoms of depression and of suicidal ideation is not appreciated. Physicians must be alert to the presence of such symptoms and to the possibility for beneficial intervention with drugs or psychotherapy on an inpatient or outpatient basis.

THE INITIATION OF PSYCHOTHERAPY

Some medical patients seek psychotherapy because of a conscious belief or unconscious wish that it will improve their health or their chances for long-term survival. This belief has been reinforced in recent years by attention in the media to the role of psychological factors in illness and to some scientific evidence that links psychological well-being with a favorable medical outcome. However, although such benefit may occur, unrealistic expectations of benefit from psychotherapy may also contribute to traumatic disappointment. Some patients harbor magical expectations that a therapist can help them even without their participation in the process. Many of these patients are unfamiliar with the process of psychotherapy and may need education about what is required and what may reasonably be expected from psychotherapy.

Some medical patients want help to modify behavior that is affecting their health adversely, eg, noncompliance with the treatment regimen for conditions such as coronary artery disease, diabetes mellitus, or end-stage renal disease. Such concerns are valid as a focus of treatment. However, the preoccupation with illness may also be an avoidance of important underlying issues. In particular, it is convenient for some patients to attribute all of their personal difficulties to their illness, even when these difficulties have antedated the onset of illness. At the other extreme, some patients exclude the illness from their consciousness altogether. This avoidance may be an attempt to deny the significance or even the existence of the illness. Although the adaptive value of denial, especially dur-

ing the acute phase of an illness, should not be underestimated, the benefits of long-term therapy will be extremely limited unless the implications of a serious illness are taken into account.

The degree to which psychotherapy in the medically ill should be extended to include aspects not directly related to the illness will depend upon a variety of factors, including the suitability of the patient for insight-oriented therapy. However, with medically ill patients, the capacity for insight and psychological change may be difficult to determine. Some issues that arise regarding determination of the depth and focus of treatment are demonstrated by the following case.

Illustrative Case

A married woman in her 30s with insulin-dependent diabetes for 2 years sought psychotherapy because she had been unable to control her eating, and she feared that poor metabolic control posed a risk to her health. Although highly disciplined in all other areas of her life, she felt frustrated by her inability to control her appetite. She viewed the problem of dietary noncompliance as distinct from the rest of her personality, and she wanted help only in dealing with her eating problem.

After a brief period of psychotherapy during which a therapeutic relationship was established, the eating problem was satisfactorily brought under control. However, by this time, the patient came to recognize that her difficulty in regulating her diet was related to a number of underlying concerns, ie, conflicts related to dependency, helplessness, and the fear of losing control. Even more distressing than her inability to control her eating was the fear that she would become unable to control her feelings. Her initial attempt to restrict the focus of the treatment process was a means of ensuring that she would not be overwhelmed by unmanageable feelings. When this fear was addressed, she felt able to participate more fully in the therapeutic process. She recalled how the onset of her diabetes 2 years earlier was a blow to her sense of self-sufficiency. She remembered lying in bed for 2 weeks, feeling depressed and experimenting with homeopathic remedies. Subsequently, she began to cope with her illness by denying to herself and to others that her diabetes was of any significance. She worried that others would regard her as incompetent if they knew about the diagnosis. As she came to trust the therapist, she experienced a sense of sadness about her illness and was able to mourn many of the losses she had suffered.

In this case, the patient's therapy began with a limited focus on a specific dietary symptom and later included a variety of issues related and unrelated to her diabetes. Restricting the treatment to the patient's initial request would have unnecessarily limited its potential benefit.

THE THERAPEUTIC PROCESS

Psychotherapy with chronically ill medical patients basically resembles therapy with patients who are physically well. Some adjustments are necessary, however, when there is a significant exacerbation of the medical disorder, in which case the need for hospitalization may disrupt the course of psychotherapy. Furthermore, when a chronically ill patient experiences marked physical deterioration, it may be necessary to shift from insight-oriented therapy to therapy that is more supportive in nature.

Psychotherapy with medically ill patients requires flexibility on the part of the therapist. When a patient is hospitalized, treatment may continue in less than optimal circumstances. It is sometimes necessary to conduct psychotherapy at the bedside, even when there are other patients in the room. Although the patient's right to privacy must be respected, involvement of the therapist through all phases of an illness may be crucial in maintaining the therapeutic alliance. For many patients, the medical illness has already created feelings of isolation from the "normal" or "healthy" world. A therapist who discontinues treatment when the medical condition worsens may contribute to these feelings of isolation.

THE PROCESS OF THERAPY

The Expression of Grief

Medical patients frequently enter psychotherapy in a state of distress because their usual coping mechanisms have been eroded by the physical and psychological effects of illness. Following the discovery of a new illness or of an ominous complication of a chronic illness, a state of shock, disbelief, or numbness may be present. This state is similar to the grief response that follows bereavement. In the case of a medical illness, the grief is commonly related to the anticipated or actual loss of competence and bodily integrity and to the disruption in the expected trajectory of life span and accomplishments. Oscillations are common initially between denying the implications of the illness and feeling overwhelmed by it. The first phase of psychotherapy of such patients involves listening to the patient and allowing thoughts and feelings related to the illness to emerge in a gradual and tolerable fashion. This may involve providing support and reassurance with patients who are flooded with feelings and gentle exploration when they have become closed off. The following case illustrates this and other phases of psychotherapy in a patient who was referred after cervical cancer was diagnosed.

Illustrative Case

A 32-year-old married woman was referred for psychotherapy after being told that a cervical smear and subsequent biopsy indicated the presence of a malignancy. She reported feeling enraged, hopeless, and wanting to commit suicide. She described a recent dream of a woman being murdered. She believed that this dream reflected her own experience of being assaulted and even destroyed by the illness. On subsequent exploration in the weekly sessions that were arranged, it became apparent that her suicidal wishes reflected not only her hopelessness and anger but also her wish to numb herself and to avoid thinking or feeling anything about her condition. For similar reasons, she refused even to consider any of the medical or surgical treatments that were being recommended.

The therapeutic task in the initial phase of therapy was to facilitate the gradual expression of feelings related to the illness. The therapist needed to proceed flexibly and to be guided in each session by the patient's willingness and capacity to explore her feelings. During this phase of acute grief, patients are commonly unable to be introspective or to make use of psychological insight. The most important goal at this point is to provide an environment in which thoughts and feelings related to the illness can be safely discussed. The stabilizing effect of the therapeutic relationship is more often beneficial at this stage than are any specific interpretations. Indeed, the process of understanding cannot begin until the acute period of grief has passed and the patient feels less overwhelmed. In the case presented, the patient felt more hopeful after the fifth session and said to the therapist that she had "combined my strength with yours." She also felt able to consider medical treatment options and had begun to discuss them with her family doctor.

Meaning & Mourning

The meaning of an illness is determined by a complex interaction among a variety of factors—including the nature of the illness—and individual factors such as the patient's premorbid personality, developmental stage, life experiences, and personal conflicts and vulnerabilities. For example, although damage to the sense of self is a common consequence of a serious medical illness, this effect is likely to be most pronounced in those whose self-esteem has been fragile or particularly dependent upon physical health or appearance. Similarly, although a sense of loss may be common following the onset of a serious medical illness, this experience may be most profound in those who have previously experienced traumatic or recurrent losses.

In the case described, the diagnosis of cancer revived long-standing feelings of defectiveness and unacceptability. The site of the cancer undermined her sense of femininity, which was important for her self-worth. She reported a dream in which she was a teenager who was accepted at a desirable school but then received a notice informing her that she could not continue. This dream represented for her both the opportunities and plans she felt the illness had stolen from her as well as her underlying sense of having been damaged and made undesirable to others. She felt more aware of her vulnerabilities than ever before, and she worried that she could be easily injured, as if she had "no skin . . . no defenses." Setbacks in her work now made her feel like an "idiot" or a "failure." She felt in great need of involvement from the therapist and easily felt rejected and hopeless when she perceived him to be less than constantly available. The experience of her illness had brought her much closer to underlying feelings of dependency and abandonment. At this time, she reported a fantasy of being a needy, colicky baby whose mother could not cope with her and revealed for the first time to anyone her belief that her mother never really wanted her.

Although some of her feelings at this stage of therapy were evident earlier, she was now able to be reflective and to understand her feelings. The therapist could now be of assistance to her in integrating and working through the mourning process associated with the illness. Feelings of sadness could now more safely be expressed in the presence of a firmly established therapeutic relationship. Providing meaning and organization of her experience in this phase helped to diminish her feelings of helplessness and isolation. This process of understanding depended upon the empathic involvement of the therapist, whom the patient felt was able to "live the experience with me."

Mastery

Serious medical illness often represents a threat to an individual's sense of competence. An important goal of psychotherapeutic treatment is to restore the sense of competence and mastery. Earlier unsuccessful attempts to achieve mastery by denying the illness or by warding off its significance may now be replaced by a greater capacity to experience safely a broader range of feelings related to the illness. This change is particularly important in the medically ill, whose sense of competence has been undermined.

As treatment progressed in the case described, the patient became more able to tolerate feelings of vulnerability without feeling overwhelmed. She now felt motivated to examine her previous tendency to conceal feelings of insecurity and dependency beneath a veneer of self-sufficiency. In this respect, she felt that the illness "removed a crutch." She now said that her awareness of her vulnerabilities was not so threatening and, in fact, now allowed her to "love and to be loved." She felt more able to accept her illness and to consider and select appropriate treatment. She no longer felt the need to affirm her strength by denying her illness, refusing treatment, or taking her life.

Terminal Illness

All human beings are faced with the possibility of death, but this becomes more imminent with a serious or terminal illness. Kübler-Ross identified the following five stages of adaptation to a terminal illness: (1) denial, or the temporary feeling of "no, it can't be me"; (2) anger, and the feeling of "why me?"; (3) bargaining, or attempting to postpone the inevitable; (4) depression and mourning; and (5) acceptance and relinquishing the struggle to overcome the illness. Of course, individual patients do not necessarily proceed through these stages in an orderly, predictable, or complete manner, and mixed states are common. Furthermore, much of the task of living with a terminal illness involves adjusting not to death but to continually altering circumstances as the illness progresses. This adjustment is an active process that requires realignment of goals and possibilities so that they are realistic but still meaningful.

Patients in the final stages of a terminal illness may focus on the finality of death. However, prior to this stage, patients are more often concerned with how to live with the condition than with how to die from it. The therapeutic relationship may assist in the process and decrease the likelihood that unremitting feelings of hopelessness or depression will supervene. Indeed, for some patients, increased awareness of the brevity of life leads to an affirmation of its meaning and value. When the patient described above experienced a heightened sense of the passage of time, she found herself engaging more fully in her work and in her professional relationships. She said, "In spite of my anger, I now get more enjoyment from everything I do." She added, "I don't have time to waste. I am looking for meaningful relationships and I have a hunger to accomplish." This increased pressure of time may also facilitate the process of psychotherapy and diminish resistance that otherwise might develop.

The last phase of adjustment to a terminal illness, referred to by Kübler-Ross as acceptance, has been described as a process of withdrawal from relationships and responsibilities. In the final states of succumbing to cancer of the oropharynx, Sigmund Freud described this mental state as "a small island of pain floating on an ocean of indifference." This psychological process of withdrawal may act to diminish emotional distress that might otherwise occur. It may also arise owing to the effects of the disease, medical treatment, and analgesics on brain function. A therapist who has maintained a relationship with a patient up to this point, must now accept a more passive role in which his or her physical presence may be more important to the patient than any verbal intervention.

THERAPIST-PATIENT RELATIONSHIPS

Transference

In the case described above, the therapist was at times perceived as an idealized figure. Such idealization is common during the course of psychotherapy arid may facilitate the treatment process. Idealization of the primary physician is also common among medical patients and is frequently therapeutic. This tendency to idealize authority figures is especially prominent in persons who have had difficulty maintaining self-esteem and have relied on "powerful others" in order to feel secure.

In general, physicians and psychotherapists need to accept being idealized by their patients. Optimally, idealization of the therapist during psychotherapy is tempered gradually by the minor disappointments that inevitably occur. This process of disillusionment is tolerable when it is gradual and when it is associated with a more realistic perception of the therapist and a greater ability to maintain self-esteem without such external support. Premature or excessive disappointment in the therapist or primary physician may precipitate a sense of despair. Such extreme disappointment is more likely to occur when patients with progressive medical disorders have had initial unrealistic expectations of their physicians. These patients may be filled with rage and feelings of hopelessness when their expectations prove unrealistic. Nonpsychiatric physicians and therapists should be cautious about accepting without reservation the omnipotent role conferred upon them by some patients with progressive medical conditions. The idealizations of such patients may need to be interpreted and clarified early in treatment in order to minimize traumatic disillusionment.

Intense feelings of anger and helplessness are common among medical patients and may be projected onto the therapist or primary physician, who is then perceived as hostile or ineffectual. During psychotherapy, such projections must be recognized and interpreted as part of the transference. However, the therapist must also consider to what extent his or her own stance contributes to these negative feelings in the patient. At times, transference feelings are difficult to identify when they are diluted by the patient's involvement with several people on the medical staff who are or are perceived to be of life-sustaining importance.

Countertransference

Medically ill patients may provoke a variety of emotional reactions in the therapist. Some patients elicit overconcern; others arouse feelings of hostility and rejection. The therapist must identify such feelings in order to understand the patient better and to maintain an attitude of therapeutic neutrality. Neutrality in this context does not mean a lack of concern for the patient but refers to an attitude which is consistent and empathic with the patient's feelings without undue distortion by the personal reactions of the therapist. Interventions that arise from the needs of the therapist, even when well intended, may not be useful to the patient. An overly supportive attitude may develop when the therapist identifies with the patient's helplessness or attempts to counteract his or her own underlying feelings of frustration and impotence. Such support may deprive some patients of the opportunity to develop greater autonomy and self-sufficiency. Hostile feelings toward the patient may also arise for various reasons. In some cases, such negative feelings on the part of the therapist serve to maintain an emotional distance from a patient whose distress threatens to be overwhelming. In other cases, patients wish to provoke hostility in the therapist. Patients with intense rage may achieve a greater sense of control over their feelings when they can provoke similar feelings in the therapist. Both primary physicians and therapists who care for the medically ill must be able to tolerate intense feelings in themselves and in their patients in order to maintain a helpful attitude.

Collaboration With the Primary Care Physician

Psychotherapy with medically ill patients places special emotional and practical demands on the therapist, such as the need to collaborate with the physicians who retain responsibility for medical management of the patient. The therapist must remain aware of the patient's current medical status without assuming responsibility for it. Therapists must acknowledge resentment and other feelings toward the primary care physician but should be careful not to collude with such feelings.

Some patients attempt to form special relationships that split the medical staff and create tension among them. This can be prevented only by frequent communication among all members of the medical staff. Because of the need for such communication, it is generally unwise for the therapist to promise absolute confidentiality. Therapists should avoid unnecessary disclosure of personal information about the patient to medical staff but should be free to communicate about matters that affect the medical course. Some issues regarding collaboration with the medical staff are depicted in the following case:

Illustrative Case

A 21-year-old single diabetic woman was referred for psychiatric consultation during a hospital admission at a time when her vision was deteriorating rapidly. She agreed to the consultation, although she did not feel in need of assistance. In fact, as her vision failed, she resented the increased protectiveness of her family and others and decided to move out of the family home. From the time of onset of her diabetes at age 6 years, she believed that her parents experienced it as a burden. She felt unable to rely on them for support and withdrew from emotional contact with them.

The patient began weekly psychotherapy cautiously. Whenever she felt neglected or abused by any of her physicians, she experienced resentment that was generalized to include everyone she was involved with, including the therapist. Specifically, she objected to the medical staff's communicating with one another about her and knowing that she was seeing a psychiatrist. She was angry that communication between the therapist and the rest of the medical team about her physical status had been established as a condition of her psychotherapy.

Although the patient's concerns about confidentiality were acknowledged to be valid, the importance of the therapist's ongoing contact with the medical staff became increasingly apparent. It was sometimes difficult to determine to what extent her emotional state was affected by alterations in her metabolic control. At other times, when the factitious administration of insulin or sedative drugs was suspected, discussion and collaboration with the medical staff were essential.

The therapeutic relationship provided the patient with a limited and restricted means by which she could begin to develop some degree of trust in others. The intimacy and dependency that resulted were frightening for her, and she responded initially with detachment and attempts to split the medical staff. Only later did deep-seated fears of her unacceptability and her potential destructiveness to others emerge. Although she was sometimes able to accept interpretations about her anger, it was often necessary to let her simply ventilate her feelings.

OUTCOME & COST-BENEFIT ANALYSIS OF PSYCHOTHERAPY WITH THE MEDICALLY ILL

Psychotherapy is often underestimated by medical practitioners as a means of improving the quality of life of medical patients. Although the benefit of psychotherapy has often been difficult to demonstrate, some of the clearest evidence has been obtained from studies of the medically ill. This benefit has been measured not only by the improvement in psychological well-being but also by the reduced utilization of medical resources. Medical patients who participate in psychotherapy have been shown to require fewer medical investigations and treatments, either because of the effect of psychotherapy on overall health status or because of the more appropriate allocation of medical and psychological resources. There are also some reports that psychotherapy may result in prolonged survival in patients with cancer and other serious medical conditions.

SUMMARY

Medical illness is a stressful event in the life of any patient, although the specific meaning of the illness and the psychological response to it may depend on a variety of factors. Supportive psychotherapy as an adjunct to treatment may be an important function of the primary care practitioner. A small proportion of medical patients may benefit from expressive (insight-oriented) psychotherapy. This should be conducted by a specially trained psychotherapist with suitable patients. Psychotherapy may assist patients in working through feelings associated with the multiple losses produced by a medical illness and with the possibility of death. This treatment may diminish the likelihood of persistent depression or of a premature giving up on the possibilities of life. However, insight-oriented therapy may be contraindicated with some medical patients because of physical debilitation or cognitive impairment.

It is common (and often therapeutic) for patients to idealize physicians and others in the helping professions. However, the stress of illness may predispose the patient to an early and fragile idealization of the therapist or primary physician. It may be necessary to interpret this idealization early in treatment to avoid traumatic disappointment and disillusionment. Mourning may also be an important feature early in therapy. Patients must grieve for anticipated losses as well as for those that have already occurred.

Medical complications or hospitalizations may disrupt the therapeutic process. The ability of the patient to tolerate affective arousal may fluctuate widely, and therapeutic interventions at any point must take this into account. In some cases, the painful reality of the physical condition interferes with the ability of the patient to form a therapeutic relationship. The transference relationship may be diluted by the need to rely on various medical staff who may have life-sustaining significance for the patient. Furthermore, the therapeutic relationship may be affected by other factors such as the breach of confidentiality that occurs when therapists work in collaboration with the medical treatment team.

Although psychotherapy may in some cases be the most important feature of management of a medically ill patient, psychotherapists more often play a secondary role. The treatment of medical complications must often assume the most urgent priority. Physical illness may also impose realistic limitations that cannot be overcome by psychological treatment. In these and other respects, medical illness may present an ongoing challenge to the sense of competence of the therapist as well as to that of the patient.

REFERENCES

Cassel EJ: The nature of suffering and the goals of medicine. N Engl J Med 1982;306:639.

Forester B, Kornfeld DS, Fleiss JL: Psychotherapy during radiotherapy: Effects on emotional and physical distress. Am J Psychiatry 1985;142:22.

Freyberger H: Psychotherapeutic possibilities in medically extreme situations. Psychother Psychosom 1975;26:337.

Karasu TB: Psychotherapy with physically ill patients. In: *Specialized Techniques in Individual Psychotherapy*. Karasu TB, Bellak L (editors). Brunner/Mazel, 1980.

Köhle K, Simons C: Integrations of the psychosomatic approach into the management of the severely and fatally ill. Psychother Psychosom 1975;26:357.

Kübler-Ross E: *On Death and Dying*. Macmillan, 1969.

Moos RH, Schaefer JA: The crisis of physical illness: An overview and conceptual approach. In: *Coping With Physical Illness*. Vol 2: *New Perspectives*. Moos RH (editor). Plenum Press, 1984.

Murphy GE: The physician's responsibility for suicide. 2. Errors of omission. Ann Intern Med 1975;82:305.

Psychotherapy Research: Methodological and Efficacy Issues. American Psychiatric Association Commission on Psychotherapies, 1982.

Rodin GM: Expressive psychotherapy in the medically ill: Resistance and possibilities. Int J Psychiatry Med 1984;14:99.

Rodin GM, Littlefield C: *Depression in the Medically Ill: An Integrated Approach*. Brunner/Mazel. [In press.]

Sifneos P: *Short-Term Psychotherapy and Emotional Crisis*. Harvard Univ Press, 1972.

Sourkes BM: *The Deepening Shade: Psychological Aspects of Life-Threatening Illness*. Univ of Pittsburgh Press, 1982.

Spiegel D: Can psychotherapy prolong cancer survival? Psychosomatics 1990,31:361.

Stein EH, Murdaugh J, MacLeod JA: Brief psychotherapy of psychiatric reactions to physical illness. Am J Psychiatry 1969;125:1040.

Geriatric Psychiatry

40

Gary L. Gottlieb, MD, MBA

Long life is desirable if adequate physical function and, especially, intellectual function can be maintained. Many people face the aging process with apprehension. Fears about cognitive decline are heightened by increasing awareness that pathologic processes accompany aging. Older adults are concerned that they will lose their autonomy and personal identity. The aging process may threaten the ability to think, love, and communicate. Early recognition by the physician of behavioral disorders in aging patients may allow rapid treatment of reversible causes and fuller exploitation of retained assets in chronic and deteriorating conditions. Optimization of mental abilities can be expected to favorably influence the outcome of aging-related problems of many kinds and perhaps to avoid the need for long-term custodial or nursing home care.

DEMOGRAPHIC ISSUES

Just 30 years ago, only one of every 11 Americans was over 65 years of age. Today, slightly less than one in eight have reached that age. The United States Census Bureau (1987) expects that the elderly population will have grown by 23% to nearly 31 million during the 1980s. As a result of relatively small depression era birth rates, the older population should grow by only about 10% in the 1990s and by 12% in the first decade of the next century. This rate of growth will yield about 39 million older Americans by 2010. Shortly thereafter, the aging of the post-World War II "baby boom" cohort will cause a dramatic growth in the over-65 population segment. By 2030, about one-fourth of the population—about 66 million people—will be over 65. By the year 2000, 45% of the older population will be at least 75 years old, with the number of those over 85 growing at a faster rate than any other segment of the population (Soldo and Agree, 1988).

Sex differences in life expectancy and the distribution of minorities among the elderly have important health-related consequences. There are approximately three women for every two men over age 65 and five women for every two men over age 85. Ethnic minorities comprise a growing segment of the older population. In 1980, about 10% of persons over age 65 were nonwhite. By the year 2025, about 15% of the elderly are projected to be members of minority groups (National Center for Health Statistics, 1988). While life expectancy at birth for Caucasians exceeds that for African Americans by about 8%, at age 75, mortality rates for the latter are lower than those for Caucasians. However, very old African Americans have considerably higher rates of poverty and illness than Caucasians in the same age group. Economic and social discrimination and underprivilege associated with minority status are exaggerated by the socioeconomic realities of older age: Accrued social and financial resources are limited, barriers to preventive and acute health care are harder to breach, and the need for non-health care governmental services is greater, including housing, transportation, food, and income maintenance. Cultural differences may also affect the expression of illness and the ways in which health care is accessed and delivered.

In 1986, one in eight people over age 65—or about 3.5 million Americans—had an income below the poverty level. About 10% of the younger population were in that income category. Indigence appears to increase with age: about one-fifth of people who live past the age of 85 have incomes at or below the poverty level. These rates are even more dramatic for women and for minorities. For example, 60% of black women over age 65 not living with their families were below the poverty level in 1986.

ORGAN SYSTEM FUNCTION & AGING

Over the past century, numerous theories have been offered to explain biological aging, or the normative decline in the quantity of active metabolic cells and the reduction in cellular function that occur throughout the life cycle (Busse, 1989). Some of these theories are partially supported by documented aging changes in cell and tissue structure and function. However, a truly useful and empirically demonstrated theory of the aging process is as yet unavailable.

Diminished reserve and ability to respond to stress and insults reflect a reduction in functional and regenerative capacity. Individual aging can be thought of as the manifestation of a person's genetic vulnerability to disease. Aging affects every organ system. Cells are lost and enzymatic and messenger systems within cells reach a state of reduced productivity or responsiveness.

Age-related changes in body composition result in a decrease of as much 80% in total muscle mass and an average increase of 35% in total body fat. Body fat is also redistributed, accumulating within the viscera and diminishing at or near the body surface. In both sexes, the lungs, kidneys, and skin age more rapidly than the heart and liver. Bone mineralization in women after menopause declines eight to ten times more rapidly than in men of the same age, which means that women are at risk for osteoporosis-related fractures about 10 years earlier than men. Ovarian function declines in middle age, and production of estrogens and progesterone ceases. This results not only in menopause but in loss of the protective effects of these hormones, increasing the risk of atherosclerotic cardiovascular disease and stroke as well as osteoporosis. In contrast, testicular function and hormonal production and secretion persist in men with little alteration until at least the eighth decade.

The central nervous system undergoes a somewhat selective loss of neurons during aging. While there is constant cell loss throughout the brain over the life span, total age-related cortical neuronal degeneration is minimal. There is random loss of neurons throughout the cortex and disproportionately greater loss of cells in the locus ceruleus, the substantia nigra, the cerebellum, and the olfactory bulbs.

Brain changes associated with aging could suggest that cognitive decline is also inevitable. However, a growing neuropsychology literature suggests that aging affects certain aspects of cognition while sparing others and that global decline, such as that seen in dementia, is certainly not normal. Individual factors such as intelligence, education, and environment affect cognitive ability and test performance in aging individuals. Therefore, generalizations regarding changes in cognitive function with aging should be made cautiously.

Memory is the component of cognition that concerns practitioners and patients most. Older adults fear that memory loss will contribute to loss of autonomy. Furthermore, memory loss is the symptom that we most strongly associate with progressive dementia, particularly Alzheimer's disease. Numerous studies have evaluated memory function in older adults compared with younger people. Most of these investigations indicate that there is a decline in the speed with which information is retrieved from memory stores associated with aging and that acquisition and retrieval of new information are most profoundly affected by the aging process. Memory for entrenched learning and personal information does not appear to be affected by aging.

Certain aspects of general intellectual function appear to be unaffected by aging. Knowledge acquired in the course of socialization and development tends to remain stable into older adulthood. However, the abilities required for the solution of complex new problems decline slowly through the life span. Poor physical health and overall loss of personal well-being also affect intellectual function adversely.

MENTAL HEALTH & THE OLDER ADULT

Over 18% of older adults are thought to be suffering with significant mental health problems at any given time (Myers et al, 1984). These people (and their families) depend almost exclusively on primary care physicians to recognize and manage complaints related to intellectual and emotional function—specifically, depression and dementia. Inasmuch as the elderly consume a substantial proportion of general medical services, prevention and early detection of disorders of high prevalence in this population are essential. The subtlety of mental impairment in this population unfortunately limits the ability of most primary care physicians to diagnose and treat the disorders.

Mental function influences all other areas of individual function. While the ability to interact and communicate with others and to manage one's personal affairs are controlled by higher-order cortical functions, virtually all activities of daily living are adversely influenced by disturbances in cognitive or emotional status.

Similarly, medical well-being and hygienic lifestyle are severely undermined by psychiatric disorders. Compliance with medical regimens is poor among older adults. Older patients with even mild symptoms of depression express a negative perception of their own health status, have more physical complaints, and make more physician visits than do normal elderly patients (Waxman, Carner, and Blum, 1983).

Early recognition of mental disorders is important for a number of reasons. Older adults are more vulnerable than others to the central nervous system effects of somatic illnesses and their treatments. For example, urinary tract infections and surgical repair of hip fracture are associated with delirium in the elderly. Similarly, treatment of chronic pain with opioids may impair mood and cognition. The assumption that changes in mental well-being are normal features of the aging process may make the practitioner less aggressive than would be optimal in determining the origin of a change in cognition, affect, or thought content. This may prevent possible improvements in function and quality of life. For example, Larson et al (1985) found that almost 28% of 200 patients carefully evaluated for suspected dementia showed some improvement in response to appropriate medical or psychiatric intervention. Numerous studies indicate that between 55% and 80% of elderly depressives will respond to psychotherapeutic or somatic treatments. However, reversibility apparently depends on early recognition and treatment—ie, delayed intervention imposes a risk of chronic deterioration. Improvement in symptoms may prolong productive and autonomous function and postpone or avoid altogether the need for acute or long-term institutionalization.

Mental disorders are the most frequently diagnosed problems in nursing homes. Families report that difficulty in managing the behavior of an impaired older adult is of substantial importance in the decision to seek nursing home placement. Early intervention by the physician can potentially prolong an individual's ability to remain in the less restrictive and more affordable home environment.

Community surveys estimate that severe forms of dementing illness affect more than 5% of people over 65 years of age. Another 10–15% of elderly adults are thought to suffer mild to moderate dementia (Schneck, Reisberg, and Ferris, 1982). Prevalence rates for dementia jump to 23–47% in adults over age 85 (Evans et al, 1989). Nearly 70% of patients who present with evidence of significant cognitive impairment probably have Alzheimer's disease.

The prevalence of symptoms of depression among the elderly is similarly impressive. Two groups of investigators found a 13–18% point prevalence of depression in large samples of community-resident elderly (Gurland, Dean, and Cross, 1980; Murrell, Himmelfarb, and Wright, 1983). Studies of elderly medical patients reveal an even higher prevalence of this disorder (about 27%). Suicide rates among the elderly are disproportionately high. This population comprises only 11.9% of the population but accounts for nearly one-fourth of all suicides. For example, while the suicide rate for the general population is approximately 13 per 100,000, the rate for men in their 80s is close to three times that number (Frederick, 1978). Older depressives have more somatic symptoms and visit primary care providers more frequently than their nondepressed counterparts, and they rarely are treated by mental health specialists. For that reason, identification and treatment of depression in older adults—or referral for management by a psychiatrist—becomes a major responsibility of the primary physician.

RISK FACTORS ASSOCIATED WITH AGING

Losses and adverse life events are now recognized as major determinants of psychiatric illness in the elderly. Losses are the price of aging as friends and loved ones die or move away, so that social isolation may replace established support networks. Retirement or loss of primary function in the home, especially when it is unplanned or unwanted, has been correlated with apathy, involution, and depression. Grief and bereavement are probably the most important threats to emotional well-being of old people. Loss of a child or, more commonly, a spouse is an important risk factor for major depression, hypochondriasis, and decline in function. While these environmental and psychosocial stressors are unavoidable in the process of normal aging, their identification by the physician is important in order to prevent morbid outcomes.

The consequences of grief and bereavement can be eased by establishment of at least one intimate and confiding relationship. Murphy (1982) has shown that such a relationship can protect against depression. The physician who is aware of a recent or impending loss in the life of a patient can help by fostering a relationship with a friend or relative. Family members may need to be instructed about the need for this level of intimacy and support. Isolated elderly people must be repeatedly encouraged to participate in church or community senior activities and, if necessary, support groups for the bereaved. If no network of support or relationship can be established, referral for supportive psychotherapy during the period of acute loss may be necessary.

Retirement is associated with a one-third to one-half reduction in personal income (Soldo and Agree, 1988). Role changes will also have direct effects on self-esteem. Many individuals retire in their late 50s or early 60s. Close to 90% of men in their early 50s are in the labor force, while only about 45% of men between the ages of 62 and 64 work (Schulz, 1988). The employment rate declines rapidly with advancing age; after age 70, only about 10% of men and 4% of women are still working. Elimination of mandatory retirement and shifting of the American economy from heavy industry to less physically demanding kinds of employment may extend the working longevity of the population in the near future.

The physician should envision retirement as a period of loss in the patient's life history. However, appropriate planning can mitigate its adverse effects. Individuals who undertake retirement with plans to do what they enjoy and value are least likely to become depressed. As soon as the physician is aware of a patient's retirement plans, a process should be put in motion for prevention of adverse consequences. Social workers, activities counselors, and occupational therapists as well as career counselors can for example suggest opportunities for skilled volunteer work, part-time employment, and structured recreational activities. Activities planned for the retirement period must be considered meaningful and serve to replace and compensate for the patient's narcissistic investment in work roles.

Functional disability resulting from multiple medical illnesses and orthopedic and neurologic disabilities must be perceived as a major loss. However, education about the severity of illness, prognosis, and the usefulness of medication can allow the patient to maintain control and self-esteem when fears about dependency become dominant. As disability becomes evident, assessment of patient function becomes necessary in two general areas: (1) in the basic activities of daily living (ADL)—eating, bathing and grooming, toileting, ambulation and transportation; and (2) the instrumental activities of daily living (IADL)—functions required to maintain independent community living, including managing finances, using public transportation, shopping, using the telephone, etc. After these assessments, the physician will have adequate data to help the patient improve function while maintaining retained assets.

Sensory function must be assessed carefully, and attempts to correct deficits must be made aggressively. Auditory and visual impairments are common in older adults. These disabilities heighten isolation and may be mistaken for cognitive or emotional disorders. Sensory losses are associated with both paranoid disorders and depression. Paraphrenic disorders (late life paranoia) are highly correlated with hearing loss and, to a lesser extent, with blindness. Audiometric screening and appropriate use of a hearing aid have been shown to reverse some of these symptoms. Deafness may accentuate alienation and discrimination, which may be reversible with the use of an aid. Similarly, cataracts and glaucoma commonly impair vision in the elderly. However, psychiatric symptoms, including confusion, anxiety, fearfulness, and depression, may precede complaints of visual impairment. Improvement of sensory function may eradicate these symptoms without the need for psychiatric intervention.

EVALUATING CLINICAL COMPLAINTS

Although the prevalence of chronic illness peaks in older adulthood, most older people enjoy relatively good health. Even so, older adults consume approximately 30% of all health care resources though they comprise only about 12% of the population. The aging-related challenges and losses described above have been shown to increase somatic symptoms and medical care utilization. Furthermore, older adults are likely to suffer at least mild chronic pain and some alteration in baseline physical health and functional ability. Therefore, it may be difficult to distinguish reality-based complaints and preoccupations from psychiatric symptoms. Similarly, psychiatric and neurological syndromes in geriatric patients are often accompanied by somatic preoccupation.

Preoccupation with physical health and fear of illness cause many older people to describe symptoms for which no organic cause can be found. They may be subjected to uncomfortable, risky, and expensive workups from numerous physicians serially or even simultaneously. Even though aggressive evaluation is essential and somatic complaints should never be ignored, medical workups may have substantial health risks in frail older patients. Geriatric health care there-

fore should include communication between all treating physicians and efforts to minimize redundancy and overlap. The care of older patients includes the need to obtain all available records from hospitals, other physicians, and reliable informants.

History Taking

All of the risk factors described in the previous section can be documented in the process of routine medical history taking. The description of medical symptoms and the related systems review form the core of the patient interview. The same rapport required to obtain a good medical history will allow essential psychosocial data to be obtained. However, the interaction of medical and psychiatric disorders in the elderly requires painstaking assessment and special clinical skill to discriminate somatic and behavioral complaints.

Mental Status Examination; Assessing Cognitive Function & Depression

The prevalence of behavioral disorders of the elderly requires that a brief examination of mental status be part of every evaluation. Observation of appearance, affect, mood, psychomotor function (ie, retardation or agitation), speech, and thought processes and content (including suicidal and homicidal ideation) should be part of routine history taking. Attention to these details will improve sensitivity to mood disorders, symptoms of anxiety and panic, paranoid thinking, hallucinosis, other elements of psychosis, and cognitive impairment. The review of systems should garner data about sleep patterns, appetite, concentration, memory, and sexual function.

Retained social skills, the subtlety of findings, and patient and family denial may make routine screening for changes in **cognitive function** a difficult task. The lack of clear age-related norms for intellectual ability hampers efforts to distinguish normal aging from diseases of old people. However, inasmuch as cognitive impairment is highly prevalent in the elderly and because many conditions that impair cognition can be palliated, it is essential that physicians have the ability to rapidly screen for dysfunction. The Mini-Mental State Examination (MMSE) (Folstein, Folstein, and McHugh, 1975) is used widely both in clinical research and in practice to screen for problems with orientation, memory, concentration, language, and comprehension. It has been correlated with sophisticated psychometric testing, and cut-off scores for "normal" and impaired function have been established. Orientation, registration, calculating ability (concentration), recall, naming, figure copying, graphic ability, and ability to follow complex commands are superficially screened in only a few minutes. The MMSE is a simple method for determining the need for further evaluation and quickly reassessing cognitive status.

Depression can be difficult to discern in older adults. Nearly 20% of older adults with depression present with complaints of physical illness, and depressive symptoms are easily confused with numerous medical conditions (Busse and Simpson, 1983). Subjectively depressed mood, guilt, and suicidal ideation are rarely expressed. Somatic complaints, disturbances of sleep and appetite, anxiety, and apathy often predominate. Patients often insist that their difficulties are physical in origin. Diffuse pain and gastrointestinal discomfort are common. These complaints, as well as apathy, fatigue, and weight loss are an indication for an extensive workup. Again, aggressive evaluation is necessary to rule out disorders that present with depressed mood, including occult cancer, infections (eg, viral pneumonia or hepatitis), endocrine disorder (eg, hypothyroidism, apathetic hyperthyroidism, Cushing's disease, Addison's disease, panhypopituitarism), central nervous system disease (eg, Parkinson's disease, early Alzheimer's disease), intracranial mass lesions, stroke, major systemic illnesses (eg, congestive heart failure), dehydration, renal disease, and early pulmonary disease. These disorders often affect mood and function and can give rise to symptoms similar to those of major depression. However, even completely negative exhaustive workups rarely convince patients that symptoms are primarily "mental."

Careful scrutiny of patient medication regimens may uncover an iatrogenic origin for changes in function and perceived quality of life. Many drugs given for medical disorders in the elderly have adverse central nervous system side effects. Depressive symptoms are not uncommonly associated with antihypertensives, including reserpine, methyldopa, beta-blockers, and hydralazine. Histamine H_2 antagonists, digoxin, oral hypoglycemics, steroids, and cytotoxic agents may cause depression. Almost any central nervous system depressant, including barbiturates, benzodiazepines, neuroleptics, and alcohol, may also precipitate these symptoms and cognitive changes.

Somatic complaints, vegetative symptoms, apathy, and lethargy often persist even after extensive medical evaluation and changes of drug regimens. Despite the patient's rejection of the diagnosis, major depression is then a likely diagnosis. Similarly, a patient who has recently suffered an acute illness or injury (eg, myocardial infarction, stroke, or hip fracture) who is unable to recover premorbid function should be examined closely. If depression screening and formal mental status examination reveal anorexia, insomnia, fatigue, constricted affect, inability to experience pleasure, hopelessness, and apathy, treatment of depression should be considered. Many depressives have "good reasons" for being depressed. Support alone, therefore, is unlikely to remedy the situation or induce recovery from the primary medical or surgical illness. Depression and depressive symptoms have been shown to cause disability similar to that imposed by major chronic illnesses. Appropriate treatment of the depression will enhance rehabilitation and permit prompt return to the premorbid functional level. Accurate diagnosis may prevent the need for supervised care.

Much has been written about cognitive impairment in the presentation of depression in the elderly. The **dementia of depression,** or **pseudodementia,** causes substantial cognitive impairment and can easily be mistaken for parenchymal dementia. Memory impairment associated with major depression in older adults may be partially or completely reversible. Controversy continues while evidence suggests but does not prove that cognitive capacity will recover somewhat with improvement in depression even in patients with mild to moderate organic dementias. Discrimination of dementia of depression from a primary degenerative dementia can be quite difficult. In the dementia of depression, onset of symptoms is usually more sudden, and patients may admit to awareness of impairment, classically responding with "I don't know" rather than confabulating. Psychomotor retardation is prominent, as are constriction of affect and classical vegetative signs. On cognitive screening, disorders of concentration and long-term memory are more prominent than the deficits in recall and registration associated with dementias such as Alzheimer's disease and multi-infarct dementia (MID).

The Workup for Dementia

The prevalence of impairment in intellectual ability among the elderly dictates the importance of appropriate assessment of complaints of memory loss, confusion, and deteriorating functional ability. The purpose of a comprehensive evaluation is to determine the presence of dementia and its potential "reversibility" and to slow deterioration as much as possible. The recommended workup is based on numerous reports that between 10% and 30% of cognitively impaired patients have treatable problems. Equally convincing are data indicating that as many as 30% of geriatric patients, when properly evaluated, may have more than one illness contributing to the dementia. In the well-controlled study of Larson et al (1985), treatment of concomitant medical, neurological, and psychiatric disorders provided at least temporary improvement in 27.5% of patients and sustained gains in 14%. While reversibility was usually not possible, improvement in quality of life was reported by patients and their families.

The dementia evaluation includes a complete medical and psychiatric history, a review of all medications, physical examination, a complete neurological examination, and a mental status examination, including rating with an instrument such as the MMSE (see above). Laboratory screening includes a complete blood count, serum electrolytes and liver function tests, VDRL (or RPR), serum vitamin B_{12} and folate levels, CT scan or MRI of the head, and a chest x-ray. Admittedly, this is a costly workup. However, the cost savings associated with improvement in intellectual ability and prolongation of relative autonomy are estimated to be considerable as well.

In the Larson study cited above, the most common treatable illnesses associated with or causing dementia were drug toxicity, hypothyroidism and other metabolic diseases, and depression. In all, more than 250 medical illnesses were recognized in 60% of the 200 patients studied. Treatment of many of these entities improved outcome.

The vulnerability of older adults to even the rarest toxic effects of medications must be recognized. The sparsest possible drug regimen—particularly the withholding of direct central nervous system toxins—is recommended for all older patients and especially for those with cognitive impairment. All medications should be considered suspect, and questionably necessary agents should be withdrawn when feasible.

Treatment of other medical illness that may cause or complicate dementia—including thyroid disease, neurosyphilis, vitamin B_{12} or folate deficiencies, azotemia, hypercalcemia, iron deficiency anemia, substance (including alcohol) use disorders, thiamine deficiency, subdural hematoma, central nervous system tumor, normal pressure hydrocephalus, and depression—should be undertaken in standard fashion but with as much cooperation from caregivers as possible.

Most dementias are due to irreversible causes. Between 60% and 70% of elderly patients with global cognitive disability suffer from Alzheimer's disease. Another 10–20% probably have multi-infarct dementia (Larson et al, 1984). Early recognition of these dementias is important in preventing unnecessary rapid deterioration and in helping families and caregivers to make short- and long-term plans. By definition, the clinical diagnosis of Alzheimer's disease is one of exclusion. Because of the uncertain nature of the diagnosis and the unpredictable duration of its course, clinicians must be cautious about labeling possibly affected individuals. Patients with dementia are extremely susceptible to alterations in cognition and function when they become medically ill. Infections, metabolic disturbances, and changes in drug regimens can cause rapid changes in mental status. Any rapid change in function in a patient with a slowly progressive dementia should arouse a suspicion of the presence of a secondary medical process. Aggressive management of medical illnesses is likely to lead to elimination of "excess disability." Similarly, discontinuation of potentially toxic medications can improve function to the patient's baseline level of disability. Examples are anticholinergics, antidepressants [anticholinergic effects may cause confusion or delirium], sedative-hypnotics, some antihypertensives and antiarrhythmics, digitalis, antiparkinsonism drugs, analgesics, antineoplastics, and histamine H_2 antagonists).

ISSUES IN PSYCHIATRIC MANAGEMENT OF BEHAVIORAL DISORDERS IN THE ELDERLY

General Issues in Psychotherapy

Psychotherapy is as appropriate for the elderly as it is in younger populations. However, older adults tend to perceive a stigma associated with care from mental health specialists and may for that reason resist referral. Longer term interventions may not be appropriate in frail populations with chronic and terminal illnesses.

Several types of psychotherapy have been shown to improve mood in older adult depressives. Psychodynamic, behavioral, cognitive, and supportive psychotherapy can be useful either in group or individual settings. As in other populations, therapies must be tailored to individual needs. The major losses and stressors associated with aging are frequently a focus for adaptive strategies. Psychotherapy often attempts to address the major Eriksonian challenge of the final stage of the life cycle: the struggle to maintain ego integrity and hold the line against despair.

Pharmacotherapeutic Issues

Decisions about drug therapy for older adult patients should be made in spirit of thoughtful conservatism. While all classes of psychotropics that are useful in younger adults can be used effectively in the elderly, age-related pharmacokinetic and pharmacodynamic changes dictate modifications in therapeutic approach. Every drug-related decision demands evaluation of potential risks and benefits. The physician must be aware of all prescribed and over-the-counter medications the patient is taking, the patient's history of previous responses and adverse effects, and the potential effects of a medication on overall function. Adverse drug effects may be more important in the older adult than in younger patients. For example, psychotropic use has been shown to be an important risk factor for hip fracture in the elderly. Similarly, constipating effects of anticholinergic drugs may be an inconvenience in a younger person but could cause fecal impaction or even paralytic ileus in an immobilized frail older adult. Therefore, the primary maxim of geriatric pharmacology is always to "start low and go slow."

Although gastric pH and motility and total intestinal surface area and blood flow decrease with age, drug absorption does not appear to be affected by aging in the absence of gastrointestinal disease. Diminished hepatic blood flow and decreased microsomal enzyme activity may slow metabolic pathways in the elderly, causing increased serum levels of some psychotropics (eg, tertiary amine tricyclic antidepressants). Drug distribution is affected largely by lipid solubility. Increased proportions of body fat to water in older adults increase the volume of distribution of psychotropics, most of which are highly lipid-soluble. Decreases in plasma proteins, including albumin and glycoproteins, can affect protein binding and drug distribution. Decreased renal function reduces clearance of hydrophilic metabolites of tricyclics and other psychotropic agents and of lithium in the elderly. Moreover, physical illnesses can alter all aspects of pharmacokinetics, as can interactions with other medications.

Medical illnesses and interactions with other agents alter the therapeutic and toxic effects of psychotropics in the elderly. Changes in neurotransmitters may change the effects of psychotropics, but outcomes have not been well demonstrated. Numerous reports have described the increased vulnerability of the elderly to adverse psychotropic effects, particularly to central nervous system toxicity of these agents. However, systematic scientific studies of changes in pharmacodynamics with age have not been undertaken. Needless to say, suggested treatment with psychotropics is based largely on experience in younger adults. Therefore, cautious titration of dosage is always advised.

Antidepressant pharmacotherapy is the mainstay of treatment for major depression in the elderly. Tricyclics have been used extensively. However, anticholinergic and cardiac side effects, including delayed conduction through the His-Purkinje system and postural hypotension, may limit their utility. Secondary amine tricyclics, particularly desipramine and nortriptyline, are less anticholinergic and less sedating than tertiary amines. Nortriptyline may be less likely to cause orthostatic hypotension. These agents should be titrated slowly and serum levels employed to guide dosing and to allow patients to become accustomed to side effects. Similarly, monoamine oxidase inhibitors can be used safely in the elderly. Gradual dose increases and particular attention to hypotensive effects are necessary. Trazodone has little anticholinergic effect and does not prolong cardiac conduction. However, this agent is quite sedating and may cause orthostatic hypotension, premature ventricular contractions, and priapism, all of considerable concern in the elderly. Fluoxetine and bupropion are newer antidepressants with less anticholinergic and cardiac side effects (see Chapter 32), but clinical trials in the older population are not yet available. There is evidence that antidepressant efficacy may require longer trials in the elderly. A full 6-week trial of any agent is recommended.

Anxiolytics and sedative-hypnotics should be used with caution in older adults. Even in relatively low doses, they can cause sedation, cognitive impairment, and ataxia. While the indications for benzodiazepine use are similar to those in younger populations, effects on function must always weigh heavily in the decision to treat. Pharmacokinetic and pharmacodynamic changes with aging suggest that short-acting agents with few or no active metabolites (eg, lorazepam,

oxazepam, temazepam, triazolam) are superior to long-acting agents with active metabolites (eg, diazepam, flurazepam, chlordiazepoxide). Overall, these agents should be used with extreme caution and only upon clear indications. Short trials and "as needed" dosing are recommended.

All of the principles of neuroleptic use in younger populations (see Chapter 32) apply, perhaps with greater force, to the elderly. For example, older adults appear to be more vulnerable to tardive dyskinesia. Jeste and Wyatt (1987) concluded that as many as 40% of older adult inpatients with histories of prolonged neuroleptic exposure have tardive dyskinesia. This risk is even greater in patients with dementia. Treatment with neuroleptics always requires a balancing of the sedative and anticholinergic properties of low-potency agents (eg, thioridazine and chlorpromazine) with the increased risk of extrapyramidal side effects associated with higher-potency drugs (eg, haloperidol and fluphenazine). Use of any of these agents in the elderly—and in patients with dementia in particular—requires slow titration and low dosage regimens.

Psychiatric symptoms often complicate cognitive decline. In the earliest phases of dementia, moderate anxiety and depression are not uncommon. As the illness progresses, paranoia, hallucinosis, agitation, and insomnia may become prominent. These latter symptoms may be the most difficult for families to manage and may serve as an impetus to hospitalization or institutionalization. Any psychiatric symptoms in these patients must be managed holistically. Medical and toxic contributions must be ruled out prior to intervention. Remaining "excess" psychiatric symptoms may respond to drug treatment. While good studies demonstrating efficacy are sparse, very low dose neuroleptic medications can be employed successfully. Benzodiazepines and other sedative hypnotics should be employed only transiently, as they may promote more confusion and even agitation. Other agents, including trazodone, propranolol, and carbamazepine, have also been suggested for management of agitation in dementia. However, clinical trials demonstrating their safety and efficacy have not been conducted.

Family Issues

The physician is apt to be a most important source of information and support for patients and their families. The physician can be assisted in this task by well-informed nonphysician care providers. Demented individuals often deny their symptoms and are unable to "take in" the implications of the diagnosis. Family members and other caregivers can benefit greatly from education about the illness, its possible course, associated symptoms, and available community resources. Appropriate family support can prolong care in noninstitutional settings, protect financial resources, and enhance prevention and early detection of medical or psychiatric illnesses. Family members should be encouraged to attend support groups. Family meetings held by the primary physician or other closely involved providers can educate "en masse" all potential caregivers and provide direction for optimal care. Respite for caregivers should be encouraged.

Community senior adult programs or day care settings can supplement available family care. Where resources are available, companions and other home health aides may also be employed. Long-term care provided by family caregivers is not without substantial cost. Depending upon the level of support necessary, home health and respite care may approach institutionalization in actual dollar costs. Family members may miss days of work, be forced to elect early retirement, and endure stress. Renovations of the home environment and the purchase of medical equipment can be quite expensive. As dementia progresses, these problems must be weighed against the costs of institutionalization.

CONCLUSION

Prevention and early detection of disorders impairing mental function in older adults can be accomplished to a great extent in the primary care setting. The investigative style and personal rapport intrinsic to primary care practice are important tools in screening for risk factors and mental disorder. Treatment of medically and behaviorally complex patients often requires psychiatric consultation or primary psychiatric care.

Geriatric psychiatry is a field whose growth is fueled by the needs and size of the older adult population. Advances in neuroscience, in psychotherapy, and psychopharmacology are supporting the development of a specialty that can respond to the enormity of the demands it faces. However, it is the rich experience and wisdom of the older adult, challenged by the attendant changes of the aging process, that makes holistic and thoughtful geriatric care exciting and rewarding for the practitioner.

REFERENCES

Arie T: Prevention of mental disorders of old age. J Am Geriatr Soc 1984;32:460.

Busse EW: The myth, history, and science of aging. In: *Geriatric Psychiatry*. Busse EW, Blazer DG (editors). American Psychiatric Press, 1989.

Busse EW, Simpson D: Depression and antidepressants and the elderly. J Clin Psychiatry 1983;44:5(Sec 2):35.

Cath SH, Sadavoy J: Psychosocial aspects. In: Sadavoy J, Lazarus LW, Jarvik LF (editors): *Comprehensive Review of Geriatric Psychiatry*. American Psychiatric Press, 1991.

Evans DA et al: Prevalence of Alzheimer's disease in a community population of older persons: Higher than previously reported. JAMA 1989;262:2551.

Folstein MF, Folstein SE, McHugh PR: Mini-Mental State: A practical method for grading the cognitive state of patients for the clinician. J Psychiatr Res 1975;12:189.

Frederick CJ: Current trends in suicidal behavior in the United States. Am J Psychother 1978;32:172.

Georgotas A et al: How effective and safe is continuation therapy in elderly depressed patients? Arch Gen Psychiatry 1988;45:929.

Georgotas A et al: Comparative efficacy and safety of MAOIs versus TCAs in treating depression in the elderly. Biol Psychiatry 1986;21:1155.

Gurland B, Dean L, Cross B: The epidemiology of depression and dementia in the elderly: The use of multiple indicators of these conditions. In: *Psychopathology in the Aged*. Cole JD, Barrett JE (editors). Raven Press, 1980.

Hazzard WR: Geriatric medicine: Life in the crucible of the struggle to contain health care costs. In: *The Medical Cost Containment Crisis*. McCue JD (editor). Health Administration Press, 1989.

Hyer L et al: Depression, anxiety, paranoid reactions, crisis and cognitive decline of later-life inpatients. Gerontology, 1987;42:92.

Jeste DV, Wyatt RJ: Aging and tardive dyskinesia. In: *Schizophrenia and Aging*. Miller NE, Cohen GD (editors). Guilford, 1987.

Kenney AR: *Physiology of Aging: A Synopsis*, 2nd ed. Year Book, 1989.

Larson EB et al: Dementia in elderly outpatients: A prospective study. Ann Intern Med 1984;100:417.

Larson EB et al: Diagnostic evaluation of 200 elderly outpatients with suspected dementia. J Gerontol 1985;40:536.

Lazarus LW, Sadavoy J, Langsley PR: Individual psychotherapy. In Sadavoy J, Lazarus LW, Jarvik LF (editors): *Comprehensive Review of Geriatric Psychiatry*. American Psychiatric Press, 1991.

Leventhal EA: Biological aspects. In: Sadavoy J, Lazarus LW, Jarvik LF: *Comprehensive Review of Geriatric Psychiatry*. American Psychiatric Press, 1991.

Lipowski ZJ: Transient cognitive disorders in the elderly. Am J Psychiatry 1983;140:1426.

Manton KG, Siegler IC, Woodbury MA: Patterns of intellectual development in later life. J Gerontol 1986;41:486.

McAllister TW, Price TR: Severe depressive pseudodementia with and without dementia. Am J Psychiatry 1982;139:626.

McKhann G et al: Clinical diagnosis of Alzheimer's disease: Report for the NINCDS-ADRDA work group under the auspices of the Department of Health and Human Services Task Force on Alzheimer's Disease. Neurology 1984;34:939.

Meyers B, Kalayam B: Update in geriatric psychopharmacology. In: *Advances in Psychosomatic Medicine*, vol 19. Karger, 1988.

Murphy E: Social origins of depression in old age. Brit J Psychiatry 1982;141:135.

Murrell SA, Himmelfarb S, Wright K: Prevalence of depression and its correlates in older adults. Am J Epidemiol, 1983;117:173.

Myers JK et al: Six month prevalence of psychiatric disorders in three communities. Arch Gen Psychiatry 1984;41:959.

National Center for Health Statistics: Health United States, 1987. (DHHS Pub. No. [PHS] 88–1232). U.S. Government Printing Office, 1988.

Poon LW, Siegler IC: Psychological aspects of normal aging. In: Sadavoy J, Lazarus LW, Jarvik LF (editors): *Comprehensive Review of Geriatric Psychiatry.* American Psychiatric Press, 1991.

Raskind MA, Risse SC, Lampe TH: Dementia and antipsychotic drugs. J Clin Psychiatry 1987;485(Suppl):16.

Riggs BL et al: Dietary calcium intake and rates of bone loss in women. J Clin Invest 1987;80:979.

Rovner BW, Kafonek S, Filipp L: Prevalence of mental illness in a community nursing home. Am J Psychiatry 1986;143:1446.

Schaie KW: Intellectual development in adulthood. In: *Handbook of the Psychology of Aging,* 3rd ed. Birren JE, Schaie KW (editors). Academic Press, 1990.

Schneck MK, Reisberg B, Ferris SH: An overview of current concepts of Alzheimer's disease. Am J Psychiatry 1982;139:165.

Schulz J: *Economics of Aging,* 4th ed. Auburn House, 1988.

Secretary's Task Force on Alzheimer's Disease: U.S. Department of Health and Human Services, DHHS Publication No. (ADM) 84-1323, 1984.

Soldo BJ, Agree EM: America's elderly population. Population Bulletin (March) 1988;43:1.

Terry RD, De Teresa R, Hansen LAS: Neocortical cell counts in normal adult aging. Ann Neurol 1987;21:530.

U.S. Bureau of the Census: An aging world. International Population Reports. Series P–95, No. 78. U.S. Government Printing Office, 1987.

Waxman HM, Carner EA, Blum A: Depressive symptoms and health service utilization among community elderly. J Am Geriatr Soc 1983;31:145.

Waxman HM, Carner EA, Klein M: Underutilization of mental health professionals by community elderly. The Gerontologist 1984;24:23.

Waxman HM, Carner EA: Physicians' recognition, diagnosis and treatment of mental disorders in elderly medical patients. The Gerontologist 1984;24:593.

Winograd CH, Jarvik L: Physician management of the demented patient. J Am Geriatr Soc 1986;34:295.

Young RC, Myers BS: Psychopharmacology. In Sadavoy J, Lazarus LW, Jarvik LF (editors): *Comprehensive Review of Geriatric Psychiatry.* American Psychiatric Press, 1991.

41

Consultation Psychiatry in the General Hospital

Richard J. Goldberg, MD

Consultation psychiatry is the practical application of psychiatric knowledge and techniques to the care of medical patients in a general hospital. While commonly assumed to be synonymous with psychosomatic medicine, consultation psychiatry is actually more diverse and requires a knowledge of general psychiatry as well as familiarity with medical and surgical diseases and their treatments, neuroanatomy and neurobehavioral disorders, pharmacology, and systems theory.

As the bridge between psychiatry and medicine, consultation psychiatry has always occupied a strategic position. At present, while psychiatry reenters the mainstream of medicine, this strategic position is more critical than ever. Consultation psychiatry provides a scientific understanding and effective management of the emotional and cognitive problems of medical and surgical patients. It also participates in the training of medical students, medical residents, and psychiatric residents.

The Need for Consultation

In clinical practice, consultation psychiatrists treat medical and surgical patients with emotional, behavioral, and cognitive problems. Epidemiological studies (vonAmmon Cavanaugh, 1983) show that 30–65% of medical inpatients have significant psychiatric symptoms, with the most frequent diagnoses being anxiety, depression, and organic mental disorder. Contributing further to the incidence of psychiatric problems in medical patients is the high rate of physical illness in psychiatric patients (Hoffman and Koran, 1984), who may represent a disproportionately large segment of the population seeking medical treatment (Hankin et al, 1982).

With the recent development and application of brief cognitive screening tests (see Chapter 11), there is increasing appreciation that medical and surgical patients have a high rate of cognitive impairments. For example, about 30% of patients in acute medical inpatient units have cognitive deficits (Lipowski, 1989). The rate may be twice as high on neurology inpatient units. However, since many brief cognitive screening examinations do not systematically assess constructional or language skills, the true prevalence

of cognitive impairment in medical populations is probably greater than reported.

Despite a high incidence of emotional and cognitive disturbances, a small percentage (approximately 2%) of medical and surgical patients are evaluated by a psychiatric consultant (Steinberg, 1980; Craig, 1982). The reasons for this are not completely clear, but a number of factors may be at work. If the psychiatric symptoms seem understandable in the context of the patient's illness, the primary physician may feel no need to request a psychiatric consultation. For example, when a patient with cancer develops depressive symptoms, the primary physician may feel the reaction is appropriate and that no treatment is required—or that if treatment is required, the primary physician should be able to provide it. Primary physicians may also believe that a psychiatric consultant might have nothing positive to offer and might even upset the patient. Another critical factor is that in many cases, primary physicians simply fail to recognize emotional and cognitive problems in their patients.

This chapter focuses on inpatient consultation psychiatry and is intended to make the primary physician a better consumer of the services. Eight common clinical problems for which psychiatric consultation is indicated will be discussed: organic mental disorder, depression, patient management problems, symptoms of obscure origin, pain, substance abuse, management of medical and surgical patients with major psychiatric disorders, and forensic issues. The roles of the various professionals that make up the psychiatric consultation team will then be briefly described.

CONSULTATION PROCEDURE

A primary care physician may request a consultation by making a personal call to the consultant or by written request. Optimally, the patient would be informed of the request for psychiatric consultation and the reason for the request, but in practice this is often not done.

After the primary physician's request for consultation, the consultant's first task is to define as precisely as possible the questions being asked. Sometimes this is quite easy, as with the patient who has attempted suicide and may require evaluation of the need for suicide precautions or further psychiatric treatment. At other times the questions asked are quite vague— eg, the consultee may believe that the patient's emotional response to the medical illness is inappropriate but is unable to state the problems more precisely. A preliminary discussion with the consultee can sharpen the focus of the consultation. Following this, the consultant reviews the chart to understand the medical context of the problem. Discussion with the nursing staff and the family often provides important supplemental information.

The consultant then interviews the patient, preferably in private. Consultants must make it clear at the outset that they are psychiatrists and discuss any feelings the patient has about being interviewed by a psychiatrist. Patients are then asked to verbalize their understanding of the medical or surgical problem and the difficulties it has created. During the interview, a formal mental status examination should be performed. The essence of the consultation process, however, is to gather information about the problems that led to the consultation request. While this may seem obvious, it is not uncommon for inexperienced consultants to gather extensive information about the patient's life and psychodynamics without investigating the "chief complaint" identified by the referring physician.

The consultant should then formulate a differential diagnosis and discuss it with the primary physician along with whatever has been learned about the specific issues for which the consultation was requested. These issues should also be discussed with the nursing staff. For example, a depressed medical patient with suicidal ideation should be discussed at length with the nursing staff so that they will understand the context of the patient's depression and the specific precautions to be taken.

The Consultation Note

The consultation note (Garrick and Stotland, 1982) should be brief and specifically labeled as a psychiatric consultation, with date, time, and sources of information. Details of the history and information about the specific problem for which the consultation was requested should be stated. Discretion is called for, since medical records have less privacy protection than psychiatric records. It is critical to omit superfluous information that may be embarrassing or lead to inappropriate labeling of the patient. The mental status examination should be recorded in detail, since it represents the most objective information in the note. It is particularly helpful as baseline information that can be referred to when the patient is seen later. Finally, a working diagnosis and a differential diagnosis are recorded.

The heart of the consultation note is the recommendations, and these must address the consultee's questions. The recommendations should be stated as specifically as possible. It is not sufficient to state that the patient should be evaluated for certain conditions and started on certain medications. Rather, the specific tests recommended and details of the proposed drug regimen should be stated, along with the target symptoms and potential adverse effects. Follow-up examination by the consultant is an integral part of all consultations. This allows the patient, consultee, and consultant to evaluate the impact of the initial recommendations and to make appropriate modifications.

PSYCHIATRIC CONSULTATION

The eight categories discussed below do not necessarily reflect traditional diagnostic categories, and most are not medical or psychiatric syndromes. All can be considered complex clinical situations that include the interaction of biological, psychological, and social factors. The consultant also needs a working knowledge of how to assess a patient's personality type and how this personality interacts with a particular medical situation to create a behavioral management problem (see Chapter 26). Despite the psychologically traumatic nature of most medical catastrophes, the capacity of people to adjust is remarkably high. Problem patients usually have a history of personality or emotional difficulties. As a basic principle of consultation psychiatry, the patient's psychological defenses should be supported whenever possible and psychotropic medications used appropriately when needed. Coping skills and strengths should be discovered and reinforced.

Organic Mental Disorders

A significant number of hospital patients have an organic mental disorder that remains unrecognized or masquerades as some other problem such as depression or noncompliant behavior. Organic mental disorder should be the first consideration in any evaluation of impaired mood, thought, or behavior. In its most dramatic form, gross delirium is easily recognized by noting the patient's impaired attention, perceptual disturbances, agitation, and disorientation. Visual hallucinations, which many clinicians associate with schizophrenia, are actually more common in organic mental disorders such as delirium tremens and toxic encephalopathy. It is not uncommon for consultees to mistakenly ascribe even obvious organic delirium to some psychogenic cause. There are, of course, many less severe cases in which mild delirium or dementia is characterized by impaired intellect, memory deficits, or personality change. In many situations, the consultant will recognize the presence of organic mental disorder only by performing a specific mental status examination (see Chapter 11). Assessment of language and other higher functioning is often neglected but critical for the detection of aphasia, apraxia, and agnosia.

The recognition of organic mental disorder is important because it often has a specific cause and treatment. Furthermore, failure to provide treatment may lead to permanent deficits and mislabeling of the patient's symptoms. The common denominator in organic mental disorder is impairment of cerebral function. Specific causes include metabolic derangements, drug toxicity or withdrawal, vascular compromise, infections, intracranial tumors, and neuronal degeneration. The consultant must be prepared to review the medical evaluation of the patient with special emphasis on the presence of neurological findings. The psychiatric consultant must also review all laboratory evaluations and neurodiagnostic tests, such as lumbar puncture, electroencephalography, and cranial CT or MRI scans and be prepared to make recommendations for further tests. In the hospital setting, most cases of organic mental disorder are either partially or entirely reversible. The most frequent cause is metabolic imbalance due to alterations in renal, pancreatic, hepatic, cardiovascular, or pulmonary function. A comprehensive drug review is crucial because of the high prevalence of psychiatric symptoms secondary to medication (Abramowicz, 1989). This may be supplemented by toxicology screening and serum levels of potentially psychoactive substances. Although a great many drugs may produce psychiatric symptoms as adverse side effects, the most common offenders are the central nervous system depressants and stimulants, cimetidine, levodopa, corticosteroids, and antihypertensive and cholinergic agents.

Primary treatment of delirium consists of correction of the underlying medical abnormality. In addition, certain adjunctive measures are useful. Neuroleptics in small doses may be useful in controlling the agitation of the confused patient and are often superior to benzodiazepines, which may further confuse patients with organic mental disorder. Environmental changes can minimize patient confusion. Such manipulations include providing calendars, clocks, nightlights (to minimize "sundowning"), familiar objects from home, and frequent orientation by staff and family. Clear, straightforward, and consistent communication from the staff and family also helps patients organize their experience. Precautions must also be instituted for individuals at risk for hurting themselves (eg, by falling out of bed, getting lost) as a result of their cognitive impairment.

Depression

Depressed mood is probably the most common reason for psychiatric consultations. When such depression is a response to the stresses of medical illness, it may respond to improvement in the patient's clinical condition or to reassurance by the primary physician. However, when symptoms become severe and interfere with the patient's activities or participation in treatment, psychiatric evaluation should be requested. Aside from depressed mood or crying, the depressed medical patient may be noncompliant with treatment, functioning at a more severely impaired level than is warranted by the medical condition, or preoccupied with somatic symptoms.

There is a tendency to assume that depressed mood in a medical patient represents an understandable adjustment reaction that does not warrant treatment. ('Wouldn't you be depressed if you had cancer?") This may lead to needless suffering, since the depression may respond to treatment. For example, approximately 50% of patients are persistently depressed following stroke. Although it might be reasonable to think that the degree of disability is the main risk factor for the development of depression, in fact it is not. The location of the lesion plays a much greater role. Patients with left hemispheric stroke, especially involving the anterior pole, are at greatest risk for developing depression, which can often be treated with antidepressant medication.

While depression is often neglected in the medical setting, it can also be overdiagnosed in medical patients since its cardinal features may be due to other causes. For example, sleep disturbances may be due to pain; appetite disturbance to nausea; fatigue to anemia; and impaired concentration to the effects of drugs such as theophylline.

As in other settings, the treatment of depression in medically ill patients involves both psychotherapy and antidepressant medications. Supportive psychotherapy assists many patients and their families in coping with the illness. Antidepressant drugs are useful in treating depressed medical patients and can improve mood, appetite, and sleep patterns. Tricyclic agents must be used cautiously in patients with cardiac conduction abnormalities (especially bundle branch blocks); in patients with organic mental disorder, who may become more confused; and in those for whom anticholinergic side effects would be detrimental. Many of these drugs cause orthostatic hypotension and must be used carefully in patients who cannot tolerate a decrease in blood pressure. The nontricyclic agents, including central nervous system stimulants (Woods et al, 1986), may cause fewer adverse effects in the medically ill. Monoamine oxidase inhibitors should be used with extreme caution in this population, because the drugs have numerous interactions with food substances and with other drugs.

The evaluation and documentation of suicidal potential (Goldberg, 1987) is a major function of the psychiatric consultant. The possibility of suicide must be evaluated in all depressed medical patients. The consultant must decide whether the patient requires suicide precautions (constant observation, plastic dining utensils, etc) and what type of psychiatric follow-up is indicated after recovery in cases of self-inflicted medical or surgical problems (Goldberg, 1989).

Patient Management Problems

Psychiatric consultation may be requested to assist in management of (1) the agitated, disruptive patient; (2) the patient whose noncompliance may have serious consequences (eg, the patient who insists upon leaving the hospital against medical advice); and (3) the patient whose personality problems interfere with clinical management (eg, patients who are excessively demanding, seductive, or paranoid) (see Chapter 26). The psychiatric consultant is not an alternative to the hospital security personnel, though this sometimes seems to be a prevailing expectation. The physically threatening patient is better managed initially by a specially trained team, if available, by calling upon properly trained security officers or, if necessary, police officers from the community.

The evaluation of patient management problems involves consideration of biological, psychological, and social factors as they interact in a particular clinical setting. Since many patient management problems arise out of some underlying medical process, recognition and correction of that problem are of primary concern. Metabolic imbalance, drug intoxication, and drug withdrawal syndromes are frequent causes of agitation. The consultant should make specific recommendations for immediate management, including the indications and contraindications for use of restraints or medications to control agitation. The consultant should decide whether antipsychotic drugs or benzodiazepines are indicated and in what dosages (Goldberg et al, 1989). The consultant is also expected to offer guidelines regarding the legal implications (if any) of treating such patients (see Chapter 42).

The consultant must assess to what extent a patient's personality style might be contributing to a dysfunctional response to illness (Goldberg, 1983). At times, brief psychiatric intervention helps the patient adjust to the situation by identification of specific anxieties concerning illness and hospitalization. Specific issues, if pertinent, should be discussed with the staff along with appropriate management guidelines (eg, limit-setting for regressed patients). For many patients, control is a major concern. These patients often engage in power struggles with the staff over their own diagnosis and treatment. Conceding to these patients as much "control" as possible if it does no harm (eg, letting the patient decide which arm the blood is drawn from) minimizes conflict over more critical matters (eg, agreeing to take medications or consent to surgical procedures). Schizophrenia and bipolar affective disorder are not frequent causes of problems in medical patient management.

Social dysfunction contributes to patient management problems in many cases. The psychiatric consultant must often function as a social system consultant by suggesting ways in which medical treatment protocols can be modified to avoid or overcome management problems. When several specialists are involved in the care of the patient, poor communication, diffu-

sion of clinical responsibility, and some mismanagement may result. If patients know that there are conflicting opinions about what should be done for them, they may become anxious, angry, or depressed. One solution is for the psychiatric consultant to suggest that a consensus be reached and executed by the primary physician in charge of the case.

In this section, for the sake of discussion, we have distinguished biological, personality, and social systems. However, it is important to consider how interactions of these factors operate in disruptive or excessively anxious patients. Many instances of abrupt departure against medical advice (and other problems with disruptive patients) emerge through the interplay of an underlying organic mental disorder (eg, drug withdrawal) and dysfunction of the interaction between the patient and the treatment team (Goldberg, 1983). Evaluation and intervention in all three systems is frequently required to resolve such problems without interfering with clinical care.

Symptoms With No Apparent Medical Cause

Psychiatric consultation is often requested for evaluation of patients who have chronic somatic complaints or impaired sensory, motor, or autonomic function for which no medical explanation can be found. The frustration such a patient engenders in the primary clinician is often what prompts the consultation request. The consultant may be asked whether the patient has a conversion disorder. Conversion disorder is characterized by the presence of a psychological conflict out of the patient's awareness that produces anxiety and the unconscious "conversion" of this anxiety into a somatic sign or symptom that symbolically expresses and resolves the psychological conflict. Hypnosis or amobarbital interviews may be useful both in evaluating and in treating this condition.

Other categories of psychiatric illness may also lead to physical signs and symptoms with no apparent medical basis. Both depressed and schizophrenic patients may present with somatic preoccupations that are quite confusing until the psychiatric diagnosis is made. Certain patients, usually women, have lifelong patterns of multiple somatic complaints, sometimes called **Briquet's syndrome** or **somatization disorder** (See Chapter 24). Patients with factitious disorders consciously simulate a medical illness or a specific sign or symptom (see Chapter 29). This simulation may represent a life-style devoted to simulating medical illness (Munchausen's syndrome, or chronic factitious illness). These patients differ from malingerers, who pretend to have medical problems to achieve a specific conscious goal (eg, to obtain narcotics or disability compensation). Recognition of these psychological conditions should alert the staff to withhold invasive diagnostic and therapeutic efforts. Treatment can then be focused on psychosocial issues.

The consultation psychiatrist should watch for medical illnesses presenting as psychiatric syndromes. Systemic lupus erythematosus, multiple sclerosis, seizure disorders, and degenerative central nervous system diseases (eg, emotional lability associated with multi-infarct dementia) may be puzzling because the somatic signs and symptoms and the associated emotional symptoms are often wrongly attributed to psychiatric illness. Although treatment must be directed first toward the medical condition, it is occasionally necessary to treat the psychiatric symptoms as well (eg, antipsychotic medication for the psychosis associated with systemic lupus erythematosus).

In the course of psychiatric evaluation of these patients, two recurrent issues need clarification. The first is "secondary gain" (eg, sympathy, or exemption from social expectations or responsibilities). Since all illnesses offer some degree of secondary gain, this mechanism should not be assumed uncritically to "explain" the signs or symptoms. The psychiatric consultant should help the patient and the family prevent secondary gain from impeding recovery.

The second issue is the diagnosis of "histrionic personality disorder" (Chapter 26). It is not true that patients with this disorder are more likely than others to have conversion disorders. The problem is that these histrionic and seductive patients present their somatic signs and symptoms (which may in fact have a medical explanation) in a less-than-believable fashion. Long-term follow-up of patients with the diagnosis of conversion reaction reveals that about 25% have a medical disorder that accounts for the symptoms (Watson and Buranen, 1979). Presumably, the initial presentation of these patients is in the early stages of the medical disease when it is difficult to make the diagnosis.

Pain

Patients may continue to complain of pain despite analgesic management that is usually effective. This difficult clinical problem may give rise to requests for psychiatric consultation. Such consultation requires an awareness that pain is a complex phenomenon involving an interplay of biological and psychosocial factors. Optimally, the psychiatrist would participate as a member of a multidisciplinary pain assessment team.

The consultant should review these patients with the primary physician, with emphasis on the potential biological basis for the pain and the current treatment strategies. The patient is then evaluated for certain psychiatric disorders that are associated with unusual or refractory pain syndromes. Depression should be considered, since its association with chronic pain may lead to increased preoccupation with the pain and louder complaints. Other syndromes to consider include schizophrenia, somatoform pain disorder, and factitious disorders (see above).

Psychosocial factors may also play a role in refractory pain syndromes. Pain may have a special meaning for the patient or may be "modeled" after the pain of a person who was emotionally close to the patient. At times it may mimic the pain a close relative experienced in a terminal illness. Cultural background, unresolved mourning, and secondary gain may play a role in the pain syndrome (see Chapter 24).

Patients with chronic pain often increase their demands for pain medication in a way that make primary physicians uncomfortable. Although it has been estimated that iatrogenic "addiction" is relatively rare in medical patients, physicians often perceive these demands as evidence of drug dependency and request consultation. Because physicians wish to avoid having their patients become "addicted" to opioids, pain is often undertreated. Undermedication often leads to increased protestations of pain. If the patient's complaint has a "dramatic" emphasis, the physician and staff may discount its true nature, so that a vicious cycle may ensue with the patient receiving less and less analgesic medication in spite of increasing complaints. The psychiatric consultant must have a thorough knowledge of analgesic management and be able to recognize pain problems due to undermedication. Cases of "refractory pain" are often adequately managed by simply increasing the analgesic dosage. This is especially true in the case of acute pain or the pain of terminal cancer. Another mechanism is patient-controlled analgesia, which results in relief of pain often with lower total dosages of opioids.

Over the past few years, techniques for pain control other than opioid analgesics have been developed for chronic pain. Nonsteroidal anti-inflammatory agents are effective alternatives to narcotics for many patients. Tricyclic antidepressants, often in lower doses than used to treat depression, have been effective for chronic pain. The mechanism of their action is unknown, but it appears to be distinct from their antidepressant effects. Supportive psychotherapy, guided imagery, and hypnosis can also be effective for about one-fourth of patients (see Chapters 23, 35, and 38).

For many years, placebos had a role in the evaluation and treatment of chronic pain. The basis for their use was the mistaken notion that response to placebos indicated a functional (nonorganic) cause. In fact, the only thing response to a placebo tells the physician is that the patient is a placebo responder. Evidence that analgesia produced by placebos can be reversed by the narcotic antagonist naloxone suggests that placebos act at least in part through physiological mechanisms (see Chapter 5).

Substance Abuse

The consultation psychiatrist has a role in the evaluation, treatment, and referral of patients with substance abuse problems who are being treated in a medical setting. Narcotic abusers are not uncommon on surgical wards, where they are usually being treated for abscesses, cellulitis, or injuries. These patients tolerate pain poorly and are quite demanding of the staff's attention. It is helpful to remember that 10–20 mg of methadone twice a day is sufficient to block withdrawal symptoms in most of these patients. After recovery from their medical or surgical problems, referral to a substance abuse treatment facility is indicated.

Withdrawal from alcohol or sedative drugs (especially barbiturates) is more life-threatening than withdrawal from narcotics. The psychiatric consultant must be prepared to help in the assessment of patients with nonnarcotic substance abuse and to assist in the pharmacological management of delirium tremens and other sedative drug withdrawal syndromes (see Chapter 18).

Inasmuch as patients with alcohol-related medical problems account for up to 25% of admissions to hospitals (Lange and Schacter, 1989), it is surprising how poorly this problem is evaluated and treated. Other than quantifying the incoming patient's alcohol consumption over the recent past, no other inquiries are usually made. However, it is important to ask about the circumstances at onset or recurrence of drinking, periods of abstinence, attempts at treatment and their outcome, and any history of blackouts or delirium tremens. Referral to alcohol treatment programs should be vigorously pursued.

Management of Other Psychiatric Disorders

A patient with a major psychiatric disorder may be admitted for management of a medical or surgical illness. Since these patients (those with schizophrenia and major affective or anxiety disorders) may be taking a number of psychotropic medications (antipsychotic drugs, antidepressants, lithium carbonate), the psychiatrist should offer consultation on drug interactions and medically relevant side effects. Specific advice on patient management may allow the staff and the patient to become more comfortable with each other. Psychotic patients, for example, need to have reality pointed out to them and their misperceptions corrected (eg, that the antibiotic medication is treating their pneumonia, not poisoning them). The consultant may also act as the liaison between the hospital and other psychiatric referral facilities to provide useful information about the patient's previous psychiatric history and treatment.

Forensic Issues

The psychiatric consultant is often asked to make a judgment about the competence of a patient to refuse or consent to a medical or surgical procedure. Part of this process consists of evaluating whether the patient has a psychiatric disorder (emotional or cognitive) that impairs judgment. Competence is the ability to give informed consent, ie, to understand the nature, benefits, and risks of treatment and the consequences of refusing it. The standard of competence varies with the risk/benefit ratio of the procedure. A patient with moderate organic mental disorder may be competent to consent to a CT scan but not to major surgery. The determination of competence is a judicial decision, though psychiatric opinion often serves as the basis for decisions.

Most "forensic" cases for which the consultant is called represent patient management problems. For example, the problem of the cancer patient refusing chemotherapy can usually be dealt with by a clinical approach to the patient's experience rather than by seeking to declare the patient incompetent, appointing a guardian, or imposing treatment on an unwilling patient. Patients refusing treatment should be evaluated for the presence of organic mental disorder and depression and asked about concerns regarding their life situation. Court permission is usually required before a patient's medical condition can be treated without consent (beyond provision of emergent, life-saving measures). The ethical issues in such cases often pose a dilemma for the clinician, usually untrained in ethics or the law.

While the laws differ in some jurisdictions, commitment is not generally a recourse for patients who refuse medical treatment. Patients can be committed if there is a present risk that they will harm themselves or others because of a mental disorder. However, this means being actively suicidal, not simply refusing medical treatment. Even in the rare instance when refusal of medical treatment is an active suicide attempt, commitment may allow the physicians to treat the mental condition against the patient's will but not the medical condition. Psychiatric consultants should become familiar with the state laws and court decisions in regard to competence, commitment, and obligations regarding the management of dangerousness.

PSYCHIATRIC CONSULTATION TEAM

Consultation psychiatrists may work alone or in conjunction with other mental health professionals. While such collaboration is not new, there remains much confusion over the shared and unique contributions of the psychiatrist, psychologist, social worker, and nurse in hospital consultation.

One model that integrates various disciplines involves formation of a multidisciplinary team. The concept of the team, however, implies a coordinated interdisciplinary effort. The interdisciplinary team concept does not imply simply that there are four professions (psychiatry, psychology, social work, and nursing) competing for overlapping territory and role functions. When the unique contributions of each team member have not been properly identified, there are strained feelings, competitiveness, political hostility, and confusion—all affecting patient care adversely. While it is true that some of the same clinical functions can be performed as well by one professional as another, it is by understanding the unique contributions of each team member that an effective clinical force is created and directed toward helping patients.

SUMMARY

Consultation psychiatry in the general hospital involves the comprehensive evaluation and treatment of medical and surgical patients. Psychiatrists in this field are in the unique position of being able to consider the interaction of biological, psychological, and social factors. As the major link between psychiatry and medicine, consultation psychiatrists are playing a major role in the establishment of a biopsychosocial model of medical care. Finally, by identifying and treating psychiatric comorbidity in medical patients, consultation psychiatry may have a positive effect on the cost of medical care (Ackerman et al, 1988; Fulop et al, 1989).

REFERENCES

Abramowicz M (editor): Drugs that cause psychiatric symptoms. Med Lett Drugs Ther 1989;31:113.

Ackerman AD et al: The Impact of coexisting depression and timing of psychiatric consultation on medical patients' length of stay. Hosp Community Psychiatry 1988;39:173.

Craig TJ: An epidemiological study of a psychiatric liaison service. Gen Hosp Psychiatry 1982;4:131.

Fulop G et al: Medical disorders associated with psychiatric comorbidity and prolonged hospital stay. Hosp Community Psychiatry 1989;40:80.

Garrick TR, Stotland NL: How to write a psychiatric consultation. Am J Psychiatry 1982;139:849.

Goldberg RJ: The assessment of suicide risk in the general hospital. Gen Hosp Psychiatry 1987;9:446.

Goldberg RJ: The use of constant observation in general hospitals. Int J Psychiatry Med 1989;19:193.

Goldberg RJ, Dubin WR, Fogel BS: Behavioral emergencies: assessment and psychopharmacologic management. Clin Neuropharm 1989;12:233.

Goldberg RJ: Personality types and personality disorders. Chapter 4 in: *Psychiatry in the Practice of Medicine.* Leigh H (editor.) Addison-Wesley, 1983.

Hankin JR et al: Use of general medical care services by persons with mental disorders. Arch Gen Psychiatry 1982;39:225.

Hoffman RS, Koran LM: Detecting physical illness in patients with mental disorders. Psychosomatics 1984; 25:654.

Lange DE, Schacter B: Prevalence of alcohol related admissions to general medical units. Int J Psychiatry Med 1989;19:371.

Lipowski ZJ: Delirium (acute confusional states). JAMA 1987;258:1989.

Steinberg H, Torem M, Saravay SM: An analysis of physician resistance to psychiatric consultations. Arch Gen Psychiatry 1980;37:1007.

vonAmmon Cavanaugh S: The prevalence of emotional and cognitive dysfunction in a general medical population: Using the MMSE, GHQ, and BDI. Gen Hosp Psychiatry 1983;5:15.

Watson CG, Buranen C: The frequency and identification of false-positive conversion reactions. J Nerv Ment Dis 1979;167:243.

Woods SW, Tesar GE, Murray GB, Cassem NH: Psychostimulant treatment of depressive disorders secondary to medical illness. J Clin Psychiatry 1986;47:12.

Forensic Psychiatry

42

Bernard L. Diamond, MD

Forensic psychiatry is a general term that denotes the interface between law and psychiatry. This chapter will discuss the field of forensic psychiatry under the following headings: the psychiatric expert witness; criminal law and psychiatry, including insanity, the guilty but mentally ill offender, and competency to stand trial; involuntary hospitalization and conservatorship; the rights of patients, including informed consent, the right to treatment, the right to refuse treatment, confidentiality and privileged communication; and special issues.

THE PSYCHIATRIC EXPERT WITNESS

The law and its institutions function in society as decision-making and dispute-resolving instruments. Depending on the nature of the disputed issue, the decisions may be made by the executive (administrative), legislative, or judicial branch of government, and in some cases by direct vote of the people. Certain kinds of judicial decisions call for input of technical information beyond the scope of knowledge of the layperson.

Information required for legal fact finding is most commonly obtained from witnesses. **Ordinary witnesses** at trial are called to provide factual information about which they have direct personal knowledge; generally speaking (there are exceptions), they are not permitted to express their opinions. When specialized or technical information is needed, the parties must call **expert witnesses** to provide technical data and to express their relevant opinions.

The psychiatrist called on to present clinical testimony should be willing to testify if the patient wishes the psychiatrist to do so, or if the privilege of confidentiality has been waived by the patient, or if the psychiatrist is legally required to testify. The psychiatrist should maintain adequate records and properly prepare to give testimony. Preparation should include close familiarity with the details of the patient's clinical condition and treatment and some knowledge of the pertinent legal issues. A preliminary conference with the attorney acting for the patient is often useful. The attorney may wish a written report before the court appearance.

The psychiatrist may be required to give testimony in the form of a **deposition.** A deposition is a device for taking sworn testimony before trial for use at trial. Its purpose is to preserve testimony for later use in cases where the witness might not be available at trial for any reason. A deposition may take place in the doctor's own office or at any convenient place. Usually, only the opposing attorney and a court reporter are present. However, witnesses giving deposition testimony are under oath just as if they were in court. They may or may not be required to give testimony again in court before a judge and jury. It is important that there be no discrepancies between the testimony in the deposition and that given later in the trial court.

A **subpoena** is an order, backed by the authority of a judge, for the witness to appear at a deposition or in court. It usually also requires that the physician produce the patient's clinical records, or that the records be made available to the attorney, in which case a personal appearance is not required. Failure to comply with a subpoena is punishable as contempt of court. A subpoena to appear at a deposition or in court will specify a particular time and place. In the case of depositions, reasonable requests for changes in time and place of appearance will usually be granted by the attorney for the requesting party. The psychiatrist may not have to be subpoenaed if there is an agreement to testify voluntarily. The arrangements for time and place can then be agreed on between the attorney and the doctor.

The psychiatrist who testifies as an expert in court or in a deposition or who prepares a report for any legal purpose is entitled to a reasonable fee. In all cases it should be understood clearly how much will be paid, when payment will be made, and who is responsible for payment. Although lawyers are permitted to take most civil cases on a contingent fee basis, it is not ethical for doctors to agree to a contingent fee for professional services and testimony. It is not improper, if circumstances warrant, to request partial payment in advance.

Expert witnesses should be prepared to give their professional qualifications. A prepared resume is helpful, including education, postgraduate training, licensing, specialty board certification, membership in professional organizations, publications, honors and awards, and any other information relevant to establishing the psychiatrist's credentials as an expert.

In providing forensic psychiatric testimony, psychiatrists are in quite a different role. They may or may not have performed a clinical examination of the litigant, or if they did, the examination was performed solely for legal purposes. Usually it is not the patient who seeks the examination, and control over the findings is not retained by either the psychiatrist or the subject of the examination. It is generally preferable to perform an appropriate clinical examination whenever possible. However, a forensic psychiatrist may sometimes be called on to provide testimony on purely hypothetical issues or to give opinions about scientific or clinical issues relevant to the legal questions.

Forensic expert testimony requires much more legal knowledge than ordinary clinical testimony. Special training is advisable, and it is now possible to obtain certification as an expert witness from the American Board of Forensic Psychiatry. In order to sit for the board examinations, the candidate must first be certified in psychiatry by the American Board of Psychiatry and Neurology and must have additional training, experience, and specialized practice in forensic work.

Difficult ethical problems may arise in the practice of forensic psychiatry. A person being examined by a "doctor" may be confused about the function of the forensic specialist and may assume the existence of a traditional clinical relationship, believing that the examination is for the patient's benefit or that what the patient and specialist say is confidential. It is imperative that the psychiatrist in such a situation explain his or her role to the subject and disclose the purposes of the examination, the limits of confidentiality, what is likely to happen to the information derived, and what may be the possible consequences. There have been instances where psychiatrists have attempted to obtain incriminating information from suspects, sometimes coercing or eliciting confessions under the guise of therapy. Psychiatrists have deliberately deceived defendants by concealing their role and giving false assurances of confidentiality. Such conduct is not only unethical and unprofessional, but it may form the basis of successful appeal of the defendant's conviction.

In 1985, the US Supreme Court made an important decision in *Ake v Oklahoma,* holding that when a state allows the defense of insanity, the state must provide funds for the employment of a psychiatric expert for an indigent defendant. In its discussion of the role of the psychiatric expert, the Court made it clear that such an expert is part of the defense team and may participate actively in the trial on behalf of the defense, rejecting the concept of the expert as an uninvolved and impartial participant in the legal process.

The psychiatric expert witness should strive toward objectivity, honesty, and a high standard of ethical practice. Because expert witnesses are important participants in our adversary system of justice, they can-

not avoid being placed in an adversarial position and should not claim an attitude of impartiality that does not exist. Often the public reputation of the forensic psychiatrist is that of the "hired gun," willing to accommodate opinions and testimony to the needs of the lawyer who pays the most. This image, and the consequent detriment to the psychiatric profession as a whole, can only be avoided by the most scrupulous ethical and professional integrity.

CRIMINAL LAW & PSYCHIATRY

Insanity

Many of the decisions that must be made in the area of criminal law depend upon the psychological attributes of the defendant. Traditionally, Anglo-American systems of criminal justice rely heavily on blameworthiness. Persons who commit criminal acts are held responsible only to the extent that they deserve blame for what they have done. Blameworthiness implies that the criminal act was the result of a willful decision by one exercising a power of free will. Hence, a crime must consist of the union of the guilty act *(actus reus)* and the guilty mind or intent *(mens rea)*.

This basically theological system of criminal responsibility has been gradually modified, so that today in the USA, a mental element—*mens rea*—in its original free-will sense is not a necessary feature of the definition of every crime. However, in the case of most common-law crimes such as murder, robbery, and theft, American law follows the traditional model. To convict a defendant of a crime it must be proved, beyond a reasonable doubt, that the defendant committed the criminal act and possessed, at the time of the act, the mental state or "criminal intent" required by the statutory definition of the crime charged.

This system of criminal law is often called *mens rea* law. A system of law in which people are held responsible for their acts without consideration of their mental state or blameworthiness is known as "strict liability" law. One may challenge the relevancy, utility, and efficiency of *mens rea* law in modern society. However, it is deeply rooted in our religious, social, and political heritage, and it is not likely to be replaced in the foreseeable future with a system of criminal law dominated by strict liability.

Accordingly, in every criminal trial, a decision must be made concerning this psychological element of the crime. An insane defendant is deemed to be incapable, because of mental disease or defect, of possessing any degree of *mens rea;* hence, an insane person is not capable of committing any crime, regardless of what he or she has done—thus the verdict, "Not guilty by reason of insanity." In short, an insane person is not to be blamed for his or her actions, which are the result of mental disease rather than exercise of free will, and he or she cannot be held criminally responsible.

Juries are reluctant to find a defendant not guilty by reason of insanity even though the evidence might indicate that to be a just and proper verdict. Most insanity acquittals have been in trials to a judge without a jury, where the prosecution has agreed with the defense lawyer that the defendant was insane.

In ancient law, only the most obviously deranged persons were considered to be insane. The terms *furiosus, non compos mentis,* etc, denoted total deprivation of reason and will. Insanity was thought to be recognizable by any layperson, and no expert testimony was needed.

The good and evil test was introduced into English law as early as the 14th century, when it was used to define the criminal responsibility of children. By the 16th century, it was applied as a criterion for the criminal responsibility of adults. By the early 19th century, the good and evil test had been recast into the "knowledge of right and wrong" test. There is nothing to indicate that the change represented a substantive alteration.

In January 1843, a young Scotsman, Daniel M'Naghten, assassinated the secretary to the Prime Minister of England. He had intended to kill the Prime Minister, Sir Robert Peel, but shot the secretary instead. In a sensational trial, M'Naghten was declared not guilty by reason of insanity. Queen Victoria, the Prime Minister, the press, and the public could not accept what seemed to be exculpation of a defendant they were convinced was a political assassin. An investigation by the House of Lords culminated in the summoning of the 15 Chief Justices of England to Parliament. The justices were asked to respond to a series of questions about the laws of England relevant to the acquittal by reason of insanity of defendants such as M'Naghten. Their response to these questions has been immortalized in the criminal law throughout the English-speaking world as the "M'Naghten rules of insanity."

The principal rule incorporated into the criminal laws of the USA and most countries that derive their legal systems from English common law is as follows (West and Walk, 1977:79):

> . . . [T]o establish a defense on the ground of insanity, it must be clearly proved that, at the time of the committing of the act, the party accused was labouring under such a defect of reason, from disease of the mind, as not to know the nature and quality of the act he was doing, or, if he did know it, that he did not know he was doing what was wrong. The mode of putting the latter part of the question to the jury on these occasions has generally been whether the accused at the time of doing the act knew the difference between right and wrong. . . .

Although this formula presented to the House of Lords did not carry the legal authority of an appellate decision, it fitted in so well with traditional concepts of morality and responsibility that it was almost immediately adopted by most American states and has tended to dominate all legal concepts of criminal responsibility of the mentally ill. The concepts that went into the M'Naghten rules were not new, as has sometimes been thought; they simply restated in contemporary language legal principles already established in the USA and England.

Even by 1843 standards, knowledge of right and wrong as a criterion of criminal responsibility was outdated by existing concepts of psychopathology, since it considered only abnormalities of cognition, ignoring defects of will and impulse control. Most of the efforts subsequently to broaden the applicability of the insanity defense have consisted of adding some type of volitional factor as an alternative to the purely cognitive principle of the M'Naghten formula. The volitional test was at first defined as "irresistible impulse" and later as "ability to adhere to the right" or as "ability to conform one's actions to the requirements of the law." In 1869 and 1871, the New Hampshire Supreme Court held that if the jury determines, as issues of fact, that the defendant is suffering from a mental disease or defect and that the criminal act is a result or product of the mental disease or defect, the defendant must be found not guilty by reason of insanity. In 1895 and 1897, the United States Supreme Court held that a defendant is insane if, because of mental disease or defect, he or she was unable at the time of the offense to distinguish right from wrong or if, though able to make that distinction, the defendant's powers of will were so destroyed that he or she could not control the actions. The Supreme Court also ruled that when the issue of insanity is raised by the defendant, the prosecutor has the burden of proving beyond a reasonable doubt that the defendant is sane. Later, in 1952, the Court held that these decisions were binding only on federal courts and need not be followed by the states.

In 1954, Judge David Bazelon of the District of Columbia Court of Appeals wrote the famous *Durham* decision:

> The rule . . . is not unlike that followed by the New Hampshire court since 1870. It is simply that an accused is not criminally responsible if his unlawful act was the product of mental disease or mental defect.

Although hailed at the time as a great advance of the law, other jurisdictions were reluctant to follow. This was especially so after the District of Columbia Court of Appeals held that this rule applied to defendants with a diagnosis of antisocial personality who were not otherwise mentally ill. A substantial number of defendants were found insane in the District who would not have been deemed so elsewhere.

The American Law Institute (ALI) developed in the 1950s a "Model Penal Code" in an attempt to bring some uniformity to the widely disparate criminal law codes of the states. Included was a proposal for a rule of responsibility of the mentally ill that included both cognitive and volitional factors:

> A person is not responsible for criminal conduct if at the time of such conduct as a result of mental disease or defect he lacks substantial capacity either to appreciate the criminality [wrongfulness] of his conduct or to conform his conduct to the requirements of law.

To prevent the so-called sociopathic (antisocial) personality from using the defense of insanity, there is a clause that has not always been accepted in jurisdictions where the ALI rule has been adopted:

> The terms "mental disease or defect" do not include an abnormality manifested only by repeated criminal or otherwise antisocial conduct.

Although the psychiatrists who participated in the drafting of the ALI rule would have preferred the *Durham* rule, many state and federal courts adopted ALI as the standard, and finally, in 1972, the District of Columbia Court of Appeals relinquished *Durham* in favor of a slightly modified ALI rule. Public and legislative outcry after the insanity acquittal of John Hinckley for the attempted assassination of President Reagan has prompted both the American Psychiatric Association and the American Bar Association to retreat from their former support of the ALI rule. Both organizations have now recommended the adoption of the "Bonnie rule" (after Professor Richard J. Bonnie of the University of Virginia, who first proposed it):

> A person is not responsible for criminal conduct if, at the time of such conduct, and as a result of mental disease or defect, that person was unable to appreciate the wrongfulness of such conduct.

In 1984, Congress enacted the Insanity Defense Reform Act of 1985, which applies to all federal crimes and is essentially the same as the Bonnie rule:

> It is an affirmative defense to a prosecution under any federal statute that, at the time of the commission of the acts constituting the offense, the defendant, as a result of a severe mental disease or defect, was unable to appreciate the nature and quality or the wrongfulness of his acts. Mental disease or defect does not otherwise constitute a defense. 18 USCA Sect. 20(a) (Supp 1986).

For the first time, a uniform rule of responsibility for all federal jurisdictions was established by legislative action rather than judicial decision. The trend in most state laws, since the Hinckley verdict, is away from liberalization and toward the original M'Naghten rule. Thus, most of the 20th century liberal reforms of the insanity defense have been discarded.

A persistent concern of the public is the possibility of early release of a dangerously mentally ill person after he or she has been acquitted by reason of insanity. It is widely feared that such persons will kill again, and sometimes the fear proves justified. In the 19th century, a verdict of not guilty by reason of insanity resulted in confinement for life in a mental institution. But with the development of modern treatment methods, including psychotropic drugs, periods of hospital confinement generally have been greatly shortened. The difficulties of making accurate predictions of potential for future violent behavior have aggravated this problem.

It is not possible to return to the old system of indefinite confinements, for appellate courts have generally held that the period of hospital confinement of a defendant who has been committed after having been found not guilty by reason of insanity can be no longer than the period of imprisonment for the crime charged. If a defendant recovers from his or her illness and is evaluated as not dangerous by the time the trial is completed, the defendant must be set free after his or her acquittal on grounds of insanity at the time of the offense. Generally, release from confinement after an insanity acquittal is contingent on recovery to the point of no longer being dangerous rather than recovery from the mental illness itself.

Guilty But Mentally Ill

Alaska, Connecticut, Georgia, Illinois, Indiana, Kentucky, Michigan, and New Mexico have adopted a new verdict of "guilty but mentally ill" while still retaining the verdict of not guilty by reason of insanity.

Although the guilty but mentally ill verdict may suggest by its terms that the convicted offender will receive treatment for the mental illness, such treatment is not mandatory. Furthermore, this verdict does not mitigate the sentence and may even enhance the sentence, since a parole or release board may be reluctant to release an offender with a record of mental illness after a minimum period of imprisonment.

Many who advocate this verdict hope that it will reduce or eliminate successful insanity defenses, since it gives the jury an alternative verdict. However, experience in Michigan with the guilty but mentally ill verdict has not been associated with a decrease in the number of acquittals based on insanity.

Despite the popular appeal of this verdict, both the American Psychiatric Association (in 1982) and the American Bar Association (in 1986) expressed their opposition to the addition of guilty but mentally ill to the possible verdicts of the criminal law. If such a verdict does not provide assurance of psychiatric care and treatment and does not mitigate the severity of the criminal sentence, it is difficult to see what value it has other than to create the false appearance that some special consideration is being given to a mentally ill defendant.

Competency to Stand Trial

Due process in criminal trials requires that the defendant be able to understand what is happening and to participate in a meaningful way in the trial process. Competency to stand trial is assumed unless the issue is raised before the trial starts. Although the issue of insanity can be raised only by the defense, the question of competency can be raised by the defense, the prosecution, or the judge. When the issue is raised, the judge will either appoint psychiatrists to examine the defendant or will commit the defendant to a hospital for evaluation.

A hearing is then held to determine if the defendant is competent to be tried. The defendant is entitled to a jury trial on this issue if he or she wishes. In contrast to the legal issues concerned with criminal responsibility, the criteria for determining competency to stand trial are identical in all jurisdictions in the USA. In *Dusky v United States*, 362 US 402 (1960), the United States Supreme Court ruled as follows:

> . . . [T]he test must be whether he has sufficient present ability to consult with his lawyer with a reasonable degree of rational understanding—and whether he has a rational as well as factual understanding of the proceedings against him.

If found to be incompetent to stand trial, the defendant is then usually committed to a mental institution for treatment. When competency is restored, the defendant may then go to trial and may be found guilty unless it is determined that the defendant was insane at the time of the offense.

Because determining incompetency is simpler than a full-scale criminal trial and no proof is required that the defendant actually committed the crime, there has been a tendency to use competency procedures as a permanent disposition of offenders who might otherwise have been found to be insane. The defendant would be committed to a state hospital and, if never reevaluated as competent, could be involuntarily hospitalized indefinitely.

In *Jackson v Indiana*, 406 US 715, 738 (1972), the United States Supreme Court radically altered this situation. The appeal concerned a mentally retarded deaf-mute with limited ability to communicate who had been charged with two trivial offenses. Although he was harmless, Indiana law required that he be committed to a state hospital for the criminally insane until he became competent. In his case, that meant confinement for life for trivial offenses he might not even have committed. The Court stated, as a matter of law:

> . . . [A] person charged by a State with a criminal offense who is committed solely on account of his incapacity to proceed to trial cannot be held more than the reasonable period of time necessary to determine whether there is a substantial probability that he will attain that capacity in the foreseeable future.

The *Jackson* decision has required revision of most state laws on the commitment of incompetent defendants, including limiting the period of confinement to no longer than the maximum period that could be imposed after a guilty verdict or plea of guilty. No longer can a determination of incompetency be used as a means of permanent disposition of a defendant, and institutions are under pressure to restore competency by adequate treatment and return the defendant for trial at the earliest possible time.

INVOLUNTARY HOSPITALIZATION & CONSERVATORSHIP

Until the 1960s, the involuntary hospitalization of mental patients was accomplished by complex formal legal proceedings that resulted in near-total loss of the civil, legal, and personal rights of ordinary citizens. Commitments were indefinite and remained in effect until the patient was restored to competency by a second legal procedure.

Because of the expense and complexity of the legal requirements, the actual proceedings were often greatly foreshortened in the interest of convenience. Judges sometimes served as "rubber stamps," indiscriminately approving whatever recommendations were made by examining physicians who may have had no training or experience in psychiatry and may have obtained their appointment to the "lunacy commission" as a political reward.

Most patients, especially if they were depressed or passive, received little legal guidance or protection. A paranoid, demanding, or aggressive patient might demand a jury trial, which would involve protracted legal proceedings. In many cases, to avoid that expense, commitment proceedings simply would be dropped and the patient released.

By the mid 1960s, new forms of commitment procedures were being devised. The leading example was the Lanterman-Petris-Short Mental Health Act of California, which became effective in 1969. The goals of the new laws were as follows: (1) to eliminate altogether, or to reduce to the absolute minimum, legal procedures for short-term commitments; (2) to eliminate all involuntary hospitalizations based solely on the existence of a mental disease or the need for care and treatment; (3) to permit involuntary hospitalization only if the patient is dangerous to self or others or is unable to provide for basic living requirements; (4) to eliminate all indefinite, purely custodial commitments; and (5) to maximize opportunities for effective treatment and early restoration of patients to their communities.

Where previous commitment periods were measured in months and years, these new procedures spoke only of hours and days of involuntary confinement. Furthermore, the patient was not to be deprived of any legal or civil rights and was not automatically assumed to be incompetent.

After an initial 72-hour period of observation, patients could be involuntarily detained for 2 weeks if found to be dangerous to themselves or others or to be gravely disabled. This 2-week extension required no legal procedures and was accomplished solely on the certification of the staff of the mental health facility. A patient who continued to be actively suicidal could be detained for an additional 2-week period. But after that, the patient must consent to voluntary treatment or be released.

No commitment provisions were made for long-term hospitalization for disabled patients. Instead, the concept of conservatorship was developed. A conservatorship differs from a guardianship in important ways. When made the ward of a guardian, one loses all rights of self-determination. One becomes like a child whose parent assumes responsibility for care and decisions. A conservator, however, acquires only limited powers over the conservatee. In a mental health conservatorship, the conservator usually has the authority to admit the conservatee to a mental hospital as a voluntary patient and to act as a substitute decision maker in consenting for treatment. The period of conservatorship is limited by statute; in California, it is 1 year, and the patient is entitled to legal counsel and a jury trial in superior court. The only ground for granting a mental health conservatorship is that the patient be gravely disabled. Grave disability is defined as inability, because of mental disease, to provide food, clothing, and shelter for oneself. The fact of grave disability must be proved beyond a reasonable doubt.

Most mental health laws permit commitment for longer periods for persons found to be dangerous to others.

Some states have additional commitment procedures for the involuntary hospitalization of special types of cases. There are (or have been) commitment procedures for sexual psychopaths (mentally disordered sex offenders) and so-called psychopathic delinquents. The national trend is away from such specialized commitments.

Commitments of all types were originally for indefinite periods of time. But one by one, each type of commitment has been subject to time limitations either by legislative or judicial action. Today in some states in the USA, no indeterminate commitments of any kind are permitted.

THE RIGHTS OF PATIENTS

The Right to Treatment

Although commitments for involuntary hospitalization are usually for the purpose of providing treatment,

until recently there was no way to require a state to provide such treatment. Many state institutions for the mentally ill and the mentally retarded provided neither adequate treatment nor humane physical facilities for their involuntary patients.

Dr Morton Birnbaum, a lawyer and physician in general practice, first suggested, in 1960, that involuntarily institutionalized patients have a constitutional right to treatment and that this could be a means of forcing states to meet at least the minimum standards for care and treatment.

It was not until 1972 that this constitutional right to treatment was established in federal court. In the leading class-action case of *Wyatt v Stickney,* 314F Supp 373 (1972), it was held that the physical conditions and lack of treatment in both the state hospital and the institution for the mentally retarded in Alabama were so bad that the constitutional rights of the inmates were being violated.

The *Wyatt* decision was upheld on appeal, so the constitutional right to treatment for involuntary patients is now established throughout the USA. Unfortunately, this decision does not establish a right to treatment for *voluntary* patients.

The United States Supreme Court accepted for review a somewhat parallel case, that of *O'Connor v. Donaldson,* 422 US 563 (1975), upholding the principle that mental illness alone can never justify restricting a person's liberty. There must always be something more, such as a condition dangerous to oneself or others. However, the Court found that it was not necessary to reach the issue of the constitutionality of the right to treatment in Donaldson's case. Chief Justice Burger, in a separate opinion, made it clear that he did not believe there is a legal right to treatment that can be enforced on the states.

Although the constitutional right to treatment is now incorporated into existing law, there is concern that should it come before the United States Supreme Court and the views of former Chief Justice Burger should prevail, this progressive concept will be destroyed.

Informed Consent & the Right to Refuse Treatment

It is a basic principle of law that adults of sound mind must consent to medical or surgical procedures. They have the right to refuse all treatment even when their refusal is foolish and contrary to the judgment of their physicians and families.

In recent years, there has been considerable emphasis on the right of informed consent. Without adequate information on which to base a decision, consent is without legal force, and it is a professional obligation of physicians to provide their patients with the information required to make rational decisions. To perform a medical or surgical procedure on a patient without consent is a battery, a misdemeanor (although the consent in low-hazard procedures may be implied by the patient's cooperation). To obtain consent without properly informing a patient may constitute negligence.

The leading cases on medical informed consent are *Canterbury v Spence,* 464 F 2d 772 (DC Cir 1972), and *Cobbs v Grant,* 8 Cal 3d 229 (1972). Both courts insist that informed consent is a legal duty and its fulfillment is to be judged by legal standards instead of by the standards of practice of the medical community. This represents a significant change whose implications are still not fully appreciated by the medical profession, for many doctors unwittingly fail to provide the legal minimum of information to their patients.

The patient must be given adequate information about the nature, risks, and benefits of the proposed treatment. For the patient to make a rational choice, he or she must also be given similar information about alternative treatments. Hazards of extremely low incidence need not be mentioned. If the patient does not wish to be informed and says so to the doctor, he or she need not be given further information.

Denial of the opportunity to weigh the risks and alternatives for oneself and to make a personal decision is proper only when the patient is a minor, is incompetent, or is in a condition of emergency. If competency is questioned, the court must be petitioned to so state and to appoint a conservator to make the required decision.

For a minor, informed consent must be obtained from the parent or guardian unless there is a specific statutory exception. The exceptions—such as the minor's right to consent to obstetric care or to treatment for communicable disease, or to receive information about use of contraceptives—vary greatly from state to state, and *it is of critical importance that psychiatrists be familiar with the consent laws of the state in which they practice.* A few states have special provisions for minors to consent, in certain limited circumstances, to psychotherapy or drug or alcohol treatment without their parents' knowledge.

Emergencies are generally defined by the law as life-and-death situations that demand immediate action. If a patient is unconscious and requires immediate treatment, consent is not necessary.

If a patient is mentally incompetent, the right of informed consent generally passes to the nearest available relative or to a designated substitute decision maker, such as a conservator. A serious problem exists with many modern commitment laws. Accepting the principle that involuntary hospitalization should not also result in unlimited legal disability and loss of rights, short-term commitment laws do not declare a patient incompetent. It can be argued that even though a psychotic patient is certified for involuntary hospitalization and treatment, the patient has not necessarily lost the right of informed consent and the right to refuse treatment. To override that

right may require a complicated legal procedure to adjudge the patient incompetent.

At present, hospital psychiatrists generally assume that laws authorizing involuntary hospitalization for purposes of treatment authorize that treatment to be given without informed consent and despite the patient's objection. That assumption may be incorrect.

There is a clear trend toward close legal scrutiny of the problems of consent of persons in coercive situations. In 1980, the United States Supreme Court held that a prisoner may be transferred from a prison to a mental hospital for treatment without informed consent only after a formal hearing with reasonable due process safeguards. The minimum procedural requirements are considerably stricter than some states now impose for short-term involuntary hospitalization of nonprisoners. It can be anticipated that these minimum procedures will eventually become mandatory for all persons.

Confidentiality & Privileged Communication

There is no disagreement that effective psychotherapy requires a trusting relationship between patient and therapist. The foundation of that trust is the patient's belief that the therapist will maintain the confidentiality of their communications. If the therapist is required by law to breach that confidentiality, therapy becomes difficult, if not impossible. An enforced demand for breach of confidentiality with respect to one patient's communications may affect all patients, for the others may cease to believe—and rightly—that their confidences will be kept confidential.

The obligation of confidentiality between doctor and patient is usually required by professional practice regulations and by the ethical standards of professional organizations. However, of greater importance are the statutory provisions establishing immunity to the subpoena power for certain types of confidential communications.

Neither the criminal law nor the civil law could function adequately if courts did not have the right to compel witnesses to testify. This compulsion is accomplished by means of the subpoena (meaning "under penalty"), which is an order to appear as a witness in court or at a deposition. Doctors are usually served with a *subpoena duces tecum,* which requires that they also produce their relevant records and documents. Although the power to issue subpoenas belongs to the judge (or sometimes to a legislative committee or other governmental investigative agency), it is customary to issue subpoenas routinely at the request of an attorney representing a party to the action.

It has been established since ancient times that the preservation of certain relationships requires confidentiality and that the social importance of preserving these relationships outweighs the requirements of law and justice. The confidential communications of such a protected relationship are called **privileged communications.**

Traditionally, privilege has existed for communications between priest and penitent, attorney and client, and husband and wife. Privilege for the confidential communications of physicians and patients has traditionally existed in most European countries. Contrary to what most doctors believe, it never existed in Anglo-American common law. Protection of confidential communications between physicians and patients in the USA is therefore entirely statutory. The protection provided for physician-patient communications is in many cases so slight that it is useless in the instances where it is needed most. For example, many state laws provide no protection if the patient is involved in any type of criminal proceeding.

As the practice of psychotherapy became widespread in the 1950s, it became increasingly apparent that additional protection was necessary for the psychotherapist-patient relationship. There seemed to be little possibility of strengthening the physician-patient privilege, and even if that could be accomplished, it would not help nonmedical psychotherapists. The solution was to draft special psychotherapist-patient privileged communication laws. By the 1960s, Georgia, Connecticut, California, and a few other states had enacted psychotherapist-patient privilege laws, but the privilege does not exist in federal law.

Although the psychotherapist-patient privilege is far broader than the physician-patient privilege in that it provides protection in criminal as well as civil cases, the protection is far from absolute. The statutes provide many exceptions. For example, a patient who puts his or her mental state at issue in litigation thus waives the right of privilege for relevant records and the therapist's testimony. If a patient is believed to be dangerous to the person or property of others, the therapist may be privileged or even required to breach confidentiality. In addition, statutes such as those for the reporting of child abuse, communicable disease, and gunshot or other wounds—and judicial decisions such as the result in California's *Tarasoff* case—may require breaches of confidence. It is not unusual for there to be unresolved conflicts in the law, where one law permits therapists to maintain confidentiality and another requires them to breach it.

The *Tarasoff* decision (17 Cal 3d 425 [1976]) imposes upon a psychotherapist who knows (or should know) that a patient is dangerous to a specific potential victim the duty to protect the victim by notifying the police or by warning the victim. Although commitment laws may grant immunity from suit for any action taken in connection with the involuntary hospitalization of a patient, they do not give immunity for failure to comply with the *Tarasoff* duty. New Jersey has now adopted *Tarasoff*, and other states may well follow this precedent. In 1986, the California legislature simplified the *Tarasoff* obligation to warn the victim and limited the liability of the therapist.

The right of privilege belongs solely to the patient, who may waive this right without the consent of the therapist. All attempts to provide joint control over the privilege for both therapist and patient (as exists for the priest-penitent relationship) have failed.

Increasingly, legislatures are requiring the therapist to breach confidentiality even if there is only a suspicion of child abuse or child molestation. Reporting of dependent and elderly adult abuse is required in some states.

It is of critical importance that psychotherapists familiarize themselves with the laws regulating confidentiality and privilege in the state within which they practice. There are great differences between states, and one cannot extrapolate the law of one state with the assumption that it will provide a reliable guide to the law of one's own jurisdiction.

SPECIALIZED AREAS IN FORENSIC PSYCHIATRY

There are increasing numbers of legal areas where the skills of the forensic psychiatrist are utilized. Because most of these require specialized legal and medical knowledge, the average psychiatrist is not likely to be involved in them. Hence, they will be discussed only superficially in this chapter.

The law has been hesitant to permit the recovery of damages for **emotional distress.** However, now the law is tending to become less restrictive, and all sorts of claims are being made for psychological and emotional harm alleged to have been inflicted by the negligence of others. As a result, forensic psychiatrists are frequently called on to evaluate such claims and to testify as expert witnesses in these personal injury trials. This area of tort law is still very complex, and one should not participate as such an expert unless one is thoroughly familiar with the legal issues.

Workers' compensation law is another area that has tended to attract the interest of forensic psychiatrists. It is now well settled that the stress of employment may sometimes cause or aggravate mental or emotional illness. When this occurs, the worker is entitled to be compensated in proportion to the disability as one would be for a physical injury incurred on the job. The stresses of employment may also be relevant to disability retirement claims. These cases must be carefully evaluated by a psychiatrist, the degree of disability assessed, reports written, and often testimony given in hearings.

Psychiatric malpractice is another growing field. There is a steady increase in the number of malpractice suits filed against psychiatrists. The level is not yet a cause for concern, but each case requires a specialized inquiry and often will require expert testimony on a wide variety of issues.

Child custody issues may require psychiatric expertise on questions of the "best interests of the child," the child-parent relationship, psychological needs of children at different stages of development, fitness of parents, and the impact of parental psychological disturbance on the child. As "no-fault" divorce laws become widespread, there is a tendency for legal battles that would have previously been fought on questions of morality, blame, money, and property to shift to the arena of child custody. This results in an increased need for forensic skills in child psychiatry.

As the behavioral sciences have become more involved in the justice system, there are frequent needs for experts to participate in evidentiary hearings on particular issues. Expert testimony may be needed on questions such as the validity of hypnosis for the enhancement of memory of witnesses; the ability of psychiatrists to predict dangerousness; the psychology

of entrapment; the effects of racial discrimination; the stress of combat in the armed forces; and many other issues.

Despite the serious problem of credibility of psychiatric expert testimony in criminal trials, there seems to be an endless need for the expertise of the forensic psychiatrist. In the complex modern world, it is inevitable that the processes of the law will require an ever-increasing input of technical expertise. In the past, psychiatry has tended to dominate forensic behavioral science. This is changing rapidly: Psychologists with proper credentials and experience are accepted as experts on insanity, child custody, and other legal issues; and sociologists, anthropologists, linguists, criminologists, and penologists are all beginning to appear in court to offer useful opinion for the benefit of the trier of fact in reaching difficult decisions. However, the basic principle of expert testimony remains unchanged: that the witness be truly an expert in training, experience, and knowledge.

REFERENCES

American Bar Association: Criminal justice mental health standards. Chapter 7 in: *American Bar Association Standards for Criminal Justice*. Little, Brown, 1986.

American Medical Association Committee on Medicolegal Problems: Insanity defense in criminal trials and limitation of psychiatric testimony. (Committee report.) JAMA 1984;251:2967.

American Psychiatric Association: Statement on the insanity defense. Am J Psychiatry 1983;140:681.

Bimbaum M: The right to treatment. J Am Bar Assoc 1960;46:499.

Brooks AD: *Law, Psychiatry and the Mental Health System.* Little, Brown, 1974. [Supplement, 1980.]

Diamond BL: The fallacy of the impartial expert. Arch Crim Psychodynamics 1959;3:221. [Reprinted in: Allen RC, Ferster EZ, Rubin JG: *Readings in Law and Psychiatry,* rev ed. Johns Hopkins Press, 1975.]

Diamond BL: Isaac Ray and the trial of Daniel McNaughten. Am J Psychiatry 1954;112:39.

Goldstein J, Freud A, Solnit AJ: *Before the Best Interests of the Child.* Free Press, 1979.

Goldstein J, Freud A, Solnit AJ: *Beyond the Best Interests of the Child.* Free Press, 1973.

Platt A, Diamond BL: The origins of the "right and wrong" test of criminal responsibility and its subsequent development in the United States: An historical survey. Calif Law Rev 1966;54:1227.

West DJ, Walk A (editors): *Daniel McNaughton. His Trial and the Aftermath.* Gaskell, 1977.

Legal Cases

Addington v Texas, 441 US 418 (1979).

Ake v Oklahoma, 407 US 68 (1985).

Brawner v United States, 471 F 2d 969 (DC Cir 1972).

Canterbury v Spence, 464 F 2d 772 (DC Cir 1972).

Cobbs v Grant, 8 Cal 3d 229, 104 Cal Rptr 505, 502 P 2d 1 (1972).

Davis v United States, 160 US 469 (1895) and 165 US 373 (1897).

Durham v United States, 214 F 2d 862 (DC Cir 1954).

Dusky v United States, 362 US 402 (1960).

Frye v United States, 293 F 1013 (DC App 1923).

Jackson v Indiana, 406 US 715, 738 (1972).

O'Connor v Donaldson, 422 US 563 (1975).

Rennie v Klein, 653 F 2d 836 (3d Cir 1981).

Roger v Okin, 634 F 2d 650 (1st Cir 1980).

State of New Hampshire v Jones, 50 NH 3269 (1871)

State of New Hampshire v Pike, 49 NH 399 (1869).

Tarasoff v Regents of the University of California, 17 Cal 3d 425, 131 Cal Rptr 14, 551 P 2d 334 (1976).

Vitek v Jones, 445 US 480 (1980).

Wyatt v Stickney, 314 F Supp 373 (MD Ala ND 1972); *Wyatt v Aderholt,* 503 F 2d 1305 (5th Cir 1974).

Roland Levy, MD, & Beth Goldman, MPH, MD

Every physician must be prepared to make a prompt diagnosis and provide efficient treatment for psychiatric emergencies. This chapter emphasizes actual or attempted homicide and suicide, since these are the most serious psychiatric emergencies the physician is called upon to deal with. Careful assessment and prompt institution of appropriate management may significantly affect the outcomes in such cases and may prevent harm to the medical staff. Other psychiatric emergencies are mentioned, and cross-references are made to more complete discussions in other chapters in this text.

The physician should be familiar with the state or local reporting requirements relating to self-injury or injuries to others by means of a weapon.

SUICIDE

In the USA in 1988, suicide ranked as the seventh major cause of death, with over 25,000 recorded suicides each year. It was the third leading cause of death among 15- to 24-year-olds, taking almost 5000 lives in 1987. Conservative estimates are that attempted suicide is eight times more frequent than successful suicide. These figures do not include unconsciously motivated fatal "accidents" or other self-destructive behaviors (eg, alcoholism).

Those who attempt suicide and succeed differ demographically from those who make unsuccessful attempts. Successful suicide is about three times more common in men than in women and increases with advancing age. More recently, in the USA, there has been an increased incidence of successful suicide attempts in persons aged 15–24 years. Suicide is also more common in persons who are not married and in those who are isolated, uprooted, or lonely. Protestants are more likely to commit suicide than Catholics or Jews, and foreign-born immigrants are at greater risk also. Guns are the most commonly used means of successful suicide (50% of men and 25% of women), and men are more likely than women to commit suicide by violent means. Unsuccessful suicide attempts are three times more common in women than in men. They are most common in the

20- to 24-year age group. Unsuccessful attempts commonly involve nonviolent means, such as cutting, poisoning, or carbon monoxide. (See Table 43–1.)

The clinician evaluating the risk of suicide should try to determine whether the patient has formed a definite plan for suicide—eg, Has the patient made out a will, changed an insurance policy, or decided on the method, time, and place for the act? The clinician must assess previous suicide attempts and obtain a family history of suicide. In evaluating mental status, the clinician should ask about feelings of rejection and uselessness and whether the patient is working. The patient should be asked if he is hearing voices telling him to harm himself (command hallucinations). Coexisting depression with associated anxiety or acute worsening of depression is a danger signal, as is a rapid superficial improvement in depression, which may be a sign that a plan for suicide has been devised. Increasing hostility may also be a clue to impending suicide. Financial worries (real or imagined) with ideas of impending poverty are often associated with suicide. People with painful illnesses, particularly if associated with prolonged sleep disturbance, are at greater risk of suicide. Individuals with a recent history of alcoholism or drug abuse—especially recent use of cocaine—are also definite suicidal risks. Patients are at high risk for suicide while intoxicated on alcohol.

Clues to Suicide

People who are contemplating suicide often provide clues that must be carefully assessed.

A. Verbal Clues: The individual may sometimes make direct statements about wanting to die or "end it all." Less direct ways of expressing suicidal ideation are, "It's too much to bear!" "You'd be better off without me!" "I'd be better off dead!" A patient who asks, "How does one leave his body to science?" or who says, "I have a friend who's real depressed and talks about suicide a lot" is sending messages in very simple code.

B. Behavioral Clues: A direct behavioral clue is ingestion of a small amount of some potentially lethal drug. Prematurely or inappropriately "putting one's affairs in order," arranging for a casket, and giving away prized possessions are indirect clues.

C. Situational Clues: Situational clues are inherent in life experiences associated with major stress, eg, an impending surgical procedure, a diagnosis of

Table 43–1. Risk categories for suicide.[1]

Factor	High-Risk Category	Low-Risk Category
Age	45 years and older	Under 45 years of age
Sex	Male	Female
Race	White	Nonwhite
Marital status	Separated, divorced, widowed	Single, married
Living arrangements	Alone	With others
Employment status[2]	Unemployed, retired	Employed[3]
Physical health	Poor (acute or chronic condition in the 6 months preceding the attempt)	Good[3]
Mental condition	Nervous or mental disorder, mood or behavioral symptoms, including alcoholism	Presumably normal, including brief situational reactions[3]
Medical care (within 6 months)	Yes	No[3]
Method	Hanging, firearms, jumping, drowning	Cutting or piercing, gas or carbon monoxide, poisoning, combination of other methods, other
Season	Warm months (April to September)	Cold months (October to March)
Time of day	6:00 AM to 5:59 PM	6:00 PM to 5:59 AM
Where attempt was made	Own or someone else's home	Other type of premises, out of doors
Time interval between attempt and discovery	Almost immediately; reported by person making attempt	Later
Intent to commit suicide (self report)	No[3]	Yes
Suicide note	Yes	No[3]
Previous attempt or threat	Yes	No[3]

[1] Modified and reproduced, with permission, from Tuckman J, Youngman WF: A scale for assessing suicide risk of attempted suicides. J Clin Psychol 1968;24:17.
[2] Does not include homemakers and students.
[3] Includes cases for which information on this factor was not given in the police report.

chronic fatal illness, or a recent loss—the death of a loved one, loss of a job, eviction, retirement, etc.

D. Syndromic Clues: Syndromic clues are certain constellations of emotions that are commonly associated with suicide. Depression is the most common one, but there are others. Suicide also occurs in people who are not depressed but are disoriented— eg, in acute delirium, suicidal behavior may be an attempt to flee some imagined threat. Individuals with psychotic disorders associated with impaired impulse control may attempt suicide in response to hallucinations commanding them to do so. Suicide also occurs in defiant people, who may view suicide as a means of taking an active, resistive stance in the face of some real or imagined threat to their self-esteem. Suicide by a dependent, dissatisfied individual is often a masked hostile gesture toward some other individual or group perceived as not having fulfilled dependency needs. ("Now you'll feel sorry!")

ASSESSING THE RISK OF SUICIDE

The physician must stay alert to the possibility of suicide in patients presenting for treatment. Most people who attempt suicide have been seen by a physician a few months before, and most successful suicides have signaled their intent to loved ones and others and have expressed a need for help, often in the preceding 24 hours. The physician must regard suicide attempts or verbalized suicidal thoughts as emergencies, since even so-called "hysterical" and "manipulative" patients may succeed in self-destructive acts.

A number of factors influence the assessment suicide risk: the patient's usual level of functioning, past history of suicide attempts and mental illness, current social and economic circumstances, and cognitive/affective state.

Useful questions that might be considered in any evaluation for suicidal risk can be formulated as follows:

> How has the patient reacted to stress in the past, and how effective are his or her typical coping strategies?
>
> Has the patient contemplated or attempted suicide in the past? If so, how frequently and under what circumstances? If the patient has made attempts in the past, how serious were they?
>
> What are the patient's current social and economic circumstances and how similar are they to past situations when suicide was attempted?

What is the patient's current cognitive state? Hopeless, helpless, powerless? Angry? Oriented, hallucinating, delusional?

Does the patient have somatic manifestations of depression such as constipation, insomnia, fatigue, loss of appetite, diminished libido, anxiety, or menstrual irregularities?

When suicide is suspected, the clinician must ask the patient directly about the nature and extent of suicidal thinking. The following types of suicidal thoughts and the feelings associated with them are discussed in order of increasing risk:

(1) Transient thoughts about dying. People with transient ideas of death may entertain fantasies such as, "They'll miss me when I'm gone." Such common notions are usually of little significance. Concern and caution are warranted, however, if the patient is an adolescent or an emotionally unstable adult.

(2) Sustained thoughts about dying and recurrent wishes for death. Sustained ideas about death and recurrent death wishes may function as a painful habit that enables the individual to deal with stress. Suicidal gestures such as superficial wrist cutting or nonlethal ingestion of drugs may occur occasionally.

(3) Frustrated feelings and impulsive behavior. A patient may have little hope for support from the environment and may feel that most forms of relief have been exhausted. The patient is therefore frustrated and close to anger much of the time. The anger may be turned inward or outward, leading to the possibility of a suicidal or homicidal act.

(4) Court of last resort. A person may feel depleted of all emotional resources. Such an individual no longer feels rage, frustration, or despair, and death is viewed as a way of avoiding further anguish.

(5) The logical decision to die. A person may approach suicide from a logical and philosophical point of view. Such a person sees death as inevitable and asks, "So why not now?" This type of individual is at the highest risk of suicide, but the patient's decision rarely comes to the attention of the physician.

If suicide is being seriously considered, the lethality of the method chosen—as well as its availability—must be assessed. A person considering a well thought out, concrete plan is at higher risk than one who has no particular plan in mind.

Finally, the nature and extent of the patient's support system must be assessed.

Patients presenting after an unsuccessful suicide attempt must also be assessed. Some patients no longer feel suicidal once they have gotten the message of their distress across by making a suicidal gesture. Again, the lethality of the method as well as the likelihood of intervention and rescue are taken into account when evaluating patients who have "tried to commit suicide."

SUICIDE PREVENTION

The concept underlying and justifying suicide prevention efforts is that people contemplating suicide may nonetheless want to be prevented from doing so. Even those who do not want to be "rescued" or dissuaded from their suicidal purpose should be, since proper treatment and environmental adjustments can often restore such people to better health. Astute observation can almost always uncover clues to suicidal intentions. Almost all suicidal behavior stems from a sense of isolation and anguish. The function of suicide is to terminate unbearable existence. A single significant relationship may be sufficient to sustain an individual in an otherwise intolerable situation.

Many persons considered to be suicidal risks do not require hospitalization. Those in high-risk categories should be hospitalized. In doubtful cases, the decision about hospitalization is based on the physician's assessment of the adequacy of the patient's external support system and the integrity of the patient's impulse control mechanism. Lack of an effective support system and poor impulse control in patients otherwise at low risk for suicide may call for hospitalization. Conversely, appropriate crisis intervention in the emergency room may obviate the need for hospitalization of some individuals who have presented after making a suicidal gesture.

People with suicidal ideas should not be offered the means of acting on them. When such a patient is hospitalized with suicide precautions, there should be no access to an unsecured window, stairwell, etc. Potential instruments of suicide such as shoelaces, belts, coat hangers, caustic cleansers, and cutlery should be kept from the patient. Some patients need constant close observation.

Although some general measures apply to the management of all suicidal persons, specific measures depend on the specific underlying diagnosis, since treatment differs depending on whether the patient has a major affective disorder, schizophrenia, delirium, or dysthymic disorder. Appropriate treatment may include psychotherapy, pharmacological therapy, and, in some cases, electroconvulsive therapy.

Illustrative Case No. 1

A 20-year-old unmarried college student living at home with her parents and younger siblings was brought to the emergency room after a nearly fatal drug overdose. The family had come to the USA from a Middle Eastern country 3 years previously. The patient stated that her suicide attempt was in response to her father's demands that she maintain the cultural values of their native country rather than adopt those of the new culture. She resented his "dictatorial'' approach and envied the freedom of her American peers. The patient showed no evidence of psychosis and was felt to be suffering from adjustment disorder.

Treatment centered on several emergency family sessions. The father was approached as the head of the family and was helped to express his concerns and fears about the family's exposure to new cultural attitudes. He was able to see how his attitudes were reflected in his children's conflicts, and he reluctantly agreed to allow them greater freedom. The children learned to view their father not as a tyrant but rather as a man in culture shock still trying to be a good father. After the initial hostility had subsided, an agreement was reached that both ''sides'' were able to feel comfortable with. The patient was discharged after 1 day in the hospital, and the family was referred to an outpatient psychiatric clinic for further family therapy.

Illustrative Case No. 2

A 58-year-old divorced surgeon experienced a manic episode. He had a history of depression that began in late adolescence, and his last episode of depression had occurred 10 years before. During the manic episode, he lost all of his hospital affiliations, incurred several malpractice suits, and accumulated huge debts, all in several weeks. He was hospitalized and treated with lithium, and his excitement subsided. He then became suicidally depressed. The depression responded favorably to the addition of tricyclic antidepressant medication to the regimen. After the patient was discharged from the hospital, the dosage of the tricyclic antidepressant was reduced and finally discontinued. Maintenance treatment with lithium alone was subsequently successful.

Illustrative Case No. 3

A 72-year-old retired married man had experienced the onset of depression 2 years previously. He was agitated and had regressed, and his wife could not cope with him. Antidepressant medications were tried but had to be stopped because of their side effects. The patient consented to electroconvulsive therapy and underwent a series of nine treatments that resulted in complete remission of symptoms.

SUICIDE IN ADOLESCENTS

In recent years, the rate of suicide among adolescents in the United States has risen at an alarming rate—150% between 1960 and 1980. More than 5000 adolescents kill themselves each year. This rise has not been paralleled in other age groups. Research has indicated that the rise in the suicide rate may result in part from changes in our society, including child-rearing practices and loss of stability in the home. The increase in the suicide rate closely parallels the increase in the divorce rate. The association between suicide and parental divorce is statistically significant. Other factors associated with suicide in adolescents include antisocial behavior and substance abuse.

Adolescents generally tend to be more impulsive than adults, and the suicidal adolescent is less likely to be suffering from depression than an adult. Although behavioral changes often precede a suicide attempt, they are less likely to be the classical neurovegetative signs of depression. Symptoms such as social withdrawal, preoccupation with bizarre ideas, or decline in academic performance may precede a suicide attempt in an adolescent suffering from early symptoms of schizophrenia.

Illustrative Case

A 16-year-old boy was admitted to the hospital after swallowing several of his mother's antihypertensive pills. The history revealed progressive social withdrawal over the past year, and school records showed a significant decline in academic performance for 2 years. The patient admitted having auditory hallucinations in the form of derogatory voices, and he also had ideas of reference. Antipsychotic medications relieved both his hallucinations and his suicidal ideation.

HOMICIDE

Homicide is the killing of a human being by another human being. Murder, as defined by California Penal Code Section 187, is ''the unlawful killing of a human being, or a fetus, with malice aforethought.'' In this discussion, the term ''homicide'' is used without regard to legal distinctions (justifiable, excusable, with or without malice, etc).

Most homicides occur at night, with the highest incidence between 8:00 PM Saturday and 2:00 AM Sunday. Fifty percent of homicides occur on weekends or holidays; most of them occur in the home; the victim and perpetrator are frequently members of the same family; and the victim may be the perpetrator. Homicide is committed five times more often by men than by women, though in recent years the incidence of homicides perpetrated by women has been increasing.

The risk of homicide is increased in persons with psychosis characterized by persecutory delusions, and the risk is especially high when the delusions have come to focus on one individual. The homicide risk is increased also in individuals with a history of violence, hatred of authority, or antisocial personality traits. Other significant risk factors are any evidence of rivalry, jealousy, or sexual conflicts; a recent history of withdrawal, brooding, and moodiness; and a history of alcoholism or drug abuse.

Most homicidal acts are not premeditated but occur during periods of heightened emotional tension that coincide with the ready availability of some sort of weapon. Anything that impairs impulse control increases the risk of violent assault, eg, ''premedicated'' murder after the use of alcohol or street drugs by the perpetrator.

Illustrative Case

A 54-year-old municipal employee believed that his supervisor and fellow workers were ridiculing him by making sexual gestures and remarks and creating obstacles to performance of his job. He drank alcohol to excess for many year, and recently began using cocaine. His wife was aware of his misuse of alcohol and street drugs but did not notify his physician. After a negative performance review one day, the patient shot his supervisor and two coworkers. Medical testimony at the patient's trial emphasized impaired judgment resulting from his state of chronic intoxication. He was found guilty of second-degree murder.

GENERAL APPROACH TO VIOLENT OR ACUTELY EXCITED PATIENTS

The physician attempting to deal with a violent patient should use a calm, systematic approach. The patient's behavior should be accepted as a symptom of the illness, and no patient should ever be ridiculed. Patients who become violent in the emergency room are often those who have been kept waiting—these patients interpret the wait as a sign that others do not consider them important or do not feel they need immediate treatment. The physician should act promptly and decisively, introduce himself or herself, and explain the plan of treatment: ''Mr Allen, I'm Dr Rodriguez of the emergency department staff. I'd like to talk to you for a few minutes and then do a physical examination.'' The physician should then obtain a history and perform the examination. Information from friends and relatives is often needed in order to develop an appropriate plan of treatment.

The physician should make sure that backup help is available for management of patients who are obviously psychotic or aggressive. The area should be free of objects that could be used as weapons. The medical staff should never turn their backs or let the patient come between them and the door; the door should be readily accessible both to the patient and the interviewer. If a violent patient escapes security guards, the police should be called immediately.

Threatening calls or letters from patients should never be ignored, since doing so may actually encourage the caller or writer to escalate the activity.

When a violent patient presents in the office or emergency room, it is appropriate to acknowledge realistic fear but not panic. The physician must exercise self-control in order to control the patient and the situation. Facing the patient at a discreet distance with arms crossed is a nonthreatening stance that nevertheless enables the physician to avoid or deflect blows. The physician should not attempt to deal unaided with a violent patient. Agitated patients confronted with ample force are less likely to become assaultive.

Potentially assaultive patients should be discreetly searched for weapons in the emergency room by being asked to change to hospital clothing.

If restraints are needed, they should be used promptly and applied as gently as possible. An early show of authority and control may prevent injuries and allow the physician to proceed with treatment. Destructive behavior must be prevented not only because of the property damage or personal injuries to others that might result but also because of the guilt feelings and lowered self-esteem the patient inevitably faces when self-control is restored.

The physician should never threaten a patient, never openly disagree with a hostile patient, never make insincere promises, never ridicule a patient, and never do anything that would hurt a patient's pride. If the physician intends to obtain psychiatric consultation, medication should be avoided, if possible, so that the psychiatric staff can better assess the patient's baseline condition. It is best not to assume that a violent patient has a psychogenic problem until various organic causes of the psychological disturbance have been appropriately investigated.

OTHER PSYCHIATRIC EMERGENCIES

ACUTE NONPSYCHOTIC DISORDERS

Emergencies may occur in three types of nonpsychotic disorders: anxiety disorders, including panic attacks and conversion reactions of a dissociative type, as well as fugue states; personality disorders; and antisocial states, in which aggressive behavior occurs frequently (see Chapters 23, 24, and 26).

Illustrative Case No. 1

An 18-year-old man was brought to the emergency room after he threatened his mother with a knife when she refused to give him money. He had a long history of depression and antisocial behavior—theft, assault, robbery—and had been incarcerated in juvenile facilities several times. He was released after a brief period of observation, since his mother refused to press charges and he was neither psychotic nor depressed.

Illustrative Case No. 2

A 22-year-old male college student was brought to the emergency room for evaluation after a sudden onset of paralysis and aphonia following a motor vehicle accident. The other driver had been tailgating him for a mile and then smashed his car from behind. After medical examination failed to account for the symptoms, thiopental sodium was administered intravenously, the patient was encouraged to recall the events of the accident, and the symptoms quickly disappeared. The patient then related that just before the onset of paralysis and aphonia, he had experienced a feeling of murderous rage toward the other driver.

DELIRIUM

Delirium is common in patients presenting to emergency rooms, especially in association with alcohol or drug intoxication. Any stimulant or depressant drug may cause delirium when taken in sufficient quantities. Of special importance is phencyclidine psychosis, since individuals who have ingested this drug often exhibit episodes of extreme violence, and the reaction lasts longer than those due to other hallucinogens (see Chapter 18). Delirium may also be caused by other factors, eg, head trauma, cardiovascular disorders, metabolic disorders, prescription drugs, and infections (see Chapters 17 and 41).

Illustrative Case

A 68-year-old woman was brought to the hospital by her brother, who had been called by the manager of her apartment building. She had been wandering the halls and bothering other tenants and had not been caring for herself. Laboratory studies revealed severe hypothyroidism. Thyroid hormone replacement therapy led to gradual improvement in the patient's mental status.

DEMENTIA

Persons suffering from dementia are not usually highly aggressive. They do have a lowered threshold of emotional control, however, and may become assaultive when they find themselves in situations they do not understand.

Illustrative Case

An 86-year-old man was admitted to the hospital

after he assaulted his 89-year-old sister. She reported that over the past several years, he had shown progressive deterioration in intellectual function. He completely denied his failing abilities and became assaultive when his sister tried to help him prepare a meal. Examination revealed senile dementia.

ACUTE PSYCHOTIC DISORDERS

Impulse control may be tenuous in individuals experiencing an acute psychotic episode, and they may be extremely assaultive as a result. The paranoid delusions associated with paranoid schizophrenia and other paranoid psychotic disorders may lead patients to act out, and the delusions are a special cause for concern if patients feel that a specific person in the environment is the source of the persecution.

The excitement that may erupt during a catatonic episode occurs less frequently than agitation caused by paranoid delusions, but it is unpredictable and usually associated with extreme violence.

Illustrative Case No. 1

A 40-year-old single man with a long history of paranoid schizophrenia made an appointment at a medical clinic for evaluation of chronic urologic complaints. After the examination, he was told that there were no physical abnormalities. A few minutes later, the patient thought he heard the doctor discussing his case in a demeaning way with a group of nurses. In a rage, he pulled out a gun and shot the physician.

Individuals in the manic phase of bipolar disorder may be assaultive if they feel someone is interfering with their activities. Manic patients are not always jovial and humorous and may in fact be extremely agitated and aggressive. Aggressive behavior may also occur during episodes of depression; in fact, psychotically depressed people may be homicidal. The victim is often a loved one with whom the patient has identified and onto whom the patient's misery is projected. (''You're just like me, and we're both miserable. I'll kill you and then myself, and then we'll both be free from all of this.'') The act is committed in order to save the other person from ''a life of misery.''

Illustrative Case No. 2

During a recurrent manic attack, a 31-year-old man became impatient while waiting for a bus. He approached a car stopped at an intersection, pulled the driver out, drove off at high speed, and hit another vehicle. In the emergency room, he had to be physically restrained while the physician gave treatment for severe lacerations.

Illustrative Case No. 3

A 42-year-old woman who had been married for

some time became pregnant for the first time. Three months after delivery of a healthy child, she experienced severe depression with suicidal ideation. In her state of hopelessness, she drowned the child in the bathtub and then slashed her wrists.

UNTOWARD CONSEQUENCES OF MEDICATION

Emergencies may arise as a consequence of medications being used to treat a psychiatric condition. Antipsychotic medications, particularly high-potency preparations, may cause dramatic dystonic states, catatonia, and neuroleptic malignant syndrome (see Chapters 17 and 32). Lithium therapy must be closely monitored to avoid toxicity. The heterocyclic antidepressants and fluoxetine prescribed for major depression may be used in a suicide attempt. Monoamine oxidase inhibitors may produce serious hypertensive reactions resulting from interaction with exogenous tyramine and similar sympathomimetic substances (see Chapter 32). Many antidepressant, antipsychotic, and antiparkinsonism drugs have anticholinergic properties, especially when used in combination or in high doses. Medical emergencies such as acute urinary retention or paralytic ileus may result.

ADJUSTMENT DISORDER & POSTTRAUMATIC STRESS DISORDER

Adjustment disorder represents a transient response to overwhelming environmental stress in individuals without apparent underlying psychiatric illness. Adjustment disorder is characterized by impaired social or vocational functioning and by symptoms that exceed the normally expected reaction. Such symptoms may develop in persons who suffer a major loss or in those who are victims of violence (eg, rape, spouse beating, or child abuse).

Posttraumatic stress disorder (stress response syndrome) is a reaction to an identifiable stress outside the normal range of experience (eg, car crash, natural disaster). The pattern of response consists of an initial outcry (an emotional response that is almost a reflex), followed by denial (emotional numbing, avoidance of ideas connected witho the stressor, and behavioral constriction), an intrusive phase (unbidden ideas and feelings that are difficult to dispel), and a phase of working through and completion.

In both adjustment disorder and posttraumatic stress disorder, prompt crisis intervention may facilitate resolution of symptoms and prevent development of a more chronic psychiatric disorder (see Chapters 23 and 25).

•　　•　　•

SUMMARY

Dealing with psychiatric emergencies requires considerable knowledge and skill. The physician must be able to reach an accurate diagnosis quickly and begin appropriate treatment without delay. The crisis should be resolved promptly and in a way that eases the transition to the next phase of treatment. How the physician behaves during the emergency phase will strongly influence what happens later.

REFERENCES

Bulletin of Suicidology, Vols 1–8: National Clearinghouse for Mental Health Information, Rockville, Maryland, 1967–1971.

Hayes JR, Roberts TK, Solway SS (editors): *Violence and the Violent Individual*. Spectrum, 1981.

Roy A: Psychiatric emergencies. Chapter 29 in: *Comprehensive Textbook of Psychiatry/V*, 5th edition. Kaplan HI, Sadock BJ (editors). Williams & Wilkins, 1989.

Rund DA, Hutzler JC: *Emergency Psychiatry*. Mosby, 1983.

Sandus S et al: *Violent Individuals and Families*. Thomas, 1984.

Suicide and attempted suicide. Chapter 71 in: *Psychiatry*, rev ed, 1990. Michels R et al (editors). Lippincott, 1990.

Tuckman J, Youngman WF: A scale for assessing suicide risk of attempted suicides. J Clin Psychol 1968;24:17.

Glossary of Psychiatric Signs & Symptoms

The diagnostic process in psychiatry begins with a careful history, physical examination, and mental status examination. Observations take the form of signs and symptoms. This section is a glossary of terms used to define and describe these signs and symptoms.

Affect: Emotions or feelings as they are expressed by the patient and observable by others. Affect is an objective sign observable on mental status examination—in contrast to mood (see below), which is a subjective experience reported by the patient. Affect is characterized in several ways: (1) By the type of emotion expressed and observed: anger sadness, elation etc. (2) By the intensity and the range of emotion expressed: flat, blunted, constricted, or broad. In **flat** affect, there is no expression of feeling; the face is immobile and the voice monotonous. In **blunted** affect, the expression of feeling is severely reduced. In **constricted** affect, the expression of feelings is clearly reduced but to a lesser degree than in the case of blunted affect. **Broad** affect is the normal condition in which a full range of feelings is expressed. (3) By its appropriateness: **Inappropriate** affect is apparent emotion discordant with accompanying thought or speech (eg, laughing while telling a story most people would find horrifying). (4) By consistency of emotion: **Labile** affect shifts rapidly between different emotional states such as crying, laughing, and anger.

Ambivalence: The condition of having two strong but opposite feelings or ideas. The individual cannot decide to respond one way or the other, with the result that there is difficulty in taking any action. A feature of obsessive compulsive disorder and schizophrenia.

Anhedonia: Loss of interest in pleasure-seeking activities. A feature of depressive disorder.

Anorexia: Loss of or diminished appetite. A feature of depressive disorder.

Anxiety: A dysphoric (unpleasant) state similar to fear when there is no apparent source of danger. A feeling of apprehension, anticipation, or dread of possible danger. Anxiety is sometimes defined by the physiological state of autonomic arousal, alertness, vigilance, and motor tension. Free-floating anxiety is anxiety in the absence of an identifiable object of dread. Phobia (see below) is severe anxiety aroused by a specific object or circumstance even though the subject knows the feeling "doesn't make sense."

Autistic thinking: Thought derived from fantasy. External reality is accorded subjective and fantasied meanings. Preoccupation with the private world may lead the autistic individual to withdraw from external reality.

Automatic obedience: Obedience to commands without exercising critical judgment. A feature of catatonia.

Blocking: Disruption of thought evidenced by an interruption or momentary disruption of speech. It appears as if the individual is trying to remember what he or she was thinking or saying.

Catalepsy: A condition in which the subject "freezes" in almost any abnormal posture in which he or she is placed (left arm extended, etc). A feature of catatonia.

Catatonia: A syndrome characterized by cataleptic posturing, stereotypy, mutism, stupor, negativism, automatic obedience, echolalia, and echopraxia. There are two subtypes: excited and retarded. Catatonia was formerly thought to be a subtype of schizophrenia. It is now thought to be a feature of affective disorders (chiefly mania), schizophrenia, organic mental disorder, and other psychoses.

Cerea flexibilitas ("waxy flexibility"): A specific type of catalepsy in which the examiner encounters resistance ('like bending a soft wax rod') upon attempting to move parts of the subject's body. A feature of catatonia.

Circumstantiality: A disturbance of communication in which the train of associations is interrupted by frequent digressions before the central idea is finally presented. The digressions are irrelevant or marginally relevant to what is being said. Seen in a wide variety of pathological states, or may be a normal if annoying language habit.

Clang associations: The rhyming or punning associations of one word with another with no logical connection. **Example:** "My head is rock candy. Dandy. Randy. Sandy. Piece of the rock. Mutual of Omaha." Seen in manic episodes, schizophrenia, and other psychotic states.

Clouding of consciousness: In *DSM-III-R*, impaired awareness of the environment. Defined elsewhere as the least severe impairment of consciousness on the continuum from full alertness to coma.

Compulsion: The need to repeat some action in a ritualistic, stereotyped manner, uncontrollable by an act of will. The act frequently has symbolic meaning. The subject knows there is no true connection between the motor behavior and the fantasied wish or fear. The compulsive act may seem unpleasant, tedious, or distressful, but resistance is associated with mounting anxiety that can be relieved only by performing the act. Seen in obsessive compulsive disorder and schizophrenia.

Concrete thinking: Thinking characterized by diminished capacity to form abstractions. The subject is unable to think metaphorically or hypothetically. Thought is limited to one dimension of meaning. Words and figures of speech are taken literally, and the nuances of implied meaning are not used or not appreciated. Common in organic mental disorder and schizophrenia.

Confabulation: The fabrication of events or data that either fill in gaps in a story or constitute entire fictions in response to questions that cannot be factually answered because of organic memory impairment. A feature of amnestic syndrome.

Confusion: A disturbance of consciousness with loss of orientation to person, place, or time. (See Disorientation.) Confusion may be due to impaired memory loss (as in dementia) or to deficit in attention (as in delirium).

Delirium: A disturbance of consciousness resulting from organic brain disease (usually acute) and characterized by clouding of consciousness, restlessness, confusion, psychomotor retardation or agitation, and affective lability. It has a rapid onset and a fluctuating, waxing and waning course, and there is an associated disturbance of sleep.

Delusion: (See also Hallucination, Ideas of reference, and Paranoia.) A false belief or idea firmly held despite abundant contradictory evidence. A defect of reality testing. (A belief is not delusional if it is shared by other members of a culture or large group.) A delusion is always evidence of psychosis. *Examples:* (1) Delusions of **being controlled**, ie, that thoughts, feelings, or behaviors are controlled by external forces. (2) Delusions of **grandeur,** ie, that one is influential and important, perhaps having occult powers, or that one actually is some powerful figure out of history ('Napoleonic complex'). (3) Delusions of **persecution,** ie, that one is being followed, harassed, threatened, or plotted against. (4) Delusions of **reference,** ie, that external events or "portents" have personal significance, such as special messages or commands. A person with delusions of reference believes that strangers on the street are talking about him or her, the television commentator is sending coded messages, etc.

Dementia: Deterioration (due to organic brain syndrome) from a previous level of intellectual functioning involving personality change and resulting in impairment of memory, abstract thinking, judgment, and impulse control. Clouding of consciousness does not occur. Dementia may be chronic (with insidious onset) or acute and reversible or irreversible.

Depersonalization: The experience of feeling strange, unreal, and detached from the environment or from oneself, ie, of being outside one's body, or that parts of the body are very large or very small or not under one's control, etc. Seen in a wide variety of disorders, including depression, anxiety, schizophrenia, epilepsy, and hypnagogic states. It may

be a normal finding in adolescents. (See Derealization.)

Derailment: "Getting off the track" with respect to speech, volition, or thought. Moving in random fashion from one topic, thought, or behavior to another.

Derealization: The experience of feeling that the immediate environment is unreal or changed. (Depersonalization and derealization occur together and are probably aspects of the same phenomenon.)

Dereistic thinking: Failure to take the facts of reality into account, so that thoughts derive mainly from fantasy rather than experience and logical inference.

Disorientation: (1) Not oriented to **time,** ie, not knowing what day, month, season, or year it is; (2) not oriented to **place,** ie, not knowing the name of the building one is in or the kind of building, or the city, state, or country where one is presently located; or (3) not oriented to **person,** ie, not knowing who one is. Disorientation is one of the diagnostic criteria for delirium and is seen in delirium and organic memory disturbances.

Echolalia: Repetition of another person's speech. (See next item.)

Echopraxia: Imitation of another person's movements. (Echolalia and echopraxia are seen in pervasive developmental disorders, organic mental disorders, catatonia, and other psychotic disorders.)

Flight of ideas: A series of thoughts verbalized rapidly with abrupt shifts of subject matter with no apparent logical reason. Flight of ideas is associated with pressure of speech (see below). It is often difficult to differentiate flight of ideas from loosening of associations (see below). Classically, the connections between associations in flight of ideas are thought to be more coherent than in loosening of associations. However, in its severe form, flight of ideas can result in complete disorganization and incoherence. Seen in mania as well as in organic mental disorders, schizophrenia, and other psychotic and nonpsychotic states.

Folie à deux ("madness for two"): A disorder characterized by the sharing of delusional (usually persecutory) ideas by two or more (folie à plusieurs) individuals living in close association usually in a family relationship. One member of the pair (or group) seems always to influence and dominate the others. The delusional ideas may lead to strange types of behavior such as preparing for the end of the world.

Formication: See Hallucination, tactile, below.

Fugue: Sudden, unexpected "flights" or wandering away from home or workplace and assumption of a new identity. There is amnesia for the previous identity and no memory of the fugue when it is over.

Hallucination: A false sensory perception of what is not there. An illusion (see below) differs in being a perceptual distortion of something that is there. A delusion (see above) differs in being a disorder of thought. A delusion is always a sign of psychosis, since it represents a defect in reality testing. A hallucination is not always a sign of psychosis; eg, one who "sees" pink elephants but knows they are not really there is not psychotic. One who "feels" bugs crawling on his or her skin and believes the bugs are really there is not only hallucinating but is also psychotic. **Examples:** (1) **Auditory** hallucinations—false perceptions of sounds (voices, music, buzzing, motor noises, murmuring). (2) **Gustatory** hallucinations—false perceptions of taste. (3) **Olfactory** hallucinations—false perceptions of smell. (4) **Somatic** hallucinations—false sensations of something happening in or to the body such as the sensation of knives piercing the body or a feeling of electricity in the arms. (Usually associated with a delusion consistent with the feeling.) (5) **Tactile** hallucinations—false sensations of touch. (Usually associated with a delusion consistent with the sensation.) **Formication** (from L *formica,* "ant"), a particular type of tactile hallucination, is the sensation of bugs crawling on or under the skin. (6) **Visual** hallucinations—false visual perceptions with eyes open in a lighted environment. (Visual images with the eyes closed are not true hallucinations. **Hypnagogic** and **hypnopompic** hallucinations—images experienced during the "twilight" stages while falling asleep and waking up, respectively—are not true hallucinations.)

All of the above hallucinations can occur in schizophrenia, affective disorders, and organic mental disorders. Auditory and somatic hallucinations are common in functional disorders. Visual hallucinations are suggestive of organic mental disorders but are seen in functional disorders. Gustatory, olfactory, and tactile hallucinations strongly suggest organic mental disorders. Tactile hallucinations are common in drug and alcohol withdrawal and intoxication states.

Ideas of reference: Similar to delusions of reference (see above) but held with less conviction.

Illusion: (See also Hallucination.) A distorted perception of a material object.

Incoherence: Speech that is incomprehensible because of severe loosening of associations, distortions of grammar or syntax, or the use of idiosyncratic word definitions.

Insomnia: Difficulty sleeping—either **initial insomnia,** difficulty in falling asleep; **middle insomnia,** waking up in the middle of the night and going back to sleep with difficulty; or **terminal insomnia,** awakening early without being able to go back to sleep.

Loosening of associations: (See also Flight of Ideas and Tangentiality.) A disorder of thinking and speech in which ideas shift from one subject to another with remote or no apparent reasons. The speaker is unaware of the incongruity. A classical sign of schizophrenia but may be seen also in any psychotic state.

Mood: The subjective experience of feeling or emotion as described by the patient in the history. Mood is a pervasive and sustained emotion. Distinct from affect (see above), which is a feeling state noted by the examiner during the mental status examination. Mood is characterized by the type of emotion the patient describes, eg, sadness, feeling blue, happiness, elation, anger, and anxiety. Mood is **dysphoric** if the experience is unpleasant, eg, characterized by irritability, anger, or depression. Mood can be elevated, expansive, or **euphoric,** eg, characterized by increasing feelings of well-being, energy, and positive self-regard.

Mood-congruent: A term applied to hallucinations or delusions whose content is consistent with the predominant mood. Mood-congruent hallucinations or delusions in mania, for example, typically involve grandiosity, inflated self-esteem, confidence of one's personal powers, and identifications with famous persons or deities. Mood-congruent hallucinations or delusions in depression involve themes of worthlessness, guilt, defectiveness, disease, death, nihilism, and deserved punishment.

Mood-incongruent: A term applied to hallucinations or delusions whose content has no apparent relationship to the predominant mood. Examples are persecutory delusions, delusions of reference, delusions of control, thought insertion, thought withdrawal, and thought broadcasting, in which the content has no apparent relation to the mood-congruent themes mentioned above. Mood-incongruent hallucinations and delusions are seen in schizophrenia and sometimes in mania and depression.

Mutism: Not speaking. A feature of catatonia.

Negativism: Extreme opposition, resistance to suggestion. A feature of catatonia.

Neologisms: Invented "new words," with new meanings, often formed by combining elements of other words. A feature of schizophrenia and other psychotic disorders.

Obsession: Recurring ideas, images, or wishes that dominate thought. The content may be unacceptable and actively resisted but intrudes into consciousness again and again. A feature of obsessive compulsive disorder and some cases of schizophrenia.

Panic attacks: Anxiety attacks, characterized by palpitations, a sense of imminent doom, fear of losing control, tightness in the chest, hyperventilation, lightheadedness, nausea, and peripheral paresthesias. There are no cardiopulmonary, endocrine, or other physical disorders that might account for the symptoms. Seen in a wide variety of psychotic and nonpsychotic disorders as well as in normal people subjected to sufficient stress.

Paranoia: A psychotic disorder characterized by delusions of grandeur and persecution, suspiciousness, hypersensitivity, hyperalertness, jealousy, guardedness, resentment, humorlessness, litigiousness, and sullenness. Paranoid schizophrenia is listed separately as a subtype of schizophrenia. (1) **Paranoid ideation** is a consistent finding in paranoid patients, who are convinced that people are thinking "bad thoughts" about them, that they are being followed, that they are the object of evil conspiracies, etc. It includes ideas of reference, ideas of persecution, grandiose ideas, and ideas of jealousy. Paranoid ideation differs from paranoid delusions in that the ideas are held with less conviction than delusions. (2) **Paranoid style** is a character style featuring hypervigilance, litigiousness, rigidity, humorlessness, jealousy, sullenness, suspiciousness, and hyperattention to evidence in the environment that corroborates paranoid suspicions.

Perseveration: Repetitive behavior or repetitive expression of a particular word, phrase, or concept during the course of speech. Perseveration is seen in organic mental disorders, schizophrenia, and other psychotic disorders.

Phobia: (See also Anxiety.) An admittedly irrational fear of a particular object or situation, so that the person's life is dominated by avoidance behavior.

Posturing: The assumption of various abnormal bodily positions, often a feature of catatonia.

Poverty of content of speech: Speech that is persistently vague, overly concrete or abstract, repetitive, or stereotyped.

Poverty of speech: Speech that is decreased in amount and nonspontaneous, consisting mainly of brief and unelaborated responses to questions.

Pressure of speech: (See also Flight of Ideas.) Speech that is rapid and unstoppable, as if the speaker is driven to keep speaking. Speech is often loud and emphatic and hard to interrupt. It can dominate conversations or go on when no one is listening or responding. A feature of mania and seen also in other psychotic conditions, organic mental disorders, and nonpsychotic conditions associated with stress.

Psychomotor agitation: Motor restlessness and hyperactivity associated with tension, anxiety, and irritability.

Psychomotor retardation: Decreased motor activity, slowed speech, poverty of speech, delayed response to questions, and low, monotonous voice tones associated with feelings of fatigue.

Psychosis: A level of disordered thinking in which the person is unable to distinguish reality from fantasy because of impaired ability to test reality. Psychosis may be transient (hours or days) or persistent (months or years). The characteristic deficit in psychosis is not "loss of touch with reality" but loss of the ability to process experience appropriately, ie, to differentiate what data are coming from the outside world and what information originates in one's inner world of preconceptions, expectations, and emotions. Psychosis can be defined as an impairment of reality testing. Reality sense can be impaired in the absence of psychosis. One may "sense" that people are following him or her when that is not the case, and may experience hallucinations. One may have a quite distorted view of his or her strengths or weaknesses. As long as these hypotheses, no matter how bizarre, can be tested against objective evidence and rejected or at least doubted as a result of that rational process, psychosis can be ruled out. As reality testing—the capacity to challenge bizarre perceptions—becomes further impaired, the subject becomes less able or willing to look at or be swayed by external evidence. "Ideas" solidify as delusions, which progressively become more bizarre and complex. Thought becomes more and more preoccupied with fantasy and the subjective world as external cues are progressively ignored. The boundary between nonpsychotic and psychotic ideation and perception is not sharp. There is a spectrum from minimally distorted to grossly distorted nonpsychotic thinking, from mild impairment to severe impairment of reality testing, and from mild psychosis with circumscribed delusions to the extremely bizarre and disorganized psychotic state.

Reality sense: (See Psychosis, above.) One's feelings, thoughts, and perceptions about the way things are.

Reality testing: (See Psychosis, above.) The process of testing one's thoughts or hypotheses against cues identified in the external world.

Schneiderian first-rank symptoms: Symptoms believed by Kurt Schneider (1957), a German psychiatrist, to be pathognomonic of schizophrenia in the absence of organic disease: (1) Certain kinds of auditory hallucinations—hearing one's thoughts spoken aloud, hearing voices conversing with one another, or hearing voices keeping a running commentary on one's behavior. (2) **Somatic hallucinations**—frequently of a sexual nature, accompanied by delusional beliefs consistent with the sensations. The physical sensations are commonly attributed by the person to external causes, forces, energies, or hypnotic suggestion. (3) **Thought withdrawal**—the belief that other people are taking one's thoughts away. (4) **Thought insertion**—the belief that someone else is implanting thoughts into one's head. (5) **Thought broadcasting**—the belief that one's thoughts are known by others, as if everyone else could read one's mind. (6) **Delusional perceptions**—attaching abnormal significance, usually with self-reference, to a genuine perception. For example, the subject interprets a stop sign as an exhortation from another world to "stop being such a bad person." (7) **Delusions of being controlled**—the belief that one's actions, feelings, and impulses are really derived from, influenced by, or directed by external people or forces.

Stereotypy: An isolated, purposeless movement performed repetitively. A feature of catatonia and seen also in schizophrenia. Intoxication with amphetamine-like drugs will also produce stereotypical behavior.

Stupor: Stupor is a particular level of diminished consciousness (ie, one stage more alert than coma) in which mental and physical activity is minimal as a result of organic impairment. Stupor can also refer to a functional state in which the patient appears to be unaware of the environment, unresponsive and motionless but aware of the surroundings. A feature of catatonia and seen also in severe depression and schizophrenia.

Tangentiality: A disturbance of communication in which the subject "takes off on a tangent" away from a central idea or question and does not return. It may be a digression or an introduction of a new theme. It is related to loosening of associations and speech derailment in that there is a jump from one thought or topic to another. Tangentiality has been used synonymously with loosening of associations; however, the latter is characterized by repeated derailments with many associations that seem disconnected. Tangential thinking can be quite coherent as long as it successfully evades the central theme. A feature of a wide variety of pathological and normal states.

Thought broadcasting, thought insertion, thought withdrawal: See Schneiderian first-rank symptoms, above.

Thought disorder: Any disturbance of thinking that affects language, communication, thought content, or thought process. A disorder of thought **content** is characterized by delusions or marked illogicality. A formal thought disorder is a disorder in form or process of thinking, as distinguished from content of thought. Formal thought disorder is characterized by a failure to follow semantic, syntactic, or logical rules. It may range from simple blocking and mild circumstantiality to loosening of associations and loss of reality testing. Classically, formal thought disorder is the hallmark of schizophrenia. However, because the meaning of formal thought disorder is not clearly delineated, it is not used as a descriptive term by *DSM-III*.

Vegetative signs: In describing signs of depression, the term refers to disturbances of sleep, loss of appetite, weight loss, constipation, and loss of sexual interest. Vegetative functions refer to autonomic physiological functions related to growth, nutrition, or homeostasis of the organism.

Index